The GALE
ENCYCLOPEDIA of
SURGERY

The GALE ENCYCLOPEDIA of SURGERY

A GUIDE FOR PATIENTS AND CAREGIVERS

VOLUME

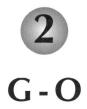

G-O

ANTHONY J. SENAGORE, M.D., EXECUTIVE ADVISOR
CLEVELAND CLINIC FOUNDATION

GALE®

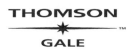

THOMSON

GALE

Detroit • New York • San Diego • San Francisco • Cleveland • New Haven, Conn. • Waterville, Maine • London • Munich

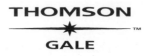

THOMSON ™
GALE

Gale Encyclopedia of Surgery: A Guide for Patients and Caregivers

Anthony J. Senagore MD, Executive Adviser

Project Editor
Kristine Krapp

Editorial
Stacey L. Blachford, Deirdre Blanchfield, Madeline Harris, Chris Jeryan, Jacqueline Longe, Brigham Narins, Mark Springer, Ryan Thomason

Editorial Support Services
Andrea Lopeman, Sue Petrus

Indexing
Synapse

Illustrations
GGS Inc.

Permissions
Lori Hines

Imaging and Multimedia
Leitha Etheridge-Sims, Lezlie Light, Dave Oblender, Christine O'Brien, Robyn V. Young

Product Design
Michelle DiMercurio, Jennifer Wahi

Manufacturing
Wendy Blurton, Evi Seoud

LIBRARY OF CONGRESS CATALOGING-IN-PUBLICATION DATA

Gale encyclopedia of surgery : a guide for patients and caregivers /
Anthony J. Senagore, [editor].
p. cm.
Includes bibliographical references and index.
ISBN 0-7876-7721-3 (set : hc) — ISBN 0-7876-7722-1 (v. 1) — ISBN 0-7876-7723-X (v. 2) — ISBN 0-7876-9123-2 (v. 3)
Surgery—Encyclopedias. 2. Surgery—Popular works. I. Senagore, Anthony J., 1958-

RD17.G34 2003
617'.91'003—dc22   2003015742

This title is also available as an e-book.
ISBN: 0-7876-7770-1 (set)
Contact your Gale sales representative for ordering information.

Printed in Canada
10 9 8 7 6 5 4 3 2 1

CONTENTS

LIST OF ENTRIES

PLEASE READ—
IMPORTANT INFORMATION

The *Gale Encyclopedia of Surgery* is a medical reference product designed to inform and educate readers about a wide variety of surgeries, tests, drugs, and other medical topics. The Gale Group believes the product to be comprehensive, but not necessarily definitive. While the Gale Group has made substantial efforts to provide information that is accurate, comprehensive, and up-to-date, the Gale Group makes no representations or warranties of any kind, including without limitation, warranties of merchantability or fitness for a particular purpose, nor does it guarantee the accuracy, comprehensiveness, or timeliness of the information contained in this product. Readers should be aware that the universe of medical knowledge is constantly growing and changing, and that differences of medical opinion exist among authorities.

INTRODUCTION

The *Gale Encyclopedia of Surgery: A Guide for Patients and Caregivers* is a unique and invaluable source of information for anyone who is considering undergoing a surgical procedure, or has a loved one in that situation. This collection of 465 entries provides in-depth coverage of specific surgeries, diagnostic tests, drugs, and other related entries. The book gives detailed information on 265 surgeries; most include step-by-step illustrations to enhance the reader's understanding of the procedure itself. Entries on related topics, including anesthesia, second opinions, talking to the doctor, admission to the hospital, and preparing for surgery, give lay readers knowledge of surgery practices in general. Sidebars provide information on who performs the surgery and where, and on questions to ask the doctor.

This encyclopedia minimizes medical jargon and uses language that laypersons can understand, while still providing detailed coverage that will benefit health science students.

Entries on surgeries follow a standardized format that provides information at a glance. Rubrics include:

Definition
Purpose
Demographics
Description
Diagnosis/Preparation
Aftercare
Risks
Normal results
Morbidity and mortality rates
Alternatives
Resources

Inclusion criteria

A preliminary list of surgeries and related topics was compiled from a wide variety of sources, including professional medical guides and textbooks, as well as consumer guides and encyclopedias. Final selection of topics to include was made by the executive adviser in conjunction with the Gale editor.

About the Executive Adviser

The Executive Adviser for the *Gale Encyclopedia of Surgery* was Anthony J. Senagore, MD, MS, FACS, FASCRS. He has published a number of professional articles and is the Krause/Lieberman Chair in Laparoscopic Colorectal Surgery, and Staff Surgeon, Department of Colorectal Surgery at the Cleveland Clinic Foundation in Cleveland, Ohio.

About the contributors

The essays were compiled by experienced medical writers, including physicians, pharmacists, nurses, and other health care professionals. The adviser reviewed the completed essays to ensure that they are appropriate, up-to-date, and medically accurate. Illustrations were also reviewed by a medical doctor.

How to use this book

The **Gale Encyclopedia of Surgery** has been designed with ready reference in mind.

- Straight **alphabetical arrangement** of topics allows users to locate information quickly.

- **Bold-faced terms** within entries and **See also terms** at the end of entries direct the reader to related articles.

- **Cross-references** placed throughout the encyclopedia direct readers from alternate names and related topics to entries.

- A list of **Key terms** is provided where appropriate to define unfamiliar terms or concepts.

- A sidebar describing **Who performs the procedure and where it is performed** is listed with every surgery entry.

- A list of **Questions to ask the doctor** is provided wherever appropriate to help facilitate discussion with the patient's physician.

- The **Resources** section directs readers to additional sources of medical information on a topic. Books, periodicals, organizations, and internet sources are listed.
- A **Glossary** of terms used throughout the text is collected in one easy-to-use section at the back of book.
- A valuable **Organizations appendix** compiles useful contact information for various medical and surgical organizations.
- A comprehensive **General index** guides readers to all topics mentioned in the text.

Graphics

The *Gale Encyclopedia of Surgery* contains over 230 full-color illustrations, photos, and tables. This includes over 160 step-by-step illustrations of surgeries. These illustrations were specially created for this product to enhance a layperson's understanding of surgical procedures.

Licensing

The Gale Encyclopedia of Surgery is available for licensing. The complete database is provided in a fielded format and is deliverable on such media as disk or CD-ROM. For more information, contact Gale's Business Development Group at 1-800-877-GALE, or visit our website at www.gale.com/bizdev.

CONTRIBUTORS

Laurie Barclay, M.D.
Neurological Consulting Services
Tampa, FL

Jeanine Barone
Nutritionist, Exercise Physiologist
New York, NY

Julia R. Barrett
Science Writer
Madison, WI

Donald G. Barstow, R.N.
Clinical Nurse Specialist
Oklahoma City, OK

Mary Bekker
Medical Writer
Willow Grove, PA

Mark A. Best, MD, MPH, MBA
Associate Professor of Pathology
St. Matthew's University
Grand Cayman, BWI

Maggie Boleyn, R.N., B.S.N.
Medical Writer
Oak Park, MIn

Susan Joanne Cadwallader
Medical Writer
Cedarburg, WI

Diane Calbrese
*Medical Sciences and Technology
  Writer*
Silver Spring, MD

Richard H. Camer
Editor
International Medical News Group
Silver Spring, MD

Rosalyn Carson-DeWitt, M.D.
Medical Writer
Durham, NC

Lisa Christenson, PhD
Science Writer
Hamden, CT

Rhonda Cloos, RN
Medical Writer
Austin, TX

Angela Costello
Medical writer
Cleveland, OH

**Esther Csapo Rastegari, RN,
  BSN, EdM**
Medical Writer
Holbrook, MA

**L. Lee Culvert, BS,
  Biochemistry**
Health Writer
Alna, ME

Tish Davidson, AM
Medical Writer
Fremont, CA

Lori De Milto
Medical Writer
Sicklerville, NJ

Victoria E. DeMoranville
Medical Writer
Lakeville, MA

Altha Roberts Edgren
Medical Writer
Medical Ink
St. Paul, MN

Lorraine K. Ehresman
Medical Writer
Northfield, Quebec, Canada

**L. Fleming Fallon, Jr., MD,
  DrPH**
Professor of Public Health
Bowling Green State University
Bowling Green, OH

Paula Ford-Martin
Freelance Medical Writer
Warwick, RI

Janie Franz
Freelance Journalist
Grand Forks, ND

Rebecca J. Frey, PhD
Freelance Medical Writer
New Haven, CT

Debra Gordon
Medical Writer
Nazareth, PA

Jill Granger, M.S.
Sr. Research Associate
Dept. of Pathology
University of Michigan Medical
  Center
Ann Arbor, MI

Laith F. Gulli, M.D.
M.Sc., M.Sc.(MedSci), M.S.A.,
  Msc.Psych, MRSNZ
FRSH, FRIPHH, FAIC, FZS
DAPA, DABFC, DABCI
*Consultant Psychotherapist in
  Private Practice*
Lathrup Village, MI

Stephen John Hage, AAAS, RT(R), FAHRA
Medical Writer
Chatsworth, CA

Maureen Haggerty
Medical Writer
Ambler, PA

Robert Harr, MS, MT (ASCP)
Associate Professor and Chair
Department of Public and Allied Health
Bowling Green State University
Bowling Green, OH

Dan Harvey
Medical Writer
Wilmington, DE

Katherine Hauswirth, APRN
Medical Writer
Deep River, CT

Caroline Helwick
Medical Writer
New Orleans, LA

Lisette Hilton
Medical Writer
Boca Raton, FL

René A. Jackson, RN
Medical Writer
Port Charlotte, FL

Nadine M. Jacobson, RN
Medical Writer
Takoma Park, MD

Randi B. Jenkins, BA
Copy Chief
Fission Communications
New York, NY

Michelle L. Johnson, M.S., J.D.
Patent Attorney and Medical Writer
ZymoGenetics, Inc.
Seattle, WA

Paul A. Johnson, Ed.M.
Medical Writer
San Diego, CA

Cindy L. A. Jones, Ph.D.
Biomedical Writer
Sagescript Communications
Lakewood, CO

Linda D. Jones, BA, PBT (ASCP)
Medical Writer
Asheboro, NY

Crystal H. Kaczkowski, MSc.
Health Writer
Chicago, IL

Beth A. Kapes
Medical Writer
Bay Village, OH

Jeanne Krob, M.D., F.A.C.S.
Physician, Writer
Pittsburgh, PA

Monique Laberge, PhD
Sr. Res. Investigator
Dept. of Biochemistry & Biophysics, School of Medicine
University of Pennsylvania
Philadelphia, PA

Richard H. Lampert
Senior Medical Editor
W.B. Saunders Co.
Philadelphia, PA

Victor Leipzig, Ph.D.
Biological Consultant
Huntington Beach, CA

Lorraine Lica, PhD
Medical Writer
San Diego, CA

John T. Lohr, Ph.D.
Assistant Director, Biotechnology Center
Utah State University
Logan, UT

Jennifer Lee Losey, RN
Medical Writer
Madison Heights, MI

Jacqueline N. Martin, MS
Medical Writer
Albrightsville, PA

Nancy F. McKenzie, PhD
Public Health Consultant
Brooklyn, NY

Mercedes McLaughlin
Medical Writer
Phoenixville, CA

Christine Miner Minderovic, BS, RT, RDMS
Medical Writer
Ann Arbor, MI

Mark A. Mitchell, M.D.
Freelance Medical Writer
Bothell, WA

Erika J. Norris, MD, MS
Medical Writer
Oak Harbor, WA

Teresa Norris, R.N.
Medical Writer
Ute Park, NM

Debra Novograd, BS, RT(R)(M)
Medical Writer
Royal Oak, MI

Jane E. Phillips, PhD
Medical Writer
Chapel Hill, NC

J. Ricker Polsdorfer, M.D.
Medical Writer
Phoenix, AZ

Elaine R. Proseus, M.B.A./T.M., B.S.R.T., R.T.(R)
Medical Writer
Farmington Hills, MI

Robert Ramirez, B.S.
Medical Student
University of Medicine & Dentistry of New Jersey
Stratford, NJ

Martha S. Reilly, OD
Clinical Optometrist/ Medical Freelance Writer
Madison, WI

Toni Rizzo
Medical Writer
Salt Lake City, UT

Richard Robinson
Freelance Medical Writer
Sherborn, MA

Nancy Ross-Flanigan
Science Writer
Belleville, MI

Belinda Rowland, Ph.D.
Medical Writer
Voorheesville, NY

Laura Ruth, Ph.D.
*Medical, Science, & Technology
  Writer*
Los Angeles, CA

Kausalya Santhanam, Ph.D.
Technical Writer
Branford, CT

Joan Schonbeck
Medical Writer
Nursing Department
Massachusetts Department of
  Mental Health
Marlborough, MA

Stephanie Dionne Sherk
Freelance Medical Writer
University of Michigan
Ann Arbor, MI

Lee A. Shratter, MD
Consulting Radiologist
Kentfield, CA

Jennifer Sisk
Medical Writer
Havertown, PA

Allison J. Spiwak, MSBME
Circulation Technologist
The Ohio State University
Columbus, OH

Kurt Sternlof
Science Writer
New Rochelle, NY

Margaret A Stockley, RGN
Medical Writer
Boxborough, MA

Dorothy Stonely
Medical Writer
Los Gatos, CA

Bethany Thivierge
Biotechnical Writer/Editor
Technicality Resources
Rockland, ME

Carol Turkington
Medical Writer
Lancaster, PA

Samuel D. Uretsky, Pharm.D.
Medical Writer
Wantagh, NY

Ellen S. Weber, M.S.N.
Medical Writer
Fort Wayne, IN

Barbara Wexler
Medical Writer
Chatsworth, CA

Abby Wojahn, RN, BSN, CCRN
Medical Writer
Milwaukee, WI

Kathleen D. Wright, R.N.
Medical Writer
Delmar, DE

Mary Zoll, Ph.D.
Science Writer
Newton Center, MA

Michael V. Zuck, Ph.D.
Medical Writer
Boulder, CO

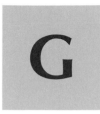

G

Gallbladder removal *see* **Cholecystectomy**

Gallbladder ultrasound *see* **Abdominal ultrasound**

Gallstone removal

Definition

Also known as cholelithotomy, gallstone removal is a procedure that rids the gallbladder of calculus buildup.

Purpose

The gallbladder is not a vital organ. It is located on the right side of the abdomen underneath the liver. The gallbladder's function is to store bile, concentrate it, and release it during digestion. Bile is supposed to retain all of its chemicals in solution, but commonly one of them crystallizes and forms sandy or gravel-like particles, and finally gallstones. The formation of gallstones causes gallbladder disease (cholelithiasis).

Chemicals in bile will form crystals as the gallbladder draws water out of the bile. The solubility of these chemicals is based on the concentration of three chemicals: bile acids, phospholipids, and cholesterol. If the chemicals are out of balance, one or the other will not remain in solution. Dietary fat and cholesterol are also implicated in crystal formation.

As the bile crystals aggregate to form stones, they move about, eventually occluding the outlet and preventing the gallbladder from emptying. This blockage results in irritation, inflammation, and sometimes infection (cholecystitis) of the gallbladder. The pattern is usually one of intermittent obstruction due to stones moving in and out of the way. Meanwhile, the gallbladder becomes more and more scarred. Sometimes infection fills the gallbladder with pus, which is a serious complication.

Occasionally, a gallstone will travel down the cystic duct into the common bile duct and get stuck there. This blockage will back bile up into the liver as well as the gallbladder. If the stone sticks at the ampulla of Vater (a narrowing in the duct leading to the pancreas), the pancreas will also be blocked and will develop pancreatitis.

Gallstones will cause a sudden onset of pain in the upper abdomen. Pain will last for 30 minutes to several hours. Pain may move to the right shoulder blade. Nausea with or without vomiting may accompany the pain.

Demographics

Gallstones are approximately two times more common in females than in males. Overweight women in their middle years constitute the vast majority of patients with gallstones in every racial or ethnic group. An estimated 10% of the general population has gallstones. The prevalence for women between ages 20 and 55 varies from 5–20%, and is higher after age 50 (25–30%). The prevalence for males is approximately half that for women in a given age group. Certain people, in particular the Pima tribe of Native Americans in Arizona, have a genetic predisposition to forming gallstones. Scandinavians also have a higher than average incidence of this disease.

There seems to be a strong genetic correlation with gallstone disease, since stones are more than four times as likely to occur among first-degree relatives. Since gallstones rarely dissolve spontaneously, the prevalence increases with age. Obesity is a well-known risk factor since overweight causes chemical abnormalities that lead to increased levels of cholesterol. Gallstones are also associated with rapid weight loss secondary to dieting. Pregnancy is a risk factor since increased estrogen levels result in an increased cholesterol secretion and abnormal changes in bile. However, while an increase in dietary cholesterol is not a risk factor, an increase in triglycerides is positively associated with a higher incidence of gallstones. Diabetes mellitus is also believed to be a risk factor for gallstone development.

Description

Surgery to remove the entire gallbladder with all its stones is usually the best treatment, provided the patient is able to tolerate the procedure. A relatively new technique of removing the gallbladder using a laparoscope has resulted in quicker recovery and much smaller surgical incisions than the 6-in (15-cm) gash under the right ribs that had previously been the standard procedure; however, not everyone is a candidate for this approach. If the procedure is not expected to have complications, laparoscopic **cholecystectomy** is performed. Laparoscopic surgery requires a space in the surgical area for visualization and instrument manipulation. The laparoscope with attached video camera is inserted. Several other instruments are inserted through the abdomen (into the surgical field) to assist the surgeon to maneuver around the nearby organs during surgery. The surgeon must take precautions not to accidentally harm anatomical structures in the liver. Once the cystic artery has been divided and the gallbladder dissected from the liver, the gallbladder can be removed.

If the gallbladder is extremely diseased (inflamed, infected, or has large gallstones), the abdominal approach (open cholecystectomy) is recommended. This surgery is usually performed with an incision in the upper midline of the abdomen or on the right side of the abdomen below the rib (right subcostal incision).

If a stone is lodged in the bile ducts, additional surgery must be done to remove it. After surgery, the surgeon will ordinarily insert a drain to collect bile until the system is healed. The drain can also be used to inject contrast material and take x rays during or after surgery.

A procedure called endoscopic retrograde cholangiopancreatoscopy (ERCP) allows the removal of some bile duct stones through the mouth, throat, esophagus, stomach, duodenum, and biliary system without the need for surgical incisions. ERCP can also be used to inject contrast agents into the biliary system, providing finely detailed pictures.

Patients with symptomatic cholelithiasis can be treated with certain medications called oral bile acid litholysis or oral dissolution therapy. This technique is especially effective for dissolving small cholesterol-composed gallstones. Current research indicates that the success rate for oral dissolution treatment is 70–80% with floating stones (those predominantly composed of cholesterol). Approximately 10–20% of patients who receive medication-induced litholysis can have a recurrence within the first two or three years after treatment completion.

Extracorporeal shock wave **lithotripsy** is a treatment in which shock waves are generated in water by lithotripters (devices that produce the waves). There are several types of lithotripters available for gallbladder removal. One specific lithotripter involves the use of piezoelectric crystals, which allow the shock waves to be accurately focused on a small area to disrupt a stone. This procedure does not generally require analgesia (or anesthesia). Damage to the gallbladder and associated structures (such as the cystic duct) must be present for stone removal after the shock waves break up the stone. Typically, repeated shock wave treatments are necessary to completely remove gallstones. The success rate of the fragmentation of the gallstone and urinary clearance is inversely proportional to stone size and number: patients with a small solitary stone have the best outcome, with high rates of stone clearance (95% are cleared within 12–18 months), while patients with multiple stones are at risk for poor clearance rates. Complications of shock wave lithotripsy include inflammation of the pancreas (pancreatitis) and acute cholecystitis.

A method called contact dissolution of gallstone removal involves direct entry (via a percutaneous transhepatic catheter) of a chemical solvent (such as methyl tertiary-butyl ether, MTBE). MTBE is rapidly removed unchanged from the body via the respiratory system (exhaled air). Side effects in persons receiving contact dissolution therapy include foul-smelling breath, dyspnea (difficulty breathing), vomiting, and drowsiness. Treatment with MTBE can be successful in treating cholesterol gallstones regardless of the number and size of stones. Studies indicate that the success rate for dissolution is well over 95% in persons who receive direct chemical infusions that can last five to 12 hours.

Diagnosis/Preparation

Diagnostically, gallstone disease, which can lead to gallbladder removal, is divided into four diseases: biliary colic, acute cholecystitis, choledocholithiasis, and cholangitis. Biliary colic is usually caused by intermittent cystic duct obstruction by a stone (without any inflammation), causing a severe, poorly localized, and intensifying pain on the upper right side of the abdomen.

These painful attacks can persist from days to months in patients with biliary colic.

Persons affected with acute cholecystitis caused by an impacted stone in the cystic duct also suffer from gallbladder infection in approximately 50% of cases. These people have moderately severe pain in the upper right portion of the abdomen that lasts longer than six hours. Pain with acute cholecystitis can also extend to the shoulder or back. Since there may be infection inside the gallbladder, the patient may also have fever. On the right side of the abdomen below the last rib, there is usually tenderness with inspiratory (breathing in) arrest (Murphy's sign). In about 33% of cases of acute cholecystitis, the gallbladder may be felt with palpation (clinician feeling abdomen for tenderness). Mild jaundice can be present in about 20% of cases.

Persons with choledocholithiasis, or intermittent obstruction of the common bile duct, often do not have symptoms; but if present, they are indistinguishable from the symptoms of biliary colic.

A more severe form of gallstone disease is cholangitis, which causes stone impaction in the common bile duct. In about 70% of cases, these patients present with Charcot's triad (pain, jaundice, and fever). Patients with cholangitis may have chills, mild pain, lethargy, and delirium, which indicate that infection has spread to the bloodstream (bacteremia). The majority of patients with cholangitis will have fever (95%), tenderness in the upper right side of the abdomen, and jaundice (80%).

In addition to a **physical examination**, preparation for laboratory (blood) and special tests is essential to gallstone diagnosis. Patients with biliary colic may have elevated bilirubin and should have an ultrasound study to visualize the gallbladder and associated structures. An increase in the white blood cell count (leukocytosis) can be expected for both acute cholecystitis and cholangitis (seen in 80% of cases). Ultrasound testing is recommended for acute cholecystitis patients, whereas ERCP is the test usually indicated to assist in a definitive diagnosis for both choledocholithiasis and cholangitis. Patients with either biliary colic or choledocholithiasis are treated with elective laparoscopic cholecystectomy. Open cholecystectomy is recommended for acute cholecystitis. For cholangitis, emergency ERCP is indicated for stone removal. ERCP therapy can remove stones produced by gallbladder disease.

Aftercare

Without a gallbladder, stones rarely recur. Patients who have continued symptoms after their gallbladder is removed may need an ERCP to detect residual stones or damage to the bile ducts caused by the original stones.

QUESTIONS TO ASK THE DOCTOR

- How long must I remain in the hospital following gallstone removal?
- How do I care for the my incision site?
- How soon can I return to normal activities following gallstone removal?

Occasionally, the ampulla of Vater is too tight for bile to flow through and causes symptoms until it is opened up.

Risks

The most common medical treatment for gallstones is the surgical removal of the gallbladder (cholecsytectomy). Risks associated with gallbladder removal are low, but include damage to the bile ducts, residual gallstones in the bile ducts, or injury to the surrounding organs. With laparoscopic cholecystectomy, the bile duct damage rate is approximately 0.5%.

Normal results

Most patients undergoing laparoscopic cholecystectomy may go home the same day of surgery, and may immediately return to normal activities and a normal diet, while most patients who undergo open cholecystectomy must remain in the hospital for five to seven days. After one week, they may resume a normal diet, and in four to six weeks they can expect to return to normal activities.

Morbidity and mortality rates

Cholecystectomy is generally a safe procedure, with an overall mortality rate of 0.1–0.3%. The operative mortality rates for open cholecystectomy in males is 0.11% for males aged 30, and 13.84% for males aged 81–90 years. Women seem to tolerate the procedure better than males since mortality rates in females are approximately half those in men for all age groups. The improved technique of laparoscopic cholecystectomy accounts for 90% of all cholecystectomies performed in the United States; the improved technique reduces time missed away from work, patient hospitalization, and postoperative pain.

Alternatives

There are no other acceptable alternatives for gallstone removal besides surgery, shock wave fragmentation, or chemical dissolution.

See also Cholecystectomy.

Resources

BOOKS

Bennett, J. Claude, and Fred Plum, eds. *Cecil Textbook of Medicine.* Philadelphia: W. B. Saunders Co., 1996.

Bilhartz, Lyman E., and Jay D. Horton. "Gallstone Disease and Its Complications." In *Sleisenger & Fordtran's Gastrointestinal and Liver Disease,* edited by Mark Feldman, et al. Philadelphia: W. B. Saunders Co., 1998.

Fauci, Anthony S., et al., editors. *Harrison's Principles of Internal Medicine.* New York: McGraw-Hill, 1997.

Feldman, Mark, editor. *Sleisenger & Fordtran's Gastrointestinal and Liver Disease,* 7th Edition. St. Louis: Elsevier Science, 2002.

Hoffmann, Alan F. "Bile Secretion and the Enterohepatic Circulation of Bile Acids." In *Sleisenger & Fordtran's Gastrointestinal and Liver Disease,* edited by Mark Feldman, et al. Philadelphia: W. B. Saunders Co., 1998.

Mulvihill, Sean J. "Surgical Management of Gallstone Disease and Postoperative Complications." In *Sleisenger & Fordtran's Gastrointestinal and Liver Disease,* edited by Mark Feldman, et al. Philadelphia: W. B. Saunders Co., 1997.

Noble, John. *Textbook of Primary Care Medicine,* 3rd Edition. St. Louis. Mosby, Inc., 2001.

Paumgartner, Gustav. "Non-Surgical Management of Gallstone Disease." In *Sleisenger & Fordtran's Gastrointestinal and Liver Disease,* edited by Mark Feldman, et al. Philadelphia: W. B. Saunders Co., 1998.

Sabiston Textbook of Surgery, 16th Edition. Philadelphia: W. B. Saunders Co., 2001.

Laith Farid Gulli, MD
Nicole Mallory, MS, PA-C
J. Polsdorfer, MD

Ganglion cyst removal

Definition

Ganglion cyst removal, or ganglionectomy, is the removal of a fluid-filled sac on the skin of the wrist, finger, or sole of the foot. The cyst is attached to a tendon or a joint through its fibers and contains synovial fluid, which is the clear liquid that lubricates the joints and tendons of the body. The surgical procedure is performed in a doctor's office. It entails aspiration, or draining fluid from the cyst with a large hypodermic needle. The cyst may also be excised (removed by cutting).

Purpose

Ganglion cysts are sacs that contain the synovial fluid found in joints and tendons. They are the most common forms of soft tissue growth on the hand and are distinguished by their sticky liquid contents. The cystic structures are attached to tendon sheaths via a long thin tube-like arm. About 65% of ganglion cysts occur on the upper surface of the wrist, with another 20%–25% on the volar (palm) surface of the hand. Most of the remaining 10%–15% of ganglion cysts occur on the sheath of the flexor tendon. In a few cases, the cysts emerge on the sole of the foot.

Ganglion cysts have appeared in medical writing from the time of Hippocrates (c. 460–c. 375 B. C.). Their exact cause is unknown. There are some indications, however, that ganglion cysts result from trauma to or deterioration of the tissue lining in the joints that secretes synovial fluid.

WHO PERFORMS THE PROCEDURE AND WHERE IS IT PERFORMED?

Aspiration or excision to treat ganglion cysts is done by primary care doctors as well as orthopedic surgeons. The procedures may be performed in the doctor's office or at an outpatient clinic.

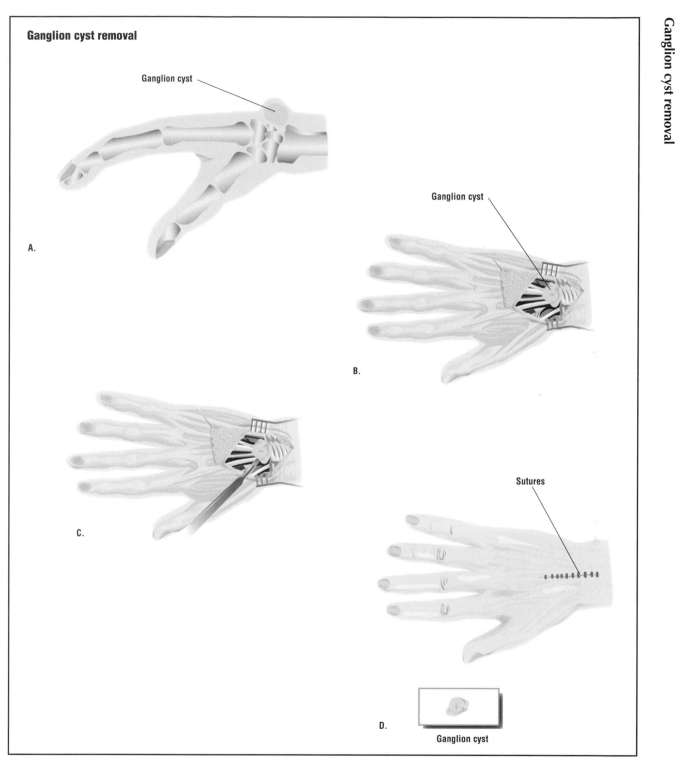

Ganglion cyst removal

A ganglion cyst is usually attached to a tendon or muscle in the wrist or finger (A). To remove it, the skin is cut open (B), the growth is removed (C), and the skin is sutured closed (D). *(Illustration by GGS Inc.)*

Ganglion cysts can emerge quite quickly, and can disappear just as fast. They are benign growths, usually causing problems in the functioning of the joints or tendons of the hand or finger only when they are large. Many people do not seek medical attention for ganglion cysts unless they cause pain, affect the move-

Excision

Some ganglion cysts are so large that the doctor recommends excision. This procedure also takes place in the physician's office with local or regional anesthetic.

Excision of a ganglion cyst is performed as follows:

- The physician palpates, or feels, the borders of the sac with the fingers and marks the sac and its periphery.

- The sac is cut away with a scalpel.

- The doctor closes the incision with sutures and applies a bandage.

- The patient is asked to remain in the office for at least 30 minutes.

Diagnosis/Preparation

Ganglion cysts are fairly easy to diagnose because they are usually visible and pliable to the touch. They are distinguished from other growths by their location near tendons or joints and by their fluid consistency. Ganglion cysts are sometimes confused with a carpal boss (a bony, non-mobile spur on the top of the wrist), but can usually be distinguished by the fact that they can be moved and are usually less painful for the patient.

The doctor may schedule one or more imaging studies of the hand and wrist. An x-ray may reveal bone or joint abnormalities. Ultrasound may be used to diagnose the presence of occult cysts.

Aftercare

Patients should avoid strenuous physical activity for at least 48 hours after surgery and report any signs of infection or inflammation to their physician. A follow-up appointment should be scheduled within three weeks of aspiration or excision. Excision may result in some stiffness after the surgery and some difficulties in flexing the hand because of scar tissue formation.

Risks

Aspiration has very few complications as a treatment for ganglion cysts; the most common aftereffects are infection or a reaction to the cortisone injection. Complications of excision include some stiffness in the hand and scar formation. Ganglion cysts recur after excision in about 5–15% of cases, usually because the cyst was not completely removed.

Normal results

Aspirated ganglion cysts disappear and cause no further symptoms in 27–67% of cases. They may, how-

ment of the nearby tendons, or become particularly unsightly.

An old traditional treatment for a ganglion cyst was to hit it with a Bible, since the cysts can burst when struck. Today, cysts are removed surgically by aspiration but often reappear. Surgical excision is the most reliable treatment for ganglion cysts, but aspiration is the more common form of therapy.

Demographics

Ganglion cysts account for 50%–70% of all soft tissue tumors of the hand and wrist. They are most likely to occur in adults between the ages of 20 and 50, with the female: male ratio being about 3: 1. Most ganglion cysts are visible; however, some are occult (hidden). Occult cysts may be diagnosed because the patient feels pain in that part of the hand or has noticed that the tendon cannot move normally. In about 10% of cases, there is associated trauma.

Description

Patients are given a local or regional anesthetic in a doctor's office. Two methods are used to remove the cysts. Most physicians use the more conservative procedure, which is known as aspiration.

Aspiration

- An 18- or 22-gauge needle attached to a 20–30-mL syringe is inserted into the cyst. The doctor removes the fluid slowly by suction.

- The doctor may inject a corticosteroid medication into the joint after the fluid has been withdrawn.

- A compression dressing is applied to the site.

- The patient remains in the office for about 30 minutes.

KEY TERMS

Aspiration—A surgical procedure in which the physician uses a thick needle to draw fluid from a joint or from a sac produced by a growth or by infection.

Cyst—An abnormal saclike growth in the body that contains liquid or a semisolid material.

Excision—Removal by cutting.

Ganglion—A knot or knot-like mass; it can refer either to groups of nerve cells outside the central nervous system or to cysts that form on the sheath of a tendon.

Ganglionectomy—Surgery to excise a ganglion cyst.

Occult—Hidden; concealed from the doctor's direct observation. Some ganglion cysts are occult.

Synovial fluid—A transparent alkaline fluid resembling the white of an egg. It is secreted by the synovial membranes that line the joints and tendon sheaths.

Volar—Pertaining to the palm of the hand or the sole of the foot.

ever, reoccur and require repeated aspiration. Aspiration combined with an injection of cortisone has more success than aspiration by itself. Excision is a much more reliable procedure, however, and the stiffness that the patient may experience after the procedure eventually goes away. The formation of a small scar is normal.

Morbidity and mortality rates

The only risks for ganglion cyst removal are infections or inflammation due to the cortisone injection. There is a small risk of damage to nearby nerves or blood vessels.

Alternatives

Alternatives to aspiration and excision in the treatment of ganglion cysts include watchful waiting and resting the affected hand or foot. It is quite common for ganglion cysts to fade away without any surgical treatment.

Resources

BOOKS

"Common Hand Disorders." Section 5, Chapter 61 in *The Merck Manual of Diagnosis and Therapy*, edited by Mark H. Beers, MD, and Robert Berkow, MD. Whitehouse Station, NJ: Merck Research Laboratories, 1999.

Ferri, Fred F. *Ferri's Clinical Advisor: Instant Diagnosis and Treatment*. St. Louis, MO: Mosby, Inc., 2003.

Ruddy, Shaun, et al. *Kelly's Textbook of Rheumatology*, 6th ed. Philadelphia, PA: W.B. Saunders, 2001.

PERIODICALS

Tallia, A. F., and D. A. Cardone. "Diagnostic and Therapeutic Injection of the Wrist and Hand Region." *American Family Physician* 67 (February 15, 2003): 745-750.

OTHER

MDConsult.com. *Ganglion Cyst Removal (Ganglionectomy).* <www.mdconsult.com.>

Nancy McKenzie, PhD

Gastrectomy

Definition

Gastrectomy is the surgical removal of all or part of the stomach.

Purpose

Gastrectomy is performed most commonly to treat the following conditions:

• stomach cancer

• bleeding gastric ulcer

• perforation of the stomach wall

• noncancerous polyps

Demographics

Stomach cancer was the most common form of cancer worldwide in the 1970s and early 1980s, and the incidence rates have always shown substantial variation in different countries. Rates are currently highest in Japan and eastern Asia, but other areas of the world have high incidence rates, including Eastern European countries and parts of Latin America. Incidence rates are generally lower in Western Europe and the United States.

Gastrointestinal diseases (including gastric ulcers) affect an estimated 25–30% of the world's population. In the United States, 60 million adults experience gastrointestinal reflux at least once a month, and 25 million adults suffer daily from heartburn, a condition that may evolve into ulcers.

Description

Gastrectomy for cancer

Removal of the tumor, often with removal of the surrounding lymph nodes, is the only curative treatment for various forms of gastric (stomach) cancer. For many patients, this entails removing not only the tumor, but part of the stomach as well. The extent to which lymph nodes should also be removed is a subject of debate, but some studies show additional survival benefits associated with removal of a greater number of lymph nodes.

Gastrectomy, either total or subtotal (also called partial), is the treatment of choice for gastric adenocarcinomas, primary gastric lymphomas (originating in the stomach), and the rare leiomyosarcomas (also called gastric sarcomas). Adenocarcinomas are by far the most common form of stomach cancer and are less curable than the relatively uncommon lymphomas, for which gastrectomy offers good chances of survival.

General anesthesia is used to ensure that the patient does not experience pain and is not conscious during the operation. When the anesthesia has taken hold, a urinary catheter is usually inserted to monitor urine output. A thin nasogastric tube is inserted from the nose down into the stomach. The abdomen is cleansed with an antiseptic solution. The surgeon makes a large incision from just below the breastbone down to the navel. If the lower end of the stomach is diseased, the surgeon places clamps on either end of the area, and that portion is excised. The upper part of the stomach is then attached to the small intestine. If the upper end of the stomach is diseased, the end of the esophagus and the upper part of the stomach are clamped together. The diseased part is removed, and the lower part of the stomach is attached to the esophagus.

After gastrectomy, the surgeon may reconstruct the altered portions of the digestive tract so that it may continue to function. Several different surgical techniques are used, but, generally speaking, the surgeon attaches any remaining portion of the stomach to the small intestine.

Gastrectomy for gastric cancer is almost always done using the traditional open surgery technique, which requires a wide incision to open the abdomen. However, some surgeons use a laparoscopic technique that requires only a small incision. The laparoscope is connected to a tiny video camera that projects a picture of the abdominal contents onto a monitor for the surgeon's viewing. The stomach is operated on through this incision.

The potential benefits of laparoscopic surgery include less postoperative pain, decreased hospitalization, and earlier return to normal activities. The use of laparoscopic gastrectomy is limited, however. Only patients with early-stage gastric cancers or those whose surgery is intended only for palliation (pain and symptomatic relief rather than cure) are considered for this minimally invasive technique. It can only be performed by surgeons experienced in this type of surgery.

Gastrectomy for ulcers

Gastrectomy is also occasionally used in the treatment of severe peptic ulcer disease or its complications. While the vast majority of peptic ulcers (gastric ulcers in the stomach or duodenal ulcers in the duodenum) are managed with medication, partial gastrectomy is sometimes required for peptic ulcer patients who have complications. These include patients who do not respond satisfactorily to medical therapy; those who develop a bleeding or perforated ulcer; and those who develop pyloric obstruction, a blockage to the exit from the stomach.

The surgical procedure for severe ulcer disease is also called an **antrectomy**, a limited form of gastrectomy in which the antrum, a portion of the stomach, is removed. For duodenal ulcers, antrectomy may be combined with other surgical procedures that are aimed at reducing the secretion of gastric acid, which is associated with ulcer formation. This additional surgery is commonly a **vagotomy**, surgery on the vagus nerve that disables the acid-producing portion of the stomach.

Diagnosis/Preparation

Before undergoing gastrectomy, patients require a variety of such tests as x rays, computed tomography (CT) scans, ultrasonography, or endoscopic biopsies (microscopic examination of tissue) to confirm the diagnosis and localize the tumor or ulcer. **Laparoscopy** may be done to diagnose a malignancy or to determine the extent of a tumor that is already diagnosed. When a tumor is strongly suspected, laparoscopy is often performed immediately before the surgery to remove the tumor; this method avoids the need to anesthetize the patient twice and sometimes avoids the need for surgery altogether if the tumor found on laparoscopy is deemed inoperable.

Aftercare

After gastrectomy surgery, patients are taken to the recovery unit and **vital signs** are closely monitored by

Gastrectomy

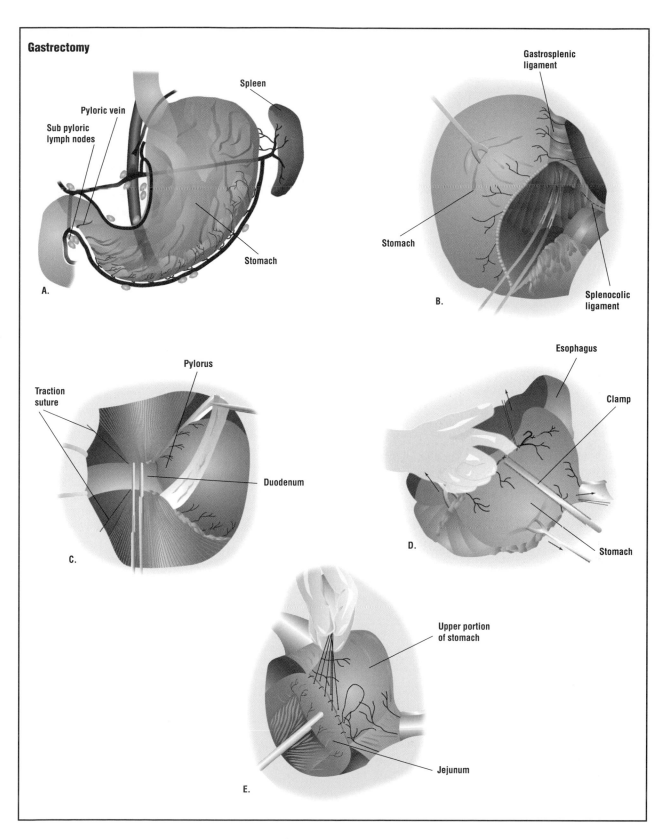

A.

Spleen
Pyloric vein
Sub pyloric lymph nodes
Stomach

B.

Gastrosplenic ligament
Stomach
Splenocolic ligament

C.

Pylorus
Traction suture
Duodenum

D.

Esophagus
Clamp
Stomach

E.

Upper portion of stomach
Jejunum

To remove a portion of the stomach in a gastrectomy, the surgeon gains access to the stomach via an incision in the abdomen. The ligaments connecting the stomach to the spleen and colon are severed (B). The duodenum is clamped and separated from the bottom of the stomach, or pylorus (C). The end of the duodenum will be stitched closed. The stomach itself is clamped, and the portion to be removed is severed (D). The remaining stomach is attached to the jejunum, another portion of the small intestine (E). *(Illustration by GGS Inc.)*

QUESTIONS TO ASK THE DOCTOR

- What happens on the day of surgery?
- What type of anesthesia will be used?
- How long will it take to recover from the surgery?
- When can I expect to return to work and/or resume normal activities?
- What are the risks associated with a gastrectomy?
- How many gastrectomies do you perform in a year?
- Will there be a scar?

the nursing staff until the anesthesia wears off. Patients commonly feel pain from the incision, and pain medication is prescribed to provide relief, usually delivered intravenously. Upon waking from anesthesia, patients have an intravenous line, a urinary catheter, and a nasogastric tube in place. They cannot eat or drink immediately following surgery. In some cases, oxygen is delivered through a mask that fits over the mouth and nose. The nasogastric tube is attached to intermittent suction to keep the stomach empty. If the whole stomach has been removed, the tube goes directly to the small intestine and remains in place until bowel function returns, which can take two to three days and is monitored by listening with a **stethoscope** for bowel sounds. A bowel movement is also a sign of healing. When bowel sounds return, the patient can drink clear liquids. If the liquids are tolerated, the nasogastric tube is removed and the diet is gradually changed from liquids to soft foods, and then to more solid foods. Dietary adjustments may be necessary, as certain foods may now be difficult to digest. Overall, gastrectomy surgery usually requires a recuperation time of several weeks.

Risks

Surgery for peptic ulcer is effective, but it may result in a variety of postoperative complications. Following gastrectomy surgery, as many as 30% of patients have significant symptoms. An operation called highly selective vagotomy is now preferred for ulcer management, and is safer than gastrectomy.

After a gastrectomy, several abnormalities may develop that produce symptoms related to food intake. They happen largely because the stomach, which serves as a food reservoir, has been reduced in its capacity by the surgery. Other surgical procedures that often accompany gastrectomy for ulcer disease can also contribute to later symptoms. These procedures include vagotomy, which lessens acid production and slows stomach emptying; and **pyloroplasty**, which enlarges the opening between the stomach and small intestine to facilitate emptying of the stomach.

Some patients experience lightheadedness, heart palpitations or racing heart, sweating, and nausea and vomiting after a meal. These may be symptoms of "dumping syndrome," as food is rapidly dumped into the small intestine from the stomach. Dumping syndrome is treated by adjusting the diet and pattern of eating, for example, eating smaller, more frequent meals and limiting liquids.

Patients who have abdominal bloating and pain after eating, frequently followed by nausea and vomiting, may have what is called the "afferent loop syndrome." This is treated by surgical correction. Patients who have early satiety (feeling of fullness after eating), abdominal discomfort, and vomiting may have bile reflux gastritis (also called bilious vomiting), which is also surgically correctable. Many patients also experience weight loss.

Reactive hypoglycemia is a condition that results when blood sugar levels become too high after a meal, stimulating the release of insulin, occurring about two hours after eating. A high-protein diet and smaller meals are advised.

Ulcers recur in a small percentage of patients after surgery for peptic ulcer, usually in the first few years. Further surgery is usually necessary.

Vitamin and mineral supplementation is necessary after gastrectomy to correct certain deficiencies, especially vitamin B_{12}, iron, and folate. Vitamin D and calcium are also needed to prevent and treat the bone problems that often occur. These include softening and bending of the bones, which can produce pain and osteoporosis, a loss of bone mass. According to one study, the risk for spinal fractures may be as high as 50% after gastrectomy.

Normal results

Overall survival after gastrectomy for gastric cancer varies greatly by the stage of disease at the time of surgery. For early gastric cancer, the five-year survival rate is as high as 80–90%; for late-stage disease, the prognosis is bad. For gastric adenocarcinomas that are amenable to gastrectomy, the five-year survival rate is 10–30%, depending on the location of the tumor. The prognosis for patients with gastric lymphoma is better, with five-year survival rates reported at 40–60%.

KEY TERMS

Adenocarcinoma—A form of cancer that involves cells from the lining of the walls of many different organs of the body.

Antrectomy—A surgical procedure for ulcer disease in which the antrum, a portion of the stomach, is removed.

Laparoscopy—The examination of the inside of the abdomen through a lighted tube, sometimes accompanied by surgery.

Leiomyosarcoma—A malignant tumor of smooth muscle origin. Can occur almost anywhere in the body, but is most frequent in the uterus and gastrointestinal tract.

Lymphoma—Malignant tumor of lymphoblasts derived from B lymphocytes, a type of white blood cell. Most commonly affects children in tropical Africa.

Sarcoma—A form of cancer that arises in such supportive tissues as bone, cartilage, fat, or muscle.

Most studies have shown that patients can have an acceptable quality of life after gastrectomy for a potentially curable gastric cancer. Many patients will maintain a healthy appetite and eat a normal diet. Others may lose weight and not enjoy meals as much. Some studies show that patients who have total gastrectomies have more disease-related or treatment-related symptoms after surgery and poorer physical function than patients who have subtotal gastrectomies. There does not appear to be much difference, however, in emotional status or social activity level between patients who have undergone total versus subtotal gastrectomies.

Morbidity and mortality rates

Depending on the extent of surgery, the risk for postoperative death after gastrectomy for gastric cancer has been reported as 1–3% and the risk of non-fatal complications as 9–18%. Overall, gastric cancer incidence and mortality rates have been declining for several decades in most areas of the world.

Resources

BOOKS

"Disorders of the Stomach and Duodenum." In *The Merck Manual*. Whitehouse Station, NJ: Merck & Co., Inc., 1992.

"Stomach and Duodenum: Complications of Surgery for Peptic Ulcer Disease." In *Sleisenger & Fordtran's Gastrointesti-nal and Liver Disease*, edited by Mark Feldman et al. Philadelphia: W. B. Saunders Co., 1998.

PERIODICALS

Fujiwara, M., et al. "Laparoscopy-Assisted Distal Gastrectomy with Systemic Lymph Node Dissection for Early Gastric Carcinoma: A Review of 43 Cases." *Journal of the American College of Surgeons* 196 (January 2003): 75–81.

Iseki, J., et al. "Feasibility of Central Gastrectomy for Gastric Cancer." *Surgery* 133 (January 2003): 75–81.

Kim, Y. W., H. S. Han, and G. D. Fleischer. "Hand-Assisted Laparoscopic Total Gastrectomy." *Surgical Laparoscopy, Endoscopy & Percutaneous Techniques* 13 (February 2003): 26–30.

Kono, K., et al. "Improved Quality of Life with Jejunal Pouch Reconstruction after Total Gastrectomy." *American Journal of Surgery* 185 (February 2003): 150–154.

ORGANIZATIONS

American College of Gastroenterology. 4900-B South 31st St., Arlington, VA 22206. (703) 820-7400. <www.acg.gi.org>.

American Gastroenterological Association (AGA). 4930 Del Ray Avenue, Bethesda, MD 20814. (301) 654-2055. <www.gastro.org>.

OTHER

Mayo Clinic Online: Gastrectomy. <www.mayohealth.com >.

Caroline A. Helwick
Monique Laberge, PhD

Gastric acid inhibitors

Definition

Gastric acid inhibitors are medications that reduce the production of stomach acid. They are different from antacids, which act on stomach acid after it has been produced and released into the stomach.

Purpose

Gastric acid inhibitors are used to treat conditions that are either caused or made worse by the presence of acid in the stomach. These conditions include gastric ulcers; gastroesophageal reflux disease (GERD); and Zollinger-Ellison syndrome, which is marked by atypical gastric ulcers and excessive amounts of stomach acid. Gastric acid inhibitors are also widely used to protect the stomach from drugs or conditions that may cause stomach ulcers. Medications that may cause ulcers include steroid compounds and **nonsteroidal anti-inflammatory drugs** (NSAIDs), which are often used to treat arthritis. Gastric acid inhibitors offer some protection against the stress ulcers that are associated with some types of illness and with surgery.

Description

There are two types of gastric acid inhibitors, H_2-receptor blockers and proton pump inhibitors. H_2-receptor blockers are a type of antihistamine. Histamine, in addition to its well-known effects in colds and allergies, also stimulates the stomach to produce more acid. The receptors (nerve endings) that respond to the presence of histamine are called H_2 receptors, to distinguish them from the H_1 receptors involved in causing allergy symptoms. The most common H_2-receptor blockers are cimetidine (Tagamet), famotidine (Pepcid), nizatidine (Axid), and ranitidine (Zantac).

The proton pump inhibitors (PPIs) are drugs that block an enzyme called hydrogen/potassium adenosine triphosphatase in the cells lining the stomach. Blocking this enzyme stops the production of stomach acid. These drugs are more effective in reducing stomach acid than the H_2-receptor blockers. The PPIs include such medications as omeprazole (Prilosec), esomeprazole (Nexium), lansoprazole (Prevacid), pantoprazole (Protonix) and rabeprazole (AcipHex).

Recommended dosages

The recommended dosage depends on the specific drug; the purpose for which it is being used; and the route of administration, whether oral or intravenous. Patients should check with the physician who prescribed the medication or the pharmacist who dispensed it. If the drug is an over-the-counter preparation, patients should read the package labeling carefully, and discuss the correct use of the drug with their physician or pharmacist. This precaution is particularly important with regard to the H_2-receptor blockers, because they are available in over-the-counter (OTC) formulations as well as prescription strength. The two are not interchangeable; OTC H_2-receptor blockers are only half as strong as the lowest available dose of prescription-strength versions of these drugs.

Patients should not use the over-the-counter preparations as an alternative to seeking professional care. For some conditions, particularly stomach ulcers, acid-inhibiting drugs may relieve the symptoms, but will not cure the underlying problems, which require both acid reduction and antibiotic therapy.

Gastric acid inhibitors work best when they are taken regularly, so that the amounts of stomach acid are kept low at all times. Patients should check the package directions or ask the physician or pharmacist for instructions on the best way to take the medicine.

Precautions

There are relatively few adverse reactions when gastric acid inhibitors are used for one to two doses before or just after surgery, The side effects listed below are most often seen with long-term use.

H_2-receptor blockers

Although the H_2-receptor blockers are very safe drugs, they are capable of causing thrombocytopenia, a disorder in which there are too few platelets in the blood. This deficiency may cause bleeding problems, since platelets are essential for blood clotting. Platelet deficiencies can only be recognized by blood tests; there are no symptoms that the patient can see or feel. In addition to affecting platelet levels, the H_2-receptor blockers may cause changes in heart rate, making the heart beat either faster or slower than normal. Patients should call a physician immediately if any of these signs occur:

- tingling of the fingers or toes
- difficulty breathing
- difficulty swallowing
- swelling of the face or lips
- rapid heartbeat
- slow heartbeat

In addition to these signs, the H_2-receptor blockers may cause the following unwanted reactions:

- headache
- diarrhea
- dizziness
- drowsiness
- nausea
- depression
- skin rash
- vomiting

In addition, cimetidine is an inhibitor of male sex hormones; it may cause loss of libido, breast tenderness and enlargement, and impotence.

Ranitidine may cause loss of hair or severe skin rashes that require prompt medical attention. In rare cases, this drug may cause a reduction in the white blood cell count.

Before using H_2-receptor blockers, people with any of these medical problems should make sure their physicians are aware of their conditions:

- kidney disease
- liver disease

• medical conditions associated with confusion or dizziness

Proton pump inhibitors

The proton pump inhibitors are also very safe, but have been associated with rare but severe skin reactions. Patients should be sure to report any rash or change in the appearance of the skin when taking these drugs. The following adverse reactions are also possible:

• stomach cramps

• weakness

• chest pain

• constipation

• diarrhea

• dizziness

• drowsiness

• gas pains

• headache

• nausea with or without vomiting

• itching

• blood in urine

The PPIs make some people feel drowsy, dizzy, lightheaded, or less alert. Anyone who takes these drugs should not drive, use heavy machinery, or do anything else that requires full alertness until they have found out how the drugs affect them.

Before using proton pump inhibitors, people with liver disease should make sure their physicians are aware of their condition.

Taking gastric acid reducers with certain other drugs may affect the way the drugs work or may increase the chance of side effects.

Side effects

The most common side effects of both types of gastric acid reducer are mild diarrhea, nausea, vomiting, stomach or abdominal pain, dizziness, drowsiness, lightheadedness, nervousness, sleep problems, and headache. The frequency of each type of problem varies with the specific drug selected and the dose. These problems usually go away as the body adjusts to the drug and do not require medical treatment unless they are bothersome.

Serious side effects are uncommon with these medications, but may occur. Patients should consult a physician immediately if they notice any of the following:

• skin rash or such other skin problems as itching, peeling, hives, or redness

• fever

• agitation or confusion

• hallucinations

• shakiness or tremors

• seizures or convulsions

• tingling in the fingers or toes

• pain at the injection site that lasts for some time after the injection

• pain in the calves that spreads to the heels

• swelling of the calves or lower legs

• swelling of the face or neck

• difficulty swallowing

• rapid heartbeat

• shortness of breath

• loss of consciousness

Other side effects may occur in rare instances. Anyone who has unusual symptoms after taking gastric acid inhibitors should get in touch with his or her physician.

Interactions

Gastric acid inhibitors may interact with other medicines. When an interaction occurs, the effects of one or both of the drugs may change or the risk of side effects may be increased. Anyone who takes gastric acid inhibitors should give their physician a list of all the other medicines that he or she is taking.

Of the drugs in this class, cimetidine has the highest number of drug interactions, and specialized reference works should be consulted for guidance about this medication.

The drugs that may interact with H_2-receptor blockers include:

• itraconazole (Sporanox)

• ketoconazole (Nizoral)

• warfarin (Coumadin)

• dofetilide (Tikosyn)

• drugs given to open the airway (bronchodilators), including aminophylline, theophylline (Theo-Dur and other brands), and oxtriphylline (Choledyl and other brands)

Drugs that may interact with proton pump inhibitors include:

• itraconazole (Sporanox)

• ketoconazole (Nizoral)

• phenytoin (Dilantin) and other anticonvulsant drugs

- cilostazol (Pletal)
- voriconazole (Vfend)

The preceding lists do not include every drug that may interact with gastric acid inhibitors. Patients should be careful to consult a physician or pharmacist before combining gastric acid inhibitors with any other prescription or nonprescription (over-the-counter) medicine.

Resources

BOOKS

"Factors Affecting Drug Response: Drug Interactions." Section 22, Chapter 301 in *The Merck Manual of Diagnosis and Therapy*, edited by Mark H. Beers, MD, and Robert Berkow, MD. Whitehouse Station, NJ: Merck Research Laboratories, 1999.

"Peptic Ulcer Disease." Section 3, Chapter 23 in *The Merck Manual of Diagnosis and Therapy*, edited by Mark H. Beers, MD, and Robert Berkow, MD. Whitehouse Station, NJ: Merck Research Laboratories, 1999.

Reynolds, J. E. F., ed. *Martindale: The Extra Pharmacopoeia*, 31st ed. London, UK: The Pharmaceutical Press, 1996.

Wilson, Billie Ann, RN, PhD, Carolyn L. Stang, PharmD, and Margaret T. Shannon, RN, PhD. *Nurses Drug Guide 2000*. Stamford, CT: Appleton and Lange, 1999.

ORGANIZATIONS

American Society of Health-System Pharmacists (ASHP). 7272 Wisconsin Avenue, Bethesda, MD 20814. (301) 657-3000. <www.ashp.org>.

United States Food and Drug Administration (FDA). 5600 Fishers Lane, Rockville, MD 20857-0001. (888) INFO-FDA. <www.fda.gov>.

OTHER

<www.nlm.nih.gov/medlineplus/druginfo/medmaster/a682256.html>.
<www.nlm.nih.gov/medlineplus/druginfo/medmaster/a601106.html>.
<www.nlm.nih.gov/medlineplus/druginfo/uspdi/500275.html>.
<www.nlm.nih.gov/medlineplus/druginfo/uspdi/202283.html>.
<www.nlm.nih.gov/medlineplus/druginfo/uspdi/202283.html>.

Samuel Uretsky, PharmD

Gastric bypass

Definition

A gastric bypass is a surgical procedure that creates a very small stomach; the rest of the stomach is removed. The small intestine is attached to the new stomach, allowing the lower part of the stomach to be bypassed.

Purpose

Gastric bypass surgery is intended to treat obesity, a condition characterized by an increase in body weight beyond the skeletal and physical requirements of a person, resulting in excessive weight gain. The rationale for gastric bypass surgery is that by making the stomach smaller a person suffering from obesity will eat less and thus gain less weight. The operation restricts food intake and reduces the feeling of hunger while providing a sensation of fullness (satiety) in the new smaller stomach.

Demographics

Obesity affects nearly one-third of the adult American population (approximately 60 million people). The number of overweight and obese Americans has steadily increased since 1960, and the trend has not slowed down in recent years. Currently, 64.5% of adult Americans (about 127 million) are considered overweight or obese. Each year, obesity contributes to at least 300,000 deaths

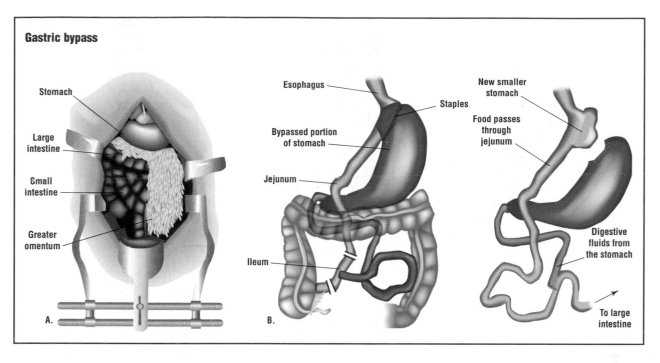

Gastric bypass

Stomach

Large intestine

Small intestine

Greater omentum

A.

Esophagus

Bypassed portion of stomach

Jejunum

Ileum

Staples

B.

New smaller stomach

Food passes through jejunum

Digestive fluids from the stomach

To large intestine

In this Roux-en-Y gastric bypass, a large incision is made down the middle of the abdomen (A). The stomach is separated into two sections. Most of the stomach will be bypassed, so food will no longer go to it. A section of jejunum (small intestine) is then brought up to empty food from the new smaller stomach (B). Finally, the surgeon connects the duodenum to the jejunum, allowing digestive secretions to mix with food further down the jejunum. *(Illustration by GGS Inc.)*

in the United States, with associated health-care costs amounting to approximately $100 billion.

In the United States, obesity occurs at higher rates in such racial or ethnic minority populations as African American and Hispanic Americans, compared with Caucasian Americans and Asian Americans. Within the minority populations, women and persons of low socioeconomic status are most affected by obesity.

Description

Several types of malabsorptive procedures, meaning procedures that are intended to lower caloric intake, may be used to perform gastric bypass surgery, including:

• gastric bypass with long gastrojejunostomy

• Roux-en-Y (RNY) gastric bypass

• transected (Miller) Roux-en-Y bypass

• laparoscopic RNY bypass

• vertical (Fobi) gastric bypass

• distal Roux-en-Y bypass

• biliopancreatic diversion

All procedures aim to restrict food intake and differ in the surgical approach used to create a smaller stomach.

Choice of procedure relies on the patient's overall health status and on the surgeon's judgement and experience.

In the **operating room**, the patient is first put under general anesthesia by the anesthesiologist. Once the patient is asleep, an endotracheal tube is placed through the mouth of the patient into the trachea (windpipe) to connect the patient to a respirator during surgery. A urinary catheter is also placed in the bladder to drain urine during surgery and for the first two days after surgery. This also allows the surgeon to monitor the patient's hydration. A nasogastric (NG) tube is also placed through the nose to drain secretions and is typically removed the morning after surgery.

In most clinics and hospitals, the operation of choice for obese people is the RNY gastric bypass, which has the endorsement of the National Institutes of Health (NIH). The surgeon starts by creating a small pouch from the patient's original stomach. When completed, the pouch will be completely separated from the remainder of the stomach and will become the patient's new stomach. The original stomach is first separated into two sections. The upper part is made into a very small pouch about the size of an egg that can initially hold 1–2 oz (30–60 ml), as compared to the 40–50 oz (1.2–1.5 l) held by a normal stomach. It is created along the more muscular side of the stomach, which makes it less likely to stretch over time. This procedure will allow food to proceed from the mouth to the esophagus, into the gastric pouch, and then immediately into the part of the small bowel called the jejunum (or Roux limb). Food no longer goes to the larger portion of the stomach. Because none of the original stomach is removed, its secretions can travel to the duodenum. The two parts of the stomach are thus completely separated and are closed by stapling and sewing to eliminate the possibility of leaks. Scar tissue eventually forms at the stapled and sewn area so that the pouch and stomach are permanently separated and sealed. Finally, the surgeon reconnects the first part of the jejunum and the duodenum containing the juices from the stomach, pancreas, and liver (the biliopancreatic limb) to the segment of small bowel that was connected to the gastric pouch (the Roux limb).

The opening between the new stomach and the small bowel is called a stoma. It has a diameter of some 0.31 in (0.8 cm). All food goes into the new small stomach and must then pass through this narrow stoma before entering the small intestine. The part of the small intestine from the upper functioning small stomach and the part of the small intestine from the initial lower stomach are joined in a Y connection so that the gastric juices can mix with the food coming from the small pouch.

The RNY can also be performed laparoscopically. The result is the same as an open surgery RNY, except that instead of opening the patient with a long incision on the stomach, surgeons make a small incision and insert a pencil-thin optical instument, called a laparoscope, to project a picture to a TV monitor. The laparoscopic RNY results in smaller scars, and usually only three to four small incisions are made. The average time required to complete the laparoscopic RNY gastric bypass is approximately two hours.

Diagnosis/Preparation

A diagnosis of obesity relies on the patient's medical history and on a body weight assessment based on the body mass index (BMI) and on waist circumference measurements. According to the American Obesity Associa-

tion (AOA), a BMI greater than 25 defines overweight and marks the point where the risk of disease increases from excess weight. A BMI greater than 30 defines obesity and marks the point where the risk of death increases from excess weight. Waist circumference exceeding 40 in (101 cm) in men and 35 in (89 cm) in women increases disease risk. Gastric bypass as a weight loss treatment is considered only for severely obese patients.

To prepare for surgery, the patient is asked to arrive at the hospital a few hours before surgery. While in the preoperative holding room, the patient meets the anesthesiologist who explains the procedure and answers any questions. An intravenous (IV) line is placed, and the patient may be given a sedative to help relax before going to the operating room.

Aftercare

In most cases, gastric bypass is a patient-friendly operation. Patients experience postoperative pain and such other common discomforts of major surgery, as the NG tube and a dry mouth. Pain is managed with medication. A large dressing covers the surgical incision on the abdomen of the patient and is usually removed by the second day in the hospital. Short showers 48 hours after surgery are usually allowed. Patients are also fitted with Venodyne boots on their legs to massage them. By squeezing the legs, these boots help the blood circulation and prevent blood clot formation. At the surgeon's discretion, some patients may have a **gastrostomy** tube (g-tube) inserted during surgery to drain secretions from the larger bypassed portion of the stomach. After a few days, it will be clamped and will remain closed. When inserted, the g-tube usually remains for another four to six weeks. It is kept in place in the unlikely event that the patient may need direct feeding into the stomach. By the evening after surgery or the next day at the latest, patients are usually able to sit up or walk around. Gradually, physical activity may be increased, with normal activity resuming three to four weeks after surgery. Patients are also taught breathing exercises and are asked to cough frequently to clear their lungs of mucus. Postoperative pain medication is prescribed to ease discomfort and initially administered by an epidural. By the time patients are discharged from the hospital, they will be given oral medications for pain. Patients are not allowed anything to eat immediately after surgery and may use swabs to keep the mouth moist. Most patients will typically have a three-day hospital stay if their surgery is uncomplicated.

Postoperative day 1

The NG tube is removed in the morning after surgery. The patient is allowed sips of water throughout the day. The patient is assisted to get out of bed and encouraged to walk. It is very important to walk as early after surgery as possible to help prevent pneumonia, blood clots in the legs, and constipation.

Postoperative day 2

If the patient has tolerated water intake on day 1, he or she may begin taking clear liquids. Patients are encouraged or helped to walk in the hallways at least three times a day and are encouraged to use the breathing machine. The urinary catheter is removed from the bladder. Patients given oral pain medications, crushed, chewed, or in liquid form.

Postoperative day 3

Patients are advanced to a more substantial diet that usually includes milk-based liquids. When the diet is tolerated, pain is well controlled on oral pain medication, and patients are able to walk independently, they are discharged from the hospital. A dietitian usually visits the patient prior to discharge to review any questions about diet. Although most patients spend three days in the hospital, they may remain longer if they have postoperative nausea, fevers, or weakness.

Additional tests are performed at a later stage to ensure that there have been no surgical complications. For example, a swallow study may be performed to make sure that there is no leak where the pouch and intestines have been joined together. Sometimes chest x rays are also performed to make sure that there are no signs of pneumonia. Blood tests may be required. These and other postoperative tests are performed on an individual basis as determined by the **surgical team**.

Risks

Gastric bypass surgery has many of the same risks associated with any other major abdominal operation. Life-threatening complications or death are rare, occurring in fewer than 1% of patients. Such significant side effects as wound problems, difficulty in swallowing food, infections, and extreme nausea can occur in 10–20% of patients. Blood clots after major surgery are rare but extremely dangerous, and if they occur may require re-hospitalization and anticoagulants (blood thinning medication).

Some risks, however, are specific to gastric bypass surgery:

• Dumping syndrome. Usually occurs when sweet foods are eaten or when food is eaten too quickly. When the food enters the small intestine, it causes cramping, sweating, and nausea.

QUESTIONS TO ASK THE DOCTOR

• How is gastric bypass surgery performed?
• What are the benefits of the surgery?
• How long will it take to recover from the surgery?
• When can I expect to return to work and/or resume normal activities?
• What are the risks associated with a gastric bypass?
• How many gastric bypasses do you perform in a year?
• What are the alternatives?

• Abdominal hernias. These are the most common complications requiring follow-up surgery. Incisional hernias occur in 10–20% of patients and require follow-up surgery.

• Narrowing of the stoma. The stoma, or opening between the stomach and intestines, can sometimes become too narrow, causing vomiting. The stoma can be repaired by an outpatient procedure that uses a small endoscopic balloon to stretch it.

• Gallstones. They develop in more than a third of obese patients undergoing gastric surgery. Gallstones are clumps of cholesterol and other matter that accumulate in the gallbladder. Rapid or major weight loss increases a person's risk of developing gallstones.

• Leakage of stomach and intestinal contents. Leakage of stomach and intestinal contents from the staple and suture lines into the abdomen can occur. This is a rare occurrence and sometimes seals itself. If not, another operation is required.

Because of the changes in digestion after gastric bypass surgery, patients may develop such nutritional deficiencies as anemia, osteoporosis, and metabolic bone disease. These deficiencies can be prevented by taking iron, calcium, Vitamin B_{12}, and folate supplements. It is also important to maintain hydration and intake of high-quality protein and essential fat to ensure healthy weight loss.

Normal results

In the years following surgery, patients often regain some of the lost weight. But few patients regain it all. Of course, diet and activity level after surgery also play a role in how much weight a patient may ultimately lose.

Results from long-term follow-up data of gastric bypass surgery show that over a five-year period, patients lost 58% of their excess weight. Over 10 years, the loss was 55%, and after 14 years, excess weight loss was 49%. While there is a tendency to slowly regain some of the lost weight, there is still a significant permanent weight loss over a long period of time.

Morbidity and mortality rates

Obesity by itself does not cause death. However, for those with a body mass index (BMI) above 44 lb/m^2 (20 kg/m^2), morbidity for a number of health conditions will increase as the BMI increases. (M^2 refers to the percent of body fat divided by height). Higher morbidity, in association with overweight and obesity, has been reported for hypertension, dyslipidemia, type 2 diabetes, coronary heart disease, stroke, gallbladder disease, osteoarthritis, sleep apnea and respiratory problems, and some types of cancer (endometrial, breast, prostate, and colon). Obesity is also associated with complications of pregnancy, menstrual irregularities, hirsutism, stress incontinence, and psychological disorders (depression).

Alternatives

Surgical alternatives

The Lap-Band gastric restrictive procedure represents an alternative to gastric bypass surgery. The Lap-Band offers another approach to weight loss surgery for patients who feel that a gastric bypass is not suitable for them. It causes weight loss by lowering the capacity of the stomach, thus restricting the amount of food that can be eaten at one time. The band is fastened around the upper stomach to create a new tiny stomach pouch. As a result, patients experience a sensation of fullness and eat less. Since there is no cutting, stapling, or stomach rerouting involved, the procedure is considered the least invasive of all weight loss surgeries. The surgeon makes several tiny incisions and uses long slender instruments to implant the band. By avoiding the large incision of open surgery, patients generally experience less pain and scarring. In addition, the hospital stay is shortened to less than 24 hours, including overnight hospitalization.

Vertical banded gastroplasty (VBG), another commonly used surgical technique also known as stomach stapling, is today considered inferior to RNY gastric bypass in inducing weight loss. It is also associated with several undesirable complications.

Non-surgical alternatives

Dietary therapy is the fundamental non-surgical alternative. It involves instruction on how to adjust a diet to reduce the number of calories eaten. Reducing calories mod-

erately is known to be essential to achieve gradual and steady weight loss and also to be important for maintenance of weight loss. Strategies of dietary therapy include teaching patients about the calorie content of different foods, food composition (fats, carbohydrates, and proteins), reading nutrition labels, types of foods to buy, and how to prepare foods. Some diets recommended for weight loss include low-calorie, very low-calorie, and low-fat regimes.

Another nonsurgical alternative is physical activity. Moderate physical activity, progressing to 30 minutes or more on most or preferably all days of the week, is recommended for weight loss. Physical activity has also been reported to be a key part of maintaining weight loss. Abdominal fat and, in some cases, waist circumference can be modestly reduced through physical activity. Strategies of physical activity include the use of such aerobic forms of **exercise** as aerobic dancing, brisk walking, jogging, cycling, and swimming and selecting enjoyable physical activities that can be scheduled into a regular routine.

Behavior therapy aims to improve diet and physical activity patterns and habits to new behaviors that promote weight loss. Behavioral therapy strategies for weight loss and maintenance include recording diet and exercise patterns in a diary; identifying such high-risk situations as having high-calorie foods in the house and consciously avoiding them; rewarding such specific actions as exercising for a longer time or eating less of a certain type of food; modifying unrealistic goals and false beliefs about weight loss and body image to realistic and positive ones; developing a social support network (family, friends, or colleagues); or joining a support group that can encourage weight loss in a positive and motivating manner.

Drug therapy is another nonsurgical alternative recommended as a treatment option for obesity. Three weight loss drugs been approved by the U.S. Food and Drug Administration (FDA) for treating obesity: orlistat (Xenical), phentermine, and sibutramine (Meridia).

See also Endotracheal intubation; Gastrostomy.

Resources

BOOKS

Flancbaum, L. *The Doctor's Guide to Weight Loss Surgery.* New York: Bantam Doubleday Dell Pub., 2003.

Thompson, B. *Weight Loss Surgery: Finding the Thin Person Hiding Inside You.* Tarentum, PA: Word Association Publishers, 2002.

Woodward, B. G. *A Complete Guide to Obesity Surgery: Everything You Need to Know About Weight Loss Surgery and How to Succeed.* New Bern, NC: Trafford Pub., 2001.

PERIODICALS

Al-Saif, O., S. F. Gallagher, M. Banasiak, S. Shalhub, D. Shapiro, and M. M. Murr. "Who Should Be Doing Laparoscopic Bariatric Surgery?" *Obesity Surgery* 13 (February 2003): 82–87.

Livingston, E. H., C. Y. Liu, G. Glantz, and Z. Li. "Characteristics of Bariatric Surgery in an Integrated VA Health Care System: Follow-Up and Outcomes." *Journal of Surgical Research* 109 (February 2003): 138–143.

Patterson, E. J., D. R. Urbach, and L. L. Swanstrom. "A Comparison of Diet and Exercise Therapy versus Laparoscopic Roux-en-Y Gastric Bypass Surgery for Morbid Obesity: A Decision Analysis Model." *Journal of the American College of Surgeons* 196 (March 2003): 379–384.

Rasheid, S., et al. "Gastric Bypass Is an Effective Treatment for Obstructive Sleep Apnea in Patients with Clinically Significant Obesity." *Obesity Surgery,* 13 (February 2003): 58–61.

Stanford A., et al. "Laparoscopic Roux-en-Y Gastric Bypass in Morbidly Obese Adolescents." *Journal of Pediatric Surgery* 38 (March 2003): 430–433.

ORGANIZATIONS

American Obesity Association. 1250 24th Street, NW, Suite 300, Washington, DC 20037. (202) 776-7711. <www.obesity.org>.

American Society for Bariatric Surgery. 7328 West University Avenue, Suite F, Gainesville, FL 32607. (352) 331-4900. <www.asbs.org>.

OTHER

"Laparoscopic Gastric Bypass Surgery." *Gastric Bypass Homepage.* [cited June 2003] <www.lgbsurgery.com/>.

"The Roux-en-Y Gastric Bypass." *Advanced Obesity Surgery Center.* [cited June 2003] <www.advancedobesitysurgery.com/gastric_bypass.htm>.

Monique Laberge, PhD

Gastroduodenostomy

Definition

A gastroduodenostomy is a surgical reconstruction procedure by which a new connection between the stomach and the first portion of the small intestine (duodenum) is created.

Purpose

A gastroduodenostomy is a gastrointestinal reconstruction technique. It may be performed in cases of stomach cancer, a malfunctioning pyloric valve, gastric obstruction, and peptic ulcers.

As a gastrointestinal reconstruction technique, it is usually performed after a total or partial **gastrectomy** (stomach removal) procedure. The procedure is also referred to as a Billroth I procedure. For benign diseases, a gastroduodenostomy is the preferred type of reconstruction because of the restoration of normal gastrointestinal physiology. Several studies have confirmed the advantages of the procedure, because it preserves the duodenal passage. Compared to a gastrojejunostomy (Billroth II) procedure, meaning the surgical connection of the stomach to the jejunum, gastroduodenostomies have been shown to result in less modification of pancreatic and biliary functions, as well as in a decreased incidence of ulceration and inflammation of the stomach (gastritis). However, gastroduodenostomies performed after gastrectomies for cancer have been the subject of controversy. Although there seems to be a definite advantage of performing gastroduodenostomies over gastrojejunostomies, surgeons have become reluctant to perform gastroduodenostomies because of possible obstruction at the site of the surgical connection due to tumor recurrence.

As for gastroduodenostomies specifically performed for the surgical treatment of malignant gastric tumors, they follow the general principles of oncological surgery,

---

WHO PERFORMS THE PROCEDURE AND WHERE IS IT PERFORMED?

A gastroduodenostomy is performed by a surgeon trained in gastroenterology, the branch of medicine that deals with the diseases of the digestive tract. An anesthesiologist is responsible for administering anesthesia, and the operation is performed in a hospital setting.

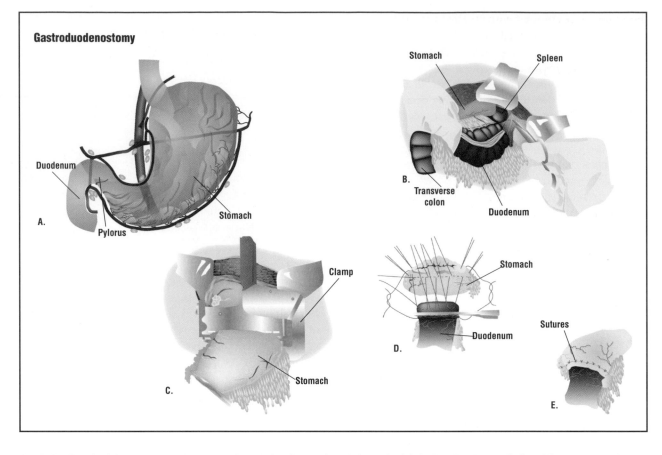

Gastroduodenostomy

An abdominal incision exposes the stomach and duodenum (small intestine) (A). The duodenum is freed from connecting materials (B), and is clamped and severed. The stomach is also clamped and severed (C). The remaining stomach is then connected to the duodenum with sutures (D and E). *(Illustration by GGS Inc.)*

aiming for at least 0.8 in (2 cm) of margins around the tumor. However, because gastric adenocarcinomas tend to metastasize quickly and are locally invasive, it is rare to find good surgical candidates. Gastric tumors of such patients are thus only occasionally excised via a gastro-duodenostomy procedure.

Gastric ulcers are often treated with a distal gastrectomy, followed by gastroduodenostomy or gastrojejunostomy, which are the preferred procedures because they remove both the ulcer (mostly on the lesser curvature) and the diseased antrum.

Demographics

Stomach cancer was the most common form of cancer in the world in the 1970s and early 1980s. The incidence rates show substantial variations worldwide. Rates are currently highest in Japan and eastern Asia, but other areas of the world have high incidence rates, including eastern Europesan countries and parts of Latin America. Incidence rates are generally lower in western European countries and the United States.

Stomach cancer incidence and mortality rates have been declining for several decades in most areas of the world.

Description

After removing a piece of the stomach, the surgeon reattaches the remainder to the rest of the bowel. The Billroth I gastroduodenostomy specifically joins the upper stomach back to the duodenum.

Typically, the procedure requires ligation (tying) of the right gastric veins and arteries as well as of the blood supply to the duodenum (pancreatico-duodenal vein and artery). The lumen of the duodenum and stomach is occluded at the proposed site of resection (removal). After resection of the diseased tissues, the stomach is closed in two layers, starting at the level of the lesser curvature, leaving an opening close to the diameter of the duodenum. The gastroduodenostomy is performed in a similar fashion as small intestinal end-to-end anastomosis, meaning an opening created between two normally separate spaces or organs. Alternatively, the Billroth I procedure may be performed with stapling equipment (ligation and thoraco-abdominal staplers).

Diagnosis/Preparation

If a gastroduodenostomy is performed for gastric cancer, diagnosis is usually established using the following tests:

- Endoscopy and barium x rays. The advantage of endoscopy is that it allows for direct visualization of abnormalities and directed biopsies. Barium x rays do not facilitate biopsies, but are less invasive and may give information regarding motility.

- Computed tomagraphy (CT) scan. A CT scan of the chest, abdomen, and pelvis is usually obtained to help assess tumor extent, nodal involvement, and metastatic disease.

- Endoscopic ultrasound (EUS). EUS complements information gained by CT. Specifically, the depth of tumor invasion, including invasion of nearby organs, can be assessed more accurately by EUS than by CT.

- Laparoscopy. This technique allows examination of the inside of the abdomen through a lighted tube.

The diagnosis of gastric ulcer is usually made based on a characteristic clinical history. Such routine laboratory tests as a complete blood cell count and iron studies can help detect anemia, which is indicative of the condition. By performing high-precision endoscopy and by obtaining multiple mucosal biopsy specimens, the diagnosis of gastric ulcer can be confirmed. Additionally, upper gastrointestinal tract radiography tests are usually performed.

Preparations for the surgery include nasogastric decompression prior to the administration of anesthesia; intravenous or intramuscular administration of **antibiotics**; insertion of intravenous lines for administration of electrolytes; and a supply of compatible blood. Suction provided by placement of a nasogastric tube is necessary if there is any evidence of obstruction. Thorough medical evaluation, including hematological studies, may indicate the need for preoperative transfusions. All patients should be prepared with systemic antibiotics, and there may be some advantage in washing out the abdominal cavity with tetracycline prior to surgery.

Aftercare

After surgery, the patient is brought to the **recovery room** where **vital signs** are monitored. Intravenous fluid and electrolyte therapy is continued until oral intake resumes. Small meals of a highly digestible diet are offered every six hours, starting 24 hours after surgery. After a few days, the usual diet is gradually introduced.

QUESTIONS TO ASK THE DOCTOR

- What happens on the day of surgery?
- What type of anesthesia will be used?
- How long will it take to recover from the surgery?
- When can I expect to return to work and/or resume normal activities?
- What are the risks associated with a gastroduodenostomy?
- How many gastroduodenostomies do you perform in a year?
- Will there be a scar?

Medical treatment of associated gastritis may be continued in the immediate postoperative period.

Risks

A gastroduodenostomy has many of the same risks associated with any other major abdominal operation performed under general anesthesia, such as wound problems, difficulty swallowing, infections, nausea, and blood clotting.

More specific risks are also associated with a gastroduodenostomy, including:

- Duodenogastric reflux, resulting in persistent vomiting.

- Dumping syndrome, occurring after a meal and characterized by sweating, abdominal pain, vomiting, lightheadedness, and diarrhea.

- Low blood sugar levels (hypoglycemia) after a meal.

- Alkaline reflux gastritis marked by abdominal pain, vomiting of bile, diminished appetite, and iron-deficiency anemia.

- Malabsorption of necessary nutrients, especially iron, in patients who have had all or part of the stomach removed.

Normal results

Results of a gastroduodenostomy are considered normal when the continuity of the gastrointestinal tract is reestablished.

Morbidity and mortality rates

For gastric obstruction, a gastroduodenostomy is considered the most radical procedure. It is recommended in the most severe cases and has been shown to provide

KEY TERMS

Adenocarcinoma—The most common form of gastric cancer.

Anastomosis—An opening created by surgical, traumatic, or pathological means between two normally separate spaces or organs.

Barium swallow—An upper gastrointestinal series (barium swallow) is an x-ray test used to define the anatomy of the upper digestive tract; the test involves filling the esophagus, stomach, and small intestines with a white liquid material (barium).

Computed tomography (CT) scan—An imaging technique that creates a series of pictures of areas inside the body, taken from different angles. The pictures are created by a computer linked to an x-ray machine.

Duodenum—The first part of the small intestine that connects the stomach above and the jejunum below.

Endoscopy—The visual inspection of any cavity of the body by means of an endoscope.

Gastrectomy—A surgical procedure in which all or a portion of the stomach is removed.

Gastroduodenostomy—A surgical procedure in which the doctor creates a new connection between the stomach and the duodenum.

Gastrointestinal—Pertaining to or communicating with the stomach and intestine.

Gastrojejunostomy—A surgical procedure in which the stomach is surgically connected to the jejunum.

Laparoscopy—The examination of the inside of the abdomen through a lighted tube, sometimes accompanied by surgery.

Lumen—The cavity or channel within a tube or tubular organ.

Small intestine—The small intestine consists of three sections: duodenum, jejunum, and ileum. All are involved in the absorption of nutrients.

good results in relieving gastric obstruction is in most patients. Overall, good to excellent gastroduodenostomy results are reported in 85% of cases of gastric obstruction. In cases of cancer, a median survival time of 72 days has been reported after gastroduodenostomy following the removal of gastric carcinoma, although a few patients had extended survival times of three to four years.

Alternatives

In the case of ulcer treatment, the need for a gastroduodenostomy procedure has diminished greatly over the past 20–30 years due to the discovery of two new classes of drugs and the presence of the responsible germ (*Helicobacter pylori*) in the stomach. The drugs are the H$_2$ blockers such as cimetidine and ranitidine and the proton pump inhibitors such as omeprazole; these effectively stop acid production. *H. pylori* can be eliminated from most patients with a combination therapy that includes antibiotics and bismuth.

If an individual requires gastrointestinal reconstruction, there is no alternative to a gastroduodenostomy.

See also Gastrectomy; Gastrostomy.

Resources

BOOKS

Benirschke, R. *Great Comebacks from Ostomy Surgery.* Rancho Santa Fe, CA: Rolf Benirschke Enterprises Inc, 2002.

Magnusson, B. E. O. *Iron Absorption after Antrectomy with Gastroduodenostomy: Studies on the Absorption from Food and from Iron Salt Using a Double Radio-Iron Isotope Technique and Whole-Body Counting.* Copenhagen: Blackwell-Munksgaard, 2000.

PERIODICALS

Kanaya, S., et al. "Delta-shaped Anastomosis in Totally Laparoscopic Billroth I Gastrectomy: New Technique of Intra-abdominal Gastroduodenostomy." *Journal of the American College of Surgeons* 195 (August 2002): 284–287.

Kim, B. J., and T. O'Connell T. "Gastroduodenostomy After Gastric Resection for Cancer." *American Surgery* 65 (October 1999): 905–907.

Millat, B., A. Fingerhut, and F. Borie. "Surgical Treatment of Complicated Duodenal Ulcers: Controlled Trials." *World Journal of Surgery* 24 (March 2000): 299–306.

Tanigawa, H., H. Uesugi, H. Mitomi, K. Saigenji, and I. Okayasu. "Possible Association of Active Gastritis, Featuring Accelerated Cell Turnover and p53 Overexpression, with Cancer Development at Anastomoses after Gastrojejunostomy. Comparison with Gastroduodenostomy." *American Journal of Clinical Pathology* 114 (September 2000): 354–363.

ORGANIZATIONS

American College of Gastroenterology. 4900-B South 31st St., Arlington, VA 22206. (703) 820-7400. <www.acg.gi.org>.

American Gastroenterological Association (AGA). 4930 Del Ray Avenue, Bethesda, MD 20814. (301) 654-2055. <www.gastro.org>.

United Ostomy Association, Inc. (UOA). 19772 MacArthur Blvd., Suite 200, Irvine, CA 92612-2405. (800) 826-0826. <http://www.uoa.org>.

OTHER

"Gastroduodenostomy After Gastric Resection for Cancer." *Nursing Hands* [cited June 2003] <www.nursinghands.com/news/newsstories/1004031.asp>.

Monique Laberge, PhD

Gastroenterologic surgery

Definition

Gastroenterologic surgery includes a variety of surgical procedures performed on the organs and conduits of the digestive system. These procedures include the repair, removal, or resection of the esophagus, liver, stomach, spleen, pancreas, gallbladder, colon, anus, and rectum. Gastroenterologic surgery is performed for diseases ranging from appendicitis, gastroesophageal reflux disease (GERD), and gastric ulcers to the life-threatening cancers of the stomach, colon, liver, and pancreas, and ulcerative conditions like ulcerative colitis and Crohn's disease.

Purpose

Scientific understanding, treatment, and diagnostic advances, combined with an aging population, have made this century the golden age of gastroenterology. Gasteroenterologic surgery's success in treating conditions of the digestive system by removing obstructions, diseased or malignant tissue, or by enlarging and augmenting conduits for digestion is now largely due to the ability to view and work on the various critical organs through video representation and by biopsy. The word abdomen is derived from the Latin *abdere*, meaning concealed or un-seeable. The use of gastrointestinal endoscopy, laproscopy, computer tomography (CT) scan, and ultrasound has made the inspection of inaccessible organs possible without surgery, and sometimes treatable with only minor surgery. With advances in other diagnostics such as the fecal occult blood test known as the Guaiac test, the need for bowel surgery can be determined quickly without expensive tests. This is especially important for colon cancer, which is the leading cause of cancer mortality in the United State, with about 56,000 Americans dying from it each year.

Some prominent surgical procedures included in gasteroentologic surgery are:

• Fundoplication to prevent reflux acids in the stomach from damaging the esophagus.

• **Appendectomy** for removal of an inflamed or infected appendix.

• **Cholecystectomy** for removal of an inflamed gallbladder and the crystallized salts called gallstones.

• Vagotomy, **antrectomy**, **pyloroplasty** are surgeries for gastric and peptic ulcers, now very rare. In the last 10 years, medical research has confirmed that gastric and peptic ulcers are due primarily to *Heliobacter pylori*, which causes more than 90% of duodenal ulcers and up to 80% of gastric ulcers. The most frequent surgeries today for ulcers of the stomach and duodenum are for complications of ulcerative conditions, largely perforation.

• **Colostomy**, **ileostomy**, and **ileoanal reservoir surgery** are done to remove part of the colon by colostomy; part of the colon as it enters the small intestine by ileostomy; and removal of part of the colon as it enters the rectal reservoir by ileonal reservoir surgery. These surgeries are required to relieve diseased tissue and allow for the continuation of waste to be removed from the body. Inflammatory bowel disease includes two severe conditions: ulcerative colitis and Crohn's disease. In both cases, portions of the bowel must be resected. Crohn's disease affects the small intestine and ulterative colitis affects the lining of the colon. Cancers in the area of the colon and rectum can also necessitate the resection of the colon, intestine, and/or rectum.

Demographics

Gasteroentologic diseases disproportionately affect the elderly, with prominent disorders including diverticulosis and other diseases of the bowel, and fecal and urinary incontinence. Many diseases, like gastrointestinal malignancies and liver diseases, occur more frequently as people age. Because the number of Americans age 65 and above is expected to rise from 35 million in 2000 to 78 million by 2050, with those over 85 rising from four million in 2000 to almost 18 million by 2050, gastroenterologic surgeries are greatly in need, not only to prolong life but to relieve suffering. It is not surprising that the elderly account for approximately 60% of health care expenditures, 35% of hospital discharges, and 47% of hospital days.

Sixty to 70 million Americans are affected by digestive diseases, according to the National Digestive Diseases Clearinghouse. Digestive diseases accounted for 13% of all hospitalizations in the United States in 1985 and 16% of all diagnostic procedures. The most costly digestive diseases are such gastrointestinal disorders as diarrhea infections ($4.7 billion); gallbladder disease ($4.5 billion); colorectal cancer ($4.5 billion); liver disease ($3.2 billion); and peptic ulcer disease ($2.5 billion). Appendectomy is the fourth most frequent intraabdominal operation performed in the United States. Appendicitis is one of the most common causes of emergency abdominal surgery in children. Appendectomies are more common in males than females, with incidence peaking in the late teens and early twenties. Each year in the United States four appendectomies are performed per 1,000 children younger than 18 years of age. Gallstones are responsible for about half of the cases of acute pancreatitis in the United States. More than 500,000 Americans have gallbladder surgery annually. The most common procedure is the laparoscopic cholecystectomy. Women 20–60 years of age have twice the rate of gallstones as men, and individuals over 60 develop gallstones at higher rates than those who are younger. Those at highest risk for gallstones are individuals who are obese and those with elevated estrogen levels, such as women who take birth control pills or hormone replacement therapy.

According to the Centers for Disease Control and Prevention, 25 million Americans suffer from peptic ulcer disease some time in their life. Between 500,000 and 850,000 new cases of peptic ulcer disease and more than one million ulcer-related hospitalizations occur each year. Ulcers cause an estimated one million hospitalizations and 6,500 deaths per year. According to the American College of Gastroenterology Bleeding Registry, patients tend to be elderly; male; and users of alcohol, tobacco, **aspirin**, non-steroidal anti-inflammatory drugs (NSAIDs), and anticoagulants. According to the National Diabetic and Digestive Diseases (NDDK), about 25–40% of ulcerative colitis patients must eventually have their colons removed because of massive bleeding, disease, rupture, or the risk of cancer. The use of **corticosteroids** to control inflammation can destroy tissue and require removal of the colon. According to the Society of American Gastrointestinal Endoscopic Surgeons, 600,000 surgical procedures alone are performed in the United States to treat a colon disease.

The incidence of gasteroenterologic diseases differs among ethnic groups. For instance, while gastroesophageal reflux disease (GERD) is common in Caucasians, its incidence is lower among African Americans. This is true for the incidence of esophageal and gastric-cardio adenocarcinoma. On the other hand, African Americans, Hispanics, and Asians have a different form of cancer of the esophagus called squamous cell carcinoma, seen also in new immigrants from northern China, India, and northern Iran. While gastric and peptic ulcerative incidence due to *Heliobacter pylori* ranges in rates from 70–80% for African Americans and Hispanics, the rate for Caucasians is only 34%. Caucasians, on the other hand, have higher rates of intestinal gastric cancer. Finally, there are differences in colon cancer mortality between African Americans and Caucasians. African Americans with colon cancer have a 50% higher mortality risk than Caucasians. Advanced cancer stage at presentation accounts for half of this increased risk. Restricted access to health care, especially screening innovations, may account for much of this disparity.

Description

Advances in **laparoscopy** allow the direct study of large portions of the liver, gallbladder, spleen, lining of the stomach, and pelvic organs. Many biopsies of these organs can be performed by laparoscopy. Increasingly, laparoscopic surgery is replacing open abdomen surgery for many diseases, with some procedures performed on an outpatient basis. Gastrointestinal applications have resulted in startling changes in surgeries for appendectomy, gallbladder, and adenocarcinoma of the esophagus, the fastest increasing cancer in North America. Significant other diseases include liver, colon, stomach, and pancreatic cancers; ulcerative conditions in the stomach and colon; and inflammations and/or irritations of the stomach, liver, bowel, and pancreas that cannot be treated with medications or other therapies. Recent research has shown that laparoscopy is useful in detecting small (< 0.8 in [< 2 cm]) cancers not seen by imaging techniques and can be used to stage pancreatic or esophageal cancers, averting surgical removal of the organ wall in a high percentage of cases. There are also recent indications, however, that some laparoscopic procedures may not have the long-lasting efficacy of open surgeries and may involve more complications. This drawback has proven true for laparoscopic fundoplication for GERD disease.

Advances in gastrointestinal fiber-optic endoscopic technology have made endoscopy mandatory for gastrointestinal diagnosis, therapy, and surgery. Especially promising is the use of endoscopic techniques in the diagnosis and treatment of bowel diseases, **colonoscopy**, and **sigmoidoscopy**, particularly with acute and chronic bleeding. Combined with laparoscopic techniques, endoscopy has substantially reduced the need for open surgical techniques for the management of bleeding.

For most gastroenterologic surgeries, whether laparoscopic or open, preoperative medications are given as well as general anesthesia. Food and drink are not allowed after midnight before the surgery the next morning. Surgery proceeds with the patient under general anesthetics for open surgery and local or regional anesthetics for laparoscopic surgery. Specific diseases require specific procedures, with resection and repair of abdomen, colon and intestines, liver, and pancreas considered more serious than other organs. The level of complication of the procedure dictates whether laparoscopic procedures may be used.

Diagnosis/Preparation

The need for surgery of the esophagus, duodenum, stomach, colon, and intestines is assessed by medical history, general physical, and x ray after the patient swallows barium for maximum visibility. Diagnosis and preparation for gasteroentological surgery involve some very advanced techniques. Upper and lower gastrointestinal endoscopies are more accurate in spotting abnormalities than x ray and can be used in treatment. Endoscopy utilizes a long, flexible plastic tube with a camera to look at the stomach and bowel. Quite often, physicians will also use a CT scan for procedures like appendectomy. Upper esophagogastroduodenal endoscopy is considered the reference method of diagnosis for ulcers of the stomach and duodenum. Colonoscopy and sigmoidoscopy are mandatory for diseases and cancers of the colon and large intestine.

Aftercare

For simple procedures like appendectomy and gallbladder surgery, patients stay in the hospital the night of surgery and may require extra days in the hospital; but they usually go home the next day. Postoperative pain is mild, with liquids strongly recommended in the diet, followed gradually with solid foods. Return to normal activities usually occurs in a short period. For more involved procedures on organs like stomach, bowel, pancreas, and liver, open surgery usually dictates a few days of hospitalization with a slow recovery period.

Risks

The risks in gastroenterologic surgery are largely confined to wounds or injuries to adjacent organs; infection; and the general risks of open surgery that involve thrombosis and heart difficulties. With some laparoscopic procedures such as fundoplication with injury or laceration of other organs, the return of symptoms within two to three years may occur. With appendectomy, the rates of infection and wound complications range between 10–18% in patients. The institution of new clinical practice guidelines that include wound guidelines and directed management of postoperative infectious complications are substantially reducing patient mortality. Gallbladder surgery, especially laparoscopic cholecystectomy, is one of the most common surgical procedures in the United States. However, injuries to adjacent organs or structures may occur, requiring a second surgery to repair it. Stomach surgical procedures carry risks, generally in proportion to their benefits. Today, surgery for peptic ulcer disease is largely restricted to the treatment of such complications as bleeding for ulcer perforation. Recent research indicates that surgery for bleeding is 90% effective using endoscopic techniques. Laparoscopic surgery for ulcer complications has not been found to be better than regular surgery. Stomach and intestinal surgery risks include diarrhea, reflux gastritis, malabsorption of nutrients, especially iron, as well as the general surgical risks associated with abdominal surgery. The risks of colon surgery are tied to both the general risks of surgical procedures—thrombosis and heart problems—and to the specific disease being treated. For instance, in Crohn's disease, resection of the colon may not be effective in the long run and may require repeated surgeries. Colon surgery in general has risks for bowel obstruction and bleeding.

Morbidity and mortality rates

According to a recent study published by the *British Journal of Surgery*, a small minority of patients undergoing gastroenterologic surgery are at high risk for postoperative complications that may lead to prolonged hospital stays. In a study of 235 patients, 47% had at least one postoperative complication, with the length of hospital stay at 11 days compared to those without complications with length of stay at six days.

Resources

PERIODICALS

Cappell, M. S. "Recent Advances in Gastroenterology." *Medical Clinics of North America* 86, no.6 (November 2002).

Cappell, M. S., J. D. Waye, J. T. Farrar, and M. H. Sleisenger. "Fifty Landmark Discoveries in Gastroenterology during the Past 50 Years" *Gastroenterology Clinics* 29, no. 2 (June 2000).

Eisen, G. M., et al. "Ethnic Issues in Endoscopy." *Gastrointestinalt Endoscopy* 53, no. 7, (June 1, 2001): 874–5.

Farrell, J. J., and L. S. Friedman. "Gastrointestinal Disorders in the Elderly." *Gastroenterology Clinics* 30, no. 2, (June, 2001).

Lang, M. "Outcome and Resource Utilization in Gastroenterological Surgery." *British Journal of Surgery* 88, no. 7 (July 1, 2001): 1006–14.

ORGANIZATIONS

Crohn's & Colitis Foundation of America, Inc. 386 Park Avenue South, 17th Floor, New York, NY 10016-8804. (800) 932-2423 or (212) 685-3440; Fax: (212) 779-4098. Email: <info@ccfa.org>. <www.ccfa.org.>.

International Foundation for Functional Gastrointestinal Disorders. P.O. Box 17864, Milwaukee, WI 53217. (414) 964-1799 or (888) 964-2001. <www.iffgd.org.>.

National Digestive Diseases Information Clearinghouse. 2 Information Way, Bethesda, MD 20892-3570. <www.niddk.nih.gov>.

OTHER

The Role of Laparoscopy in the Diagnosis and Management of Gastrointestinal Disease. Society of American Gastrointestinal Endoscopic Surgeons. <www.colonoscopy.info/>.

Nancy McKenzie, PhD

Gastroesophageal reflux scan

Definition

Gastrointestinal reflux imaging refers to several methods of diagnostic imaging used to visualize and diagnose gastroesophageal reflux disease (GERD). GERD is one of the most common gastrointestinal problems among children or adults. It is defined as the movement of solid or liquid contents from the stomach backward into the esophagus.

Purpose

The purpose of gastroesophageal reflux scanning is to allow the doctor to visualize the interior of the patient's upper stomach and lower esophagus. This type of visual inspection helps the doctor make an accurate diagnosis and plan appropriate treatment.

Description

A brief description of gastroesophageal reflux disease is helpful in understanding the scanning methods used to diagnose it. Gastroesophageal reflux disease is the term used to describe the symptoms and damage caused by the backflow (reflux) of the contents of the stomach into the esophagus. The contents of the human stomach are usually acidic. Because of their acidity, they have the potential to cause chemical burns in such unprotected tissues as the lining of the esophagus.

Gastrointestinal reflux is common in the general American population. Approximately one adult in three reports experiencing some occasional reflux, commonly referred to as heartburn. About 10% of these persons experience reflux on a daily basis. Most persons, however, have only very mild symptoms. Occasionally, someone may experience a burning sensation as a result of gastrointestinal reflux. This symptom is described as reflux esophagitis when it occurs in association with inflammation.

Gastroesophageal reflux has several possible causes:

• An incompetent lower esophageal sphincter. Acid reflux can occur when the ring of muscular tissue at the boundary of the esophagus and stomach is weak and relaxes too far. Sphincter incompetence is the most common cause of gastroesophageal reflux. The acid juices from the stomach are most likely to flow backward through a weak sphincter when a person bends, lifts a weight, or strains. People with esophageal strictures or Barrett's esophagus are more likely to experience gastroesophageal reflux than are others.

• Acid irritation. Gastric contents are acidic, with a pH lower than 3.9. This degree of acidity is very caustic to the lining of the esophagus; repeated exposures may lead to scarring. If the exposure is sufficiently severe or prolonged, strictures can develop. Occasionally, pancreatic enzymes or bile may also flow backward into the stomach and lower esophagus. These fluids are extremely acidic, with a pH lower than 2.0.

- Abnormal esophageal clearance. Clearance refers to the process of removing a substance from a part of the body, in this case the removal of stomach acid from the esophagus. Acid reflux is ordinarily washed out of the esophagus by the saliva that a person swallows over the course of a day. Saliva also contains some bicarbonate, which helps to neutralize the acidity of the stomach juices. During sleep, however, people swallow less frequently, which results in a longer period of contact between the acid contents of the stomach and the tissues that line the esophagus. The net result is a chemical injury. Sjögren's syndrome, radiation to the oral cavity, and some medications (anticholinergics) also decrease the flow of saliva and can result in chemical injury. Such other medical conditions as Raynaud's disease and scleroderma are often associated with abnormal esophageal clearance. Hiatal hernia is present in more than 90% of persons with erosive disease.

- Delayed gastric emptying. When outflow from the stomach is blocked or the stomach's contractions are weakened, the partially digested food does not leave the stomach in a timely manner. This delay makes gastric reflux more likely to occur.

Heartburn associated with gastroesophageal reflux occurs 30–60 minutes after eating. It also occurs when a person is lying down. Most people who experience gastroesophageal reflux can obtain relief from heartburn with baking soda, bismuth subsalicylate (Pepto-Bismol), or antacid tablets. A pattern of symptom relief following a dose of one of these nonprescription remedies is usually enough to make the diagnosis of gastroesophageal reflux. Under these conditions, the results of a **physical examination** and laboratory tests are usually within normal limits.

Persons with complicated GERD, or those who do not respond to nonprescription heartburn remedies, require special examinations. There are several imaging methods used in the diagnosis of GERD:

Upper endoscopy

Upper endoscopy is the standard procedure for diagnosing GERD, determining the degree of tissue damage, and documenting the findings. A barium esophagography may be performed in addition to an upper endoscopy. Between 50% and 75% of all patients diagnosed with GERD will have abnormalities in the mucous

lining of the esophagus, usually erosion, tissue fragility, and erythema. Upper endoscopy is also used to document esophageal strictures and Barrett's esophagus. Patients with such symptoms as hematemesis (vomiting blood), iron deficiency anemia, guaiac-positive stools, or dysphagia should have an upper endoscopy.

To perform this study, the doctor passes an endoscope, which is a thin instrument with a light source attached, through the patient's mouth into the esophagus. The endoscope allows the doctor to visualize the mucosal lining of the esophagus, the junction between the esophagus and the stomach, and the lining of the upper portion of the stomach. He or she can take biopsy specimens at the same time.

Ambulatory esophageal pH monitoring

This test provides information concerning the frequency and duration of episodes of acid reflux. It can also provide information related to the timing of these episodes. Ambulatory esophageal monitoring is the standard procedure for documenting abnormal acid reflux; however, it is not necessary for most persons with GERD as they can be adequately diagnosed on the basis of their history or by performing an upper endoscopy.

To perform this test, the doctor passes a tiny catheter (about 2 mm wide) with two electrodes through the patient's nose and throat. One electrode is positioned about about 2 in (5 cm) above the esophageal sphincter. The other electrode is positioned just below the esophageal sphincter. Data related to pH level are obtained every four seconds for 24 hours. The patient is instructed to keep a diary of his or her symptoms, and to record coughing episodes, meal times, bedtime, and time of rising. The electrodes are removed after 24 hours and the patients' diary is reviewed.

Barium esophagography

In a barium esophagograph, the patient is given a solution of water and barium sulfate to drink slowly. X-rays are taken at intervals as the patient swallows the mixture; the images are analyzed for signs of reflux, inflammation, dysmotility, strictures, and other abnormalities. Barium esophagography provides important information about a number of disorders involving esophageal function, including cricopharyngeal achalasia (a swallowing disorder of the throat); decreased or reverse peristalsis; and hiatal hernia.

Esophageal manometry

Esophageal manometry is a useful test for patients who may need surgery because it provides data about esophageal peristalsis and the minimum closing pressure of the esophageal sphincter by measuring the pressure within the esophagus. To perform this test, the doctor passes a thin soft tube through the patient's nose or mouth. When the patient swallows, the tip of the tube enters the esophagus and is positioned at the desired location. The patient then swallows air or water while a technician records the pressure at the tip of the tube.

Preparation

Upper endoscopy

Persons are instructed not to eat or drink for 6 hours before an upper endoscopy. A mild sedative may be given to patients who are unusually nervous.

Ambulatory esophageal pH monitoring

No special preparations are needed for this test. A short-acting anesthetic spray is sometimes used to relieve any discomfort associated with placing the electrodes.

Barium esophagography

The patient should not eat or drink for 6 hours before a barium test.

Esophageal manometry

The patient should take nothing by mouth for 8 hours prior to the test. The doctor may use an anesthetic spray to reduce the throat irritation caused by the manometry tube.

Aftercare

Upper endoscopy

After an upper endoscopy, a friend or relative should drive the patient home because of the lingering effects of the sedative.

Other esophageal scans

There are no special aftercare instructions for patients who have had ambulatory esophageal pH monitoring, barium esophagography, or esophageal manometry.

Risks

Upper endoscopy

Patients sometimes feel as if they are choking as the doctor passes the endoscope down the throat. This feeling is uncommon, however, if the patient has been given a sedative.

Ambulatory esophageal pH monitoring

There are no common complications following this test.

Barium esophagography

Constipation after the test is an infrequent side effect that is treated by giving the patient a laxative.

Esophageal manometry

Complications following this test are very rare.

Normal results

Upper endoscopy

An upper endoscopy documents the condition of the mucous lining of the lower esophagus and upper stomach, thus allowing the doctor to evaluate the progression of GERD.

Ambulatory esophageal pH monitoring

Measurements of pH are used to evaluate the degree of GERD.

Barium esophagography

Barium esophagography can detect many structural and functional abnormalities, including the presence of acid reflux, inflammation, tissue masses, or strictures in the esophagus.

Esophageal manometry

This test documents the ability of the esophageal sphincter to close adequately and keep the contents of the stomach from flowing backward into the esophagus.

Health care team roles

A family physician, pediatrician, internist, or cardiologist usually makes the initial diagnosis of GERD. A gastroenterologist usually performs the tests required for diagnosis. A radiology technologist performs the barium esophagography and a radiologist interprets it.

Resources

BOOKS

Bentley D., M. Lawson, and C. Lifschitz. *Pediatric Gastroenterology and Clinical Nutrition*. New York, NY: Oxford University Press, 2001.

Davis, M., and J.D. Houston. *Fundamentals of Gastroenterology*. Philadelphia, PA: Saunders, 2001.

Herbst, J. J. "Gastroesophageal Reflux (Chalasia)," in Richard E. Behrman et al., eds., *Nelson Textbook of Pediatrics*, 16th ed. Philadelphia, PA: Saunders, 2000.

Isselbacher, K. J., and D. K. Podolsky. "Approach to the Patient with Gastrointestinal Disease," in A. S. Fauci et al., eds., *Harrison's Principles of Internal Medicine*, 14th ed. New York, NY: McGraw-Hill, 1998.

Murry, T., and R. L. Carrau. *Clinical Manual for Swallowing Disorders*. Albany, NY: Delmar, 2001.

KEY TERMS

Barrett's esophagus—An abnormal condition of the esophagus in which normal mucous cells are replaced by changed cells. This condition is often a prelude to cancer.

Clearance—The process of removing a substance or obstruction from the body.

Dysphagia—Difficulty in swallowing.

Endoscope—An instrument with a light source attached that allows the doctor to examine the inside of the digestive tract or other hollow organ.

Erosion—A gradual breakdown or ulceration of the uppermost layer of tissue lining the esophagus or stomach.

Erythema—Redness.

Esophageal varices—Varicose veins at the lowermost portion of the esophagus. Esophageal varices are easily injured, and bleeding from them is often difficult to stop.

Esophagus—The muscular tube that connects the mouth to the stomach.

Heartburn—A sensation of warmth or burning behind the breastbone, rising upward toward the neck. It is often caused by stomach acid flowing upward from the stomach into the esophagus.

Hematemesis—Vomit that contains blood, usually seen as black specks in the vomitus.

Incompetent—In a medical context, insufficient. An incompetent sphincter is one that is not closing properly.

pH—A measure of acidity; technically, a measure of hydrogen ion concentration. The stomach contents are more acidic than the tissues of the esophagus.

Raynaud's disease—A disease of the arteries in hands or feet.

Reflux—Backflow, also called regurgitation.

Sjögren's syndrome—An autoimmune disorder characterized by dryness of the eyes, nose, mouth, and other areas covered by mucous membranes.

Sphincter—A circular band of muscle fibers that constricts or closes a passageway in the body. The esophagus has sphincters at its upper and lower ends.

Visualize—To achieve a complete view of a body structure or area.

Orlando, R. *Gastroesophageal Reflux Disease*. New York, NY: Marcel Dekker, 2000.

Owen, W. J., A. Adam, and R. C. Mason. *Practical Management of Oesophageal Disease*. Oxford, UK: Isis Medical Media, 2000.

Richter, J. E. *Gastroesophageal Reflux Disease: Current Issues and Controversies*. Basel, SWI: Karger Publishing, 2000.

Wuittich, G. R. "Diagnostic Imaging Procedures in Gastroenterology," in Lee Goldman and J. Claude Bennett, eds., *Cecil Textbook of Medicine*, 21st ed. Philadelphia, PA: W. B. Saunders, 2000.

PERIODICALS

Carr, M. M., M. L. Nagy, M. P. Pizzuto, et al. "Correlation of Findings at Direct Laryngoscopy and Bronchoscopy with Gastroesophageal Reflux Disease in Children: A Prospective Study." *Archives of Otolaryngology, Head and Neck Surgery* 127 (April 2001): 369-374.

Carr, M. M., A. Nguyen, C. Poje, et al. "Correlation of Findings on Direct Laryngoscopy and Bronchoscopy with Presence of Extraesophageal Reflux Disease." *International Journal of Pediatric Otorhinolaryngology* 54, (August 11, 2000): 27-32.

Mercado-Deane, M. G., E. M. Burton, S. A. Harlow, et al. "Swallowing Dysfunction in Infants Less Than 1 Year of Age." *Pediatric Radiology* 31 (June 2001): 423-428.

Stordal, K., E. A. Nygaard, and B. Bentsen. "Organic Abnormalities in Recurrent Abdominal Pain in Children." *Acta Paediatrica* 90 (June 2001): 638-642.

ORGANIZATIONS

American College of Gastroenterology. 4900 B South 31st Street, Arlington, VA, 22206. (703) 820-7400. <www.acg.gi.org>.

American College of Radiology. 1891 Preston White Drive, Reston, VA, 20191. (703) 648-8900. <www.acr.org>.

American Osteopathic College of Radiology. 119 East Second St., Milan, MO 63556. (660) 265-4011. <www.aocr.org>.

OTHER

American Academy of Family Physicians. <www.aafp.org/afp/990301ap/1161.html>.

American College of Gastroenterology. <www.acg.gi.org/phyforum/gifocus/2evi.html>.

American Medical Association. <www.ama-assn.org/special/asthma/library/readroom/40894.htm>.

National Digestive Diseases Clearinghouse. <www.niddk.nih.gov/health/digest/pubs/heartbrn/heartbrn.htm>.

L. Fleming Fallon, Jr., MD, DrPH

Lee A. Shratter, M.D.

Gastroesophageal reflux surgery

Definition

Gastroesophageal reflux surgery is typically performed in patients with serious gastroesophageal reflux disease that does not respond to drug therapy. Gastroesophageal reflux is classified as the symptoms produced by the inappropriate movement of stomach contents back up into the esophagus. Nissen fundoplication is the most common surgical approach in the correction of gastroesophageal reflux. The laparoscopic method of Nissen fundoplication is becoming the standard form of surgical correction.

Purpose

Gastroesophageal reflux surgery, including Nissen fundoplication and laparoscopic fundoplication, has two essential purposes: heartburn symptom relief and reduced backflow of stomach contents into the esophagus.

Heartburn symptom relief

Because Nissen fundoplication is considered surgery, it is usually considered as a treatment option only when drug treatment is only partially effective or ineffective. Nissen fundoplication is often used in patients with a particular anatomic abnormality called hiatal hernia that causes significant gastroesophageal reflux. In some cases, Nissen fundoplication is also used when the patient cannot or does not want to take reflux medication. Surgery is also more likely to be considered when it is obvious that the patient will need to take reflux drugs on a permanent basis. Reflux drugs, like virtually all drugs, may produce side effects, especially when taken over a period of years.

One of the biggest problems in diagnosing and controlling gastroesophageal reflux disease is that the severity of disease is not directly related to the presence or intensity of symptoms. There is also no consistent relationship between the severity of disease and the degree of tissue damage in the esophagus. When reflux occurs, stomach acid comes into contact with the cells lining the esophagus. This contact can produce a feeling of burning in the esophagus and is commonly called heartburn. Some of the other symptoms associated with this condition include:

- chest pain
- swallowing problems
- changes in vocal qualities

Reduced reflux

The reduction or elimination of reflux is as important, and sometimes more important, than the elimination of symptoms. This necessity leads to one of the most important points in gastroesophageal reflux disease. Long-term exposure to acid in the esophagus tends to produce changes in the cells of the esophagus. These changes are usually harmful and can result in very serious conditions, such as Barrett's esophagus and cancer of the esophagus. Because of this, all persons with gastroesophageal reflux disease symptoms need to be evaluated with a diagnostic instrument called an endoscope. An endoscope is a long, flexible tube with a camera on the end that is inserted down the throat and passed all the way down to the esophageal/stomach region.

All gastroesophageal reflux surgery, including Nissen fundoplication, attempts to restore the normal function of the lower esophageal sphincter (LES). Malfunction of the LES is the most common cause of gastroesophageal reflux disease. Typically, the LES opens during swallowing but closes quickly thereafter to prevent the reflux of acid back into the esophagus. Some patients have sufficient strength in the sphincter to prevent reflux, but the sphincter opens and closes at the wrong times. However, this is not the case in most individuals with gastroesophageal reflux disease. These individuals usually have insufficient sphincter strength. In a small number of cases, the muscles of the upper esophagus region are too weak and are not appropriately coordinated with the process of swallowing.

The development of heartburn does not necessarily suggest the presence of gastroesophageal reflux disease, which is a more serious condition. Gastroesophageal reflux disease is often defined as the occurrence of heartburn more than twice per week on a long-term basis. Gastroesophageal reflux disease can lead to more serious health consequences if left untreated. The primary symptoms of gastroesophageal reflux disease are chronic heartburn and acid regurgitation, or reflux. It is important to note that not all patients with gastroesophageal reflux disease have heartburn. Gastroesophageal reflux disease is most common in adults, but it can also occur in children.

The precise mechanism that causes gastroesophageal reflux disease is not entirely known. It is known that the presence of a hiatal hernia increases the likelihood that gastroesophageal reflux disease will develop. Other factors that are known to contribute to gastroesophageal reflux disease include:

- smoking
- alcohol ingestion
- obesity
- pregnancy

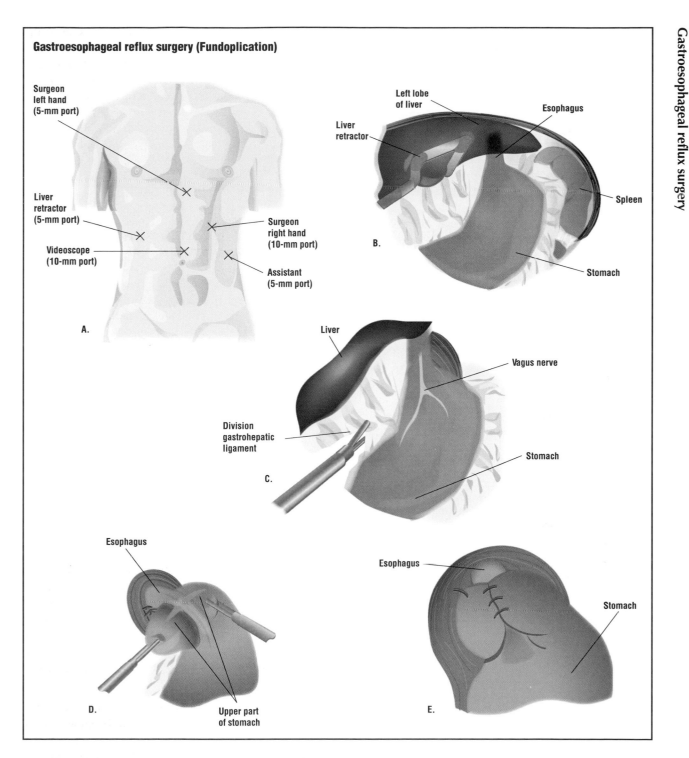

Gastroesophageal reflux surgery (Fundoplication)

In a laparoscopic surgery to alleviate gastroesophageal reflux, the surgeon makes several incisions to gain access to the stomach and esophagus (A). Using the videoscope, the stomach is visualized (B), and the ligament connecting the stomach to the liver is divided (C). The upper part of the stomach is brought up around the base of the esophagus (D), and stitched into place (E). *(Illustration by GGS Inc.)*

The following foods and drinks are known to increase the production of stomach acid and the resulting reflux into the esophagus:

- caffeinated drinks
- high-fat foods
- garlic

- onions
- citrus fruits
- chocolate
- fried foods
- foods that contain tomatoes
- foods that contain mint
- spicy foods

Most patients take over-the-counter antacids initially to relieve the symptoms of acid reflux. If antacids do not help, the physician may prescribe drugs called H_2 blockers, which can help those with mild-to-moderate disease. If these drugs are not effective, more powerful acid-inhibiting drugs called proton-pump inhibitors may be prescribed. If these drugs are not effective in controlling gastroesophageal reflux disease, then the patient may require surgery.

Demographics

It has been estimated that heartburn occurs in more than 60% of adults. About 20% of the population take antacids or over-the-counter H_2 blockers at least once per week to relieve heartburn. In addition, about 80% of pregnant women have significant heartburn. Hiatal hernia is believed to develop in more than half of all persons over the age of 50 years. Hiatal hernia is present in about 70% of patients with gastroesophageal reflux disease, but the majority of patients with hiatal hernia do not have symptoms of gastroesophageal reflux disease. In addition, about 7-10% of the population has daily episodes of heartburn. It is these individuals who are likely to be classified as having gastroesophageal reflux disease.

Description

The most common type of gastroesophageal reflux surgery to correct gastroesophageal reflux disease is Nissen fundoplication. Nissen fundoplication is a specific technique that is used to help prevent the reflux of stomach contents back into the esophagus. When Nissen fundoplication is successful, symptoms and further damage to tissue in the esophagus are significantly reduced. Prior to Nissen fundoplication, open surgery was required to gain access to the lower esophageal region. This approach required a large external incision in the abdomen of the patient.

Fundoplication involves wrapping the upper region of the stomach around the lower esophageal sphincter to increase pressure on the LES. This procedure can be understood by visualizing a bun being wrapped around a hot dog. The wrapped portion is then sewn into place so that the lower part of the esophagus passes through a small hole in the stomach muscle. When the surgeon performs the fundoplication wrap, a large rubber dilator is usually placed inside the esophagus to reduce the likelihood of an overly tight wrap. The goal of this approach is to strengthen the sphincter; to repair a hiatal hernia, if present; and to prevent or significantly reduce acid reflux.

Fundoplication was greatly improved with the development of the laparoscope. The laparoscope is a long thin flexible instrument with a camera and tiny surgical tools on the end. Laparoscopic fundoplication (sometimes called "telescopic" or "keyhole" surgery) is performed under general anesthesia and usually includes the following steps:

- Several small incisions are created in the abdomen.
- The laparoscope is passed into the abdomen through one of the incisions. The other incisions are used to admit instruments to manipulate structures within the abdomen.
- The abdomen is inflated with carbon dioxide. The contents of the abdomen can now be viewed on a video monitor that receives its picture from the laparoscopic camera.
- The stomach is freed from its attachment to the spleen.
- An esophageal dilator is passed through the mouth into the esophagus. This dilator keeps the stomach from being wrapped too tightly around the esophagus.

- The portion of the esophagus in the abdomen is freed of its attachments.

- The top portion of the stomach (the fundus) is passed behind the esophagus, wrapped around it 360°, and sutured in place.

- If a hiatal hernia is present, the hiatus (the hole in the diaphragm through which the esophagus passes) is made smaller with one to three sutures so that it fits around the esophagus snugly. The sutures keep the fundoplication from protruding into the chest cavity.

- The laparoscope and instruments are removed and the incisions are closed.

Diagnosis/Preparation

The diagnosis of gastroesophageal reflux disease can be straightforward in cases where the patient has the classic symptoms of regurgitation, heartburn, and/or swallowing difficulties. Gastroesophageal reflux disease can be more difficult to diagnose when these classic symptoms are not present. Some of the less common symptoms associated with reflux disease include asthma, nausea, cough, hoarseness, and chest pain. Such symptoms as severe chest pain and weight loss may be an indication of disease more serious than gastroesophageal reflux disease.

The most accurate test for diagnosing gastroesophageal reflux disease is ambulatory pH monitoring. This is a test of the pH (a measurement of acids and bases) above the lower esophageal sphincter over a 24-hour period. Endoscopies can be used to diagnose such complications of gastroesophageal reflux disease, as esophagitis, Barrett's esophagus, and esophageal cancer, but only about 50% of patients with gastroesophageal reflux disease have changes that are evident using this diagnostic tool. Some physicians prescribe omeprazole, a proton-pump inhibiting drug, to persons suspected of having gastroesophageal reflux disease to see if the person improves over a period of several weeks.

Aftercare

Patients should be able to participate in light physical activity at home in the days following **discharge from the hospital**. In the days and weeks following surgery, anti-reflux medication should not be necessary. Pain following this surgery is usually mild, but some patients may need pain medication. Some patients are instructed to limit food intake to a liquid diet in the days following surgery. Over a period of days, they are advised to gradually add solid foods to their diet. Patients should ask the surgeon about the post-operative diet. Such normal activities, as lifting, work, driving, showering, and sexual inter-

---

QUESTIONS TO ASK THE DOCTOR

Questions to ask the primary care physician:

- What are my alternatives?
- Is surgery the answer for me?
- Can you recommend a surgeon who performs the laparoscopic procedure?
- If surgery is appropriate for me, what are the next steps?

Questions to ask the surgeon:

- How many times have you performed Nissen or laparoscopic fundoplication?
- Are you a board-certified surgeon?
- What types of outcomes have you had?
- What are the most common side effects or complications?
- What should I do to prepare for surgery?
- What should I expect following the surgery?
- Can you refer me to one of your patients who has had this procedure?
- What type of diagnostic procedures are performed to determine if patients require surgery?
- Will I need to see another specialist for the diagnostic procedures?
- Do you use endoscopy, motility studies, and/or pH studies for your pre-operative evaluation?

---

course can usually be resumed within a short period of time. If pain is more than mild and pain medication is not effective, then the surgeon should be consulted in a follow-up appointment.

The patient should call the doctor if any of the following symptoms develop:

- drainage from the incision region

- swallowing difficulties

- persistent cough

- shortness of breath

- chills

- persistent fever
- bleeding
- significant abdominal pain or swelling
- persistent nausea or vomiting

Risks

Risks or complications that have been associated with fundoplication include:

- heartburn recurrence
- swallowing difficulties caused by an overly tight wrap of the stomach on the esophagus
- failure of the wrap to stay in place so that the LES is no longer supported
- normal risks associated with major surgical procedures and the use of general anesthesia
- increased bloating and discomfort due to a decreased ability to expel excess gas

Complications, though rare, can occur during fundoplication. These complications can include injury to such surrounding tissues and organs, as the liver, esophagus, spleen, and stomach. One of the major drawbacks to fundoplication surgery, whether it is open or laparoscopic, is that the procedure is not reversible. In addition, some of the symptoms associated with complications are not always treatable. One study showed that about 10% to 20% of patients who receive fundoplication have a recurrence of gastroesophageal reflux disease symptoms or develop such other problems, as bloating, intestinal gas, vomiting, or swallowing problems following the surgery. In addition, some patients may develop altered bowel habits following the surgery.

Normal results

One research study found that fundoplication is successful in 50% to 90% of cases. This study found that successful surgery typically relieves the symptoms of gastroesophageal reflux disease and esophagus inflammation (esophagitis). The researchers in this study, however, provided no information on the long-term stability of the procedure. Fundoplication does not always eliminate the need for medication to control gastroesophageal reflux disease symptoms. A different study found that 62% of patients who received fundoplication continued to need medication to control reflux symptoms. However, these patients required less medication than before fundoplication.

Two studies demonstrated that laparoscopic fundoplication improved reflux symptoms in 76% and 98% of the treated populations, respectively. In an additional study, researchers evaluated 74 patients with reflux disease who received Nissen fundoplication after failure of medical therapy. The researchers concluded that 93.8% of the patients had complete resolution of symptoms and did not require anti-reflux medications approximately 14 months after fundoplication. Researchers have found that when fundoplication is successful, the resting pressure in the LES increases. This increase reflects a return to more normal LES functioning where the LES keeps stomach acid in the stomach through increased pressure.

Overall, studies have suggested that the vast majority of patients who receive laparoscopic reflux surgery have positive results. These patients are either symptom-free or have significant improvements in reflux symptoms. The laparoscopic approach has a few advantages over other forms of fundoplication. These advantages include:

- decreased postoperative pain
- more rapid return to work
- decreased hospital stay
- better cosmetic results

Morbidity and mortality rates

Mortality is extremely rare during or following fundoplication. Complications and side effects are not common following fundoplication, especially using the laparoscopic approach, and are usually mild. A review of 621 laparoscopic fundoplication procedures performed in Italy found no cases of mortality and complications in 7.3% of cases. The most serious complication was acute dysphagia (difficulty swallowing) that required a re-operation in 10 patients. In general, long-term complications resulting from this procedure are uncommon.

Alternatives

There are several variations of fundoplication that may be performed. In addition, laparoscopic fundoplication may require conversion to an open, or traditional, surgical fundoplication in a small percentage of cases. The most common alternative to fundoplication is simply a continuation of medical therapy. Typically, patients receive medication for a period prior to being evaluated for surgery. A review of nine studies found that omeprazole, a proton-pump inhibitor, was as effective as surgery. This same review, however, found that the other commonly used anti-reflux drugs, histamine H_2-antagonists, were not as effective as surgery.

Resources

BOOKS

Current Medical Diagnosis & Treatment. New York: McGraw-Hill, 2003.

Ferri, Fred F. *Ferri's Clinical Advisor.* St. Louis, MO: Mosby, 2001.

PERIODICALS

Allgood, P. C., and M. Bachmann. "Medical or Surgical Treatment for Chronic Gastroesophageal Reflux: A Systematic Review of Published Effectiveness." *European Journal of Surgery* 166 (2000): 9.

Kahrilas, P. J. "Management of GERD: Medical vs. Surgical." *Seminars in Gastrointestinal Disease* 12 (2001): 3–15.

Scott, M., et al. "Gastroesophageal Reflux Disease: Diagnosis and Management." *American Family Physician* 59 (March 1, 1999): 1161–1172.

Society of American Gastrointestinal Endoscopic Surgeons. "Guidelines for Surgical Treatment of Gastroesophageal Reflux Disease (GERD)." *Surgical Endoscopy* 12 (1998): 186–188.

Spechler, S. J., et al. "Long-term Outcome of Medical and Surgical Therapies for Gastroesophageal Reflux Disease: Follow-Up of a Randomized Controlled Trial." *Journal of the American Medical Association* 285 (May 9, 2001): 2331–2338.

Triadafilopoulos, G., et al. "Radiofrequency Energy Delivery to the Gastroesophageal Junction for the Treatment of GERD." *Gastrointestinal Endoscopy* 53 (2001): 407–415.

Zaninotto, G., D. Molena, and E. Ancona. "A Prospective Multicenter Study on Laparoscopic Treatment of Gastroesophageal Reflux in Italy." *Surgical Endoscopy* 14 (2000): 282–288.

OTHER

National Digestive Diseases Information Clearinghouse. *Heartburn, Hiatal Hernia, and Gastroesophageal Reflux Disease (GERD).* 2003.

Society of American Gastrointestinal Endoscopic Surgeons. *Patient Information from Your Surgeon and SAGES.* 1997.

Mark Mitchell, M.D., M.P.H., M.B.A.

Gastrostomy

Definition

Gastrostomy is a surgical procedure for inserting a tube through the abdomen wall and into the stomach. The tube, called a "g-tube," is used for feeding or drainage.

Purpose

Gastrostomy is performed because a patient temporarily or permanently needs to be fed directly through a tube in the stomach. Reasons for feeding by gastrostomy include birth defects of the mouth, esophagus, or stomach, and neuromuscular conditions that cause people to eat very slowly due to the shape of their mouths or a weakness affecting their chewing and swallowing muscles.

Gastrostomy is also performed to provide drainage for the stomach when it is necessary to bypass a long-standing obstruction of the stomach outlet into the small intestine. Obstructions may be caused by peptic ulcer scarring or a tumor.

Demographics

In the United States, gastrostomies are more frequently performed on older persons. The procedure occurs most often in African-American populations.

Description

Gastrostomy, also called gastrostomy tube (g-tube) insertion, is surgery performed to give an external opening into the stomach. Surgery is performed either when the patient is under general anesthesia—the patient feels as if he or she is in a deep sleep and has no awareness of what is happening—or under local anesthesia. With local anesthesia, the patient is awake, but the part of the body cut during the operation is numbed.

Fitting the g-tube usually requires a short surgical operation that lasts about 30 minutes. During the surgery, a hole (stoma) about the diameter of a small pencil is cut in the skin and into the stomach; the stomach is then carefully attached to the abdominal wall. The g-tube is then fitted into the stoma. It is a special tube held in place by a disc or a water-filled balloon that has a valve inside allowing food to enter, but nothing to come out. The hole can be made using two different methods. The first uses a tube called an endoscope that has a light at the end, which is inserted into the mouth and fed down

Gastrostomy

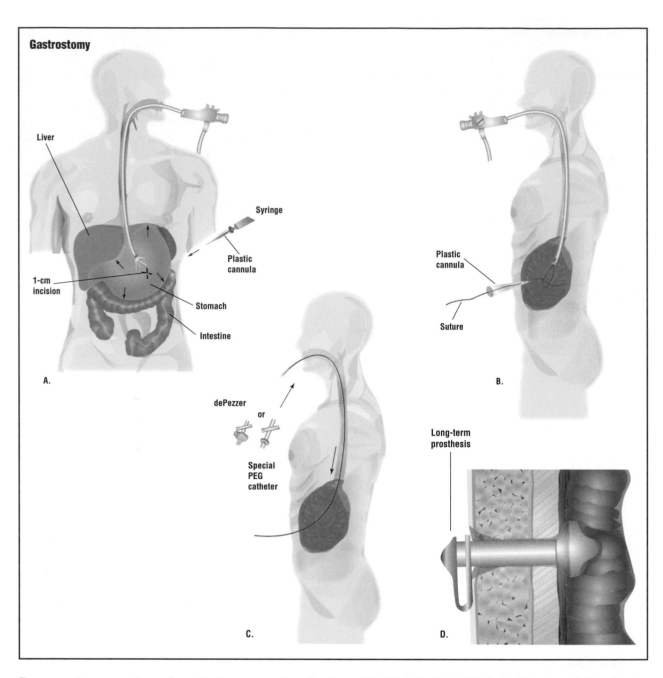

Liver

Syringe

Plastic
cannula

1-cm
incision

Stomach

Intestine

A.

Plastic
cannula

Suture

B.

dePezzer

or

Special
PEG
catheter

Long-term
prosthesis

C.

D.

For a percutaneous endoscopic gastrostomy procedure, the stomach is inflated with air (A). An incision is made into the abdomen and the stomach, and a plastic cannula is inserted (B). A catheter is inserted into the patient's mouth, pulled down the esophagus, and into the stomach (C). When the catheter is in place, access to the stomach is maintained (D). *(Illustration by GGS Inc.)*

the gullet (esophagus) into the stomach. The light shines through the skin, showing the surgeon where to perform the incision. The other procedure does not use an endoscope. Instead, a small incision is made on the left side of the abdomen; an incision is then made through the stomach. A small flexible hollow tube, usually made of polyvinylchloride or rubber, is inserted into the stomach. The stomach is stitched closely around the tube, and the incision is closed.

The length of time the patient needs to remain in the hospital depends on the age of the patient and the patient's general health. In some cases, the hospital stay can be as short as one day, but often is longer. Normally, the stomach and abdomen heal in five to seven days.

The cost of the surgery varies, depending on the age and health of the patient. Younger patients are usually sicker and require more intensive, and thus more expensive, care.

Preparation

Prior to the operation, the doctor will perform an endoscopy and take x rays of the gastrointestinal tract. Blood and urine tests will also be performed, and the patient may meet with the anesthesiologist to evaluate any special conditions that might affect the administration of anesthesia.

Aftercare

Immediately after the operation, the patient is fed intravenously for at least 24 hours. Once bowel sounds are heard, indicating that the gastrointestinal system is working, the patient can begin clear liquid feedings through the tube. The size of the feedings is gradually increased.

Patient education concerning use and care of the gastrostomy tube is very important. Patients and their families are taught how to recognize and prevent infection around the tube; how to insert food through the tube; how to handle tube blockage; what to do if the tube pulls out; and what normal activities can be resumed.

Risks

There are few risks associated with this surgery. The main complications are infection, bleeding, dislodgment of the tube, stomach bloating, nausea, and diarrhea.

Gastrostomy is a relatively simple procedure. As with any surgery, however, patients are more likely to experience complications if they are smokers, obese, use alcohol heavily, or use illicit drugs. In addition, some prescription medications may increase risks associated with anesthesia.

Normal results

The patient is able to eat through the gastrostomy tube, or the stomach can be drained through the tube.

Morbidity and mortality rates

A study performed in 1998 on hospitalized **Medicare** beneficiaries aged 65 years or older who underwent gastrostomy revealed substantial mortality rates. The in-hospital mortality rate was 15.3%. Cerebrovascular disease, neoplasms, fluid and electrolyte disorders, and aspiration pneumonia were the most common primary diagnoses. The overall mortality rate at 30 days was 23.9%, reaching 63% at one year and 81.3% at three years.

Alternatives

There are no alternatives to a gastrostomy because the decision to perform it is made when a person is un-

---

QUESTIONS TO ASK THE DOCTOR

- What happens on the day of surgery?
- What type of anesthesia will be used?
- What happens after g-tube insertion?
- What are the risks associated with the procedure?
- How is the g-tube insertion done?
- Will there be a scar?
- Will I be able to eat normal food?
- Will people notice that I have a g-tube?
- Will it be there forever?

---

able to take in enough calories to meet the demands of his or her body.

Resources

BOOKS

Griffith, H. Winter. *Complete Guide to Symptoms, Illness, & Surgery,* 3rd edition. New York: The Body Press/Perigee, 1995.

Ponsky, J. L. *Techniques of Percutaneous Gastrostomy.* New York: Igaku-Shoin Medical Pub., 1988.

PERIODICALS

Angus, F., and R. Burakoff. "The Percutaneous Endoscopic Gastrostomy Tube. Medical and Ethical Issues in Placement." *American Journal of Gastroenterology* 98 (February 2003): 272–277.

Ciotti, G., R. Holzer, M. Pozzi, and M. Dalzell. "Nutritional Support Via Percutaneous Endoscopic Gastrostomy in Children with Cardiac Disease Experiencing Difficulties with Feeding." *Cardiology of the Young* 12 (December 2002): 537–541.

Craig, G. M., G. Scambler, and L. Spitz. "Why Parents of Children with Neurodevelopmental Disabilities Requiring Gastrostomy Feeding Need More Support." *Developments in Medical Child Neurology* 45 (March 2003): 183–188.

Niv, Y., and G. Abuksis. "Indications for Percutaneous Endoscopic Gastrostomy Insertion: Ethical Aspects." *Digestive Diseases* 20 (2002): 253–256.

ORGANIZATIONS

American Gastroenterological Association (AGA). 4930 Del Ray Avenue, Bethesda, MD 20814. (301) 654-2055. <http://www.gastro.org>.

United Ostomy Association, Inc. (UOA). 19772 MacArthur Blvd., Suite 200, Irvine, CA 92612-2405. (800) 826-0826. <http://www.uoa.org>.

KEY TERMS

Anesthesia—A combination of drugs administered by a variety of techniques by trained professionals that provide sedation, amnesia, analgesia, and immobility adequate for the accomplishment of a surgical procedure with minimal discomfort, and without injury, to the patient.

Endoscopy—A procedure in which an instrument containing a camera is inserted into the gastrointestinal tract so that the doctor can visually inspect the gastrointestinal system.

OTHER

"Stomach Tube Insertion." HealthAnswers. [cited July 6, 2003]. <http://www.healthanswers.com>.

Tish Davidson, AM
Monique Laberge, PhD

GE surgery *see* **Gastroenterologic surgery**

General anesthetic *see* **Anesthesia, general**

General surgery

Definition

General surgery is the treatment of injury, deformity, and disease using operative procedures.

Purpose

General surgery is frequently performed to alleviate suffering when a cure is unlikely through medication alone. It can be used for such routine procedures performed in a physician's office, as **vasectomy**, or for more complicated operations requiring a medical team in a hospital setting, such as laparoscopic **cholecystectomy** (removal of the gallbladder). Areas of the body treated by general surgery include the stomach, liver, intestines, appendix, breasts, thyroid gland, salivary glands, some arteries and veins, and the skin. The brain, heart, lungs, eyes, feet, kidneys, bladder, and reproductive organs, to name only a few, are areas that require specialized surgical repair.

New methods and techniques are less invasive than older practices, permitting procedures that were considered impossible in the past. For example, **microsurgery** has been used in reattaching severed body parts by successfully reconnecting small blood vessels and nerves. Laparoscopic techniques are more efficient, promote more rapid healing, leave smaller scars, and have lower postoperative infection rates.

Demographics

All surgeons receive similar training in the first two years of their residency (post-medical school) training. General surgeons are the surgical equivalent of family practitioners. General surgeons typically differ from other surgical specialties in the operations that they perform. This difference is most easily understood by exclusion. For example, procedures involving nerves or the brain are usually performed by neurosurgeons. Surgeons having specialized training during the final three years of their residency period similarly focus on other regions of the body. General surgeons may perform such procedures in the absence of other surgeons with specialized training. Such procedures are the exception, however, rather than the rule.

In the United States, there are approximately 700,000 physicians licensed to practice medicine and surgery. Experts estimate that fewer than 5% of these physicians (approximately 35,000) restrict their practices to general surgery.

Description

In earlier times, surgery was a dangerous and dirty practice. Through the middle of the nineteenth century, the number of people who died from surgery approximately equaled the number of those who were cured. With the discovery and development of general anesthesia in the mid-nineteenth century, surgery became more humane. As knowledge about infections grew and sterile practices were introduced into the **operating room**, surgery became more successful. The last 50 years have brought continued advancements.

General surgery experienced major advances with the introduction of the endoscope. This is an instrument for visualizing the interior of a body canal or a hollow organ. Endoscopic surgery relies on this pencil-thin instrument, equipped with its own lighting system and small video camera. The endoscope is inserted through tiny incisions called portals. While viewing the procedure on a video screen, the surgeon then operates with various other small precise instruments inserted through one or more of the portals. The specific area of the body to be treated determines the type of endoscopic surgery performed. For example, **colonoscopy** uses an endoscope, which can be equipped with a device for obtaining tissue samples for visual examination of the colon. Gastroscopy uses an endoscope inserted through the mouth to examine the interior of the stomach. Arthroscopy refers to joint surgery. Abdominal procedures are called laparoscopies.

Endoscopy is frequently used in both treatment and diagnosis especially involving the digestive and female reproductive systems. Endoscopy has advantages over many other surgical procedures, resulting in a quicker recovery and shorter hospital stays. This noninvasive technique is being used for appendectomies, gallbladder surgery, hysterectomies, and the repair of shoulder and knee ligaments. However, endoscopy has such limitations as complications and high operating expense. Also, endoscopy does not offer advantages over conventional surgery in all procedures. Some literature states that, as general surgeons become more experienced in their prospective fields, additional noninvasive surgical procedures will become more common options.

One-day surgery is also termed same-day or **outpatient surgery**. Surgical procedures in this category usually require two hours or less and involve minimal blood loss and a short recovery time. In the majority of surgical cases, oral medications control postoperative pain. Cataract removal, **laparoscopy**, **tonsillectomy**, repair of broken bones, hernia repair, and a wide range of cosmetic procedures are common same-day surgical procedures. Many individuals prefer the convenience and atmosphere of one-day surgery centers, as there is less competition for attention with more serious surgical cases. These centers are accredited by the Joint Commission on Accreditation of Healthcare Organizations or the Accreditation Association for Ambulatory Health Care.

Diagnosis/Preparation

The preparation of persons for surgery has advanced significantly with improved diagnostic techniques and procedures. Before surgery, a candidate may be asked to undergo a series of tests, including blood and urine studies, x rays, and specific heart studies if the person's past medical history or **physical examination** warrants this testing. Before any surgical procedure, the physician will explain the nature of the surgery needed, the reason for the procedure, and the anticipated outcome. The risks involved will be discussed, along with the types of anesthesia to be utilized. The expected length of recovery and limitations imposed during the recovery period are also explained in detail before any surgical procedure.

Surgical procedures most often require some type of anesthetic. Some procedures require only local anesthesia, produced by injecting the anesthetic agent into the skin near the site of the operation. The person remains awake with this form of medication. Injecting anesthetic agents

near a primary nerve located adjacent to the surgical site produces block anesthesia (also known as regional anesthesia), which is a more extensive local anesthesia. The person remains conscious, but is usually sedated. General anesthesia involves injecting anesthetic agents into the blood stream or inhaling medicines through a mask placed over the person's face. During general anesthesia, an individual is asleep and an airway tube is usually placed into the windpipe (trachea) to help keep the airway open.

As part of the preoperative preparation, surgical patients will receive printed educational material and may be asked to review audio or videotapes. They will be instructed to shower or bathe the evening before or morning of surgery and may be asked to scrub the operative site with a special antibacterial soap. Instructions will also be given to eat or drink nothing by mouth for a determined period of time prior to the surgical procedure.

Precautions

Persons who are obese, smoke, have bleeding tendencies, or are over 60 need to follow special precautions, as do persons who have recently experienced such illnesses as pneumonia or a heart attack. People taking such medications as heart and blood pressure medicine, blood thinners, **muscle relaxants**, tranquilizers, anticonvulsants, insulin, or sedatives may require special laboratory tests prior to surgery and special monitoring during surgery. Special precautions may be necessary for persons using such mind-altering drugs as narcotics, psychedelics, hallucinogens, marijuana, sedatives, or cocaine since these drugs may interact with the anesthetic agents used during surgery.

Risks

One of the risks involved with general surgery is the potential for postoperative complications. These complications include but are not limited to pneumonia, internal bleeding, and wound infection as well as adverse reactions to anesthesia.

Normal results

Advances in diagnostic and surgical techniques have greatly increased the success rate of general surgery. Contemporary procedures are less invasive than those practiced a decade or more ago. The results include reduced length of hospital stays, shortened recovery times, decreased postoperative pain, and decreases in the size and extent of surgical incisions. The length of time required for a full recovery varies with the procedure.

Morbidity and mortality rates

Mortality from general surgical procedures is uncommon. The most common causes of mortality are adverse reactions to anesthetic agents or drugs used to control pain, postsurgical clot formation in the veins, and postsurgical heart attacks or strokes.

Abnormal results from general surgery include persistent pain, swelling, redness, drainage, or bleeding in the surgical area and surgical wound infection, resulting in slow healing.

Alternatives

For the removal of diseased or nonvital tissue, there is no alternative to surgery. Alternatives to general surgery depend on the condition being treated. Medications, acupuncture, or hypnosis are used to relieve pain. Radiation is an occasional alternative for shrinking growths. Chemotherapy may be used to treat cancer.

Some foreign bodies may remain in the body without harm.

See also Admission to the hospital; Anesthesia evaluation; Outpatient surgery; Reoperation.

Resources

BOOKS

Bland, K. I., W. G. Cioffi, and M. G. Sarr. *Practice of General Surgery.* Philadelphia: Saunders, 2001.

Grace, P. A., A. Cuschieri, D. Rowley, N. Borley, and A. Darzi. *Clinical Surgery,* 2nd Edition. London: Blackwell Publishers, 2003.

Schwartz, S. I., J. E. Fischer, F. C. Spencer, G. T. Shires, and J. M. Daly. *Principles of Surgery,* 7th Edition. New York: McGraw Hill, 1998.

Townsend, C., K. L. Mattox, R. D. Beauchamp, B. M. Evers, and D. C. Sabiston. *Sabiston's Review of Surgery,* 3rd Edition. Philadelphia: Saunders, 2001.

PERIODICALS

Arthur, J. D., P. R. Edwards, and L. S. Chagla. "Management of Gallstone Disease in the Elderly." *Annals of the Royal College of Surgery of England* 85, no. 2 (2003): 91–96.

Cook, R. C., K. T. Alscher, and Y. N. Hsiang. "A Debate on the Value and Necessity of Clinical Trials in Surgery." *American Journal of Surgery* 185, no. 4 (2003): 305–310.

Fraser, S. A., D. R. Klassen, L. S. Feldman, G. A. Ghitulescu, D. Stanbridge, and G. M. Fried. "Evaluating Laparoscopic Skills." *Surgical Endoscopy* 28 (2003): 17–23.

Lawrentschuk, N., M. Pritchard, P. Hewitt, and C. Campbell. "Dressing Size and Pain: A Prospective Trial." *Australia New Zealand Journal of Surgery* 73, no. 4 (2003): 217–219.

ORGANIZATIONS

American Board of Surgery. 1617 John F. Kennedy Boulevard, Suite 860, Philadelphia, PA 19103. (215) 568-4000; Fax: (215) 563-5718. <http://www.absurgery.org>.

American College of Surgeons. 633 North St. Clair Street, Chicago, IL 60611-32311. (312) 202-5000; Fax: (312) 202-5001. Web site: <http://www.facs.org>. E-mail: <postmaster@facs.org>.

American Medical Association. 515 N. State Street, Chicago, IL 60610. (312) 464-5000. <http://www.ama-assn.org>.

American Society for Aesthetic Plastic Surgery. 11081 Winners Circle, Los Alamitos, CA 90720. (800) 364-2147 or (562) 799-2356. <http://www.surgery.org>.

American Society for Dermatologic Surgery. 930 N. Meacham Road, P.O. Box 4014, Schaumburg, IL 60168-4014. (847) 330-9830. <http://www.asds-net.org>.

American Society of Plastic and Reconstructive Surgeons. 444 E. Algonquin Rd., Arlington Heights, IL 60005. (847) 228-9900. <http://www.plasticsurgery.org>.

OTHER

Archives of Surgery (American Medical Association) [cited April 5, 2003]. <http://archsurg.ama-assn.org/>.

Martindale's Health Science Guide [cited April 5, 2003]. <http://www-sci.lib.uci.edu/HSG/MedicalSurgery.html>.

KEY TERMS

Appendectomy—Removal of the appendix.

Endoscope—Instrument for visual examination of the inside of a body canal or a hollow organ such as the stomach, colon, or bladder.

Hysterectomy—Surgical removal of part or all of the uterus.

Laparoscopic cholecystectomy—Removal of the gallbladder using a laparoscope, a fiber-optic instrument inserted through the abdomen.

Microsurgery—Surgery on small body structures or cells performed with the aid of a microscope and other specialized instruments.

Portal—An entrance or a means of entrance.

National Medical Society [cited April 5, 2003]. <http://www.medical-library.org/j_surg.htm>.

Virtual Naval Hospital [cited April 5, 2003]. <http://www.vnh.org/EWSurg/EWSTOC.html>.

Wake Forest University School of Medicine [cited April 5, 2003]. <http://www.bgsm.edu/surg-sci/atlas/atlas.html>.

L. Fleming Fallon, Jr, MD, DrPH

GERD scan *see* **Gastroesophageal reflux scan**

GERD surgery *see* **Gastroesophageal reflux surgery**

Gingivectomy

Definition

Gingivectomy is periodontal surgery that removes and reforms diseased gum tissue or other gingival buildup related to serious underlying conditions. For more chronic gingival conditions, gingivectomy is utilized after other non-surgical methods have been tried, and before gum disease has advanced enough to jeopardize the ligaments and bone supporting the teeth. Performed in a dentist's office, the surgery is primarily done one quadrant of the mouth at a time under local anesthetic. Clinical attachment levels of the gum to teeth and supporting structures determine the success of the surgery. Surgery required beyond gingivectomy involves the regeneration of attachment structures through tissue and bone grafts.

Purpose

Periodontal surgery is primarily performed to alter or eliminate the microbial factors that create periodontitis, and thereby stop the progression of the disease. Periodontal diseases comprise a number of conditions that affect the health of periodontium. The factors include a variety of microorganisms and host conditions, such as the immune system, that combine to affect the gums and, ultimately, the support of the teeth. The primary invasive factor creating disease is plaque-producing bacteria. Once the gingiva are infected by plaque-making bacteria unabated due to immuno-suppression or by oral hygiene, the bacterial conditions for periodontitis or gum infections are present. Unless the microorganisms and the pathological changes they produce on the gum are removed, the disease progresses. In the most severe cases, graft surgery may be necessary to restore tissue ligament and bone tissue destroyed by pathogens.

In healthy gums, there is very little space between the gum and tooth, usually less than 0.15 in (4 mm). With regular brushing and flossing, most gums stay healthy and firm unless there are underlying hereditary or immunosuppressive conditions that affect the gums. The continuum of progressive bacterial infection of the gums leads to two main conditions in the periodontium: gingivitis and periodontitis. Such external factors as smoking, and certain illnesses such as diabetes are associated with periodontal disease and increase the severity of disease in the gum tissue, support, and bone structures. Two types of procedures are necessitated by the severity of gum retreat from the teeth, represented by periodontal pockets. Both nonsurgical and surgical procedures are designed to eliminate these pockets and restore gum to the teeth, thereby ensuring the retention of teeth.

Gingivitis

Gingivitis occurs when gum tissue is invaded by bacteria that change into plaque in the mouth due to disease-fighting secretions. This plaque resides on the gums and hardens, becoming tartar, or crystallized plaque, known also as calculus. Brushing and flossing cannot remove calculus. The gum harboring calculus becomes irritated, causing inflammation and a loss of a snug fit to the teeth. As the pockets between the gum and the teeth become more pronounced, more residue is developed and the calculus becomes resistant to the cleaning ability of brushing and flossing. Gums become swollen and begin to bleed. A dentist or periodontist can reverse this form of gum disease through the mechanical removal of calculus and plaque. This cleaning procedure is called curettage, which is a deep cleaning process that includes scraping the tartar off the teeth above and below the gum line and planing or smoothing the tooth at the root. Also known as dental **débridement**, this procedure is often accompanied by antibiotic treatment to stave off further microbe proliferation.

Periodontitis

Periodontitis is the generalized condition of the periodontium in which gums are so inflamed by bacteria-produced calculus that they separate from the teeth, creating large pockets (more than 0.23 in [6 mm] from the teeth), with increased destruction of periodontal structures and noticeable tooth mobility. Periodontitis is the stage of the disease that threatens significant ligament damage and tooth loss. If earlier procedures like scaling and root planing cannot restore the gum tissue to a healthy, firm state and pocket depth is still sufficient to warrant treatment, a gingivectomy is indicated. The comparative success of this surgery over such nonsurgical treatments as more débridement and more frequent use of **antibiotics** has not been demonstrated by research.

Demographics

According to a report by the U.S. Surgeon General in 2000, half of adults living in the United States have gingivitis, and about one in five have periodontitis. According to the same report, smokers are four times more likely than nonsmokers to have periodontitis, and three to four times more likely to lose some or all of their teeth. By region, individuals living in the Southern states have a higher rate of periodontal disease and tooth loss than other regions of the country. Severe gum disease affects about 14% of adults aged 45–54 years. One of the main risk factors for gum disease is lack of dental care. Initiatives by the Centers for Disease Control and Pre-

vention have begun to study the relation between periodontal disease and general health. There is growing acknowledgment of the public health issues related to chronic periodontal disease.

The delivery of oral surgery, or even dental care, to individuals in the United States is difficult to determine. Race, ethnicity, and poverty level stratified individuals making dental visits in a year. While 70% of white individuals made visits, only 56% of non-Hispanic black individuals and only 50% of Mexican-American individuals made visits. Seventy-two percent of individuals at or above the federal poverty level made visits, while only 50% of those below the poverty level made visits. Since it is also estimated that more than 100 million Americans lack dental insurance, it is likely that periodontal surgery among the people most likely to have periodontal disease (low-income individuals with nutritional issues, with little or no preventive dental care, and who smoke) are the least likely to have periodontal surgery.

Description

Periodontal procedures for gingivitis involve gingival curettage, in which the surgeon cuts away some of the most hygienically unhealthy tissue, reducing the depth of the pocket. This surgery is usually done under a local anesthetic and is done on one quadrant of the mouth at a time.

Gingival or periodontal flap surgery (gingivectomy) is indicated in advanced periodontal disease, in which the stability of the teeth are compromised by infection, which displaces ligament and bone. In gingivectomy, the gingival flap is resected or separated from the bone, exposing the root. The calculus buildup on the tooth, down to the root, is removed. The surgery is performed under local anesthetic.

Small incisions are made in the gum to allow the dentist to see both tooth and bone. The surrounding alveolar, or exposed bone, may require reforming to ensure proper healing. Gum tissue is returned to the tooth and sutured. A putty-like coating spread over the teeth and gums protects the sutures. This coating serves as a kind of bandage and allows the eating of soft foods and drinking of liquids after surgery. The typical procedure takes between one and two hours and usually involves only one or two quadrants per visit. The sutures remain in place for approximately one week. Pain medication is prescribed and antibiotic treatment is begun.

Diagnosis/Preparation

Many factors contribute to periodontal disease, and the process that leads to the need for surgery may occur early or take many months or years to develop. Early primary tooth mobility or early primary tooth loss in children may be due to very serious underlying diseases, including hereditary gingival fibromatosis, a fibrous enlargement of the gingiva; conditions induced by drugs for liver disease; or gum conditions related to leukemia. Patient-related factors for chronic periodontal disease include systemic health, age, oral hygiene, various presurgical therapeutic options, and the patient's ability to control plaque formation and smoking. Another factor includes the extent and frequency of periodontal procedures to remove subgingival deposits. Gum inflammation can be secondary to many conditions, including diabetes, genetic predisposition, stress, immuno-suppression, pregnancy, medications, and nutrition.

The most telling signs of early gum disease are swollen gums and bleeding. If gingivectomy is considered, consultation with the patient's physician is important, as are instruction and reinforcement with the patient to control plaque. Gingiva scaling and root planing should be performed to remove plaque and calculus to see if gum health improves.

The protective responses of the body and the use of dental practices to overcome the pathology of periodontal disease may be thwarted and the concentration of pathogens may be such that plaque below the gum line leads to tissue destruction. Refractory periodontitis, or the form of periodontal disease characterized by its resistance to repeated gingival treatments, and often also associated with diabetes milletis and other systematic diseases, may require surgery to remove deep pockets and to offer regenerative procedures like tissue and bone grafts.

The level of damage is determined by signs of inflammation and by measuring the pocket depth. Healthy pockets around the teeth are usually between 0.04–0.11 in (1–3 mm). The dentist measures each tooth and notes the findings. If the pockets are more than 0.19–0.23 in (5–6 mm), x rays may be taken to look at bone loss. After conferring with the patient, a decision will be made to have periodontal surgery or to try medications and/or more gingival scaling.

Risks for infection must be assessed prior to surgery. Certain conditions, including damaged heart valves, congenital heart defects, immunosuppression, liver disease, and such artificial joints as hip or **knee replacements**, put the oral surgery patient at higher risk for infection. Ultimately, the decision for surgery should be based upon the health of the patient, the quality of life with or without surgery, their willingness to change such lifestyle factors as smoking and bad nutrition, and the ability to incorporate oral hygiene into a daily regimen. Expense is also a factor since periodontal surgery is relatively expen-

QUESTIONS TO ASK THE DOCTOR

- How many quadrants for surgery will be performed at each visit?
- Can the gum scaling and root planing be repeated with antibiotic treatment as an alternative to gingivectomy?
- How effective have you found antibacterial, antibiotic, or anti-microbial treatment in slowing down disease progression?
- How often must I return to have periodontal cleaning after the surgery? Can my regular dentist do that?
- Besides dental care and home hygiene, what can I do to keep the disease from reoccurring after surgery?

sive. Long-term studies are still needed to determine if such medications as antibiotic treatments are superior to surgery for severe chronic periodontal disease.

Aftercare

Surgery will take place in the periodontist's office and usually takes a few hours from the time of surgery until the anesthetic wears off. After that, normal activities are encouraged. It takes a few days or weeks for the gums to completely heal. Ibuprofen (Advil) or **acetaminophen** (Tylenol) is very effective for pain. Dental management after surgery that includes deep cleaning by a dental hygienist will be put in force to maintain the health of the gums. Visits to the dentist for the first year are scheduled every three months to remove plaque and tartar buildup. After a year, periodontal cleaning is required every six months.

Risks

Periodontal surgery has few risks. There is, however, the risk of introducing infection into the bloodstream. Some surgeons require antibiotic treatment before and after surgery.

Normal results

The gold standard of periodontal treatment is the decrease of attachment loss, which is the decrease in tooth loss due to gingival conditions. Normal immediate results of surgery are short-term pain; some gum shrinkage due

KEY TERMS

Calculus—A term for plaque buildup on the teeth that has crystallized.

Gingivitis—Inflammation of the gingiva or gums caused by bacterial buildup in plague on the teeth.

Periodontitis—Generalized disease of the gums in which unremoved calculus has separated the gingiva or gum tissue from the teeth and threatens support ligaments of the teeth and bone.

Scaling and root planing—A dental procedure to treat gingivitis in which the teeth are scraped inside the gum area and the root of the tooth is planed to dislodge bacterial deposits.

to the surgery, which over time takes on a more normal shape; and easier success with oral hygiene. Long-term results are equivocal. One study followed 600 patients in a private periodontal practice for more than 15 years. The study found tooth retention was more closely related to the individual case of disease than to the type of surgery performed. In another study, a retrospective chart review of 335 patients who had received non-surgical treatment was conducted. All patients were active cases for 10 years, and 44.8% also had periodontal surgery. The results of the study showed that those who received surgical therapy lost more teeth than those who received nonsurgical treatment. The factor that predicted tooth loss was neither procedure: it was earlier or initial attachment loss.

Morbidity and mortality rates

The most common complications of oral surgery include bleeding, pain, and swelling. Less common complications are infections of the gums from the surgery. Rarer still is a bloodstream infection from the surgery, which can have serious consequences.

Alternatives

Alternatives to periodontal surgery include other dental procedures concomitant with medication treatment as well as changes in lifestyle. Lifestyle changes include quitting smoking, nutritional changes, **exercise**, and better oral hygiene. There have been some medication advances for the gum infections that lead to inflammation and disease. Medication, combined with scaling and root planing, can be very effective. New treatments include antimicrobial mouthwashes to control bacteria; a gelatin-filled antibiotic "chip" inserted into periodontal pockets; and low doses of an antibiotic medication to keep destructive enzymes from combining with the bacteria to create plaque.

Resources

PERIODICALS

"Guidelines for Periodontal Therapy." *Journal of Periodontology* 72, nos. 11 + 16 (November 2001): 1624–1628.

Delaney, J. E., amd M. A. Keels. "Pediatric Oral Health." *Pediatric Clinics of North America* 47, no. 5 (October 2000).

Matthews, D. C., et al. "Tooth Loss in Periodontal Patients." *Journal of the Canadian Dental Association,* 67 (2001): 207–10.

ORGANIZATIONS

Periodontal (Gum) Diseases. National Institute of Dental and Craniofacial Research, National Institutes of Health. Bethesda, MD 20892-2190. (301) 496-4261. <http://www.nidcrinfo.nih.gov.>.

OTHER

"Cigarette Smoking Linked to Gum Diseases." *National Center for Chronic Disease Prevention and Health Promotion.* <http://www.cdc.gov/nccdphp.>.

"Gingivectomy for Gum Disease." *WebMD Health.* <www.webmd.com>.

Nancy McKenzie, PhD

Glaucoma cryotherapy *see* **Cyclocryotherapy**

Glossectomy

Definition

A glossectomy is the surgical removal of all or part of the tongue.

Purpose

A glossectomy is performed to treat cancer of the tongue. Removing the tongue is indicated if the patient has a cancer that does not respond to other forms of treatment. In most cases, however, only part of the tongue is removed (partial glossectomy). Cancer of the tongue is considered very dangerous due to the fact that it can easily spread to nearby lymph glands. Most cancer specialists recommend surgical removal of the cancerous tissue.

Demographics

According to the Oral Cancer Foundation, 30,000 Americans will be diagnosed with oral or pharyngeal cancer in 2003, or about 1.1 persons per 100,000. Of

WHO PERFORMS THE PROCEDURE AND WHERE IS IT PERFORMED?

A glossectomy is performed in a hospital by a treatment team specializing in head and neck oncology surgery. The treatment team usually includes an ear, nose & throat (ENT) surgeon, an oral-maxillofacial (OMF) surgeon, a plastic surgeon, a clinical oncologist, a nurse, a speech therapist, and a dietician.

QUESTIONS TO ASK THE DOCTOR

- Will the glossectomy prevent the cancer from coming back?
- What are the possible complications of this procedure?
- How long will it take to recover from the surgery?
- How will the glossectomy affect my speech?
- What specific techniques do you use?
- How many new cancers of the head and neck do you treat every year?

these 30,000 newly diagnosed individuals, only half will be alive in five years. This percentage has shown little improvement for decades. The problem is much greater in the rest of the world, with over 350,000 to 400,000 new cases of oral cancer appearing each year.

The most important risk factors for cancer of the tongue are alcohol consumption and smoking. The risk is significantly higher in patients who use both alcohol and tobacco than in those who consume only one.

Description

Glossectomies are always performed under general anesthesia. A partial glossectomy is a relatively simple operation. If the "hole" left by the excision of the cancer is small, it is commonly repaired by sewing up the tongue immediately or by using a small graft of skin. If the glossectomy is more extensive, care is taken to repair the tongue so as to maintain its mobility. A common approach is to use a piece of skin taken from the wrist together with the blood vessels that supply it. This type of graft is called a *radial forearm free flap*. The flap is inserted into the hole in the tongue. This procedure requires a highly skilled surgeon who is able to connect very small arteries. Complete removal of the tongue, called a total glossectomy, is rarely performed.

Diagnosis/Preparation

If an area of abnormal tissue has been found in the mouth, either by the patient or by a dentist or doctor, a biopsy is the only way to confirm a diagnosis of cancer. A pathologist, who is a physician who specializes in the study of disease, examines the tissue sample under a microscope to check for cancer cells.

If the biopsy indicates that cancer is present, a comprehensive **physical examination** of the patient's head and neck is performed prior to surgery. The patient will meet with the treatment team before **admission to the hospital** so that they can answer questions and explain the treatment plan.

Aftercare

Patients usually remain in the hospital for seven to 10 days after a glossectomy. They often require oxygen in the first 24–48 hours after the operation. Oxygen is administered through a face mask or through two small tubes placed in the nostrils. The patient is given fluids through a tube that goes from the nose to the stomach until he or she can tolerate taking food by mouth. Radiation treatment is often scheduled after the surgery to destroy any remaining cancer cells. As patients regain the ability to eat and swallow, they also begin speech therapy.

Risks

Risks associated with a glossectomy include:

- Bleeding from the tongue. This is an early complication of surgery; it can result in severe swelling leading to blockage of the airway.
- Poor speech and difficulty swallowing. This complication depends on how much of the tongue is removed.
- Fistula formation. Incomplete healing may result in the formation of a passage between the skin and the mouth cavity within the first two weeks following a glossectomy. This complication often occurs after feeding has resumed. Patients who have had radiotherapy are at greater risk of developing a fistula.
- Flap failure. This complication is often due to problems with the flap's blood supply.

Normal results

A successful glossectomy results in complete removal of the cancer, improved ability to swallow food, and re-

KEY TERMS

Biopsy—A diagnostic procedure that involves obtaining a tissue specimen for microscopic analysis to establish a precise diagnosis.

Fistula (plural, fistulae)—An abnormal passage that develops either between two organs inside the body or between an organ and the surface of the body. Fistula formation is one of the possible complications of a glossectomy.

Flap—A piece of tissue for grafting that has kept its own blood supply.

Lymph—The almost colorless fluid that bathes body tissues. Lymph is found in the lymphatic vessels and carries lymphocytes that have entered the lymph glands from the blood.

Lymph gland—A small bean-shaped organ consisting of a loose meshwork of tissue in which large numbers of white blood cells are embedded.

Lymphatic system—The tissues and organs (including the bone marrow, spleen, thymus and lymph nodes) that produce and store cells that fight infection, together with the network of vessels that carry lymph throughout the body.

Oncology—The branch of medicine that deals with the diagnosis and treatment of cancer.

stored speech. The quality of the patient's speech is usually very good if at least one-third of the tongue remains and an experienced surgeon has performed the repair.

Total glossectomy results in severe disability because the "new tongue" (a prosthesis) is incapable of movement. This lack of mobility creates enormous difficulty in eating and talking.

Morbidity and mortality rates

Even in the case of a successful glossectomy, the long-term outcome depends on the stage of the cancer and the involvement of lymph glands in the neck. Five-year survival data reveal overall survival rates of less than 60%, although the patients who do survive often endure major functional, cosmetic, and psychological burdens as a result of their difficulties in speaking and eating.

Alternatives

An alternative to glossectomy is the insertion of radioactive wires into the cancerous tissue. This is an effective treatment but requires specialized surgical skills and facilities.

Resources

BOOKS

"Disorders of the Oral Region: Neoplasms." Section 9, Chapter 105 in *The Merck Manual of Diagnosis and Therapy*, edited by Mark H. Beers, MD, and Robert Berkow, MD. Whitehouse Station, NJ: Merck Research Laboratories, 1999.

Johnson, J. T., ed. *Reconstruction of the Oral Cavity*. Alexandria, VA: American Academy of Otolaryngology, 1994.

Shah, J. P., J. G. Batsakis, and J. Shah. *Oral Cancer*. Oxford, UK: Isis Medical Media, 2003.

PERIODICALS

Barry, B., B. Baujat, S. Albert, et al. "Total Glossectomy Without Laryngectomy as First-Line or Salvage Therapy." *Laryngoscope* 113 (February 2003): 373-376.

Chuanjun, C., Z. Zhiyuan, G. Shaopu, et al. "Speech After Partial Glossectomy: A Comparison Between Reconstruction and Nonreconstruction Patients." *Journal of Oral and Maxillofacial Surgery* 60 (April 2002): 404-407.

Furia, C. L., L. P. Kowalski, M. R. Latorre, et al. "Speech Intelligibility After Glossectomy and Speech Rehabilitation." *Archives of Otolaryngology - Head & Neck Surgery* 127 (July 2001): 877-883.

Kimata, Y., K. Uchiyama, S. Ebihara, et al. "Postoperative Complications and Functional Results After Total Glossectomy with Microvascular Reconstruction." *Plastic Reconstructive Surgery* 106 (October 2000): 1028-1035.

ORGANIZATIONS

American Academy of Otolaryngology - Head and Neck Surgery. One Prince Street, Alexandria, VA 22314. (703) 806-4444. <www.entnet.org>.

American Cancer Society. National Headquarters, 1599 Clifton Road NE, Atlanta, GA 30329. (800) ACS -2345. <www.cancer.org>

Oral Cancer Foundation. 3419 Via Lido, #205, Newport Beach, CA 92663. (949) 646-8000. <www.oralcancer. org>

OTHER

CancerAnswers.com. *Tongue Base and Tonsil Cancer.* <www.canceranswers.com/Tongue.Base.Tonsil.html >.

Cancer Information Network. *Oral Cavity Cancer.* <www.ontumor.com/oral/>.

Monique Laberge, Ph.D.

Glucose tests

Definition

Glucose tests are used to determine the concentration of glucose in blood, urine, cerebrospinal fluid (CSF), and other body fluids. These tests are used to detect increased blood glucose (hyperglycemia), decreased

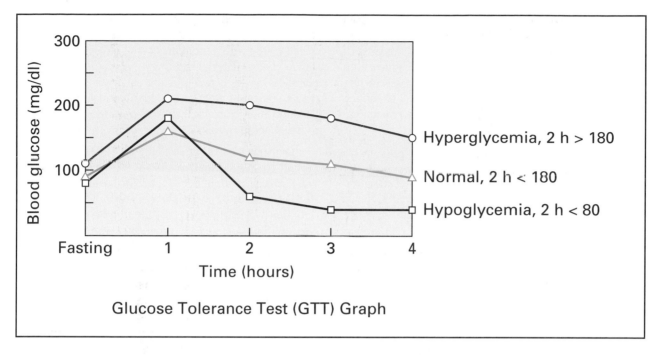

300

Blood glucose (mg/dl)

200

100

Fasting   1   2   3   4

Time (hours)

Hyperglycemia, 2 h > 180

Normal, 2 h < 180

Hypoglycemia, 2 h < 80

Glucose Tolerance Test (GTT) Graph

Glucose tolerance test (GTT) showing normal, high, and low glucose levels. *(From Fundamentals of Nursing, Standards & Practice, 1st edition by DELAUNE. (c) 1998. Reprinted with permission of Delmar Learning, a division of Thomson Learning: www.thomsonrights.com. Fax: 800-730-2215.)*

blood glucose (hypoglycemia), increased glucose in the urine (glycosuria), and decreased glucose in CSF, serous, and synovial fluid glucose.

Purpose

The results of glucose tests are used in a variety of situations, including:

• Screening persons for diabetes mellitus. The American Diabetes Association (ADA) recommends that a fasting plasma glucose (fasting blood sugar) be used to diagnose diabetes. People without symptoms of diabetes should be tested when they reach the age of 45 years, and again every three years. People in high-risk groups should be tested before the age of 45, and then more frequently. If a person already has symptoms of diabetes, a blood glucose test without fasting (a casual plasma glucose test) may be performed. In difficult diagnostic cases, a glucose challenge test called a two-hour oral glucose tolerance test (OGTT) is recommended. If the result of any of these three tests is abnormal, it must be confirmed with a second test—performed on another day. The same test or a different test can be used. However, the result of the second test must be abnormal as well to establish a diagnosis of diabetes.

• Screening for gestational diabetes. Diabetes that occurs during pregnancy is called gestational diabetes. This condition is associated with hypertension, increased birth weight of the fetus, and a higher risk for preeclampsia. Women who are at risk are screened when they are 24–28 weeks pregnant. A woman is considered at risk if she is older than 25 years; is not at her normal body weight; has a parent or sibling with diabetes; or is in an ethnic group that has a high rate of diabetes (such as Hispanic, Native American, or African-American).

• Blood glucose monitoring. Daily measurement of whole blood glucose identifies persons with diabetes who require intervention to maintain their blood glucose within an acceptable range as determined by their doctors. The Diabetes Control and Complications Trial (DCCT) demonstrated that persons with diabetes who maintained blood glucose and glycated hemoglobin (hemoglobin with glucose bound to it) at or near normal decreased their risk of complications by 50–75%. Based on results of this study, the ADA recommends routine glycated hemoglobin testing to measure long-term control of blood sugar. The most common glycated **hemoglobin test**, is the HbA_{1c}, which provides the average, overall blood glucose levels over the prior two to three month period. A DCCT randomized study found that the knowledge alone that their glycated hemoglobin results were good improved blood glucose control in some patients.

• Diagnosis and differentiation of hypoglycemia. Low blood glucose may be associated with such symptoms as confusion, memory loss, and seizures. Demonstration that such symptoms are the result of hypoglycemia requires evidence of low blood glucose at the time of symptoms and reversal of the symptoms by glucose. In documented hypoglycemia, blood glucose tests are used along with measurements of insulin and C-peptide (a fragment of proinsulin) to differentiate between fasting and postprandial (after a meal) causes.

• Analysis of glucose in body fluids. High levels of glucose in body fluids reflect a hyperglycemic state and are not otherwise clinically significant. Low body fluid glucose levels, however, indicate increased glucose utilization, often caused by infection (meningitis causes a low CSF glucose); inflammatory disease (rheumatoid arthritis causes a low pleural fluid glucose); or malignancy (a leukemia or lymphoma, such as Hodgkin's disease infiltrating the CNS or serous cavity).

Precautions

Diabetes must be diagnosed as early as possible so that treatment can begin. If left untreated, it will result in progressive vascular disease that may damage the blood vessels, nerves, kidneys, heart, and other organs. Brain damage can occur from glucose levels below 40 mg/dL and coma from levels above 450 mg/dL. For this reason, plasma glucose levels below 40 mg/dL or above 450 mg/dL are commonly used as alert values. Point-of-care and home glucose monitors measure glucose in whole blood rather than plasma. They are accurate, for the most part, within a range of glucose concentration between 40 mg/dL and 450 mg/dL. In addition, whole blood glucose measurements are generally 10% lower than those of serum or plasma glucose.

Other endocrine disorders and a number of medications can cause both hyperglycemia and hypoglycemia. For this reason, abnormal glucose test results must be interpreted by a doctor.

Glucose is affected by heat; therefore, plasma or serum must be separated from the blood cells and refrigerated as soon as possible. **Splenectomy**, for example, can result in an increase in glycated hemoglobin, but hemolytic anemia can produce a decrease in it.

There are other factors that can also affect the OGTT, such as **exercise**, diet, anorexia, and smoking. Drugs that decrease tolerance to glucose and affect the test include steroids, oral contraceptives, estrogens, and thiazide **diuretics**.

Description

The body uses glucose to produce most of the energy it needs to function. Glucose is absorbed from the gastrointestinal tract directly and is also derived from digestion of other dietary carbohydrates. It is also produced inside cells by the processes of glycogen breakdown (glycogenolysis) and reverse glycolysis (gluconeogenesis). Insulin is made by the pancreas and facilitates the movement of glucose from the blood and extracellular fluids into the cells. Insulin also increases the formation of glucose by cells.

Diabetes may result from a lack of insulin or a subnormal (below normal) response to insulin. There are three forms of diabetes: Type I or insulin-dependent (IDDM); type II or noninsulin dependent (NIDDM); and gestational diabetes (GDM). Type I diabetes usually occurs in childhood and is associated with low or absent blood insulin and production of ketones. It is caused by autoantibodies to the islet cells in the pancreas that produce insulin, and persons must be given insulin to control blood glucose and prevent ketosis. Type II accounts for 85% or more of persons with diabetes. It usually occurs after age 40, and is usually associated with obesity. Persons who have a deficiency of insulin may require insulin to maintain glucose, but those who have a poor response to insulin may not. Gestational diabetes is a form of glucose intolerance that first appears during pregnancy. It usually ends after delivery, but over a 10-year span approximately 30–40% of females with gestational diabetes go on to develop NIDDM.

There are a variety of ways to measure a person's blood glucose level.

Whole blood glucose tests

Whole blood glucose testing can be performed by a person at home or by a member of the health care team outside the laboratory. The test is usually performed using a drop of whole blood obtained by finger puncture. Care must be taken to wipe away the first drop of blood because it is diluted with tissue fluid. The second drop is applied to the dry reagent test strip or device.

Fasting plasma glucose test

The fasting plasma glucose test requires an eight-hour fast. The person must have nothing to eat or drink except water. The person's blood is usually collected by a nurse or phlebotomist (person trained to draw blood) by insertion of a needle into a vein in the patient's arm. Either serum, the liquid portion of the blood after it clots, or plasma may be used. Plasma is the liquid portion of unclotted blood that is collected. The ADA recommends a normal range for fasting plasma glucose of 55–109 mg/dL. A glucose level equal to greater than 126 mg/dL is indicative of diabetes. A fasting plasma glucose level of 110–125 gm/dL is referred to as "impaired fasting glucose."

Oral glucose tolerance test (OGTT)

The OGTT is done to see how well the body handles a standard amount of glucose. There are many variations of this test. A two-hour OGTT as recommended by the ADA is described below. The person must have at least 150 grams of carbohydrate each day for at least three days before this test. The person must take nothing but water and abstain from exercise for 12 hours before the glucose is given. At 12 hours after the start of the fast, the person is given 75 grams of glucose to ingest in the form of a drink or standardized jelly beans. A health care provider draws a sample of venous blood two hours following the dose of glucose. A glucose concentration equal to or greater than 200 mg/dL is indicative of diabetes. A level below 140 mg/dL is considered normal. A level of 140–199 mg/dL is termed "impaired glucose tolerance."

Testing for gestational diabetes

The screening test for gestational diabetes is performed between 24 and 28 weeks of pregnancy. No special preparation or fasting is required. The patient is given an oral dose of 50 grams of glucose and blood is drawn one hour later. A plasma or serum glucose level less than 140 mg/dL is normal and requires no follow-up. If the glucose level is 140 mg/dL or higher, a three-hour OGTT is performed. The same pretest preparation is followed for the two-hour OGTT described previously, except that 100 grams of glucose are given orally. Blood is drawn at the end of the fast and at one-, two-, and three-hour intervals after the glucose is ingested. Gestational diabetes is diagnosed if two or more of the following results are obtained:

• fasting plasma glucose is greater than 105 mg/dL

• one-hour plasma glucose is greater than 190 mg/dL

• two-hour plasma glucose is greater than 165 mg/dL

• three-hour plasma glucose is greater than 145 mg/dL

Glycated hemoglobin blood glucose test (G-Hgb)

The glycated (glycosylated) hemoglobin test is used to diagnose diabetes and monitor the effectiveness of treatment. Glycated hemoglobin is a test that indicates how much glucose was in a person's blood during a two- to three-month window beginning about four weeks prior to sampling. The test is a measure of the time-averaged blood glucose over the 120-day lifespan of the red blood cells (RBCs). The normal range for glycated hemoglobin measured as HbA_{1c} is 3–6%. Values above 8% indicate that a hyperglycemic episode occurred sometime during the window monitored by the test (two to three months beginning four weeks prior to the time of blood collection).

The ADA recommends that glycated hemoglobin testing be performed during a person's first diabetes evaluation, again after treatment begins and glucose levels are stabilized, then repeated semiannually. If the person does not meet treatment goals, the test should be repeated quarterly.

A related blood test, fructosamine assay, measures the amount of albumin in the plasma that is bound to glucose. Albumin has a shorter halflife than RBCs, and this test reflects the time-averaged blood glucose level over a period of two to three weeks prior to sample collection.

Preparation

Blood glucose tests require either whole blood, serum, or plasma collected by vein puncture or finger puncture. No special preparation is required for a casual blood glucose test. An eight-hour fast is required for the fasting plasma or whole-blood glucose test. A 12-hour fast is required for the two-hour OGTT and three-hour OGTT tests. In addition, the person must abstain from exercise in the 12-hour fasting period. Medications known to affect carbohydrate metabolism should be discontinued three days prior to an OGTT test if possible (the doctor should provide guidance on this), and the patient must maintain a diet of at least 150 grams of carbohydrate per day for at least three days prior to the fast.

Aftercare

After the test or series of tests is completed (and with the approval of the doctor), the person should eat and drink as normal, and take any medications that were stopped for the test.

The patient may feel discomfort when blood is drawn from a vein. Pressure should be applied to the puncture site until the bleeding stops; this will help to reduce bruising. Warm packs can also be placed over the puncture site to relieve discomfort.

Risks

The patient may experience weakness, fainting, sweating, or other reactions while fasting or during the test. If any of these reactions occur, the patient should immediately inform the doctor or nurse.

Normal results

Normal values listed below are for children and adults. Results may vary slightly from one laboratory to another depending on the method of analysis used.

• fasting plasma glucose test: 55–109 mg/dL

KEY TERMS

Diabetes mellitus—A disease in which a person can't effectively use glucose to meet the needs of the body. It is caused by a lack of the hormone insulin.

Glucose—The main form of sugar (chemical formula $C_6H_{12}O_6$) used by the body for energy.

Glycated hemoglobin—A test that measures the amount of hemoglobin bound to glucose. It is a measure of how much glucose has been in the blood during a two-to-three month period beginning approximately one month prior to sample collection.

Hyperglycemia—Abnormally increased amount of sugar in the blood.

Hypoglycemia—Abnormally decreased amount of sugar in the blood.

Ketones—Waste products in the blood that build up in uncontrolled diabetes.

Ketosis—Abnormally elevated concentration of ketones in body tissues. A complication of diabetes.

• OGTT at two hours: less than 140 mg/dL.

• glycated hemoglobin: 3%–6%

• fructosamine: 1.6–2.7 mmol/L for adults (5% lower for children)

• gestational diabetes screening test: less than 140 mg/dL

• cerebrospinal glucose: 40–80 mg/dL

• serous fluid glucose: equal to plasma glucose

• synovial fluid glucose: within 10 mg/dL of the plasma glucose

• urine glucose (random semiquantitative): negative

For the person with diabetes, the ADA recommends an ongoing blood glucose level of less than or equal to 120 mg/dL.

The following results are suggestive of diabetes mellitus, and must be confirmed with repeat testing:

• fasting plasma glucose test: greater than or equal to 126 mg/dL

• OGTT at two hours: equal to or greater than 200 mg/dL

• casual plasma glucose test (nonfasting, with symptoms): equal to or greater than 200 mg/dL

• gestational diabetes three-hour oral glucose tolerance test: two or more of the limits following are exceeded

fasting plasma glucose greater than 105 mg/dL; one-hour plasma glucose greater than 190 mg/dL; two-hour plasma glucose greater than 165 mg/dL; three-hour plasma glucose: greater than 145 mg/dL

Resources

BOOKS

Chernecky, Cynthia C., and Barbara J. Berger. *Laboratory Tests and Diagnostic Procedures,* 3rd ed. Philadelphia, PA: W. B. Saunders Company, 2001.

Henry, John B., ed. *Clinical Diagnosis and Management by Laboratory Methods,* 20th ed. Philadelphia: W. B. Saunders Company, 2001.

Kee, Joyce LeFever. *Handbook of Laboratory and Diagnostic Tests,* 4th ed. Upper Saddle River, NJ: Prentice-Hall, 2001.

Wallach, Jacques. *Interpretation of Diagnostic Tests,* 7th ed. Philadelphia, PA: Lippincott Williams & Wilkens, 2000.

ORGANIZATIONS

American Diabetes Association (ADA), National Service Center. 1660 Duke St., Alexandria, VA 22314. (703) 549-1500. <http://www.diabetes.org/main/application/commercewf<.

Centers for Disease Control and Prevention (CDC). Division of Diabetes Translation, National Center for Chronic Disease Prevention and Health Promotion. TISB Mail Stop K-13, 4770 Buford Highway NE, Atlanta, GA 30341-3724. (770) 488-5080. <http://www.cdc.gov/diabetes>.

National Diabetes Information Clearinghouse (NDIC). 1 Information Way, Bethesda, MD 20892-3560. (301) 907-8906. <http://www.niddk.nih.gov/health/diabetes/ndic.htm>.

National Institute of Diabetes and Digestive and Kidney Diseases (NIDDK). National Institutes of Health, Building 31, Room 9A04, 31 Center Drive, MSC 2560, Bethesda, MD 208792-2560. (301) 496-3583. <http://www.niddk.nih.gov>.

OTHER

National Institutes of Health. [cited April 4, 2003] <http://www.nlm.nih.gov/medlineplus/encyclopedia.html>.

Victoria E. DeMoranville
Mark A. Best

Goniotomy

Definition

A goniotomy is a surgical procedure primarily used to treat congenital glaucoma, first described in 1938. It is caused by a developmental arrest of some of the structures within the anterior (front) segment of the eye. These structures include the iris and the ciliary body, which produces the aqueous fluid needed to maintain the integrity of the eye. These structures do not develop normally in the eyes of patients with isolated congenital glaucoma. Instead, they overlap and block the trabecular meshwork, which is the primary drainage system for the aqueous fluid. As a result of this blockage, the trabecular meshwork itself becomes thicker and the drainage holes within the meshwork are narrowed. These changes lead to an excess of fluid in the eye, which can cause pressure that can damage the internal structures of the eye and cause glaucoma.

All types of congenital glaucoma are caused by a decrease in or even a complete obstruction of the outflow of intraocular fluid. The ocular syndromes and anomalies that predispose a child to congenital glaucoma include the following: Reiger's anomaly; Peter's anomaly; Axenfeld's syndrome; and Axenfeld-Rieger's syndrome. Systemic disorders that affect the eyes in ways that may lead to glaucoma include Marfan's syndrome; rubella (German measles); and the phacomatoses, which include neurofibromatosis and Sturge-Weber syndrome. Since these disorders affect the entire body as well as the eyes, the child's pediatrician or family doctor will help to diagnose and treat these diseases.

Purpose

The purpose of a goniotomy is to clear the obstruction to aqueous outflow from the eye, which in turn lowers the intraocular pressure (IOP). Lowering the IOP helps to stabilize the enlargement of the cornea and the distension and stretching of the eye that often occur in congenital glaucoma. The size of the eye, however, will not return to normal. Most importantly, once the aqueous outflow improves, damage to the optic nerve is halted or reversed. The patient's visual acuity may improve after surgery.

Goniotomies are commonly performed to treat the following eye disorders:

• Congenital glaucomas.

• Aniridia. Aniridia is a condition in which the patient lacks a visible iris. A goniotomy is performed as a preventive measure, as 50%–75% of patients with aniridia will develop glaucoma.

• Uveitic glaucoma associated with juvenile rheumatoid arthritis.

• Maternal rubella syndrome.

• JOAG.

Demographics

The congenital glaucomas affect 1: 10,000 infants, with boys affected twice as often as girls. Both eyes are affected in 75% of patients. These glaucomas are differentiated from the secondary glaucomas caused by such

> ## WHO PERFORMS THE PROCEDURE AND WHERE IS IT PERFORMED?
>
> A goniotomy is performed in a hospital by an ophthalmologist, or eye specialist, while the patient is under general anesthesia. Preoperative and postoperative evaluations are also done in a hospital setting if anesthesia is required. These evaluations can be done for older children in an office setting. An ophthalmologist qualified to perform a goniotomy has usually had advanced fellowship training in glaucoma surgery after completing a 3-year residency in ophthalmology.

medical conditions as juvenile rheumatoid arthritis (JRA), Marfan's syndrome, or diabetes; or caused by intraocular tumors, cataract surgery, or trauma. Many of the secondary glaucomas respond better to medical treatment than to surgical treatment. Ninety-five percent of developmental or congenital glaucoma appears before age three. Another type of pediatric glaucoma is usually diagnosed between ages 10 and 35 and resembles the type of glaucoma seen in adults more closely than the congenital glaucomas, although some developmental anomalies may be present. This type of glaucoma is referred to as juvenile-onset open angle glaucoma (JOAG).

Congenital glaucoma is a polygenic disorder; that is, it involves more than one gene. Since this type of glaucoma is inherited and the genes for JOAG and congenital glaucoma have been mapped, genetic testing is available to determine whether a specific child is at risk for these disorders.

Description

Before the surgeon begins the procedure, the patient is given miotics, which are drugs that cause the pupil to contract. This partial closure improves the surgeon's view of and access to the trabecular meshwork; it also protects the lens of the eye from trauma during surgery. Other drugs are administered to lower the intraocular pressure.

Once the necessary drugs have been given and the patient is anesthetized, the surgeon uses a forceps or sutures to stabilize the eye in the correct position. The patient's head is rotated away from the surgeon so that the interior structures of the eye are more easily seen. Next, with either a knife-needle or a goniotomy knife, the surgeon punctures the cornea while looking at the interior of the eye through a microscope or a loupe. An assistant uses a syringe to introduce fluid into the eye's anterior chamber through a viscoelastic tube as the surgeon performs the goniotomy.

A gonioscopy lens is then placed on the eye. As the eye is rotated by an assistant, the surgeon sweeps the knife blade or needle through 90–120 degrees of arc in the eye, making incisions in the anterior trabecular meshwork, avoiding the posterior part of the trabecular meshwork in order to decrease the risk of damage to the iris and lens.

Once the knife and tubing are removed, saline solution is introduced through the hole to maintain the integrity of the eye and the hole is closed with sutures. The surgeon then applies **antibiotics** and **corticosteroids** to the eye to prevent infection and reduce inflammation. The head is then rotated away from the incision site so that blood cannot accumulate. The second eye may be operated on at the same time. If the procedure needs to be repeated, another area of the eye is treated.

Diagnosis/Preparation

Diagnosis

The clinical signs of congenital and infantile glaucoma may be detected within a few months after birth. They include an enlarged eye, called buphthalmos; corneal swelling; decreased vision; tearing; sensitivity to light; and blepharospasm, or uncontrolled twitching of the eyes. These signs, however, are usually absent in JOAG. As a result, glaucoma in the older child may go undetected until the child loses vision.

The examiner must take some measurements in order to confirm a diagnosis of glaucoma, including measurement of the corneal diameter and the axial length of the eye. The corneal diameter is usually less then 10 mm in an infant and only 11–12 mm in a one-year-old, but can be as large as 14 mm in a child with advanced glaucoma. The axial length is measured with an A-scan, which is a type of ultrasound. The doctor will also determine the intraocular pressure with either Schiotz tonometry or a TonoPen. An elevated intraocular pressure is not always present in congenital glaucoma; unless it is extremely high, it is only one factor in the diagnosis of glaucoma. Gonioscopy, a technique used to examine the interior structures of the eye, is performed by placing a special contact lens on the eye. This lens, used in combination with a biomicroscope, allows the surgeon to evaluate the structures of the anterior part of the eye. The condition of the optic nerve is also evaluated; photos or drawings may be taken for future comparison.

Since cooperation is difficult for infants and young children, these assessments may be done either under anesthesia or with the use of a sedative. Older children are examined in a manner similar to adults.

Preparation

Once the diagnosis of glaucoma is confirmed, goniotomy is often the first line of treatment. If goniotomy is determined to be the best procedure and there is a lot of corneal haze, the surgeon may treat the patient for several days pre-operatively with azetozolamide to lower the IOP and increase the clarity of the cornea. Or, he may elect to perform another procedure called a trabeculotomy, which is the preferred surgery if the corneal diameter is greater than 14 mm. The patient is given antibiotics for several days before surgery.

Obtaining the family's **informed consent** is another important part of preparing for a goniotomy. The surgeon tells the family that the child will need general anesthesia, and that several postoperative visits with anesthesia or sedation will be necessary after the goniotomy.

Aftercare

The patient will continue to be given antibiotics, corticosteroids, and miotics for one to two weeks after surgery. If the surgeon believes that the procedure was not successful, then he or she may give the patient acetazolamide by mouth in addition to these medications for up to 10 days to lower the IOP.

The patient will be anesthetized again three to six weeks after surgery for a reevaluation of the anterior chamber of the eye. This examination is repeated every three months for the first year; every six months during the second year; and once a year thereafter. Once the child is older, usually three to four years old, the physician can perform the follow-up examination in his or her office without anesthesia or sedation. Since a visual field test is difficult or impossible to do on an infant or young child, the doctor measures the cornea to assess progression of the disease. An increase in corneal diameter indicates that the glaucoma is getting worse. Visual field testing will be performed when the child is old enough to understand it. A visual field test can establish the extent of vision loss that has occurred because of glaucoma.

An important aspect of managing glaucoma patients after surgery is assessing the degree of nearsightedness and astigmatism, both of which result from the stretching of the eye caused by increased intraocular pressure. If the child needs eyeglasses, they should be given as early in life as possible to decrease the probability of amblyopia. Amblyopia is a condition in which the vision cannot be corrected completely, even with glasses, and is common for pediatric glaucoma patients. Although almost 80% of children with congenital glaucoma can have their vision corrected to 20/50 or better, patching of an eye and vision therapy is often required to achieve this level of correction.

About 10% of goniotomy patients will experience a recurrence of the glaucoma or have it develop in the unaffected eye. As a result, the patient will need periodic eye examinations for the rest of his/her life. If glaucoma does recur later in life, then either medical or surgical treatment is instituted depending on the cause.

Risks

Since goniotomy is performed under general anesthesia, there is some risk of a reaction to the anesthetic. The most common risk of general anesthesia in infants is cardiorespiratory arrest. This complication is not life-threatening, however, and occurs in fewer than 2% of goniotomies.

A hyphema (bleeding and formation of a blood clot in the anterior chamber) is the most common complication of a goniotomy. In most cases, however, the blood clots resolve within a few days.

If the cornea is not clear during surgery, the surgeon may accidentally sever the iris from the ciliary body or separate the ciliary body from the sclera of the eye. Both of these complications can lead to hypotony, a condition in which the integrity of the eye is compromised because of insufficient intraocular fluid.

Other complications of goniotomy are cataract formation; inflammation in the anterior chamber; scarring of the cornea; subluxation or dislocation of the lens; and retinal detachment. The risk of damage to the lens is greater when the patient is aniridic.

The intraocular pressure may increase in spite of, or due to complications of the procedure, and the goniotomy may have to be repeated. If the goniotomy is not successful after two or three attempts, the surgeon will perform a trabeculotomy.

Normal results

Goniotomy is considered to be successful when the measured IOP is below 21 mm/Hg, or below 16 mm/Hg if the patient is under anesthesia; when there is no increase in corneal diameter; and when damage to the optic nerve is stabilized or even reversed. Goniotomy is successful in about 94% of patients with primary congenital glaucoma in decreasing IOP, corneal haze, and corneal diameter. Tearing, sensitivity to light, and blepharospasm all decrease over time.

If a goniotomy is successful it will be apparent within three to six weeks. A repeat goniotomy is required for 50%

of patients. Goniotomy is most successful when the child is between one month and three years of age; it is successful only a quarter of the time in patients younger than one month. It is also more successful when the corneal diameter is less than 14 mm and when the IOP is not extremely high. Even if the IOP has been lowered, anti-glaucoma medication or drops may still be needed after the goniotomy.

When a goniotomy is performed on patients with uveitic glaucoma, the success rate is 75%–83%, although most of these patients need ongoing medication for glaucoma, and 30% require a repeat procedure.

Morbidity and mortality rates

Fifteen years after a goniotomy, one in seven patients will have such serious complications as corneal decompensation or detachment of the retina. Vision loss occurs in 50% of children with congenital glaucoma in spite of surgical and medical intervention. This is particularly true of infants diagnosed with glaucoma before two months of age. About 50% of children who undergo goniotomy require a repeat procedure. Complications are more common for patients treated as young infants and as older children.

Alternatives

Congenital glaucoma does not respond well to medical treatment, so the first line of treatment is usually surgical. Medical therapy is often initiated as adjunct therapy after surgery.

One alternative to goniotomy is trabeculotomy. Goniotomy has been the preferred procedure for treatment of congenital glaucoma, but trabeculotomy has been favored in recent years because of the surgeon's difficulty in seeing the structures in the eye when the cornea is hazy. A clear view of the cornea is required for goniotomy. In a trabeculotomy, the surgeon inserts a probe into the eye, passes it through Schlemm's canal, and rotates it

KEY TERMS

Anomaly—A marked deviation from normal structure or function, particularly as the result of congenital defects.

Anterior chamber—The anterior part of the eye, bound by the cornea in front and the iris in the back, filled with aqueous fluid. The trabecular meshwork is located in a channel of the anterior chamber referred to as the angle.

Ciliary body—The structure of the eye, located behind the iris, that produces the aqueous fluid.

Congenital—Present at birth.

Cornea—The clear structure on the front of the eye that allows light to enter the eye.

Intraocular pressure (IOP)—A measurement of the degree of pressure exerted by the aqueous fluid in the eye. Elevated IOP is usually 21 mm/Hg or higher, but glaucoma can be present when the pressure is lower.

Miotics—Medications that cause the pupil of the eye to contract.

Optic nerve—A large nerve found in the posterior part of the eye, through which all the visual nerve fibers leave the eye on their way to the brain.

Schlemm's canal—A reservoir deep in the front part of the eye where the fluid drained from the trabecular meshwork collects prior to being send out to systemic or general circulation.

Trabecular meshwork—Canals of the eye through which the aqueous fluid is drained before it collects in Schlemm's canal.

inside the anterior chamber in order to tear a hole in the trabecular meshwork. This maneuver creates an alternative passageway for the aqueous fluid to leave the anterior chamber of the eye. In some cases the surgeon will perform a **trabeculectomy**, a procedure in which part of the trabecular meshwork is removed by cutting, at the same time as the trabeculotomy.

Another alternative procedure involves placement of a filtering shunt to direct the intraocular fluid out of the eye. A shunt is often placed if Schlemm's canal cannot easily be located, as in the case with infants. The safety profile for trabeculotomy and filtering surgery are comparable to goniotomy, but there is a higher rate of long-term success with goniotomies and trabeculotomies.

A newer variation of surgical goniotomy is laser goniotomy, in which the surgeon uses a Yag:Nd laser to cut into the trabecular meshwork. Laser goniotomies appear to be less effective than surgical goniotomies, but if a patient responds well to a laser procedure, then surgical goniotomy may be considered.

Other alternative treatments for pediatric glaucoma are the cyclodestructive techniques, which include cyclophotocoagulation, and the more commonly performed **cyclocryotherapy**. These procedures involve destruction of the ciliary body by using either freezing temperatures or lasers. These procedures have lower success rates and a higher risk of complications; they are usually performed as a last resort when other techniques have failed.

Resources

BOOKS

Albert, Daniel M., MD, MS, et al. *Principles and Practice of Ophthalmology*, 2nd ed. Philadelphia, PA, W.B. Saunders Company, 2000.

Azuara-Blanco, Augusto, MD, PhD, et al. *Handbook of Glaucoma*. London, UK: Martin Dunitz Ltd., 2002.

Charlton, Judie F., MD, and George W. Weinstein, MD. *Ophthalmic Surgery Complications: Prevention and Management*. Philadelphia, PA: J. B. Lippincott Company, 1995.

Epstein, David L., MD, et al. *Chandler and Grant's Glaucoma*, 4th ed. Baltimore, MD: Williams and Wilkins, 1997

Kanski, Jack, MD, MS, FRCS, FRCOphthal, et al. *Glaucoma: A Colour Manual of Diagnosis and Treatment*, 2nd ed. Oxford, UK: Butterworth Heinemann, 1996.

Krupin, Theodore, MD, and Allan E. Kolker, MD. *Atlas of Complications in Ophthalmic Surgery*. London, UK: Wolfe, 1993.

Ritch, Robert, MD, et al. *The Glaucomas*. St. Louis, MO: Mosby, 1996.

Shields, M. Bruce, MD. *Textbook of Glaucoma*. Baltimore, MD: Williams and Wilkins, 1998.

Weinreb, Robert, et al. *Glaucoma in the 21st Century*. London, UK: Mosby International, 2000.

PERIODICALS

Bayraktar, Sukru, MD, and Taylan Koseoglu, MD. "Endoscopic Goniotomy with Anterior Chamber Maintainer: Surgical Technique and One-Year Results." *Ophthalmic Surgery and Lasers* 32 (November-December 2001): 496-502.

Beck, Allen D. "Diagnosis and Management of Pediatric Glaucoma." *Ophthalmology Clinics of North America* 32 (September 2001): 501-512.

Freedman, Sharon F., MD, et al. "Goniotomy for Glaucoma Secondary to Chronic Childhood Uvicitis." *American Journal of Ophthalmology* 133 (May 2002): 617-621.

Kiefer, Gesine, et al. "Correlation of Postoperative Axial Length Growth and Intraocular Pressure in Congenital Glaucoma— A Retrospective Study in Trabeculotomy and Goniotomy." *Graefe's Archive for Clinical and Experimental Ophthalmology* 239 (December 2001): 893-899.

ORGANIZATIONS

American Academy of Ophthalmology. P. O. Box 7424, San Francisco, CA 94120-7424. (415) 561-8500. <www.aao.org>.

Canadian Ophthalmological Society (COS). 610-1525 Carling Avenue, Ottawa ON K1Z 8R9. <www.eyesite.ca>.

National Eye Institute. 2020 Vision Place, Bethesda, MD 20892-3655. (301) 496-5248. <www.nei.nih.gov>.

OTHER

Nova Southeastern University. *Congenital and Developmental Glaucoma.* <www.nova.edu/~jsowka/congenglauc.html>.

Martha Reilly, OD

Grafts and grafting *see* **Bone grafting; Coronary artery bypass graft surgery; Skin grafting**

Gum disease surgery *see* **Gingivectomy**

Gynecologic sonogram *see* **Pelvic ultrasound**

Gynecologic surgery *see* **Obstetric and gynecologic surgery**

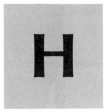

H

H$_2$ reception blockers *see* **Gastric acid inhibitors**

Hair transplantation

Definition

Hair transplantation is a surgical procedure used to treat baldness or hair loss (alopecia). Typically, tiny patches of scalp are removed from the back and sides of the head and implanted in the bald spots in the front and top of the head.

Purpose

Hair transplantation is a cosmetic procedure performed on men and occasionally on women who have significant hair loss, thinning hair, or bald spots where hair no longer grows. In men, hair loss and baldness are most commonly due to genetic factors and age. Male pattern baldness, in which the hairline gradually recedes to expose more and more of the forehead, is the most common form. Men may also experience a gradual thinning of hair at the crown, or very top of the skull. For women, hair loss is more commonly due to hormonal changes and is more likely to be a thinning of hair from the entire head. Transplants can also be performed to replace hair lost due to burns, injury, or diseases of the scalp.

Demographics

An estimated 50,000 men receive hair transplants each year.

Description

Hair transplantation surgery is performed by a physician with specialty training in plastic surgery or, less commonly, dermatology. Each surgery lasts two to

three hours during which approximately 250 grafts will be transplanted. A moderately balding man may require up to 1,000 grafts to get good coverage of a bald area; consequently, a series of surgeries scheduled three to four months apart is usually required. Individuals may be completely awake during the procedure with just a local anesthetic drug applied to numb the areas of the scalp. Some persons may be given a drug to help them relax or may be given an anesthetic drug that puts them to sleep.

The most common transplant procedure uses a thin strip of hair and scalp from the back of the head. This strip is cut into smaller clumps of five or six hairs. Tiny slits are made in the balding area of the scalp, and a clump is implanted into each slit. The doctor performing the surgery will attempt to recreate a natural-looking hairline along the forehead. Minigrafts, micrografts, or implants of single hair follicles can be used to fill in between larger implant sites and can provide a more natural-looking hairline. The implants will also be arranged so that thick and thin hairs are interspersed and the hair will grow in the same direction.

Another type of hair replacement surgery is called scalp reduction. This involves removing some of the skin from the hairless area and "stretching" some of the nearby hair-covered scalp over the cut-away area.

Health insurance will not pay for hair transplants that are performed for cosmetic reasons. Insurance plans

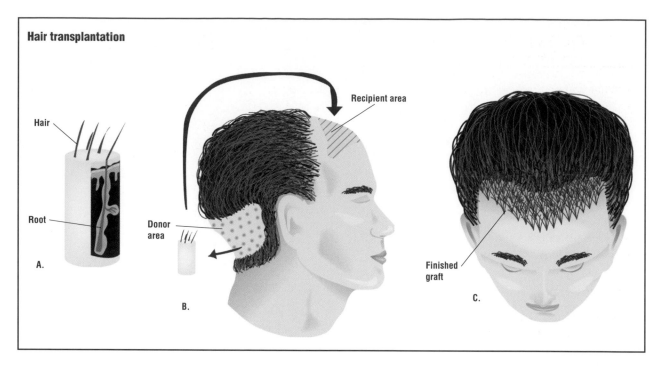

Hair transplantation

In a hair transplant, plugs of hair and supporting tissues are removed from a donor area at the back of the head (A and B). Pieces of skin are removed at the front of the head, and grafts are placed (C). *(Illustration by GGS Inc.)*

may pay for hair replacement surgery to correct hair loss due to accidents, burns, or disease.

It is important to be realistic about what the final result of a hair transplant will look like. This procedure does not create new hair. Rather, it simply redistributes the hair that an individual still has. Chest hair has been experimentally transplanted onto the scalp. As of 2003, this procedure has not been widely used.

Diagnosis/Preparation

Although hair transplantation is a fairly simple procedure, some risks are associated with any surgery. It is important to inform the physician about any medications currently being used and about previous allergic reactions to drugs or anesthetic agents. People with blood-clotting disorders also need to inform their physician before the procedure is performed.

It is important to find a respected, well-established, experienced surgeon and discuss the expected results prior to the surgery. The candidate may need blood tests to check for bleeding or clotting problems and is usually asked not to take **aspirin** products before the surgery. The type of anesthesia used will depend on how extensive the surgery will be and the setting in which it will be performed. The candidate may be awake during the procedure, but is usually given medication to cause relax-

ation. A local anesthetic drug that numbs the area will be applied or injected into the skin at the surgery sites.

Aftercare

The areas involved in transplantation may need to be bandaged overnight. People can return to normal activities within a day. Strenuous activities should be avoided in the first few days after the surgery. On rare occasions, the implants can be ejected from the scalp during vigorous **exercise**. There may be some swelling, bruising, headache, and discomfort around the graft areas and around the eyes. These symptoms can usually be controlled with a mild pain reliever such as aspirin. Scabs may form at the graft sites and should not be scraped off. There may be some numbness at the sites, but it will diminish within two to three months.

Risks

Although there are rare cases of infection or scarring, the major risk is that the grafted area might not look the way the patient expected it to look.

Normal results

The transplanted hair will fall out within a few weeks; however, new hair will start to grow in the graft

QUESTIONS TO ASK THE DOCTOR

- What will be the resulting appearance?
- Is the doctor board certified in plastic and reconstructive surgery or dermatology?
- How many hair transplantation procedures has the doctor performed?
- What is the doctor's complication rate?

KEY TERMS

Alopecia—Hair loss or baldness.

Hair follicle—A tube-like indentation in the skin from which a single hair grows.

Minigraft or micrograft—Transplantation of a small number of hair follicles, as few as one to three hairs, into a transplant site.

Transplantation—Surgically cutting out hair follicles and replanting them in a different spot on the head.

sites within about three months. A normal rate of hair growth is about 0.25–0.5 in (6–13 mm) per month.

Morbidity and mortality rates

Major complications as a result of hair transplantation are extremely rare. Occasionally, a person may have problems with delayed healing, infection, scarring, or rejection of the graft; but these are uncommon.

Alternatives

There are several alternatives to hair transplantation. The two most common include lotions containing drugs and wigs.

As of 2003, only lotions containing Minoxidil or Finasteride actually grow any new hair. This does not occur for all users. The new hair Minoxidil grows is usually only a light fuzz on the crown of the head. When Minoxidil treatment is discontinued, the fuzz disappears, in addition to any hairs that were supposed to die during treatment. In some cases, Finasteride does grow thick, strong, long-growing hair on the crown.

Wigs and hairpieces have been used for centuries. They are available in a wide price range, the more expensive ones providing more realistic appearance than less expensive models.

See also Plastic, reconstructive, and cosmetic surgery.

Resources

BOOKS

Buchwach, K. A., and R. J. Konior. *Contemporary Hair Transplant Surgery.* New York: Thieme, 1997.

Man, Daniel and L. C. Faye. *New Art of Man: Faces of Plastic Surgery: Your Guide to the Latest Cosmetic Surgery Procedures, 3rd edition.* New York: BeautyArt Press, 2003.

Maritt, Emanual. *Hair Replacement Revolution: A Consumer's Guide to Effective Hair Replacement Techniques.* Garden City Park, NY: Square One Publishers, 2001.

Papel, I. D., and S. S. Park. *Facial Plastic and Reconstructive Surgery, 2nd edition.* New York: Thieme Medical Publishers, 2000.

PERIODICALS

Bernstein, R. M., W. R. Rassman, N. Rashid, and R. C. Shiell. "The Art of Repair in Surgical Hair Restoration—Part I: Basic Repair Strategies." *Dermatologic Surgery,* 28(9) 2002: 783–794.

Bernstein, R. M., W. R. Rassman, N. Rashid, and R. C. Shiell. "The Art of Repair in Surgical Hair Restoration—Part II: The Tactics of Repair." *Dermatolical Surgery,* 28(10) 2002: 873–893.

Epstein, J. S. "Hair Transplantation in Women: Treating Female Pattern Baldness and Repairing Distortion and Scarring from Prior Cosmetic Surgery." *Archives of Facial Plastic Surgery,* 5(1) 2003: 121–126.

Epstein, J. S. "Hair Transplantation for Men with Advanced Degrees of Hair Loss." *Plastic and Reconstructive Surgery,* 111(1) 2003: 414–421.

Swinehart, J. M. "Local Anesthesia in Hair Transplant Surgery." *Dermatolical Surgery,* 28(12) 2002: 1189–1190.

ORGANIZATIONS

American Academy of Cosmetic Surgery. 401 N. Michigan Ave., Chicago, IL 60611-4267. (313) 527-6713. <http://www.cosmeticsurgeryonline.com>.

American Academy of Dermatology. 930 N. Meacham Road, P.O. Box 4014, Schaumburg, IL 60168-4014. (847) 330-0230, Fax: (847) 330-0050. <http://www.aad.org/>.

American Academy of Facial Plastic and Reconstructive Surgery. 1110 Vermont Avenue NW, Suite 220, Washington, DC 20005. (800) 332-3223.

American Board of Plastic Surgery. Seven Penn Center, Suite 400, 1635 Market Street, Philadelphia, PA 19103-2204. (215) 587-9322. <http://www.abplsurg.org/>.

American College of Plastic and Reconstructive Surgery. <http://www.breast-implant.org>.

American College of Surgeons. 633 North Saint Claire Street, Chicago, IL 60611. (312) 202-5000. <http://www.facs.org/>.

American Society for Aesthetic Plastic Surgery. 11081 Winners Circle, Los Alamitos, CA 90720. (800) 364-2147 or (562) 799-2356. <http://www.surgery.org/>.

American Society for Dermatologic Surgery. 930 N. Meacham Road, P.O. Box 4014, Schaumburg, IL 60168-4014. (847) 330-9830. <http://www.asds-net.org>.

American Society of Plastic and Reconstructive Surgeons. 444 E. Algonquin Rd., Arlington Heights, IL 60005. (847) 228-9900. <http://www.plasticsurgery.org>.

American Society of Plastic Surgeons. 444 E. Algonquin Rd., Arlington Heights, IL 60005. (888) 475-2784. <http://www.plasticsurgery.org/>.

OTHER

Columbia University College of Physicians and Surgeons [cited March 23, 2003]. <http://cpmcnet.columbia.edu/dept/derm/hairloss/>.

CosmeticSurgeryFYI.com [cited March 23, 2003]. <http://www.cosmeticsurgeryfyi.com/surgeries/hair_transplantation.html>.

How Stuff Works [March 23, 2003]. <http://people.howstuffworks.com/hair-replacement6.htm>.

University of Washington School of Medicine [cited March 23, 2003]. <http://faculty.washington.edu/danberg/bergweb/page3.htm>.

L. Fleming Fallon, Jr, MD, DrPH

Hammer, claw, and mallet toe surgery

Definition

Hammer, claw, and mallet toe surgery refers to a series of surgical procedures performed to correct deformed toes.

Purpose

There are three main forms of toe abnormalities in the human foot: hammer toes, claw toes, and mallet toes. A hammer toe, also called contracted toe, bone spur, rotated toe, or deformed toe, is a toe curled as the result of a bend in the middle joint. It may be either flexible or rigid, and may affect any of the four smaller toes. The joints in the toe buckle due to tightening of the ligaments and tendons, which points the toe upward at an angle. The patient's shoes then put pressure on the prominent portion of the toe, leading to inflammation, bursitis, corns, and calluses. Mallet toes and claw toes are similar to hammer toes, except that different joints on the toe are affected. The joint at the end of the toe buckles in a mallet toe, while a claw toe involves abnormal positions of all three joints in the toe.

Toe deformities are caused by a variety of factors:

- Genetic. All three toe deformities may be hereditary.

- Poorly fitted shoes. Claw toes are usually the result of wearing shoes that are too short. Many people have second toes that are longer than their big toes; if they wear shoes sized to fit the big toe, the second toe has to bend to fit into the shoe. High-heeled shoes with pointed toes are also a major cause of claw toes.

- Bunions. A bunion is an abnormal prominence of the first joint of the big toe that pushes the toe sideways toward the smaller toes. Hammer toes often develop together with bunion deformities, and they are often treated together.

- Flat feet. This condition is due to poor biomechanics of the foot and may lead to hammer toes.

- Highly arched feet.

- Rheumatoid arthritis.

- Tendon imbalance. When the foot cannot function normally, the tendons may stretch or tighten to compensate and lead to toe deformities.

- Traumatic injuries of the toes.

When the toe deformity is painful or permanent, surgical repair is performed to relieve pain, correct the problem, and provide a stable, functional toe.

Demographics

As of 2002, the incidence of claw and hammer toe deformities ranges from 2–20% of the population in the United States, with the frequency gradually increasing in the older age groups. Claw and hammer toes are most often seen in patients in the seventh and eight decades of life. Women are affected four to five times more often than men. Little is known about the incidence of these deformities among people who usually wear sandals or go barefoot.

Description

Some of the most common surgical procedures used to repair hammer, claw, and mallet toes include:

- Tenoplasty and capsulotomy. These procedures release or lengthen tightened tendons and ligaments that have caused the toe joints to contract. In some patients with flexible hammer toes, the toe straightens out after these soft tissue structures are lengthened or relaxed.

- Tendon transfer. This procedure is used to correct a flexible hammer toe deformity. It involves the repositioning of a tendon to straighten the toe.

- Bone **arthroplasty**. In this procedure, the surgeon removes some bone and cartilage to correct the toe deformity. A small segment of bone is removed at the joint to eliminate pressure on the toe, relieve pain, and straighten the toe. The tendons and ligaments surrounding the joint may also be reconstructed.

- Derotation arthroplasty. In this technique, the surgeon removes a small wedge of skin and realigns the deformed toe. The surgeon may also remove a small section of bone, and repair tendons and ligaments if necessary.

- Implant arthroplasty. In this procedure, the surgeon inserts a silicone rubber or metal implant specially designed for the toe to replace the gliding surfaces of the joint and act as a joint spacer.

Diagnosis/Preparation

Patients usually consult a doctor about toe deformities because of pain or discomfort in the foot when walking or running. The physician takes several factors into consideration when examining a patient who may require surgery to correct a toe deformity. Some surgical procedures require only small amounts of cutting or tissue removal while others require extensive dissection. The blood supply in the affected toe is an important factor in planning surgery. It determines not only whether the toe will heal fully but also whether the surgeon can perform more than one procedure on the toe. In addition to a visual examination of the patient's foot, the doctor will ask the patient to walk back and forth in the office or hallway in order to evaluate the patient's gait (habitual pattern of walking). This part of the office examination allows the doctor to identify static or dynamic forces that may be causing the toe deformity. Imaging tests are also performed, usually x-ray studies.

If the doctor considers it necessary to rule out systemic disorders, he or she may order the following laboratory tests: a fasting glucose test to evaluate or rule out diabetes, and a sedimentation rate test to evaluate the possibility of an underlying infection in the foot.

Before surgery, the patient receives an appropriate local anesthetic, and the foot is cleansed and draped.

Aftercare

The patient can expect moderate swelling, stiffness and limited mobility in the operated foot following toe surgery, sometimes for as long as eight to 12 weeks. Patients are advised to keep the operated foot elevated above heart level and apply ice packs to reduce swelling during the first few days after surgery. Many patients are able to walk immediately after the operation, although the podiatric surgeon may restrict any such activity for at least 24 hours. Crutches or walkers are not usually needed. There is no cast on the foot, but only a soft gauze dressing. Wearing a splint for the first two to four weeks after surgery is usually recommended. Special surgical shoes are also available to protect the foot and help to redistribute the patient's body weight. If the surgeon has used sutures, they must be kept dry until they are removed, usually seven to 10 days after the operation.

The patient's physician may also suggest exercises to be done at home or at work to strengthen the toe muscles. These exercises may include picking up marbles with the toes and stretching the toe muscles.

Risks

Risks associated with hammer, claw, and mallet toe surgery include:

- swelling of the toes for one to six months following surgery
- recurrence of the deformity
- infection
- persistent pain and discomfort
- nerve injury

KEY TERMS

Arthroplasty—The surgical repair of a joint.

Bunion—A swelling or deformity of the big toe, characterized by the formation of a bursa and a sideways displacement of the toe.

Bursa (plural, bursae)—A pouch lined with joint tissue that contains a small quantity of synovial fluid. Bursae are located between tendons and bone, or between bones and muscle tissue.

Bursitis—Inflammation of a bursa.

Callus—A localized thickening of the outer layer of skin cells, caused by friction or pressure from shoes or other articles of clothing.

Corn—A horny thickening of the skin on a toe, caused by friction and pressure from poorly fitted shoes or stockings.

Gait—A person's habitual manner or style of walking.

Orthopedics—The branch of medicine that deals with bones and joints.

Orthotics—Shoe inserts that are intended to correct an abnormal or irregular gait or walking pattern. They are sometimes prescribed to relieve gait-related foot pain.

Podiatrist—A physician who specializes in the care and treatment of the foot.

Normal results

All corrective toe procedures usually have good outcomes in relieving pain and improving toe mobility. They restore appropriate toe length and anatomy while realigning and stabilizing the joints in the foot.

Morbidity and mortality rates

There are no reported cases of death following corrective surgery on the toes.

Alternatives

Conservative treatments may be tried by patients with minor discomfort or less serious toe deformities. These treatments include:

• trimming or wearing protective padding on corns and calluses

• wearing supportive custom-made plastic or leather shoe inserts (orthotics) to help relieve pressure on toe deformities. Orthotics allow the toes and major joints of the foot to function more efficiently

• using splints or small straps to realign the affected toe

• wearing shoes with a wider toe box

• injecting anti-inflammatory medications to relieve pain and inflammation

See also Arthroplasty.

Resources

BOOKS

Adelaar, R. S., and R. B. Anderson, eds. *Disorders of the Great Toe.* Rosemont, IL: American Academy of Orthopaedic Surgeons, 1997.

Holmes, G. B. *Surgical Approaches to the Foot and Ankle.* New York: McGraw-Hill, 1994.

Marcinko, D. E. *Medical and Surgical Therapeutics of Foot and Ankle.* Baltimore: Williams & Wilkins, 1992.

PERIODICALS

American College of Foot and Ankle Surgeons. "Hammer Toe Syndrome." *Journal of Foot and Ankle Surgery* 38 (March-April 1999): 166-178.

Coughlin, M. J., J. Dorris, J, and E. Polk. "Operative Repair of the Fixed Hammertoe Deformity." *Foot Ankle International* 21 (February 2000): 94-104.

Harmonson, J. K., and L. B. Harkless. "Operative Procedures for the Correction of Hammertoe, Claw Toe, and Mallet Toe: A Literature Review." *Clinical Podiatric Medical Surgery* 13 (April 1996): 211-220.

Hennessy, M. S., and T. S. Saxby. "Traumatic Mallet Toe of the Hallux: A Case Report. A Thirty-Year Follow-Up." *Foot Ankle International* 22 (December 2001): 977-978.

Miller, S. J. "Hammer Toe Correction by Arthrodesis of the Proximal Interphalangeal Joint Using a Cortical Bone Allograft Pin." *Journal of the American Podiatric Medical Association* 92 (November-December 2002): 563-569.

"What is a Hammer Toe, and What Causes It?" *Mayo Clinic Health Letter* 20 (July 2002): 8.

ORGANIZATIONS

American Academy of Orthopaedic Surgeons (AAOS). 6300 North River Road, Rosemont, Illinois 60018-4262. (847) 823-7186. <www.aaos.org>

American College of Foot and Ankle Surgeons (ACFAS). 515 Busse Highway, Park Ridge, IL, 60068. (847) 292-2237 or (800) 421-2237. <www.cmeonline.com/index.html>

American Podiatric Medical Association (APMA). 9312 Old Georgetown Road, Bethesda, MD, 20814. (301) 571-9200 or (800) ASK-APMA. <www.apma.org>.

OTHER

ACFAS. *Digital Disorders and Treatments.* <www.acfas.org/brdigdis.html>.

Foot Pain and Podiatry Online. *Hammertoe Deformity.* <www.footpain.org/hammertoes.html>.

OhioHealth. *Hammertoe and Mallet Toe.* <www.ohiohealth.com/healthreference/reference/E655C4AD-F921-4C63-9B76434A5D565643.htm?category=diseases>.

Monique Laberge, Ph.D.

Hand surgery

Definition

Hand surgery refers to procedures performed to treat traumatic injuries or loss of function resulting from such diseases as advanced arthritis of the hand.

Purpose

The purpose of hand surgery is the treatment of a broad range of problems that affect the hand, whether they result from cuts, burns, crushing injuries to the hand, or disease processes. Hand surgery includes procedures that treat traumatic injuries of the hands, including closed-fist injuries; congenital deformities; repetitive stress injuries; deformities caused by arthritis and similar disorders affecting the joints; nail problems; and **tendon repair**.

The central priority of the hand surgeon is adequate reconstruction of the skin, bone, nerve, tendon, and joint(s) in the hand. Proper repair of any cuts, tears, or burns in the skin will help to ensure a wound free of infection and will provide cover for the anatomical structures beneath the skin. Early repair and grafting is an essential component of hand surgery. Nerve repair is important because a delay in reconnecting the nerve fibers may affect the recovery of sensation in the hand. Restoration of sensation in the hand is necessary if the patient is to recover a reasonable level of functionality. Next, the bones in the hand must be stabilized in a fixed position before the surgeon can repair joints or tendons. Joint mobility may be restored by specific tendon repairs or grafts. In some cases, the patient's hand may require several operations over a period of time to complete the repair.

Demographics

The demographics of hand injuries and disorders depend on the specific injury or disorder in question. Repetitive stress injuries (RSIs) of the hands are often related to occupation; for example, nurse anesthetists, dental hygienists, keyboard instrumentalists, word processors, violinists, and some assembly line workers are at relatively high risk of developing carpal tunnel syndrome or tendinitis of the fingers related to their work. Nearly 17% of all disabling work injuries in the United States involve the fingers, most often when the finger strikes or is jammed against a hard surface. Over 25% of athletic injuries involve the hand or wrist.

In terms of age groups, children under the age of six are the most likely to be affected by crushing or burning injuries of the hand. Closed-fist injuries, which frequently involve infection of the hand resulting from a human bite,

are almost entirely found in males between the ages of 15 and 35. Pain or loss of function in the hands resulting from osteoarthritis, however, is found most often in middle-aged or older adults, and affects women as often as men.

Some specific categories of conditions that may require hand surgery include:

Congenital malformations. The most common congenital hand deformity is syndactyly, in which two or more fingers are fused together or joined by webbing; and polydactyly, in which the person is born with an extra finger, often a duplication of the thumb.

Infections. Hand surgeons treat many different types of infections, including paronychia, an infection resulting from a penetrating injury to the nail; felon, an inflammation of the deeper tissue under the fingertip resulting in an abscess; suppurative tenosynovitis, an infection of the flexor tendon sheath of the fingers or thumb; and deeper infections that often result from human or animal bites.

Tumors. The most common tumor of the hand is the ganglion cyst, which is a mass of tissue fluid arising from a joint or tendon space. Giant cell tumors are the second most common hand tumor. These tumors usually arise from joints or tendon sheaths and are yellow-brown in color. The third type of hand tumor is a lipoma, which is a benign tumor that occurs in fatty tissue.

Nerve compression syndromes. These syndromes occur when a peripheral nerve is compressed, usually because of an anatomic or developmental problem, infection or trauma. For example, carpal tunnel syndrome develops when a large nerve in the arm called the median nerve is subjected to pressure building up inside the carpal tunnel, which is a passageway through the wrist. This pressure on the nerve may result from injury, overuse of the hand and wrist, fluid retention during pregnancy, or rheumatoid arthritis. The patient may experience tingling or aching sensations, numbness, and a loss of function in the hand. The ulnar nerve is another large nerve in the arm that runs along the little finger. Compression of the ulnar nerve at the elbow can cause symptoms that typically include aching pain, numbness and paresthesias.

Amputation. Some traumatic injuries result in the loss of a finger or the entire hand, requiring reattachment or replantation. Crushing injuries of the hand have the lowest chance of a successful outcome. Children and young adults have the best chances for recovery following surgery to repair an accidental amputation.

Fractures and dislocations. Distal phalangeal fractures (breaking the bone of a finger above the first joint towards the tip of the finger) are the most commonly encountered fractures of the hand. They often occur while playing sports.

Fingertip injury. Fingertip injuries are extremely dangerous since they comprise the most common hand injuries and can lead to significant disability. Fingertip injuries can cause damage to the tendons, nerves, or veins in the hands.

Description

There are a number of different procedures that may be involved in hand surgery, with a few general principles that are applicable to all cases: operative planning; preparing and draping the patient; hair removal; tourniquet usage; the use of special **surgical instruments**; magnification (special visualization attachments); and

postoperative care. The operative preplanning stage is vitally important since it allows for the best operative technique. The hand to be operated on is shaved and washed with an antiseptic for five minutes. A tourniquet will be placed on the patient's arm to minimize blood loss; special inflation cuffs are available for this purpose.

The four basic instruments used in hand surgery include a knife, small forceps, dissecting scissors, and mosquito hemostats. A standard drill with small steel points is used to drill holes in bone during reconstructive bone surgery. Additionally, visualization of small anatomical structures is essential during hand surgery. Frequently, the hand surgeon may use wire loupes (a special instrument held in place on top of the surgeon's head) or a double-headed binocular microscope in order to see the tendons, blood vessels, muscles, and other structures in the hand.

In most cases, the anesthesiologist will administer a regional nerve block to keep the patient comfortable during the procedure. The patient is usually positioned lying on the back with the affected arm extended on a hand platform. If the surgeon is performing a bone reconstruction, he or she may require such special instruments as a drill, metal plates and/or screws, and steel wires (K-wires). Arteries and veins should be reconnected without tension. If this cannot be done the hand surgeon must take out a piece of vein from another place in the patient's body and use it to reconstruct the vein in the hand. This process is called a venous graft. Nerves damaged as a result of traumatic finger injuries can usually be reconnected without tension, since bone reconstruction prior to nerve surgery shortens the length of the bones in the hand. The surgeon may also perform skin grafts or skin flaps. After all the bones, nerves, and blood vessels have been repaired or reconstructed, the surgeon closes the wound and covers it with a dressing.

Diagnosis/Preparation

With the exception of emergencies requiring immediate treatment, the diagnosis of hand injuries and disorders begins with a detailed history and **physical examination** of the patient's hand. During the physical examination, the doctor evaluates the range of motion (ROM) in the patient's wrist and fingers. Swollen or tender areas can be felt (palpated) by the clinician. The doctor can assess sensation in the hand by very light pinpricks with a fine sterile needle. In cases of trauma to the hand, the doctor will inspect the hand for bite marks, burns, foreign objects that may be embedded, or damage to deeper anatomical structures within the hand. The tendons will be evaluated for evidence of tearing or cutting. Broken bones or joint injuries will be tender to the touch and are easily visible on x-ray imaging.

The doctor may order special tests, including radiographic imaging (x rays), **wound culture**, and special diagnostic tests. X rays are the most common and most useful diagnostic tools available to the hand surgeon for evaluating traumatic injuries. Wound cultures are important for assessing injuries involving bites (human or animal) as well as wounds that have been badly contaminated by foreign matter. Such other special tests as a Doppler flowmeter examination can be used to evaluate the patterns of blood flow in the hand.

Before a scheduled operation on the hand, the patient will be given standard blood tests and a physical examination to make sure that he or she does not suffer from a general medical condition that would be a contraindication to surgery.

Aftercare

Aftercare following hand surgery may include one or more of the following, depending on the specific procedure: oral painkilling medications; anti-inflammatory medications; **antibiotics**; splinting; **traction**; special dressings to reduce swelling; and heat or massage therapy. Because the hand is a very sensitive part of the body, the patient may experience severe pain for several days after surgery. The surgeon may prescribe injections of painkilling drugs to manage the patient's discomfort.

Exercise therapy is an important part of aftercare for most patients who are recovering from hand surgery. A rehabilitation hand specialist will demonstrate exercises for the hand, instruct the patient in proper **wound care**, massage the hand and wrist, and perform an ongoing assessment of the patient's recovery of strength and range of motion in the hand.

Risks

According to the American Society of Plastic Surgeons, the most common complications associated with hand surgery are the following:

• infection

• poor healing

• loss of sensation or range of motion in the hand

• formation of blood clots

• allergic reactions to the anesthesia

Complications are relatively infrequent with hand surgery, however, and most can be successfully treated.

Normal results

Normal results for hand surgery depend on the nature of the injury or disorder being treated.

KEY TERMS

Congenital—Present at birth.

Felon—A very painful abscess on the lower surface of the fingertip, resulting from infection in the closed space surrounding the bone in the fingertip. It is also known as whitlow.

Hemostat—A small surgical clamp used to hold a blood vessel closed.

Lipoma—A type of benign tumor that develops within adipose or fatty tissue.

Loupe—A convex lens used to magnify small objects at very close range. It may be held on the hand, mounted on eyeglasses, or attached to a headband.

Paresthesia—An abnormal touch sensation, such as a prickling or burning feeling, often in the absence of an external cause.

Paronychia—Inflammation of the folds of tissue surrounding the nail.

Polydactyly—A developmental abnormality characterized by an extra digit on the hand or foot.

Skin flap—A piece of skin with underlying tissue that is used in grafting to cover a defect and that receives its blood supply from a source other than the tissue on which it is laid.

Syndactyly—A developmental abnormality in which two or more fingers or toes are joined by webbing between the digits.

Morbidity and mortality rates

Mortality following hand surgery is virtually unknown. The rates of complications depend on the nature of the patient's disorder or injury and the specific surgical procedure used to treat it.

Alternatives

Some disorders that affect the hand, such as osteoarthritis and rheumatoid arthritis, may be managed with such nonsurgical treatments as splinting, medications, physical therapy, or heat. Fractures, amputations, burns, bite injuries, congenital deformities, and severe cases of compression syndromes usually require surgery.

Resources

BOOKS

"Common Hand Disorders." Section 5, Chapter 61 in *The Merck Manual of Diagnosis and Therapy*, edited by Mark

H. Beers, MD, and Robert Berkow, MD. Whitehouse Station, NJ: Merck Research Laboratories, 1999.

Townsend, Courtney, et al., eds. *Sabiston Textbook of Surgery*, 16th ed. Philadelphia, PA: W. B. Saunders Company, 2001.

PERIODICALS

Chu, M. M. "Splinting Programmes for Tendon Injuries." *Hand Surgery* 7 (December 2002): 243-249.

Diaz, J. H. "Carpal Tunnel Syndrome in Female Nurse Anesthetists Versus Operating Room Nurses: Prevalence, Laterality, and Impact of Handedness." *Anesthesia and Analgesia* 93 (October 2001): 975-980.

Johnstone, B. R. "Proximal Interphalangeal Joint Surface Replacement Arthroplasty." *Hand Surgery* 6 (July 2001): 1-11.

Perron, A. D., M. D. Miller, and W. J. Brady. "Orthopedic Pitfalls in the ED: Fight Bite." *American Journal of Emergency Medicine* 20 (March 2002): 114-117.

Rettig, A. C. "Wrist and Hand Overuse Syndromes." *Clinics in Sports Medicine* 20 (July 2001): 591-611.

ORGANIZATIONS

American Association for Hand Surgery. 20 North Michigan Avenue, Suite 700, Chicago, IL 60602. (321) 236-3307. <www.handsurgery.org>.

American Society of Plastic Surgeons (ASPS). 444 East Algonquin Road, Arlington Heights, IL 60005. (847) 228-9900. <www.plasticsurgery.org>.

American Society for Surgery of the Hand. 6300 North River Road, Suite 600. Rosemont, IL 60018. (847) 384-1435. <www.assh.org>.

OTHER

American Society of Plastic Surgeons. *Procedures: Hand Surgery*. [June 29, 2003]. <www.plasticsurgery.org/public_education/procedures/HandSurgery.cfm>.

Laith Farid Gulli, M.D., M.S.
Bilal Nasser, M.D., M.S.
Robert Ramirez, B.S.
Nicole Mallory, M.S., PA-C

HCT *see* **Hematocrit**

Head and neck surgery *see* **Ear, nose, and throat surgery**

Health care proxy

Definition

A health care proxy, or health care proxy form, is a legal document that allows a person to choose someone to make medical decisions on their behalf when they are unable to do so. In some states the person who is authorized may be called a proxy; in others the person may be called an agent.

Description

A health care proxy form is part of a set of legal documents that allows a person to appoint someone to make medical decisions for them if or when they cannot act on their own behalf, and to make sure that health care professionals follow their wishes regarding specific medical treatments at the end of life. These documents are referred to as advance directives. The document naming the person appointed to make the decisions is called a health care proxy. The document that lists acceptable and unacceptable measures of artificial life support is called a **living will**. Most states have passed laws that authorize people to draw up living wills, but it is important to get specific information about the laws in one's own state.

Any competent adult can appoint a health care proxy or agent. It is not necessary to hire a lawyer to draw up or validate the form; most states, however, require two adult witnesses to sign a proxy form. Many hospitals provide proxy forms on request.

It is important to have a health care proxy in order to be able to choose the person who will be making medical decisions on one's behalf. In addition to naming the specific person who will make those decisions, one should think about what life-sustaining treatments one would be willing to undergo in the event of a medical emergency or terminal illness.

A health care proxy form does not deprive a person of the right to make decisions about medical treatment as long as he or she is able to do so. It is put into effect only when the patient's health care team determines that the patient is unable to make decisions on his or her own. For example, a person may be in a coma following an automobile accident. The physician would document in the patient's medical record that the patient is unable to make his or her own medical decisions; the circumstances that led to the patient's present condition; the nature of the disease or injury; and the expected length of the patient's incapacitation.

The person named as proxy makes health care decisions only as long as the patient is unable to make them for him- or herself. If the person regains the ability to make his or her own decisions, the proxy will no longer make them. If the incapacitation is permanent, the proxy will continue to make health care decisions on the patient's behalf as long as the patient is alive, or until the proxy is no longer able to carry the responsibility.

Any trusted adult can be named as a health care proxy. Most married people name their spouse, but it is not necessary to do so. In addition, it is important to select an alternate proxy, in the event that the person first named is unable to fulfill the responsibility. For example, if the spouse has been named as proxy, and both members of the couple were incapacitated in a house fire, then someone else should be empowered to act on their behalf. A married couple does not need to name the same individual as a proxy or as the alternate. It is best to choose someone who lives close enough to carry out the responsibilities of a proxy without having to travel across state lines.

One should consider whether a potential proxy will be able to ask the necessary questions of medical personnel in order to obtain information needed to make a decision. It is important to discuss with the proxy his or her own value system, and whether he or she could make a decision for someone else that he or she would not make for him- or herself. It is a good idea to carry the name and contact information of the proxy in one's wallet in the event of an emergency or sudden incapacitation.

The purpose of a living will is to give specific instructions about emergency or end-of-life health care. In some states a living will may be part of the health care proxy document. But because it is impossible to plan for all possible situations, the health care proxy can interpret one's wishes to members of the health care team and make decisions that one could not foresee at the time of making a living will. This is why it is important for the proxy to understand one's value system, so that the proxy can use his or her judgment as to what one would want. The proxy should be given a written copy of all advance directives. Even if a living will is not legal in the state in which one resides, writing such a will is an opportunity to think through one's beliefs and health care preferences. The proxy or agent can then can use the living will as a guide in making health care decisions as need arises.

Completing a health care proxy form and living will is useful because it helps one to think through one's value system and one's definition of quality of life. Some areas to consider are:

• What makes my life meaningful?

• What religious or personal beliefs do I hold that affect my health care decisions?

• Do I want my proxy to make health care decisions on his or her own, or are there other people I would want him or her to consult? If so, who are these people? Is there anyone who should *not* be consulted?

• Who besides myself will be affected by these decisions? Are they aware of my value system? Would they try to interfere with the proxy's decisions?

• What do I want to do about organ donation?

• Have I informed my physician of my wishes?

KEY TERMS

Advance directive—A general term for two types of documents, living wills and medical powers of attorney, that allow people to give instructions about health care in the event that they cannot speak for themselves.

Proxy—A person authorized or empowered to act on behalf of another; also, the document or written authorization appointing that person.

Appointing a health care proxy is not an irrevocable decision. One can change or revoke the proxy at any time, usually by filling out a new form. In some states, one can specify that the health care proxy will expire on a certain date or if certain events occur. If one has named one's spouse as an agent, the proxy is no longer in effect in the event of separation or divorce. People who want a former spouse to continue as their agent must complete a new proxy form.

In addition to keeping a copy of the proxy form in one's own file of important documents, one should give copies to the proxy, the alternate, and one's physicians.

Resources

ORGANIZATIONS

American Association of Retired Persons (AARP). 601 E. Street NW, Washington, DC 20049. (800) 424-3410. <www.aarp.org>.

American Medical Association. 515 N. State Street, Chicago, IL 60610. (312) 464-5000. <www.ama-assn.org>.

National Cancer Institute (NCI). NCI Public Inquiries Office, Suite 3036A, 6116 Executive Boulevard, MSC8322 Bethesda, MD 20892-8322. (800) 422-6237. <www.cancer.gov>.

National Library of Medicine. <www.nlm.nih.gov>.

Partnership for Caring. 1620 Eye Street NW, Suite 202, Washington, DC 20006. (202) 296-8071. <www.partnershipforcaring.org>.

Esther Csapo Rastegari, R.N., B.S.N., Ed.M.

Health history

Definition

The health history is a current collection of organized information unique to an individual. Relevant aspects of the history include biographical, demographic,

HEALTH HISTORY

Name_____   Date_____   Time_____

Demographic Data: Date of birth_____   Gender_____   Marital status_____

Reason for Seeking Health Care:_____
_____

Perception of Health Status:_____
_____

Previous Illness/Hospitalization/Surgeries:_____
_____

Client/Family Medical History:
Addiction(drugs/alcohol)_____   Diabetes_____   Mental disorders_____
Arthritis_____   Heart disease_____   Sickle cell anemia_____
Cancer_____   Hypertension_____   Stroke_____
Chronic lung disease_____   Kidney disease_____   Other_____

Immunizations/Exposure to Communicable Disease:_____
_____

Allergies:_____
_____

Home Medications:_____
_____

Developmental Level:_____
_____

Psychosocial History:
Alcohol use:_____
Tobacco use:_____
Drug use:_____
Caffeine intake:_____

Self-perception/Self-concept:_____
_____

Sociocultural History:
Family structure_____
Role in family_____
Cultural/ethnic group_____
Occupation/work role_____
Relationships with others_____

Activities of Daily Living:
Nutrition: Type of diet_____   Usual weight_____
Eating patterns_____
Types of snacks_____
Food likes/dislikes_____
Fluid intake: Type_____   Amount_____
Elimination (usual patterns): Urinary_____   Bowel_____
Sleep/Rest:
Usual sleep patterns_____
Relaxation techniques/patterns_____
Activity/Exercise:
Usual exercise patterns_____
Ability to perform self-care activities_____

Review of Systems:
Respiratory_____
Circulatory_____
Integumentary_____
Musculoskeletal_____
Neurosensory_____
Reproductive/Sexuality_____

Health Maintenance Activities:
Usual source of health care_____
Date of last exam(physical, dental, eye)_____
Other health maintenance activities_____

Health history form. *(From Fundamentals of Nursing, Standards & Practice, 1st edition by DELAUNE. (c) 1998. Reprinted with permission of Delmar Learning, a division of Thomson Learning: www.thomsonrights.com. Fax: 800-730-2215.)*

physical, mental, emotional, sociocultural, sexual, and spiritual data.

Purpose

The health history aids both individuals and health care providers by supplying essential information that will assist with diagnosis, treatment decisions, and establishment of trust and rapport between lay persons and medical professionals. The information also helps determine an individual's baseline, or what is normal and expected for that person.

Demographics

Every person should have a thorough health history recorded as a component of a periodic **physical examination**. These occur frequently (monthly at first) in infants and gradually reach a frequency of once per year for adolescents and adults.

Description

The clinical interview is the most common method for obtaining a health history. When a person or a designated representative can communicate effectively, the clinical interview is a valuable means for obtaining information.

The information that comprises the health history may be obtained from a person's previous records, the individual, or, in some cases, significant others or caretakers. The depth and length of the history-taking process is affected by factors such as the purpose of the visit, the urgency of the complaint or condition, the person's willingness or ability to contribute information, and the environment in which information is sought. When circumstances allow, a history may be holistic and comprehensive, but at times only a cursory review of the most pertinent facts is possible. In cases where the history-gathering process needs to be abbreviated, the history focuses on a person's medical experiences.

Health histories can be organized in a variety of ways. Often an organization such as a hospital or clinic will provide a form, template, or computer database that serves as a guide and documentation tool for the history. Generally, the first aspect covered by the history is identifying data.

Identifying or basic demographic data includes facts such as:

- name
- gender
- age
- date of birth

- occupation
- family structure or living arrangements
- source of referral

Once the basic identifying data is collected, the history addresses the reason for the current visit in expanded detail. The reason for the visit is sometimes referred to as the chief complaint or the presenting complaint. Once the reason for the visit is established, additional data is solicited by asking for details that provide a more complete picture of the current clinical situation. For example, in the case of pain, aspects such as location, duration, intensity, precipitating factors, aggravating factors, relieving factors, and associated symptoms should be recorded. The full picture or story that accompanies the chief complaint is often referred to as the history of present illness (HPI).

The review of systems is a useful method for gathering medical information in an orderly fashion. This review is a series of questions about the person's current and past medical experiences. It usually proceeds from general to specific information. A thorough record of relevant dates is important in determining relevance of past illnesses or events to the current condition. A review of systems typically follows a head-to-toe order.

The names for categories in the review of systems may vary, but generally consists of variations on the following list:

- head, eyes, ears, nose, throat (HEENT)
- cardiovascular
- respiratory
- gastrointestinal
- genitourinary
- integumentary (skin)
- musculoskeletal, including joints

QUESTIONS TO ASK THE DOCTOR

- What are your interpretations of my history, both normal and abnormal?
- What has changed since the last health history was obtained?
- What do you recommend as a result of your interpretation of the information obtained in this health history?
- When do you want to repeat the health history?

- endocrine

- nervous system, including both central and peripheral components

- mental, including psychiatric issues

Past and current medical history includes details on medicines taken by the person, as well as allergies, illness, hospitalizations, procedures, pregnancies, environmental factors such as exposure to chemicals, toxins, or carcinogens, and health maintenance habits such as breast or testicular self-examination or immunizations.

An example of a series of questions might include the following:

- How are your ears?

- Are you having any trouble hearing?

- Have you ever had any trouble with your ears or with your hearing?

If an individual indicates a history of auditory difficulties, this would prompt further questions about medicines, surgeries, procedures, or associated problems related to the current or past condition.

In addition to identifying data, chief complaint, and review of systems, a comprehensive health history also includes factors such as a person's family and social life, family medical history, mental or emotional illnesses or stressors, detrimental or beneficial habits such as smoking or **exercise**, and aspects of culture, sexuality, and spirituality that are relevant to each individual. The clinicians also tailor their interviewing style to the age, culture, educational level, and attitudes of the persons being interviewed.

Diagnosis/Preparation

Because the information obtained from the interview is subjective, it is important that the interviewer as-

sess the person's level of understanding, education, communication skills, potential biases, or other information that may affect accurate communication. Thorough training and practice in techniques of interviewing such as asking open-ended questions, listening effectively, and approaching sensitive topics such as substance abuse, chemical dependency, domestic violence, or sexual practices assists a clinician in obtaining the maximum amount of information without upsetting the person being questioned or disrupting the interview. The interview should be preceded by a review of the chart and an introduction by the clinician. The health care professional should explain the scope and purpose of the interview and provide privacy for the person being interviewed. Others should only be present with the person's consent.

Aftercare

Once a health history has been completed, the person being queried and the examiner should review the relevant findings. A health professional should discuss any recommendations for treatment or follow-up visits. Suggestions or special instructions should be put in writing. This is also an opportunity for persons to ask any remaining questions about their own health concerns.

Risks

There are virtually no risks associated with obtaining a health history. Only information is exchanged. The risk is potential embarrassment if confidential details are inappropriately distributed. Occasionally, a useful piece of information or data may be overlooked. In a sense, complications may arise from the findings of a health history. These usually trigger further investigations or initiate treatment. They are usually far more beneficial than negative as they often begin a process of treatment and recovery.

Normal results

Normal results of a health history correspond to the appearance and normal functioning of the body. Abnormal results of a health history include any findings that indicate the presence of a disorder, disease, or underlying condition.

Morbidity and mortality rates

Disease and disability are identified during the course of obtaining a health history. There are virtually no risks associated with the verbal exchange of information.

Alternatives

There are no alternatives that are as effective as obtaining a complete health history. The only real alternative is to skip the history. This allows disease and other pathologic or degenerative processes to go undetected. In the long run, this is not conducive to optimal health.

See also Physical examination.

Resources

BOOKS

Bickley, L. S., P. G. Szilagyi, and J. G. Stackhouse. *Bates' Guide to Physical Examination & History Taking, 8th edition.* Philadelphia: Lippincott Williams & Wilkins, 2002.

Chan, P. D., and P. J. Winkle. *History and Physical Examination in Medicine, 10th ed.* New York, NY: Current Clinical Strategies, 2002.

Seidel, Henry M. *Mosby's Physical Examination Handbook, 4th ed.* St. Louis, MO: Mosby-Year Book, 2003.

Swartz, Mark A., and William Schmitt. *Textbook of Physical Diagnosis: History and Examination, 4th edition.* Philadelphia, PA: Saunders, 2001.

PERIODICALS

Berridge, V., and K. Loughlin. "Public Health History." *Journal of Epidemiology and Community Health,* 57(3) 2003: 164–165.

Burnham, B. R., D. F. Thompson, and W. G. Jackson. "Positive Predictive Value of a Health History Questionnaire." *Military Medicine,* 167(8) 2002: 639–642.

Meurer, L. N., P. M. Layde, and C. E. Guse. "Self-rated Health Status: A New Vital Sign for Primary Care?" *Western Medical Journal,* 100(7) 2001: 35–39.

Nusbaum, M. R., and C. D. Hamilton. "The Proactive Sexual Health History." *American Family Physician,* 66(9) 2002: 1705–1712.

ORGANIZATIONS

American Academy of Family Physicians. 11400 Tomahawk Creek Parkway, Leawood, KS 66211-2672. (913) 906-6000. E-mail: <fp@aafp.org>. <http://www.aafp.org>.

American Academy of Pediatrics. 141 Northwest Point Boulevard, Elk Grove Village, IL 60007-1098. (847) 434-4000, Fax: (847) 434-8000. E-mail: <kidsdoc@aap.org>. <http://www.aap.org/default.htm>.

American College of Physicians. 190 N. Independence Mall West, Philadelphia, PA 19106-1572. (800) 523-1546, x2600, or (215) 351-2600. <http://www.acponline.org>.

American Medical Association. 515 N. State Street, Chicago, IL 60610. (312) 464-5000. <http://www.ama-assn.org>.

OTHER

Genealogy Today [cited March 1, 2003]. <http://www.genealogytoday.com/articles/genogram.html>.

Huntington's Disease Support Information [March 1, 2003]. <http://endoflifecare.tripod.com/hdhelpfulforms/id5.html>.

John C. Lincoln Hospital [March 1, 2003]. <http://www.jcl.com/mothersday>.

Parenting.Com [cited March 1, 2003]. <http://www.parenting.com/parenting/checklists/family_health.html>.

L. Fleming Fallon, Jr, MD, DrPH

Health maintenance organizations *see* **Managed care plans**

Heart-lung machines

Definition

The heart-lung machine is medical equipment that provides cardiopulmonary bypass, or mechanical circulatory support of the heart and lungs. The machine may consist of venous and arterial cannula (tubes), polyvinyl chloride (PVC) or silicone tubing, reservoir (to hold blood), bubbler or membrane oxygenator, cardiotomy (filtered reservoir), heat exchanger(s), arterial line filter, pump(s), flow meter, inline blood gas and electrolyte analyzer, and pressure-monitoring devices. Treatment provides removal of carbon dioxide from the blood, oxygen delivery to the blood, blood flow to the body, and/or temperature maintenance. Pediatric and adult patients both benefit from this technology.

Purpose

In the **operating room**, the heart-lung machine is used primarily to provide blood flow and respiration for the patient while the heart is stopped. Surgeons are able to perform coronary artery bypass grafting (CABG), open-heart surgery for valve repair or repair of cardiac anomalies, and aortic aneurysm repairs, along with treatment of other cardiac-related diseases.

The heart-lung machine provides the benefit of a motionless heart in an almost bloodless surgical field. Cardioplegia solution is delivered to the heart, resulting in cardiac arrest (heart stoppage). The heart-lung machine is invaluable during this time since the patient is unable to maintain blood flow to the lungs or the body.

In critical care units and **cardiac catheterization** laboratories, the heart-lung machine is used to support

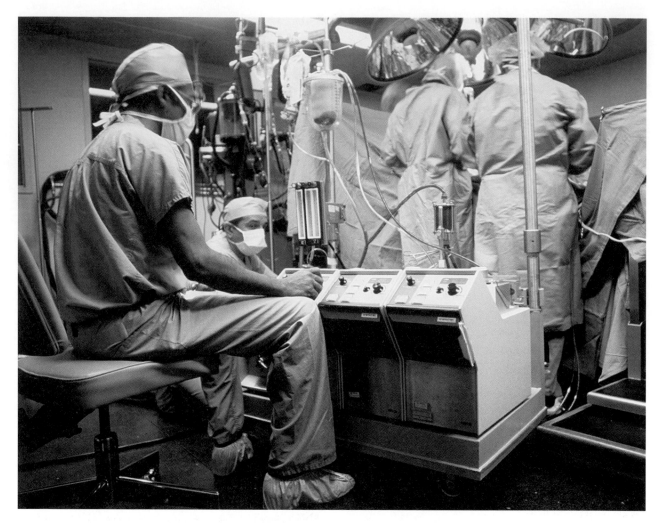

A heart-lung machine. *(Photograph by Albert Paglialunga. Phototake NYC. Reproduced by permission.)*

and maintain blood flow and respiration. The diseased heart or lung(s) is replaced by this technology, providing time for the organ(s) to heal. The heart-lung machine can be used with venoarterial extracorporeal membrane oxygenation (ECMO), which is used primarily in the treatment of lung disease. Cardiopulmonary support is useful during percutaneous transluminal coronary **angioplasty** (PTCA) and stent procedures performed with cardiac catheterization. Both treatments can be instituted in the critical care unit when severe heart or lung disease is no longer treatable by less-invasive conventional treatments such as pharmaceuticals, intra-aortic balloon pump (IABP), and **mechanical ventilation** with a respirator.

Use of this treatment in the emergency room is not limited to patients suffering heart or lung failure. In severe cases of hypothermia, a patient's body temperature can be corrected by extracorporeal circulation with the heart-lung machine. Blood is warmed as it passes over the heat exchanger. The warmed blood returns to the body, gradually increasing the patient's body temperature to normal.

Tertiary care facilities are able to support the staffing required to operate and maintain this technology. Level I trauma centers have access to this specialized treatment and equipment. Being that this technology serves both adult and pediatric patients, specialized children's hospitals may provide treatment with the heart-lung machine for venoarterial ECMO.

Description

The pump oxygenator had its first success on May 6, 1953. Continued research and design have allowed the heart-lung machine to become a standard of care in the treatment of heart and lung disease, while supporting other non-conventional treatments.

Foreign surfaces of the heart-lung machine activate blood coagulation, proteins, and platelets, which lead to clot formation. In the heart-lung machine, clot formation would block the flow of blood. As venous and arterial cannulas are inserted, medications are administered to provide anticoagulation of the blood which prevents clot formation and allows blood flow through the heart-lung machine.

Large vessels (veins and arteries) are required for cannulation, to insert the tubes (cannulas) that will carry the blood away from the patient to the heart-lung machine and to return the blood from the heart-lung machine to the patient. Cannulation sites for venous access can include the inferior and superior vena cava, the right atrium (the upper chamber of the heart), the femoral vein (in the groin), or internal jugular vein. Oxygen-rich blood will be returned to the aorta, femoral artery, or carotid artery (in the neck). By removing oxygen-poor blood from the right side of the heart and returning oxygen-rich blood to the left side, heart-lung bypass is achieved.

The standard heart-lung machine typically includes up to five pump assemblies. A centrifugal or roller head pump can be used in the arterial position for extracorporeal circulation of the blood. The four remaining pumps are roller pump in design to provide fluid, gas, and liquid for delivery or removal to the heart chambers and surgical field. Left ventricular blood return is accomplished by roller pump, drawing blood away from the heart. Surgical suction created by the roller pump removes accumulated fluid from the general surgical field. The cardioplegia delivery pump is used to deliver a high potassium solution to the coronary vessels. The potassium arrests the heart so that the surgical field is motionless during surgical procedures. An additional pump is available for emergency backup of the arterial pump in case of mechanical failure.

A pump is required to produce blood flow. Currently, roller and centrifugal pump designs are the standard of care. Both modern designs can provide pulsatile (pulsed, as from a heartbeat) or non-pulsatile blood flow to the systemic circulation.

The roller assembly rotates and engages the tubing, PVC or silicone, which is then compressed against the pump's housing, propelling blood ahead of the roller head. Rotational frequency and inner diameter of the tubing determine blood flow. Because of its occlusive nature, the pump can be used to remove blood from the surgical field by creating negative pressure on the inflow side of the pump head.

The centrifugal pump also has a negative inlet pressure. As a safety feature, this pump disengages when air bubbles are introduced. The centrifugal force draws blood into the center of the device. Blood is propelled and released to the outflow tract tangential to the pump housing. Rotational speed determines the amount of blood flow, which is measured by a flowmeter placed adjacent to the pump housing. If rotational frequency is too low, blood may flow in the wrong direction since the system is non-occlusive in nature. Magnetic coupling links the centrifugal pump to the control unit.

A reservoir collects blood drained from the venous circulation. Tubing connects the venous cannulae to the reservoir. Reservoir designs include open or closed systems. The open system displays graduated demarcations corresponding to blood volume in the container. The design is open to atmosphere, allowing blood to interface with atmospheric gasses. The pliable bag of the closed system eliminates the air-blood interface, while still being exposed to atmospheric pressure. Volume is measured by weight or by change in radius of the container. The closed reservoir collapses when emptied, as an additional safety feature.

Bubble oxygenators use the reservoir for ventilation. When the reservoir is examined from the exterior, the blood is already oxygen rich and appears bright red. As blood enters the reservoir, gaseous emboli are mixed directly with the blood. Oxygen and carbon dioxide are exchanged across the boundary layer of the blood and gas bubbles. The blood will then pass through a filter that is coated with an antifoam solution, which helps to remove fine bubbles. As blood pools in the reservoir, it has already exchanged carbon dioxide and oxygen. From here, tubing carries the blood to the rest of the heart-lung machine.

In opposition to this technique is the membrane oxygenator. Tubing carries the oxygen-poor blood from the reservoir through the pump to the membrane oxygenator. Oxygen and carbon dioxide cross a membrane that separates the blood from the ventilation gasses. As blood leaves the oxygenator, it is oxygen rich and bright red in color.

When blood is ready to be returned from the heart-lung machine to the patient, the arterial line filter will be encountered. This device is used to filter small air bubbles that may have entered, or been generated by, the heart-lung machine. Following this, filter tubing completes the blood path as it returns the blood to the arterial cannula to enter the body.

Fluid being returned from the left ventricle and surgical suction require filtration before the blood is reintroduced to the heart-lung machine. Blood enters a filtered reservoir, called a cardiotomy, which is connected with tubing to the venous reservoir. Other fluids such as blood products and medications are also added into the cardiotomy for filtration of particulate.

Heat exchangers allow body and organ temperatures to be adjusted. The simplest heat exchange design is a bucket of water. As the blood passes through the tubing placed in the bath, the blood temperature will change. A more sophisticated system separates the blood and water interface with a metallic barrier. As the water temperature is changed, so is the blood temperature, which enters the body or organ circulation, which changes the tissue temperature. Once the tissue temperature reaches the desired level, the water temperature is maintained. Being able to cool the blood helps to preserve the organ and body by metabolizing fewer energy stores.

Because respiration is being controlled, and a machine is meeting metabolic demand, it is necessary to monitor the patient's blood chemical makeup. Chemical sensors placed in the blood path are able to detect the amount of oxygen bound to hemoglobin. Other, more elaborate sensors can constantly trend the blood pH, partial pressure of oxygen and carbon dioxide, and electrolytes. This constant trending can quickly analyze the metabolic demands of the body.

Sensors that communicate system pressures are also a necessity. These transducers are placed in areas where pressure is high, after the pump. Readings outside of normal ranges often alert the operator to obstructions in the blood-flow path. The alert of high pressure must be corrected quickly as the heart-lung machine equipment may disengage under the stress of abnormally elevated pressures. Low-pressure readings can be just as serious, alerting the user to faulty connections or equipment. Constant monitoring and proper alarms help to protect the integrity of the system.

Constant scanning of all components and monitoring devices is required. Normal values can quickly change due to device failure or sudden mechanical constrictions. The diagnosis of a problem and quick troubleshooting techniques will prevent additional complications.

Normal results

Continuous scanning of all patient monitors is necessary for proper treatment and troubleshooting. Documentation of patient status is obtained every 15–30 minutes. This information allows the physician and nursing staff to follow trends that will help better manage the patient once treatment is discontinued. At the termination of device support, the perfusionist or ECMO specialist must communicate clearly to the physician all changes in support status. This allows the entire team to assess changes in patient parameters that are consistent with the patient be-

---

KEY TERMS

Anticoagulant—Pharmaceuticals to prevent clotting proteins and platelets in the blood to be activated to form a blood clot.

Cannula—Tubes that provide access to the blood are inserted into the heart or blood vessels.

Cardiopulmonary bypass—Diversion of blood flow away from the right atrium and return of blood beyond the left ventricle, to bypass the heart and lungs.

Extracorporeal—Circulation of blood outside of the body.

---

coming less dependent on the device, while the patient's heart and lungs meet the metabolic demands of the body.

It is the responsibility of the perfusionist or ECMO specialist to be at the device controls at all times.

Resources

BOOKS

Gravelee, Glenn P., Richard F. Davis, Mark Kurusz, and Joe R. Utley. *Cardiopulmonary Bypass: Principles and Practice,* 2nd edition. Philadelphia: Lippincott Williams & Wilkins, 2000.

ORGANIZATIONS

American Society of Extra-corporeal Technology. 503 Carlisle Dr., Suite 125, Herndon, VA 20170. (703) 435-8556. <http://www.amsect.org>.

Commission on Accreditation of Allied Health Education Programs. 1740 Gilpin Street, Denver, CO 80218. (303) 320-7701. <http://www.caahep.org>.

Extracorporeal Life Support Organization (ELSO). 1327 Jones Drive, Suite 101, Ann Arbor, MI 48105. (734) 998-6600. <http://www.elso.med.umich.edu/>.

Joint Commission on Accreditation of Health Organizations. One Renaissance Boulevard, Oakbrook Terrace, IL 60181. (630) 792-5000. <http://www.jcaho.org/>.

Allison J. Spiwak, MSBME

Heart-lung transplantation

Definition

Heart-lung transplantation is the replacement of the native diseased heart and lungs by transplant of donor heart and lungs.

Heart-lung transplantation

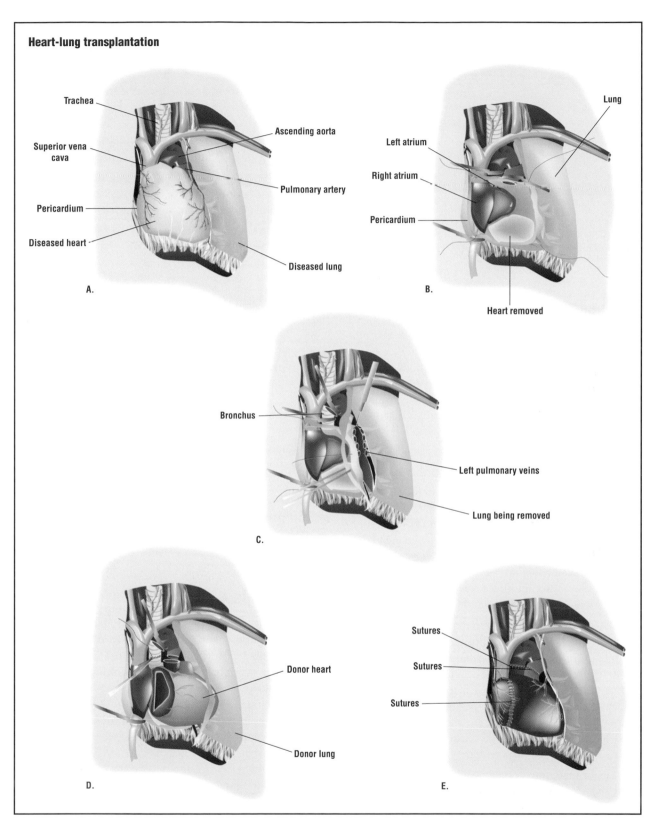

Trachea

Superior vena cava

Pericardium

Diseased heart

Ascending aorta

Pulmonary artery

Diseased lung

A.

Lung

Left atrium

Right atrium

Pericardium

Heart removed

B.

Bronchus

Left pulmonary veins

Lung being removed

C.

Donor heart

Donor lung

D.

Sutures

Sutures

Sutures

E.

Chest is opened to expose the diseased heart and lung to be removed (A). Heart and lung function is taken over by a heart-lung machine. Major blood vessels are severed, and the heart is removed (B). Bronchus and blood vessels leading to the lung are severed, and the lung is removed (C). Donor heart and lung are placed in the patient's the chest cavity (D). They are sutured to their appropriate connections, and the heart is restarted before the patient is taken off the heart-lung machine (E). *(Illustration by GGS Inc.)*

Purpose

Heart-lung transplantation is required when blood ventilation (air exchange) is inhibited. Inhibited oxygen and carbon dioxide transfer prevents the delivery of oxygen to the tissue and results in carbon dioxide levels in the blood that are higher than normal. Additionally, pulmonary hypertension can cause compromised cardiac function.

Demographics

There are factors which absolutely contraindicate (rule out) heart-lung transplantation, including multiple organ system dysfunction, current substance abuse, bone marrow failure, active malignancy, and HIV infection. Other relative contraindications include age greater than 55, anorexia, obesity, peripheral and coronary vascular disease, ventilator support, steroid dependency, chest wall deformity, and resistant infections by bacterial and fungal agents. Mental health status should be addressed, as well.

Patients who are limited in daily activity, as defined by their doctors, and have a limited life expectancy, are candidates for heart-lung transplantation. These patients suffer from untreatable end-stage pulmonary, organ, and/or vascular disease. Most often, the diagnosis includes primary pulmonary hypertension brought on by congenital blood vessel defects that include malformations in the lung. Congenital cardiac defects and other diseases may also be responsible.

Donor matching is managed by the Organ Procurement and Transplantation Network (OPTN), in which all organ centers must participate according to Federal **Medicare** and **Medicaid** programs. Established criteria for donor organ matching include the following: anatomic and immunologic compatibility between the donor and recipient; medical urgency; efficiency in organ dis-

tribution for improved organ viability; and ethical considerations. After a match for anatomic and blood group compatibility with the patients on the donor list, the organs are distributed on the basis of seniority in list standing among suitable recipients. Patients with IPF are provided special consideration on organ donor waiting lists. The average waiting time on the heart-lung transplant list is 795 days.

Description

Cardiac monitoring is a necessary part of heart-lung transplantation. Under general cardiac anesthesia, an incision is made in the patient's chest to access the heart and lungs. Anticoagulation (anti-clotting) medications are provided, and cardiopulmonary bypass to a heart-lung machine is instituted. Blood flow is discontinued through the heart by application of a clamp across the aorta. The surgeon removes the diseased organs: in the heart, the native right and left atriums are left intact, along with the native aorta beyond the coronary arteries. This provides large suture lines that allow decreased surgical time and result in fewer bleeding complications.

The donor heart is dissected to match the remaining native heart and aorta. The sutures are made to join the structures. Once completed, the cardiac chambers are de-aired as the organs fill with the patient's blood that is diverted away from the heart and lung machine. **Mechanical ventilation** of the donor lungs helps to purge any remaining air from the cardiac and pulmonary structures and inflate the lung tissue.

Diagnosis/Preparation

History, examination, and laboratory studies are performed prior to referral to a transplant center. These records are reviewed on-site for qualification to be placed on the United Network for Organ Sharing (UNOS) national waiting list. Procedures necessary for evaluation include a **chest x ray**, arterial blood samples, spirometric and respiratory flow studies, ventilation and perfusion scanning, and **cardiac catheterization** of both the right and left heart.

Aftercare

The patient will be treated in the **intensive care unit** upon completion of the surgery, and cardiac monitoring will be continued. Medications for cardiac support will be continued until cardiac function stabilizes. Mechanical circulatory support may be continued until cardiac and respiratory functions improves. Ventilator support will be continued until the patient is able to breathe independently. Medications to prevent organ rejection will be continued indefinitely, as will medications to prevent infection. The patient will be evaluated before discharge and provided with specific instructions to recognize infection and organ rejection. The patient will be given directions to contact the physician after discharge, along with criteria for emergency room care.

Risks

General anesthesia and cardiopulmonary bypass carry certain risks unassociated with the heart-lung transplant procedure. Graft rejection and technical failure are a result of lung injury sustained during the stoppage and restarting of the organ. Infection by cytomegalovirus (CMV) occurs in the first year, but is usually treatable. Immunosuppressive drugs to prevent rejection have side effects associated with malignancies; lymphomas or tumors of the skin and lips being most common. Osteoporosis and nephrotoxicity are also associated with the immunosuppressive therapies.

Normal results

Lung and cardiac function are drastically improved after transplantation. Strenuous **exercise** may still be limited, but quality of life is greatly improved. Of all heart-lung transplant recipients, 90% are satisfied with their de-

---

KEY TERMS

Congenital defect—A defect present at birth that occurs during the growth and development of the fetus in the womb.

Coronary vascular disease—Or cardiovascular disease; disease of the heart or blood vessels, such as atherosclerosis (hardening of the arteries).

Native—Refers to a patient's own organs before transplant.

Nephrotoxicity—A building up of poisons in the kidneys.

Osteoporosis—Loss of bone mass, causing bones to break easily.

Pulmonary hypertension—Increased blood pressure in the circulation around the lungs.

Resistant infections—Infections caused by bacteria that become resistant to most antibiotics.

---

cisions to undergo the transplantation procedure. The patient will continue with medical visits frequently throughout the first year, including required tissue biopsies and cardiac catheterizations. The frequency of medical visits will decrease after the first year, but invasive medical procedures will still be necessary. Medications to suppress rejection of the organs and prevent infection are continued.

Morbidity and mortality rates

Systemic hypertension is common in almost half the patients at one year after surgery and can be relieved with medical treatment. Chronic bronchiolitis is expected in one-third of patients at five years. Hyperlipidemia (high lipid concentration in blood), diabetes mellitus, and kidney dysfunction are also seen in some patients within the first year of transplantation and continue to affect an increasing number of patients each year. Malignancies that include lymphoma and lip and skin tumors are seen at a higher rate than in general populations.

Death within the first 30 days is usually associated with technical and graft failure of the transplanted organ. Rejection of the cardiac organ includes chronic coronary artery disease affecting a small percentage of patients, while bronchiolitis (inflammation caused by rejection of the lung) is responsible for the death of 60% of patients between the first and fifth years. Untreatable infections are a persistent complication in the initial 30 days and continue to affect patients into the fifth year, and result in death. Acute rejection is uncommon, but it is a complication that can also lead to death.

Five-year mortality is higher for patients with ventilator dependence, retransplantation, congenital disease, and in recipients over 60 years of age.

Alternatives

Heart-lung transplants are becoming less common. Since 1990, only 40 to 60 of these procedures are performed every year in the United States. The outcomes of single- and double-lung transplantation have provided good success for pathologies where the cardiac function is not jeopardized.

Resources

BOOKS

Hensley, Frederick A., Martin Donald E., Gravlee Glenn P., ed. *A Practical Approach to Cardiac Anesthesia,* 3rd ed. Philadelphia: Lippincott Williams & Wilkins Philadelphia, 2003.

PERIODICALS

Turlock, Elbert P. "Lung and Heart-Lung Transplantation: Overview of Results." *Seminars in Respiratory and Critical Care Medicine* 22, no.5 (2001): 479–488.

Allison Joan Spiwak, MSBME

Heart catheterization *see* **Cardiac catheterization**

Heart defect surgery *see* **Heart surgery for congenital defects**

Heart resection *see* **Myocardial resection**

Heart sonogram *see* **Echocardiography**

Heart surgery for congenital defects

Definition

Heart surgery for congenitaal defects consists of a variety of surgical procedures that are performed to repair the many types of heart defects that may be present at birth and can go undiagnosed into adulthood.

Purpose

Heart surgery for congenital defects is performed to repair a defect, providing improved blood flow to the pulmonary and systemic circulations and better oxygen delivery to the body. Congenital heart defects that are

---

WHO PERFORMS THE PROCEDURE AND WHERE IS IT PERFORMED?

Pediatric cardiologists and cardiac surgeons specialize in treatment of congenital defects. Hospitals dedicated to the care of children may provide cardiac surgery services. Congenital defects diagnosed at birth may require immediate transport of the infant to a facility that can provide timely treatment.

---

symptomatic at birth must be treated with palliative or complete surgical repair. Defects that are not symptomatic at birth may be discovered later in life, and will be treated to relieve symptoms by palliative or complete surgical repair. Surgery is recommended for congenital heart defects that result in a lack of oxygen, a poor quality of life, or when a patient fails to thrive. Even lesions that are asymptomatic may be treated surgically to avoid additional complications later in life.

Demographics

Congenital heart disease is estimated to involve less than 1% of all live births. As some defects are not found until later in life, or may never be diagnosed, this number may actually be higher. Many congenital defects are often incompatible with life leading to miscarriage and stillbirths. During a child's first year of life, the most common defects that are symptomatic include ventricular septal defect (VSD), transposition of the great vessels (TGV), tetralogy of Fallot, coarctation of the aorta, and hypoplastic left heart syndrome. Premature infants have an increased presentation of VSD and patent ductus arteriosus. Diabetic mothers have infants with a higher incidence of congenital heart defects than non-diabetic mothers. Abnormal chromosomes increase the incidence of congenital heart defects. Specific to trisomy 21 (Down syndrome), 23–56% of infants have a congenital heart defect.

Description

Congenital heart defects can be named by a number of specific lesions, but may have additional lesions. Classification best describes lesions by the amount of pulmonary blood flow (increased or decreased pulmonary blood flow) or the presence of an obstruction to blood flow. The dynamic circulation of the newborn as well as the size of the defect will determine the symptoms. Recommended ages for surgery for the most common congenital heart defects are:

Heart surgery for congenital defects

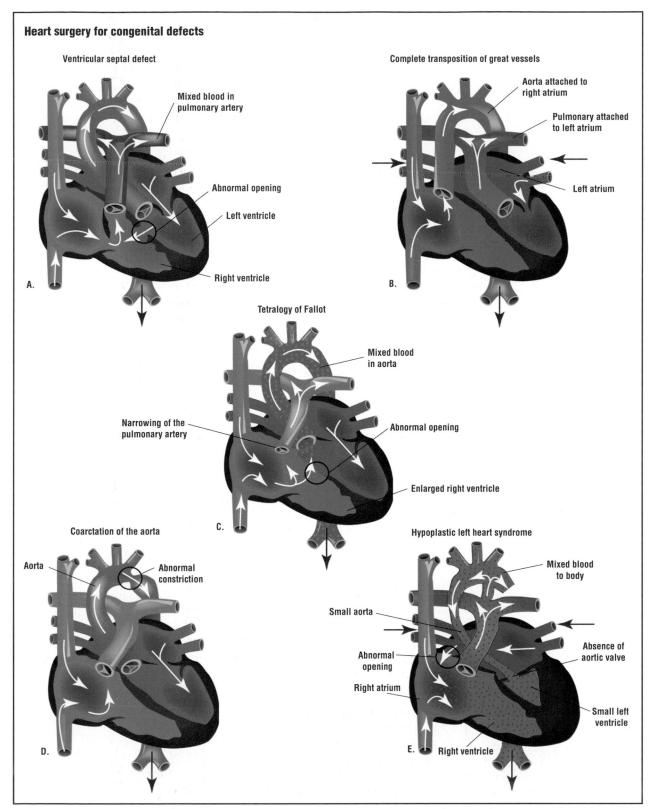

Ventricular septal defect

Mixed blood in pulmonary artery

Abnormal opening

Left ventricle

Right ventricle

A.

Complete transposition of great vessels

Aorta attached to right atrium

Pulmonary attached to left atrium

Left atrium

B.

Tetralogy of Fallot

Mixed blood in aorta

Narrowing of the pulmonary artery

Abnormal opening

Enlarged right ventricle

C.

Coarctation of the aorta

Aorta

Abnormal constriction

D.

Hypoplastic left heart syndrome

Mixed blood to body

Small aorta

Absence of aortic valve

Abnormal opening

Right atrium

Small left ventricle

E. Right ventricle

The most common types of congenital heart defects are ventricular septal defect (A), complete transposition of the great vessels (B), tetralogy of Fallot (C), coarctation of the aorta (D), and hypoplastic left heart syndrome (E). *(Illustration by GGS Inc.)*

QUESTIONS TO ASK THE DOCTOR

• What type of congenital defect has been diagnosed?

• What type of palliative and corrective surgical options are available, and what are the risks associated with each?

• Where can more information about the congenital defect and its surgical procedures be found?

• When will the repair be made?

• How many procedures of this type has the surgeon completed, and what are the surgeon-specific outcome statistics?

• What type of care will the child require until the repair can be made?

• What types of limitations are expected prior to and after the surgical procedure?

• What type of mental health support is provided for parents or caregivers?

• What type of continued care is provided for after the hospital stay?

• What type of financial support is available for the family and caregivers?

• atrial septal defects: during the preschool years

• patent ductus arteriosus: between ages one and two

• coarctation of the aorta: in infancy, if it is symptomatic, at age four otherwise

• tetralogy of Fallot: age varies, depending on the patient's symptoms

• transposition of the great arteries: often in the first weeks after birth, but before the patient is 12 months old

Surgical procedures seek to repair the defect and restore normal pulmonary and systemic circulation. Sometimes, multiple, serial surgical procedures are necessary.

Many congenital defects are often associated so that the surgical procedures described may be combined for complete repair of a specific congenital defect.

Repair for simple cardiac lesions can be performed in the **cardiac catheterization** lab. Catheterization procedures include balloon atrial septostomy and **balloon valvuloplasty**. Surgical procedures include arterial switch, Damus-Kaye-Stansel procedure, Fontan proce-

dure, Ross procedure, shunt procedure, and venous switch or intra-atrial baffle.

Catheterization procedures

Balloon atrial septostomy and balloon valvuloplasty are cardiac catheterization procedures. Cardiac catheterization procedures can save the lives of critically ill neonates and, in some cases, eliminate or delay more invasive surgical procedures. It is expected that catheterization procedures will continue to replace more types of surgery for congenital heart defects in the future. A thin tube called a catheter is inserted into an artery or vein in the leg, groin, or arm and threaded into the area of the heart that needs repair. The patient receives a local anesthetic at the insertion site. General anesthetic or sedation may be used.

BALLOON ATRIAL SEPTOSTOMY. Balloon atrial septostomy is the standard procedure for correcting transposition of the great arteries; it is sometimes used in patients with mitral, pulmonary, or tricuspid atresia. (Atresia is lack of or poor development of a structure.) Balloon atrial septostomy enlarges the atrial septal opening, which normally closes in the days following birth. A special balloon-tipped catheter is inserted into the right atrium and passed into the left atrium. The balloon is inflated in the left atrium and pulled back across the septum to create a larger opening in the atrial septum.

BALLOON VALVULOPLASTY. Balloon valvuloplasty uses a balloon-tipped catheter to open a stenotic (narrowed) heart valve, improving the flow of blood through the valve. It is the procedure of choice in pulmonary stenosis and is sometimes used in aortic and mitral stenosis. A balloon is placed beyond the valve, inflated, and pulled backward across the valve.

Surgical procedures

These procedures are performed under general anesthesia. Some require the use of a heart-lung machine, which takes over for the heart and lungs during the procedure, providing cardiopulmonary bypass. The heart-lung machine can cool the body to reduce the need for oxygen, allowing deep hypothermic circulatory arrest (DHCA) to be performed. DHCA benefits the surgeon by creating a bloodless surgical field.

ARTERIAL SWITCH. Arterial switch is performed to correct transposition of the great vessels, where the position of the pulmonary artery and the aorta are reversed. The procedure involves connecting the aorta to the left ventricle and the pulmonary artery to the right ventricle.

DAMUS-KAYE-STANSEL PROCEDURE. Transposition of the great vessels can also be corrected by the Damus-

Kaye-Stansel procedure, in which the pulmonary artery is cut in two and connected to the ascending aorta and right ventricle.

VENOUS SWITCH. For transposition of the great vessels, venous switch creates a tunnel inside the atria to redirect oxygen-rich blood to the right ventricle and aorta and venous blood to the left ventricle and pulmonary artery. This procedure differs from the arterial switch and Damus-Kaye-Stansel procedures in that blood flow is redirected through the heart.

FONTAN PROCEDURE. For tricuspid atresia and pulmonary atresia, the Fontan procedure connects the right atrium to the pulmonary artery directly or with a conduit, and the atrial septal defect is closed.

PULMONARY ARTERY BANDING. Pulmonary artery banding is narrowing the pulmonary artery with a band to reduce blood flow and pressure in the lungs. It is used for temporary repair of ventricular septal defect, atrioventricular canal defect, and tricuspid atresia. Later, the band can be removed and the defect corrected with a complete repair once the patient has grown.

ROSS PROCEDURE. To correct aortic stenosis, the Ross procedure grafts the pulmonary artery to the aorta.

SHUNT PROCEDURE. For tetralogy of Fallot, tricuspid atresia, or pulmonary atresia, the shunt procedure creates a passage between blood vessels, directing blood flow into the pulmonary or systemic circulations.

OTHER TYPES OF SURGERY. Surgical procedures are also used to treat common congenital heart defects. To close a medium to large ventricular or atrial septal defect, it is recommended that it be sutured or covered with a Dacron patch. For patent ductus arteriosus, surgery consists of dividing the ductus into two and tying off the ends. If performed within the child's first few years, there is practically no risk associated with this operation. Surgery for coarctation of the aorta involves opening the chest wall, removing the defect, and reconnecting the ends of the aorta. If the defect is too long to be reconnected, a Dacron graft is used to replace the missing piece.

Diagnosis/Preparation

Before surgery for congenital heart defects, the patient will receive a complete evaluation, which includes a physical exam, a detailed family history, a **chest x ray**, an electrocardiogram, an echocardiogram, and usually, cardiac catheterization. Blood tests will be performed to measure formed blood elements, electrolytes, and blood glucose. Additional tests for sickle cell and digoxin levels may be performed, if applicable. For six to eight hours before the surgery, the patient cannot eat or drink anything.

Aftercare

After heart surgery for congenital defects, the patient goes to an **intensive care unit** for continued cardiac monitoring. The patient may also require continued ventilator support. Chest tubes allow blood to be drained from inside the chest as the surgical site heals. Pain medications will be continued, and the patient may remain under general anesthetic. Within 24 hours, the chest tubes and ventilation may be discontinued. Any cardiac drugs used to help the heart perform better will be adjusted appropriate with the patient's condition.

For temporary procedures, additional follow-up with the physician will be required to judge timing for complete repair. In the meantime, the patient should continue to grow and thrive normally. Complete repair requires follow-up with the physician initially to judge the adequacy of repair, but thereafter will be infrequent with good prognosis. The child should be made aware of any procedure to be communicated for future medical care in adulthood.

Risks

Depending on the institution and the type of congenital defect repair, many risks can be identified, including shock, congestive heart failure, lack of oxygen or too much carbon dioxide in the blood, irregular heartbeat, stroke, infection, kidney damage, lung blood clot, low blood pressure, hemorrhage, cardiac arrest, and death. These risks should not impede the surgical procedure, as death is certain without surgical treatment. Neurological dysfunction in the postoperative period occurs in as much as 25% of surgical patients. Seizures are expected in 20% of cases, but are usually limited with no long-term effects. Additional risks include blood **transfusion** reactions and blood-borne pathogens.

Morbidity and mortality rates

Use of cardiopulmonary bypass has associated risks not related to the congenital defect repair. Procedures performed in association with cardiac catheterization have excellent long-term results, with an associated mortality of 2–4% of procedures. The Fontan procedure carries a survival rate of over 90%. Surgical procedures to repair coarctation of the aorta, in uncomplicated cases, has a risk of operative mortality from 1–2%.

Alternatives

Alternatives are limited for this patient population. Cardiac transplant is an option, but a limited number of organ donors restrict this treatment. Ventricular-assist devices and total artificial heart technology are not yet a suitable option. Temporary procedures do allow

KEY TERMS

Atresia—Lack of development. In tricuspid atresia, the triscuspid valve has not developed. In pulmonary atresia, the pulmonary valve has not developed.

Coarctation of the aorta—A congenital defect in which severe narrowing or constriction of the aorta obstructs the flow of blood.

Congenital heart defects—Congenital (conditions that are present at birth) heart disease includes a variety of defects that occur during fetal development.

Cyanotic—Inadequate oxygen in the systemic arterial circulation.

Mitral valve—The heart valve connecting the left atrium and left ventricle.

Patent ductus arteriosus—A congenital defect in which the temporary blood vessel connecting the left pulmonary artery to the aorta in the fetus fails to close in the newborn.

Pulmonary valve—The heart valve connecting the left atrium with the pulmonary arteries.

Septal defects—Openings in the septum, the muscu-lar wall separating the right and left sides of the heart. Atrial septal defects are openings between the two upper heart chambers and ventricular septal defects are openings between the two lower heart chambers.

Stenosis—A narrowing of the heart's valves.

Tetralogy of Fallot—A cyanotic defect in which the blood pumped through the body has too little oxygen. Tetralogy of Fallot includes four defects: a ventricular septal defect, narrowing at or beneath the pulmonary valve, infundibular pulmonary stenosis (obstruction of blood flow out of the right ventricle through the pulmonary valve), and over-riding aorta (the aorta crosses the ventricular septal defect into the right ventricle).

Transposition of the great vessels—A cyanotic defect in which the blood pumped through the body has too little oxygen because the pulmonary artery receives its blood incorrectly from the left ventricle and the aorta incorrectly receives blood flow from the right ventricle.

Tricuspid valve—The heart valve connecting the right atrium and right ventricle.

additional growth of the patient prior to corrective surgery, allowing them to gain strength and size before treatment.

Resources

BOOKS

"Congenital Heart Disease." In *Current Medical Diagnosis and Treatment*, 37th edition, edited by Stephen McPhee, et al. Stamford: Appleton & Lange, 1997.

Davies, Laurie K., and Daniel G. Knauf. "Anesthetic Management for Patients with Congenital Heart Disease." In *A Practical Approach to Cardiac Anesthesia*, 3rd edition, edited by Frederick A. Hensley, Jr., Donal E. Martin, and Glenn P. Gravlee. Philadelphia, PA: Lippincott Williams & Wilkins, 2000.

DeBakey, Michael E., and Antonio M. Gotto Jr. "Congenital Abnormalities of the Heart." In *The New Living Heart*. Holbrook, MA: Adams Media Corporation, 1997.

Park, Myung K. *Pediatric Cardiology for Practitioners*, 3rd edition. St. Louis: Mosby, 1996.

Texas Heart Institute. "Congenital Heart Disease." In *Texas Heart Institute Heart Owners Handbook*. New York: John Wiley & Sons, 1996.

PERIODICALS

Hicks, George L. "Cardiac Surgery." *Journal of the American College of Surgeons*, 186, no. 2 (February 1998): 129–132.

Rao, P. S. "Interventional Pediatric Cardiology: State of the Art and Future Directions." *Pediatric Cardiology*, 19 (1998): 107–124.

ORGANIZATIONS

American Heart Association. 7320 Greenville Ave., Dallas, TX 75231. (214) 373-6300. <http://www.americanheart.org>.

Children's Health Information Network. 1561 Clark Drive, Yardley, PA 19067. (215) 493-3068. <http://www.tchin.org>.

Congenital Heart Anomalies Support, Education & Resources, Inc. 2112 North Wilkins Road, Swanton, OH 43558. (419) 825-5575. <http://www.csun.edu/~hfmth006/chaser>.

Texas Heart Institute. Heart Information Service. P.O. Box 20345, Houston, TX 77225-0345. <http://www.tmc.edu/thi>.

Lori De Milto
Allison J. Spiwak, MSBME

Heart transplantation

Definition

Heart transplantation, also called cardiac transplantation, is the replacement of a patient's diseased or injured heart with a healthy donor heart.

Purpose

Heart transplantation is performed on patients with end-stage heart failure or some other life-threatening heart disease. Before a doctor recommends heart transplantation for a patient, all other possible treatments for his or her disease must have been attempted. The purpose of heart transplantation is to extend and improve the life of a person who would otherwise die from heart failure. Most patients who have received a new heart were so sick before transplantation that they could not live a normal life. Replacing a patient's diseased heart with a healthy, functioning donor heart often allows the recipient to return to normal daily activities.

Demographics

Patients are not limited by age, sex, race, or ethnicity. In 1999, the primary diagnoses of adult patients receiving cardiac transplantation include coronary artery disease, cardiomyopathy, congenital diseases, and re-transplantation associated with organ rejection. Characteristics of patient presentation include cardiomegaly, severe dyspnea, and peripheral edema.

Adults with end-stage heart failure account for 90% of heart transplant recipients. Pediatric patients make up the remaining 10%, with 50% of those going to patients under the age of five. In the United States, patients that receive heart transplant are 73% male, 77% are white, 19% are ages 35–49, and 51% are ages 50–64.

Because healthy donor hearts are in short supply, strict rules dictate criteria for heart transplant recipients. Patients who may be too sick to survive the surgery or the side effects of immunosuppressive therapy would not be good transplant candidates.

These conditions are contraindications for heart transplantation:

- active infection
- pulmonary hypertension
- chronic lung disease with loss of more than 40% of lung function
- untreatable liver or kidney disease
- diabetes that has caused serious damage to vital organs
- disease of the blood vessels in the brain, such as a stroke
- serious disease of the arteries
- mental illness or any condition that would make a patient unable to take the necessary medicines on schedule
- continuing alcohol or drug abuse

Description

Patients with end-stage heart disease unresponsive to medical treatment may be considered for heart transplantation. Potential candidates must have a complete medical examination before they can be put on the transplant waiting list. Many types of tests are done, including blood tests, x rays, and tests of heart, lung, and other organ function. The results of these tests indicate to doctors how serious the heart disease is and whether or not a patient is healthy enough to survive the **transplant surgery**.

Organ waiting list

A person approved for heart transplantation is placed on the heart transplant waiting list of a heart transplant center. All patients on a waiting list are registered with the United Network for Organ Sharing (UNOS). UNOS has organ transplant specialists who run a national computer network that connects all the transplant centers and organ-donation organizations.

When a donor heart becomes available, information about the donor heart is entered into the UNOS computer and compared to information from patients on the waiting list. The computer program produces a list of patients ranked according to blood type, size of the heart, and how urgently they need a heart. Because the heart must be transplanted as quickly as possible, a list of local patients is checked first for a good match. After that, a regional list and then a national list are checked. The patient's transplant team of heart and transplant specialists makes the final decision as to whether a donor heart is suitable for the patient.

The transplant procedure

When a heart becomes available and is approved for a patient, it is packed in a sterile cold solution and rushed to the hospital where the recipient is waiting. The recipient will be contacted to return to the hospital if chronic care occurs outside of the hospital.

A description of the procedure follows:

- General anesthesia is provided by an anesthesiologist experienced with cardiac patients.
- Intravenous **antibiotics** will prevent bacterial wound infections.
- The patient is put on a heart/lung machine, which performs the functions of the heart and lungs by pumping the blood to the rest of the body during surgery. This procedure is called cardiopulmonary bypass.
- Once the donor heart has arrived to the **operating room**, the patient's diseased heart is removed.

Heart transplantation

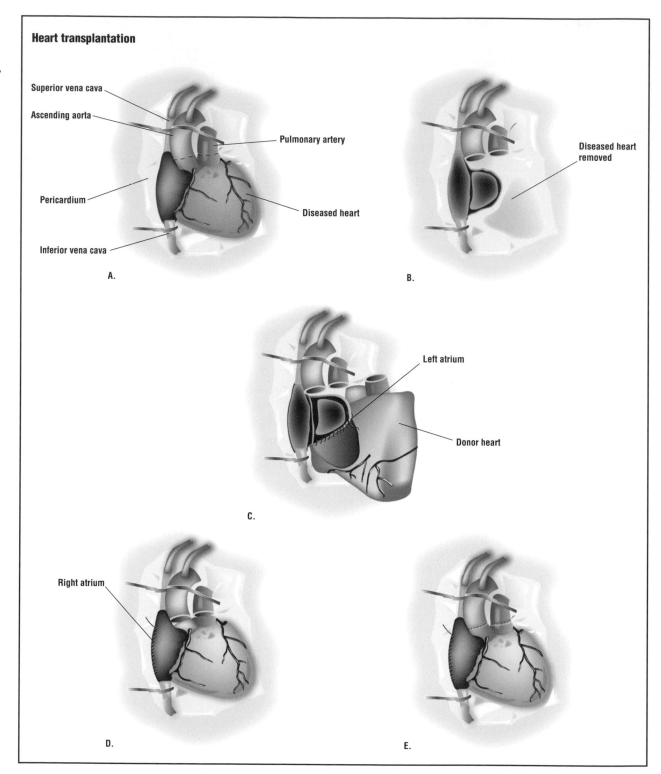

Superior vena cava

Ascending aorta

Pulmonary artery

Pericardium

Diseased heart

Inferior vena cava

A.

B.

Diseased heart removed

Left atrium

Donor heart

C.

Right atrium

D.

E.

For a heart transplantation, the area around the heart is exposed through a chest incision (A). The blood vessels leading to the heart are clamped, and the heart function is replaced by a heart-lung machine. The diseased heart is removed (B). The donor heart is placed in the chest, and the left atrium is attached (C). The right atrium is connected (D), and the aorta and pulmonary artery are finally attached (E). *(Illustration by GGS Inc.)*

- The donor heart is attached to the patient's blood vessels, including the atrium(s), pulmonary artery, and aorta.

- After the blood vessels are connected, the new heart is perfused with the patient's blood and begins beating. If the heart does not begin to beat immediately, the surgeon may use **defibrillation** to gain a productive rhythm.

- The patient is taken off the heart-lung machine.

- The new heart is stimulated to maintain a regular beat with medications and/or a pacemaker for two to five days after surgery, until the new heart functions normally on its own.

Heart transplant recipients are given immunosuppressive drugs to prevent the body from rejecting the new heart. These drugs are usually started before or during the heart transplant surgery. Immunosuppressive drugs keep the body's immune system from recognizing and attacking the new heart as foreign tissue. Normally, immune system cells recognize and attack foreign or abnormal cells such as bacteria, cancer cells, and cells from a transplanted organ. The drugs suppress the immune cells and allow the new heart to function properly. However, they can also allow infections and other adverse effects to occur to the patient.

Because the chance of rejection is highest during the first few months after the transplantation, recipients are usually given a combination of three or four immunosuppressive drugs in high doses during this time. Afterwards, they must take maintenance doses of immunosuppressive drugs for the rest of their lives.

Cost and insurance coverage

The total cost for heart transplantation varies, depending on where it is performed, whether transportation and lodging are needed, and whether there are any complications. The costs for the surgery and first year of care are estimated to be about $250,000. The medical tests and medications after the first year cost about $21,000 per year.

Insurance coverage for heart transplantation varies, depending on the policy. Most commercial insurance companies pay a certain percentage of heart transplant costs. **Medicare** pays for heart transplants if the surgery is performed at Medicare-approved centers. **Medicaid** pays for heart transplants in 33 states and in the District of Columbia.

Diagnosis/Preparation

Before patients are put on the transplant waiting list, their blood type is determined so a compatible donor heart can be found. The heart must come from a person

WHO PERFORMS THE PROCEDURE AND WHERE IS IT PERFORMED?

According to the American Heart Association, there are currently 196 centers performing cardiac transplant surgery in the United States. To meet criteria to be listed with UNOS, centers must perform 12 cardiac transplants per year with a one-year survival of 70%. A cardiac surgeon with additional training in transplant surgery will be consulted to perform the operation.

with the same blood type as the patient, unless it is blood type O negative. A blood type O negative heart is a universal donor and is suitable for any patient regardless of blood type.

A panel reactive antibodies (PRA) test is also done before heart transplantation. This test tells doctors whether or not the patient is at high risk for having a hyperacute reaction against a donor heart. A hyperacute reaction is a strong immune response against the new heart that happens within minutes to hours after the new heart is transplanted. If the PRA shows that a patient has a high risk for this kind of reaction, then a crossmatch is done between a patient and a donor heart before transplant surgery. A crossmatch checks how close the match is between the patient's tissue type and the tissue type of the donor heart. Most people are not high risk, and a crossmatch usually is not done before the transplant because the surgery must be done as quickly as possible after a donor heart is found.

While waiting for heart transplantation, patients are given treatment to keep the heart as healthy as possible. They are regularly checked to make sure the heart is pumping enough blood. Intravenous medications may be used to improve cardiac output. If these drugs are not effective, an intra-aortic balloon pump or ventricular-assist device can maintain cardiac output until a donor heart becomes available.

Aftercare

Immediately following surgery, patients are monitored closely in the **intensive care unit** (ICU) of the hospital for 24–72 hours. Most patients need to receive oxygen for four to 24 hours following surgery. Continuous cardiac monitoring is used to diagnose and treat donor heart function. Renal, liver, brain, and pulmonary functions are carefully monitored during this time.

Heart transplant patients start taking immunosuppressive drugs before or during surgery to prevent immune rejection of the heart. High doses of immunosuppressive drugs are given at this time, because rejection is most likely to happen within the first few months after the surgery. A few months after surgery, lower doses of immunosuppressive drugs usually are given, and then must be taken for the rest of the patient's life.

For six to eight weeks after the transplant surgery, patients usually come back to the transplant center twice a week for physical examinations and medical tests, which check for any signs of infection, rejection of the new heart, or other complications.

In addition to **physical examination**, the following tests may be done during these visits:

- laboratory tests to check for infection

- chest x ray to check for early signs of lung infection

- electrocardiogram (ECG) to check heart function

- echocardiogram to check the function of the ventricles in the heart

- blood tests to check liver and kidney function

- complete blood counts (CBC) to check the numbers of blood cells

- taking of a small tissue sample from the donor heart (endomyocardial biopsy) to check for signs of rejection

During the physical examination, the blood pressure is checked and the heart sounds are listened to with a **stethoscope** to determine if the heart is beating properly and pumping enough blood. Kidney and liver functions are checked because these organs may lose function if the heart is being rejected.

An endomyocardial biopsy is the removal of a small sample of the heart muscle. This is done by **cardiac catheterization**. The heart muscle tissue is examined under a microscope for signs that the heart is being rejected. Endomyocardial biopsy is usually done weekly for the first four to eight weeks after transplant surgery, and then at longer intervals after that.

Risks

The most common and dangerous complications of heart transplant surgery are organ rejection and infection. Immunosuppressive drugs are given to prevent rejection of the heart. Most heart transplant patients have a rejection episode soon after transplantation. Rapid diagnosis ensures quick treatment, and when the response is quick, drug therapy is most successful. Rejection is treated with combinations of immunosuppressive drugs given in higher doses than immunosuppressive maintenance. Most of these rejection situations are successfully treated.

Infection can result from the surgery, but most infections are a side effect of the immunosuppressive drugs. Immunosuppressive drugs keep the immune system from attacking the foreign cells of the donor heart. However, the suppressed immune cells are then unable to adequately fight bacteria, viruses, and other microorganisms. Microorganisms that normally do not affect persons with healthy immune systems can cause dangerous infections in transplant patients taking immunosuppressive drugs.

Patients are given antibiotics during surgery to prevent bacterial infection. They may also be given an antiviral drug to prevent virus infections. Patients who develop infections may need to have their immunosuppressive drugs changed or the dose adjusted. Infections are treated with antibiotics or other drugs, depending on the type of infection.

Other complications that can happen immediately after surgery are:

- bleeding

- pressure on the heart caused by fluid in the space surrounding the heart (pericardial tamponade)

- irregular heart beats

- reduced cardiac output

KEY TERMS

Anesthesia—Loss of the ability to feel pain, caused by administration of an anesthetic drug.

Angina—Characteristic chest pain that occurs during exercise or stress in certain kinds of heart disease.

Cardiopulmonary bypass—Mechanically circulating the blood with a heart-lung machine that bypasses the heart and lungs.

Cardiovascular—Having to do with the heart and blood vessels.

Complete blood count (CBC)—A blood test to check the numbers of red blood cells, white blood cells, and platelets in the blood.

Coronary artery disease—Blockage of the arteries leading to the heart.

Cross-match—A test to determine if patient and donor tissues are compatible.

Donor—A person who donates an organ for transplantation.

Echocardiogram—A test that visualizes and records the position and motion of the walls of the heart using ultrasound waves.

Electrocardiogram (ECG)—A test that measures electrical conduction of the heart.

End-stage heart failure—Severe heart disease that does not respond adequately to medical or surgical treatment.

Endomyocardial biopsy—Removal of a small sample of heart tissue to check it for signs of damage caused by organ rejection.

Graft—A transplanted organ or other tissue.

Immunosuppressive drug—Medication used to suppress the immune system.

Inotropic drugs—Medications used to stimulate the heart beat.

Pulmonary hypertension—An increase in the pressure in the blood vessels of the lungs.

• increased amount of blood in the circulatory system

• decreased amount of blood in the circulatory system

About half of all heart transplant patients develop coronary artery disease one to five years after the transplant. The coronary arteries supply blood to the heart. Patients with this problem develop chest pains called angina. Other names for this complication are coronary allograft vascular disease and chronic rejection.

Normal results

Heart transplantation is an appropriate treatment for many patients with end-stage heart failure. The outcomes of heart transplantation depend on the patient's age, health, and other factors. According to a year 2000 data from the Registry of the International Society for Heart and **Lung Transplantation** (ISHLT), 81% of transplant recipients survive one year. During the first year, infection and acute rejection are the leading causes of death. A constant 4% decrease occurs yearly after the first year as the incidence of coronary allograft vascular disease increases.

Pediatric patients less than one year of age are least likely to reject the donor heart, but 30% of older pediatric patients succumb to transplant rejection.

After transplant, most patients regain normal heart function, meaning the heart pumps a normal amount of blood. A transplanted heart usually beats slightly faster than normal because the heart nerves are cut during surgery. The new heart also does not increase its rate as quickly during **exercise**. Even so, most patients feel much better and their capacity for exercise is dramatically improved from before they received the new heart. About 90% of survivors at five years will have no symptoms of heart failure. Patients return to work and other daily activities. Many are able to participate in sports.

Alternatives

End-stage heart disease is associated with a high mortality rate even with associated medical treatment. With as many as 30,000 patients awaiting transplantation according to the ISHLT database, and only 2,196 transplants performed in 2000, viable alternatives are necessary. Additionally, 500,000 patients in the United States are diagnosed with cardiac failure, adding to the almost 4.5 million already affected. Data from the REMATCH trial, published in 2001, demonstrated ventricular assist to be a viable alternative for patients not eligible for cardiac transplant compared to medical therapy alone. After one year, quality of life was improved in patients who received **ventricular assist device** compared to medical therapy alone. Additionally, biventricular pacing and **myocardial resection** for ventricular restoration show promising results. Adding destination therapies such as the AbioCor total artificial heart and the Thoratec Heart-Mate VE may provide other alternatives for the transplant candidate.

Resources

BOOKS

Bellenir, Karen, and Peter D. Dresser, eds. *Cardiovascular Diseases and Disorders Sourcebook.* Detroit: Omnigraphics, 1995.

Texas Heart Institute. *Heart Owner's Handbook.* New York: John Wiley and Sons, 1996.

Rother, Anne L., and Charles D. Collard. "Anesthetic Management for Cardiac Transplantation." In *A Practical Approach to Cardiac Anesthesia,* 3rd edition, edited by Frederick A. Hensley, Donald E. Martin, and Glenn P. Gravlee. Philadelphia, PA: Lippincott Williams & Wilkins, 2003.

ORGANIZATIONS

American Council on Transplantation. P.O. Box 1709, Alexandria, VA 22313. (800) ACT-GIVE.

Health Services and Resources Administration, Division of Organ Transplantation. Room 11A-22, 5600 Fishers Lane, Rockville, MD 20857.

United Network for Organ Sharing (UNOS). 1100 Boulders Parkway, Suite 500, P.O. Box 13770, Richmond, VA 23225-8770. (804) 330-8500. <http://www.unos.org>.

OTHER

Craven, John, and Susan Farrow. "Surviving Transplantation." *SupportNET Publications,* 1996-1997.

"Facts About Heart and Heart/Lung Transplants." *National Heart, Lung, and Blood Institute,* November 27, 1998 [cited March 3, 1998]. <http://www.nhlbi.nih.gov/index.htm>.

"What Every Patient Needs to Know." *United Network for Organ Sharing (UNOS).* <http://www.unos.org/frame_Default.asp?Category=Patients>.

Toni Rizzo
Allison J. Spiwak, MSBME

Heart valve repair *see* **Mitral valve repair**

Heart valve replacement *see* **Mitral valve replacement; Aortic valve replacement**

Hemangioma excision

Definition

Hemangioma excision is the use of surgical techniques to remove benign tumors made up of blood vessels that are often located within the skin. Strawberry he-

> ### WHO PERFORMS THE PROCEDURE AND WHERE IS IT PERFORMED?
>
> The procedure is generally performed by plastic surgeons and, except for extremely small lesions, is done on an inpatient basis in a hospital **operating room**.

mangiomas are often called strawberry birthmarks. Hemangioma surgery involves the removal of the abnormal growth in a way that minimizes both physical and psychological scarring of the patient.

Purpose

Almost all hemangiomas will undergo a long, slow regression, known as involution, without treatment. The end result of involution is potentially worse than the scarring that would occur with surgery. Thus, surgical intervention is commonly indicated only if the growth of the tumor is life threatening or highly problematic from a medical or psychosocial point of view. For example, tumor growths that affect the ability of the eye to see, the ear to hear, or the passage of air in and out of the lungs are frequently candidates for surgical treatment. Tumors that have ulcerated are also common candidates for surgical treatment. Surgery after involution can be used to remove remaining scar tissue.

Although controversial, some surgeons also recommend surgery before or during the involution process, in an attempt to minimize the final cosmetic deformity. Small lesions that are in areas that can be excised without cosmetic or functional risk are particularly well-suited to early surgical treatment.

Demographics

Hemangiomas are the most common tumor of infancy, occurring in approximately 10–12% of all white children and are nearly twice as common in premature infants. For unknown reasons, the occurrence in children of black or Asian background is much lower, approximately 0.8–1.4%. The tumors have been reported to be from two to six times more common in females than in males. The great majority of these tumors are located in the head and neck, with the remaining appearing throughout the body, including internally.

At present, an estimated 60% of patients with hemangiomas require some form of corrective surgery sometime during recovery from the tumor surgery. The remaining 40% rely on the spontaneous involution process to resolve the lesion, although complete return to normalcy is extremely rare.

Description

Hemangiomas undergo a characteristic set of stages during the tumor development. Approximately 30% are present at birth, with the remainder appearing within the first few weeks of life, often beginning as a well-demarcated pale spot that becomes more noticeable when the child cries. The tumors are highly variable in presentation and range from flat, reddish areas known as superficial hemangiomas, to those that are bluish in color and located further under the skin, and are known as deep hemangiomas.

During the first six to 18 months of life, hemangiomas undergo a stage where they grow at an excessive rate in size due to abnormal cell division. The final size of the tumors can range from tiny, hardly noticeable red areas to large, disfiguring growths. In almost all hemangiomas, a long, slow involution process that follows the proliferation stage can take years to complete. Among the first signs of the involution process is a deepening of the red color of the tumor, a graying of the surface, and the appearance of white spots. In general, 50% of all hemangiomas are completely involuted by age five, and 75–90% have completed the process by age seven.

Once a decision to treat a hemangionma with surgery is made, the exact technique to be utilized must also be determined. The most commonly used technique for small lesions is very straightforward and involves removing the abnormal vascular tissue with a lenticular, or lens-shaped excision, that results in a linear scar. Recently, some surgeons have been advocating the use of an elliptical, circular, or irregular incision shapes, followed by a purse-string-type closure. This technique does result in a scar having radial (star-shaped) ridges that can take several weeks to flatten. However, the overall result is a shorter scar that can be followed up by removal, using the lenticular excision technique.

Larger, more extensive lesions may require **angiography**, a process that maps the path of the vessels feeding the lesion, and embolization, the deliberate blocking of these blood vessels using small particles of inert material. This process is followed by complete removal of the abnormal tissue.

Depending on the size and nature of the tumor, the excision surgery can be done on an outpatient or inpatient basis. For very small lesions, local anesthetic may be sufficient, but for the great majority, general anesthesia is necessary to keep the patient comfortable.

Diagnosis/Preparation

Initial correct diagnosis of the hemangioma is necessary for effective treatment. Generally, hemangiomas are

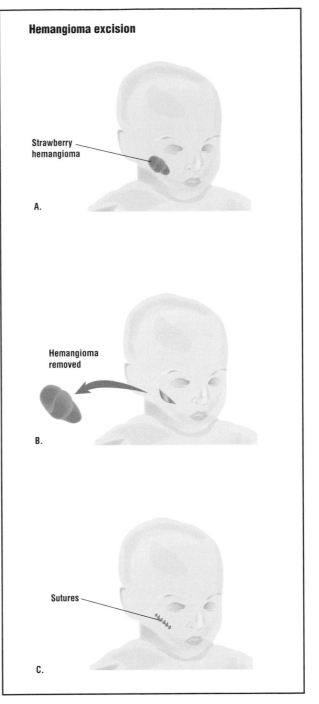

Hemangioma excision

Strawberry hemangioma

A.

Hemangioma removed

B.

Sutures

C.

To remove a hemangioma that is very large or in a troublesome area (A), the surgeon makes an incision around the mark (B), then closes the skin around it (C). *(Illustration by GGS Inc.)*

not present at birth; they proliferate during the first year of the patient's life, and then commonly begin an involution process. These clinical characteristics distinguish hemangiomas from another type of congenital vascular lesion called a vascular malformation. Vascular malformations are always present at birth, do not proliferate, and do not involute. Vascular malformations are developmental abnormalities and can involve veins, arteries, or lymphatic tissue. Because of the lack of rapid proliferation, the expectation for vascular malformations differs from those with a hemangioma, and so the precise type of lesion has a significant impact on treatment decisions.

Aftercare

Aftercare for a hemangioma excision involves **wound care** and maintenance such as changing of bandages.

Risks

The greatest risk of hemangioma excision is bleeding during the operation, as these tumors are comprised of abnormal blood vessels. Surgeons often utilize special surgical tools to reduce this risk, including thermoscalpels (an electrically heated scapel) and electrocauteries (a tool that stops bleeding using an electrical charge).

A second risk of the surgery is recurrence of the tumor, that is, an incomplete excision of the abnormally growing tissue. Surgery may also result in scarring that is at least as noticeable as what would remain after involution, if not more so. Patients and their caregivers should carefully consider this possibility when deciding to undergo surgical treatment for hemangiomas.

Other risks of the surgery are very low, and include those that accompany any surgical procedure, such as reactions to anesthesia and possible infections of the incision.

Normal results

Completely normal appearance after surgery is very rare. However, for significantly disfiguring tumors or those that impact physical function, the surgical scar may be preferable to the presence of the tumor.

KEY TERMS

Angiography—An x ray of the blood vessels after introduction of a medium that increases the contrast between the vessel path and the surrounding tissues.

Benign—Describes a tumor that is not malignant, that is unlikely to recur or spread to other areas of the body.

Embolization—The purposeful introduction of a substance into a blood vessel to stop blood flow.

Involution—The slow healing and resolution stage of a hemangioma.

Lenticular—Lens-shaped; describes a shape of a surgical excision sometimes used to remove hemangiomas.

Proliferation—The rapid growth stage of a hemangioma.

Purse-string closure—A technique used to close circular or irregularly shaped wounds that involves threading the suture through the edges of the wound and pulling it taut, bringing the edges together.

Radial—Star-shaped or radiating out from a central point; used to describe the scar-folds that results from a purse-string closure.

Morbidity and mortality rates

Morbidity and mortality resulting from this surgery is close to zero, particularly because of the new surgical techniques and tools that prevent intra-operative bleeding of the tumor.

Alternatives

Several alternatives to surgical excision include observation ("watchful waiting"), treatment with steroids during the proliferation stage to shrink the tumor and speed the involution process, and **laser surgery** techniques to alter the appearance of the tumor. Commonly, a combination of these treatment methods, including surgery, will be used to tailor a therapeutic approach for a patient's particular tumor.

Resources

BOOKS

DuFresne, Craig R. "The Management of Hemangiomas and Vascular Malformations of the Head and Neck." In *Plastic Surgery: Indications, Operations, and Outcomes,* Volume

2, edited by Craig A. Vander Kolk, et al. St. Louis, MO: Mosby, 2000.

Waner, Milton, and James Y. Suen. *Hemangiomas and Vascular Malformations of the Head and Neck.* New York: Wiley-Liss, 1999.

PERIODICALS

Mulliken, John B., Gary F. Rogers, and Jennifer J. Marler. "Circular Excision of Hemangioma and Purse-String Closure: The Smallest Possible Scar." *Plastic and Reconstructive Surgery* 109 (April 15, 2002): 1544.

ORGANIZATIONS

American Society of Plastic Surgeons. 444 E. Algonquin Rd. Arlington Heights, IL 60005. (800) 475-2784. <www.plasticsurgery.org>.

Vascular Birthmark Foundation. P.O. Box 106, Latham, NY 12110. (877) VBF-LOOK (daytime) and (877) VBF-4646 (evenings and weekends). <www.birthmark.org>.

OTHER

Sargent, Larry A. "Hemangiomas. " In *Tennessee Craniofacial Center Monographs,* 2000 [cited March 23, 2003] <www.erlanger.org/craniofacial/book>.

Michelle Johnson, MS, JD

Hematocrit

Definition

The hematocrit is a test that measures the percentage of blood that is comprised of red blood cells.

Purpose

The hematocrit is used to screen for anemia, or is measured on a person to determine the extent of anemia. An anemic person has fewer or smaller than normal red blood cells. A low hematocrit, combined with other abnormal blood tests, confirms the diagnosis. The hematocrit is decreased in a variety of common conditions including chronic and recent acute blood loss, some cancers, kidney and liver diseases, malnutrition, vitamin B_{12} and folic acid deficiencies, iron deficiency, pregnancy, systemic lupus erythematosus, rheumatoid arthritis and peptic ulcer disease. An elevated hematocrit is most often associated with severe burns, diarrhea, shock, Addison's disease, and dehydration, which is a decreased amount of water in the tissues. These conditions reduce the volume of plasma water causing a relative increase in RBCs, which concentrates the RBCs, called hemoconcentration. An elevated hematocrit may also be caused by an absolute increase in blood cells, called polycythemia. This may be secondary to a decreased amount of oxygen, called hypoxia, or the result of a proliferation of blood forming cells in the bone marrow (polycythemia vera).

Critically high or low levels should be immediately called to the attention of the patient's nurse or doctor. **Transfusion** decisions are based on the results of laboratory tests, including the hematocrit. Generally, transfusion is not considered necessary if the hematocrit is above 21%. The hematocrit is also used as a guide to how many transfusions are needed. Each unit of packed red blood cells administered to an adult is expected to increase the hematocrit by approximately 3% to 4%.

Precautions

Fluid volume in the blood affects hematocrit values. Accordingly, the blood sample should not be taken from an arm receiving IV fluid or during hemodialysis. It should be noted that pregnant women have extra fluid, which dilutes the blood, decreasing the hematocrit. Dehydration concentrates the blood, which increases the hematocrit.

In addition, certain drugs such as penicillin and chloramphenicol may decrease the hematocrit, while glucose levels above 400 mg/dL are known to elevate results. Blood for hematocrit may be collected either by finger puncture, or sticking a needle into a vein, called venipuncture. When performing a finger puncture, the first drop of blood should be wiped away because it dilutes the sample with tissue fluid. A nurse or phlebotomist usually collects the sample following cleaning and disinfecting the skin at the site of the needle stick.

Description

Blood is made up of red blood cells, white blood cells (WBCs), platelets, and plasma. A decrease in the number or size of red cells also decreases the amount of space they occupy, resulting in a lower hematocrit. Conversely, an increase in the number or size of red cells increases the amount of space they occupy, resulting in a higher hematocrit. Thalassemia minor is an exception in that it usually causes an increase in the number of red blood cells, but because they are small, it results in a decreased hematocrit.

The hematocrit may be measured manually by centrifugation. A thin capillary tube called a microhematocrit tube is filled with blood and sealed at the bottom. The tube is centrifuged at 10,000 RPM (revolutions per minute) for five minutes. The RBCs have the greatest weight and are forced to the bottom of the tube. The WBCs and platelets form a thin layer, called the buffy

KEY TERMS

Anemia—A lack of oxygen carrying capacity commonly caused by a decrease in red blood cell number, size, or function.

Dehydration—A decreased amount of water in the tissues.

Hematocrit—The volume of blood occupied by the red blood cells, and expressed in percent.

Hypoxia—A decreased amount of oxygen in the tissues.

Polycythemia—A condition in which the amount of RBCs are increased in the blood.

coat, between the RBCs and the plasma, and the liquid plasma rises to the top. The height of the red cell column is measured as a percent of the total blood column. The higher the column of red cells, the higher the hematocrit. Most commonly, the hematocrit is measured indirectly by an automated blood cell counter. It is important to recognize that different results may be obtained when different measurement principles are used. For example, the microhematocrit tube method will give slightly higher results than the electronic methods when RBCs of abnormal shape are present because more plasma is trapped between the cells.

Aftercare

Discomfort or bruising may occur at the puncture site. Pressure to the puncture site until the bleeding stops reduces bruising; warm packs relieve discomfort. Some people feel dizzy or faint after blood has been drawn, and lying down and relaxing for awhile is helpful for these people.

Risks

Other than potential bruising at the puncture site, and/or dizziness, there are no complications associated with this test.

Normal results

Normal values vary with age and sex. Some representative ranges are:

• at birth: 42-60%

• six to 12 months: 33-40%

• adult males: 42-52%

• adult females: 35-47%

Resources

BOOKS

Chernecky, Cynthia C. and Barbara J. Berger. *Laboratory Tests and Diagnostic Procedures*. 3rd ed. Philadelphia: W. B. Saunders Company, 2001.

Kee, Joyce LeFever. *Handbook of Laboratory and Diagnostic Tests*. 4th ed. Upper Saddle River, NJ: Prentice Hall, 2001.

Kjeldsberg, Carl R. *Practical Diagnosis of Hematologic Disorders*. 3rd ed. Chicago: ASCP Press, 2000.

ORGANIZATIONS

American Association of Blood Banks. 8101 Glenbrook Road, Bethesda, Maryland 20814. (301) 907-6977. Fax: (301) 907-6895. <http://www.aabb.org>.

OTHER

Uthman, Ed. *Blood Cells and the CBC*. 2000 [cited February 17, 2003]. <http://web2.iadfw.net/uthman/blood_cells.html>.

Victoria E. DeMoranville
Mark A. Best

Hemispherectomy

Definition

Hemispherectomy is a surgical treatment for epilepsy in which one of the two cerebral hemispheres, which together make up the majority of the brain, is removed.

Purpose

Hemispherectomy is used to treat epilepsy when it cannot be sufficiently controlled by medications.

The cerebral cortex is the wrinkled outer portion of the brain. It is divided into left and right hemispheres, which communicate with each other through a bundle of nerve fibers called the corpus callosum, located at the base of the hemispheres.

The seizures of epilepsy are due to unregulated electrical activity in the brain. This activity often begins in a discrete brain region called the focus of the seizure, and then spreads to other regions. Removing or disconnecting the focus from the rest of the brain can reduce seizure frequency and intensity.

In some people with epilepsy, there is no single focus. If there are multiple focal points within one hemisphere, or if the focus is undefined but restricted to one hemisphere, hemispherectomy may be indicated for treatment.

Removing an entire hemisphere of the brain is an effective treatment. The hemisphere that is removed is usually quite damaged by the effects of multiple seizures, and the other side of the brain has already assumed many of the functions of the damaged side. In addition, the brain has many "redundant systems," which allow healthy regions to make up for the loss of the damaged side.

Children who are candidates for hemispherectomy usually have significant impairments due to their epilepsy, including partial or complete paralysis and partial or complete loss of sensation on the side of the body opposite to the affected brain region.

Demographics

Epilepsy affects up to 1% of all people. Approximately 40% of patients are inadequately treated by medications, and so may be surgery candidates. Hemispherectomy is a relatively rare type of epilepsy surgery. The number performed per year in the United States is likely less than 100. Hemispherectomy is most often considered in children, whose brains are better able to adapt to the loss of brain matter than adults.

Description

Hemispherectomy may be "anatomic" or "functional." In an anatomic hemispherectomy, a hemisphere is removed, while in a functional hemispherectomy, some tissue is left in place, but its connections to other brain centers are cut so that it no longer functions.

Several variations of the anatomic hemispherectomy exist, which are designed to minimize complications. Lower portions of the brain may be left relatively intact, or muscle tissue may be transplanted in order to protect the brain's ventricles (fluid-filled cavities) and prevent leakage of cerebrospinal fluid from them.

Most surgical centers perform functional hemispherectomy. In this procedure, the temporal lobe (that region closest to the temple) and the part of the central portion of the cortex are removed. Additionally, numerous connecting fibers within the remaining brain are severed, as is the corpus callosum, which connects the two hemispheres.

During either procedure, the patient is under general anesthesia, lying on the back. The head is shaved and a portion of the skull is removed for access to the brain. After all tissue has been cut and removed and all bleeding is stopped, the underlying tissues are sutured and the skull and scalp are replaced and sutured.

Diagnosis/Preparation

The candidate for hemispherectomy has epilepsy untreatable by medications, with seizure focal points that

---

are numerous or ill defined, but localized to one hemisphere. Such patients may have one of a wide variety of disorders that have caused seizures, including:

- neonatal brain injury
- Rasmussen disease
- Hemimegalencephaly
- Sturge-Weber syndrome

The candidate for any type of epilepsy surgery will have had a wide range of tests prior to surgery. These include **electroencephalography** (EEG), in which electrodes are placed on the scalp, on the brain surface, or within the brain to record electrical activity. EEG is used to attempt to locate the focal point(s) of the seizure activity.

Several neuroimaging procedures are used to obtain images of the brain. These may reveal structural abnormalities that the neurosurgeon must be aware of. These procedures will include **magnetic resonance imaging** (MRI), x rays, computed tomography (CT) scans, or **positron emission tomography (PET)** imaging.

Neuropsychological tests may be done to provide a baseline against which the results of the surgery are measured. A Wada test may also be performed, in which a drug is injected into the artery leading to one half of the brain, putting it to sleep. This allows the neurologist to determine where in the brain language and other functions are localized, and may also be useful for predicting the result of the surgery.

Aftercare

Immediately after the operation, the patient may be on a mechanical ventilator for up to 24 hours. Patients remain in the hospital for at least one week. Physical and occupational therapy are part of the rehabilitation program to improve strength and motor function.

Risks

Hemorrhage during or after surgery is a risk for hemispherectomy. Disseminated intravascular coagulation, or blood clotting within the circulatory system, is a

---

risk that may be managed with anticoagulant drugs. "Aseptic meningitis," an inflammation of the brain's covering without infection, may occur. Hydrocephalus, or increased fluid pressure within the remaining brain, may occur in 20–30% of patients. Death from surgery is a risk that has decreased as surgical techniques have improved, but it still occurs in approximately 2% of patients.

The patient will lose any remaining sensation or muscle control in the extremities on the side opposite the removed hemisphere. However, upper arm and thigh movements may be retained, allowing adapted function with these parts of the body.

Normal results

Seizures are eliminated in 70–85% of patients, and reduced by 80% in another 10–20% of patients. Patients with Rasmussen disease, which is progressive, will not benefit as much. Medications may be reduced, and some improvement in intellectual function may occur.

Morbidity and mortality rates

Death may occur in 1–2% of patients undergoing hemispherectomy. Serious but treatable complications may occur in 10–20% of patients.

Alternatives

Corpus callosotomy may be an alternative for some patients, although its ability to eliminate seizures completely is much less. Multiple subpial transection, in which several bundles of nerve fibers are cut, is also an alternative for some patients.

See also Corpus callosotomy; Vagal nerve stimulation.

Resources

BOOKS

Devinsky, O. *A Guide to Understanding and Living with Epilepsy.* Philadelphia: EA Davis, 1994.

ORGANIZATIONS

Epilepsy Foundation. <http://www.epilepsyfoundation.org>.

Richard Robinson

Hemodialysis *see* **Kidney dialysis**
Hemodialysis fistula *see* **Arteriovenous fistula**

Hemoglobin test

Definition

Hemoglobin is a protein inside red blood cells that carries oxygen. A hemoglobin test reveals how much hemoglobin is in a person's blood. This information can be used to help physician's diagnose and monitor anemia (a low hemoglobin level) and polycythemia vera (a high hemoglobin level).

Purpose

A hemoglobin test is performed to determine the amount of hemoglobin in a person's red blood cells (RBCs). This is important because the amount of oxygen available to tissues depends upon how much oxygen is in the RBCs, and local perfusion of the tissues. Without sufficient hemoglobin, the tissues lack oxygen and the heart and lungs must work harder to compensate.

A low hemoglobin measurement usually means the person has anemia. Anemia results from a decrease in the number, size, or function of RBCs. Common causes include excessive bleeding, a deficiency of iron, vitamin B_{12}, or folic acid, destruction of red cells by antibodies or mechanical trauma, and structurally abnormal hemoglobin. Hemoglobin levels are also decreased due to cancer, kidney diseases, other chronic diseases, and excessive IV fluids. An elevated hemoglobin may be caused by dehydration (decreased water), hypoxia (decreased oxygen), or polycythemia vera. Hypoxia may result from high altitudes, smoking, chronic obstructive lung diseases (such as emphysema), and congestive heart failure. Hemoglobin levels are also used to determine if a person needs a blood **transfusion**. Usually a person's hemoglobin must be below 7–8 g/dL before a transfusion is considered, or higher if the person has heart or lung disease. The hemoglobin concentration is also used to determine how many units of packed red blood cells should be transfused. A common rule of thumb is that each unit of red cells should increase the hemoglobin by approximately 1.0–1.5 g/dL.

Precautions

Fluid volume in the blood affects hemoglobin values. Accordingly, the blood sample should not be taken from an arm receiving IV fluid. It should also be noted that pregnant women and people with cirrhosis, a type of permanent liver disease, have extra fluid, which dilutes the blood, decreasing the hemoglobin. Dehydration, a decreased amount of water in the body, concentrates the blood, which may cause an increased hemoglobin result.

Certain drugs such as **antibiotics**, **aspirin**, antineoplastic drugs, doxapram, indomethacin, **sulfonamides**, primaquine, rifampin, and trimethadione, may also decrease the hemoglobin level.

A nurse or phlebotomist usually collects the sample by inserting a needle into a vein, or venipuncture, after cleaning the skin, which helps prevent infections.

Description

Hemoglobin is a complex protein composed of four subunits. Each subunit consists of a protein, or polypeptide chain, that enfolds a heme group. Each heme contains iron (Fe^{2+}) that can bind a molecule of oxygen. The iron gives blood its red color. After the first year of life, 95-97% of the hemoglobin molecules contain two pairs of polypeptide chains designated alpha and beta. This form of hemoglobin is called hemoglobin A.

Hemoglobin is most commonly measured in whole blood. Hemoglobin measurement is most often performed as part of a **complete blood count** (CBC), a test that includes counts of the red blood cells, white blood cells, and platelets (thrombocytes).

Some people inherit hemoglobin with an abnormal structure. The abnormal hemoglobin results from a point mutation in one or both genes that code for the alpha or beta polypeptide chains. Examples of hemoglobin abnormalities resulting from a single amino acid substitution in the beta chain are sickle cell and hemoglobin C disease. Most abnormal hemoglobin molecules can be detected by hemoglobin electrophoresis, which separates hemoglobin molecules that have different electrical charges.

Preparation

No special preparation is required other than cleaning and disinfecting the skin at the puncture site. Blood is collected in a tube by venipuncture. The tube has an anticoagulant in it so that the blood does not clot in the tube, and so that the blood will remain a liquid.

Aftercare

Discomfort or bruising may occur at the puncture site. Pressure to the puncture site until the bleeding stops reduces bruising; warm packs relieve discomfort. Some people feel dizzy or faint after blood has been drawn, and lying down and relaxing for awhile is helpful for these people.

Risks

Other than potential bruising at the puncture site, and/or dizziness, there are usually no complications associated with this test.

Normal results

Normal values vary with age and sex, with women generally having lower hemoglobin values than men. Normal results for men range from 13–18 g/dL. For women the normal range is 12–16 g/dL. Critical limits (panic values) for both males and females are below 5.0 g/dL or above 20.0 g/dL.

A low hemoglobin value usually indicates the person has anemia. Different tests are done to discover the cause and type of anemia. Dangerously low hemoglobin levels put a person at risk of a heart attack, congestive heart failure, or stroke. A high hemoglobin value indicates the body may be making too many red blood cells. Other tests are performed to differentiate the cause of the abnormal hemoblogin level. Laboratory scientists perform hemoglobin tests using automated laboratory equipment. Critically high or low levels should be immediately called to the attention of the patient's doctor.

Resources

BOOKS

Chernecky, Cynthia C. and Barbara J. Berger. *Laboratory Tests and Diagnostic Procedures.* 3rd ed. Philadelphia: W. B. Saunders Company, 2001.

Kee, Joyce LeFever. *Handbook of Laboratory and Diagnostic Tests.* 4th ed. Upper Saddle River, NJ: Prentice Hall, 2001.

Kjeldsberg, Carl R. *Practical Diagnosis of Hematologic Disorders.* 3rd ed. Chicago: ASCP Press, 2000.

ORGANIZATIONS

American Association of Blood Banks. 8101 Glenbrook Road, Bethesda, Maryland 20814. (301) 907-6977. Fax: (301) 907-6895. <http://www.aabb.org>.

OTHER

Uthman, Ed. *Blood Cells and the CBC.* 2000 [cited February 17, 2003]. <http://web2.iadfw.net/uthman/blood_cells.html>.

Victoria E. DeMoranville
Mark A. Best, M.D.

Hemoperfusion

Definition

Hemoperfusion is a treatment technique in which large volumes of the patient's blood are passed over an adsorbent substance in order to remove toxic substances from the blood. Adsorption is a process in which molecules or particles of one substance are attracted to the surface of a solid material and held there. These solid materials are called sorbents. Hemoperfusion is sometimes described as an extracorporeal form of treatment because the blood is pumped through a device outside the patient's body.

The sorbents most commonly used in hemoperfusion are resins and various forms of activated carbon or charcoal. Resin sorbents are presently used in Europe but not in the United States; since 1999, all hemoperfusion systems manufactured in the United States use cartridges or columns containing carbon sorbents. A newer type of cartridge containing an adsorbent polymer has been undergoing clinical tests in the United States since the summer of 2002.

Purpose

Hemoperfusion has three major uses:

• to remove nephrotoxic drugs or poisons from the blood in emergency situations (A nephrotoxic substance is one that is harmful to the kidneys.)

• to remove waste products from the blood in patients with kidney disease

• to provide supportive treatment before and after transplantation for patients in liver failure

Hemoperfusion is more effective than other methods of treatment for removing certain specific poisons from the blood, particularly those that bind to proteins in the body or are difficult to dissolve in water. It is used to treat overdoses of **barbiturates**, meprobamate, glutethimide, theophylline, digitalis, carbamazepine, methotrexate, ethchlorvynol, and **acetaminophen**, as well as treating paraquat poisoning. Paraquat is a highly toxic weed killer that is sometimes used by people in developing countries to commit suicide.

Description

A hemoperfusion system can be used with or without a hemodialysis machine. After the patient has been made comfortable, two catheters are placed in the arm, one in an artery and one in a nearby vein. After the catheters have been checked for accurate placement, the catheter in the artery is connected to tubing leading into the hemoperfusion system, and the catheter in the vein is connected to tubing leading from the system through a pressure monitor. The patient is given heparin at the beginning of the procedure and at 15–20-minute intervals throughout the hemoperfusion in order to prevent the blood from clotting. The patient's blood pressure is also taken regularly. A typical hemoperfusion treatment takes about three hours.

Hemoperfusion works by pumping the blood drawn through the arterial catheter into a column or cartridge containing the sorbent material. As the blood passes over the carbon or resin particles in the column, the toxic molecules or particles are drawn to the surfaces of the sorbent particles and trapped within the column. The blood flows out the other end of the column and is returned to the patient through the tubing attached to the venous catheter. Hemoperfusion is able to clear toxins from a larger volume of blood than hemodialysis or other filtration methods; it can process over 300 mL of blood per minute.

Preparation

In emergency situations, preparation of the patient may be limited to cleansing the skin on the inside of the arm with an antiseptic solution and giving a local anesthetic to minimize pain caused by the needles used to insert the catheters.

The hemoperfusion system is prepared by sterilizing the cartridge containing the sorbent and rinsing it with heparinized saline solution. The system is then pressure-tested before the tubing is connected to the catheters in the patient's arm.

Normal results

Normal results include satisfactory clearance of the toxic substance or waste products from the patient's blood. The success of hemoperfusion depends in part, however, on the nature of the drug or poison to be cleared from the blood. Some drugs, such as the tricyclic antidepressants, enter the tissues of the patient's body as well as the bloodstream. As a result, even though hemoperfusion may remove as much as 80% of the drug found in the blood plasma, that may be only a small fraction of the total amount of the drug in the patient's body.

Risks

The risks associated with hemoperfusion are similar to those for hemodialysis, including infection, bleeding, blood clotting, destruction of blood platelets, an abnormal drop in blood pressure, and equipment failure. When hemoperfusion is performed by a qualified health professional, however, the risks are minor compared to the effects of poisoning or organ failure.

See also Kidney dialysis; Liver transplantation.

Resources

BOOKS

"Dialysis." Section 17, Chapter 223 in *The Merck Manual of Diagnosis and Therapy*, edited by Mark H. Beers, MD, and Robert Berkow, MD. Whitehouse Station, NJ: Merck Research Laboratories, 1999.

"Elimination of Poisons." Section 23, Chapter 307 in *The Merck Manual of Diagnosis and Therapy*, edited by Mark H. Beers, MD, and Robert Berkow, MD. Whitehouse Station, NJ: Merck Research Laboratories, 1999.

PERIODICALS

Borra, M., et al. "Advanced Technology for Extracorporeal Liver Support System Devices." *International Journal of Artificial Organs* 25 (October 2002): 939–949.

Cameron, R. J., P. Hungerford, and A. H. Dawson. "Efficacy of Charcoal Hemoperfusion in Massive Carbamazepine Poisoning." *Journal of Toxicology: Clinical Toxicology* 40 (2002): 507–512.

Hsu, H. H., C. T. Chang, and J. L. Lin. "Intravenous Paraquat Poisoning—Induced Multiple Organ Failure and Fatality—A Report of Two Cases." *Journal of Toxicology: Clinical Toxicology* 41 (2003): 87–90.

Reiter, K., et al. "In Vitro Removal of Therapeutic Drugs with a Novel Adsorbent System." *Blood Purification* 20 (2002): 380–388.

ORGANIZATIONS

American Academy of Emergency Medicine (AAEM). 611 East Wells Street, Milwaukee, WI 53202. (800) 884-2236. <http://www.aaem.org>.

Center for Emergency Medicine. 230 McKee Place, Suite 500, Pittsburgh, PA 15213. (412) 647-5300. <http://www.centerem.com>.

National Kidney Foundation. 30 East 33rd Street, Suite 1100, New York, NY 10016. (800) 622-9010 or (212) 889-2210. <http://www.kidney.org>.

Society of Toxicology (SOT). 1767 Business Center Drive, Suite 302, Reston, VA 20190. (703) 438-3115. <http://www.toxicology.org>.

OTHER

Deshpande, Girish. "Toxicity, Carbamazepine." *eMedicine.* June 21, 2002 [cited April 23, 2003]. <http://www.emedicine.com/ped/topic2732.htm>.

Horn, Alan, and Lisa Kirkland. "Toxicity, Theophylline." *eMedicine.* July 26, 2002 [cited April 23, 2003]. <http://www.emedicine.com/med/topic2261.htm>.

Rebecca Frey, Ph.D.

KEY TERMS

Adsorb—To attract and hold another substance on the surface of a solid material.

Clearance—The rate at which a substance is removed from the blood by normal kidney function or by such methods as hemoperfusion.

Extracorporeal—Occurring outside the patient's body.

Heparin—A complex sugar compound used in medicine to prevent the formation of blood clots during hemodialysis, hemoperfusion, and open-heart surgery.

Nephrotoxic—Destructive to kidney cells. Hemoperfusion can be used to remove nephrotoxic chemicals from the blood.

Paraquat—A highly toxic restricted-use pesticide. Death following ingestion usually results from multiple organ failure.

Sorbent—A material used during hemoperfusion to adsorb toxic or waste substances from the blood. Most hemoperfusion systems use resin or activated carbon as sorbents.

Hemorrhoidectomy

Definition

A hemorrhoidectomy is the surgical removal of a hemorrhoid, which is an enlarged, swollen and inflamed clus-

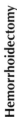

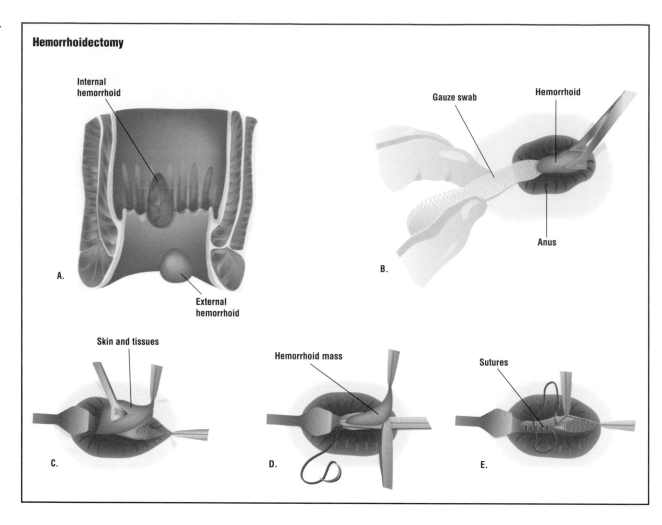

Hemorrhoidectomy

Internal hemorrhoid

External hemorrhoid

A.

Gauze swab

Hemorrhoid

Anus

B.

Skin and tissues

C.

Hemorrhoid mass

D.

Sutures

E.

Hemorrhoids can occur inside the rectum, or at its opening (A). To remove them, the surgeon feeds a gauze swab into the anus and removes it slowly. A hemorrhoid will adhere to the gauze, allowing its exposure (B). The outer layers of skin and tissue are removed (C), and then the hemorrhoid itself (D). The tissues and skin are then repaired (E). *(Illustration by GGS Inc.)*

ter of vascular tissue combined with smooth muscle and connective tissue located in the lower part of the rectum or around the anus. A hemorrhoid is not a varicose vein in the strict sense. Hemorrhoids are also known as piles.

Purpose

The primary purpose of a hemorrhoidectomy is to relieve the symptoms associated with hemorrhoids that have not responded to more conservative treatments. These symptoms commonly include bleeding and pain. In some cases the hemorrhoid may protrude from the patient's anus. Less commonly, the patient may notice a discharge of mucus or have the feeling that they have not completely emptied the bowel after defecating. Hemorrhoids are usually treated with dietary and medical measures before surgery is recommended because they are not dangerous, and are only rarely a medical emergency. Many people have hemorrhoids that do not produce any symptoms at all.

As of 2003, inpatient hemorrhoidectomies are performed significantly less frequently than they were as recently as the 1970s. In 1974, there were 117 hospital hemorrhoidectomies performed per 100,000 people in the general United States population; this figure declined to 37 per 100,000 by 1987.

Demographics

Hemorrhoids are a fairly common problem among adults in the United States and Canada; it is estimated that ten million people in North America, or about 4% of the adult population, have hemorrhoids. About a third of these people seek medical treatment in an average year; nearly 1.5 million prescriptions are filled annually for medications to relieve the discomfort of hemorrhoids. Most patients with symptomatic hemorrhoids are between the ages of 45 and 65.

Risk factors for the development of symptomatic hemorrhoids include the following:

- hormonal changes associated with pregnancy and childbirth
- normal aging
- not getting enough fiber in the diet
- chronic diarrhea
- anal intercourse
- constipation resulting from medications, dehydration, or other causes
- sitting too long on the toilet

Hemorrhoids are categorized as either external or internal hemorrhoids. External hemorrhoids develop under the skin surrounding the anus; they may cause pain and bleeding when the vein in the hemorrhoid forms a clot. This is known as a thrombosed hemorrhoid. In addition, the piece of skin, known as a skin tag, that is left behind when a thrombosed hemorrhoid heals often causes problems for the patient's hygiene. Internal hemorrhoids develop inside the anus. They can cause pain when they prolapse (fall down toward the outside of the body) and cause the anal sphincter to go into spasm. They may bleed or release mucus that can cause irritation of the skin surrounding the anus. Lastly, internal hemorrhoids may become incarcerated or strangulated.

Description

There are several types of surgical procedures that can reduce hemorrhoids. Most surgical procedures in current use can be performed on an outpatient level or office visit under local anesthesia.

Rubber band ligation is a technique that works well with internal hemorrhoids that protrude outward with bowel movements. A small rubber band is tied over the hemorrhoid, which cuts off the blood supply. The hemorrhoid and the rubber band will fall off within a few days and the wound will usually heal in a period of one to two weeks. The procedure causes mild discomfort and bleeding. Another procedure, sclerotherapy, utilizes a chemical solution that is injected around the blood vessel to shrink the hemorrhoid. A third effective method is infrared coagulation, which uses a special device to shrink hemorrhoidal tissue by heating. Both injection and coagulation techniques can be effectively used to treat bleeding hemorrhoids that do not protrude. Some surgeons use a combination of rubber band ligation, sclerotherapy, and infrared coagulation; this combination has been reported to have a success rate of 90.5%.

Surgical resection (removal) of hemorrhoids is reserved for patients who do not respond to more conserva-

> ## WHO PERFORMS THE PROCEDURE AND WHERE IS IT PERFORMED?
>
> A board certified general surgeon who has completed one additional year of advanced training in colon and rectal surgery performs the procedure. Specialists typically pass a board certification examination in the diagnosis and surgical treatment of diseases in the colon and rectum, and are certified by the American Board of Colon and Rectal Surgeons. Most hemorrhoidectomies can be performed in the surgeon's office, an outpatient clinic, or an ambulatory surgery center.

tive therapies and who have severe problems with external hemorrhoids or skin tags. Hemorrhoidectomies done with a laser do not appear to yield better results than those done with a scalpel. Both types of surgical resection can be performed with the patient under local anesthesia.

Diagnosis/Preparation

Diagnosis

Most patients with hemorrhoids are diagnosed because they notice blood on their toilet paper or in the toilet bowl after a bowel movement and consult their doctor. It is important for patients to visit the doctor whenever they notice bleeding from the rectum, because it may be a symptom of colorectal cancer or other serious disease of the digestive tract. In addition, such other symptoms in the anorectal region as itching, irritation, and pain may be caused by abscesses, fissures in the skin, bacterial infections, fistulae, and other disorders as well as hemorrhoids. The doctor will perform a digital examination of the patient's rectum in order to rule out these other possible causes.

Following the digital examination, the doctor will use an anoscope or sigmoidoscope in order to view the inside of the rectum and the lower part of the large intestine to check for internal hemorrhoids. The patient may be given a **barium enema** if the doctor suspects cancer of the colon; otherwise, imaging studies are not routinely performed in diagnosing hemorrhoids. In some cases, a laboratory test called a stool guaiac may be used to detect the presence of blood in stools.

Preparation

Patients who are scheduled for a surgical hemorrhoidectomy are given a sedative intravenously before the procedure. They are also given small-volume saline enemas to cleanse the rectal area and lower part of the large intestine. This preparation provides the surgeon with a clean operating field.

Aftercare

Patients may experience pain after surgery as the anus tightens and relaxes. The doctor may prescribe narcotics to relieve the pain. The patient should take stool softeners and attempt to avoid straining during both defecation and urination. Soaking in a warm bath can be comforting and may provide symptomatic relief. The total recovery period following a surgical hemorrhoidectomy is about two weeks.

Risks

As with other surgeries involving the use of a local anesthetic, risks associated with a hemorrhoidectomy include infection, bleeding, and an allergic reaction to the anesthetic. Risks that are specific to a hemorroidectomy include stenosis (narrowing) of the anus; recurrence of the hemorrhoid; fistula formation; and nonhealing wounds.

Normal results

Hemorrhoidectomies have a high rate of success; most patients have an uncomplicated recovery with no recurrence of the hemorrhoids. Complete recovery is typically expected with a maximum period of two weeks.

Morbidity and mortality rates

Rubber band ligation has a 30–50% recurrence rate within five to 10 years of the procedure whereas surgical resection of hemorrhoids has only a 5% recurrence rate. Well-trained surgeons report complications in fewer than

5% of their patients; these complications may include anal stenosis, recurrence of the hemorrhoid, fistula formation, bleeding, infection, and urinary retention.

Alternatives

Doctors recommend conservative therapies as the first line of treatment for either internal or external hemorrhoids. A nonsurgical treatment protocol generally includes drinking plenty of liquids; eating foods that are rich in fiber; sitting in a plain warm water bath for five to 10 minutes; applying anesthetic creams or witch hazel compresses; and using psyllium or other stool bulking agents. In patients with mild symptoms, these measures will usually decrease swelling and pain in about two to seven days. The amount of fiber in the diet can be increased by eating five servings of fruit and vegetables each day; replacing white bread with whole-grain bread and cereals; and eating raw rather than cooked vegetables.

Resources

BOOKS

"Hemorrhoids." Section 3, Chapter 35 in *The Merck Manual of Diagnosis and Therapy*, edited by Mark H. Beers, MD, and Robert Berkow, MD. Whitehouse Station, NJ: Merck Research Laboratories, 1999.

PERIODICALS

Accarpio, G., F. Ballari, R. Puglisi, et al. "Outpatient Treatment of Hemorrhoids with a Combined Technique: Results in 7850 Cases." *Techniques in Coloproctology* 6 (December 2002): 195-196.

Peng, B. C., D. G. Jayne, and Y. H. Ho. "Randomized Trial of Rubber Band Ligation Vs. Stapled Hemorrhoidectomy for Prolapsed Piles." *Diseases of the Colon and Rectum* 46 (March 2003): 291-297.

Thornton, Scott, MD. "Hemorrhoids." *eMedicine*, July 16, 2002 [June 29, 2003]. <www.emedicine.com/med/topic 2821.htm>.

ORGANIZATIONS

American Gastroenterological Association. 4930 Del Ray Avenue, Bethesda, MD 20814. (301) 654-2055; Fax: (301) 652-3890. <www.gastro.org>.

American Society of Colon and Rectal Surgeons. 85 W. Algonquin Road, Suite 550, Arlington Heights, IL 60005. <www.fascrs.org>.

National Digestive Diseases Information Clearinghouse (NIDDC). 2 Information Way, Bethesda, MD 20892-3570. <www.niddk.nih.gov>.

OTHER

National Digestive Diseases Information Clearinghouse (NDDIC). *Hemorrhoids*. Bethesda, MD: NDDIC, 2002. NIH Publication No. 02-3021. <www.niddk.nih.gov/health/digest/pubs/hems/hemords.htm>.

Laith Farid Gulli, M.D., M.S.
Bilal Nasser, M.D., M.S.
Nicole Mallory, M.S., PA-C

Hepatectomy

Definition

A hepactectomy is the surgical removal of the liver.

Purpose

Hepatectomies are performed to surgically remove tumors from the liver. Most liver cancers start in liver cells called "hepatocytes." The resulting cancer is called hepatocellular carcinoma or malignant hepatoma.

The type of cancer that can be removed by hepatectomy is called a localized resectable (removable) liver cancer. It is diagnosed as such when there is no evidence that it has spread to the nearby lymph nodes or to any other parts of the body. Laboratory tests also show that the liver is working well. As part of a multidisciplinary approach, the procedure can offer a chance of long-term remission to patients otherwise guaranteed of having a poor outcome.

WHO PERFORMS THE PROCEDURE AND WHERE IS IT PERFORMED?

A hepactectomy is performed in a hospital setting by a surgeon assisted by a full abdominal surgery team, and possibly an oncologist.

Demographics

According to the National Cancer Institute (NCI), liver cancer is relatively uncommon in the United States, although its incidence is rising, mostly as a result of the spread of hepatitis C. However, it is the most common cancer in Africa and Asia, with more than one million new cases diagnosed each year. In the United States, liver cancer and cancer of the bile ducts only account for about 1.5% of all cancer cases. Liver cancer is also associated with cirrhosis in 50–80% of patients.

Description

The extent of the hepatectomy will depend on the size, number, and location of the cancer. It also depends on whether liver function is still adequate. The surgeon may remove a part of the liver that contains the tumor, an entire lobe, or an even larger portion of the liver. In a partial hepatectomy, the surgeon leaves a margin of healthy liver tissue to maintain the functions of the liver. For some patients, **liver transplantation** may be indicated. In this case, the transplant surgeon performs a total hepatectomy, meaning that the patient's entire liver is removed, and it is replaced with a healthy liver from a donor. A liver transplant is an option only if the cancer has not spread outside the liver and only if a suitable donor liver can be found that matches the patient. While waiting for an adequate donor, the health care team monitors the patient's health while providing other therapy.

The surgical procedure is performed under general anesthesia and is quite lengthy, requiring three to four hours. The anesthetized patient is face-up and both arms are drawn away from the body. Surgeons often use a

Hepatectomy

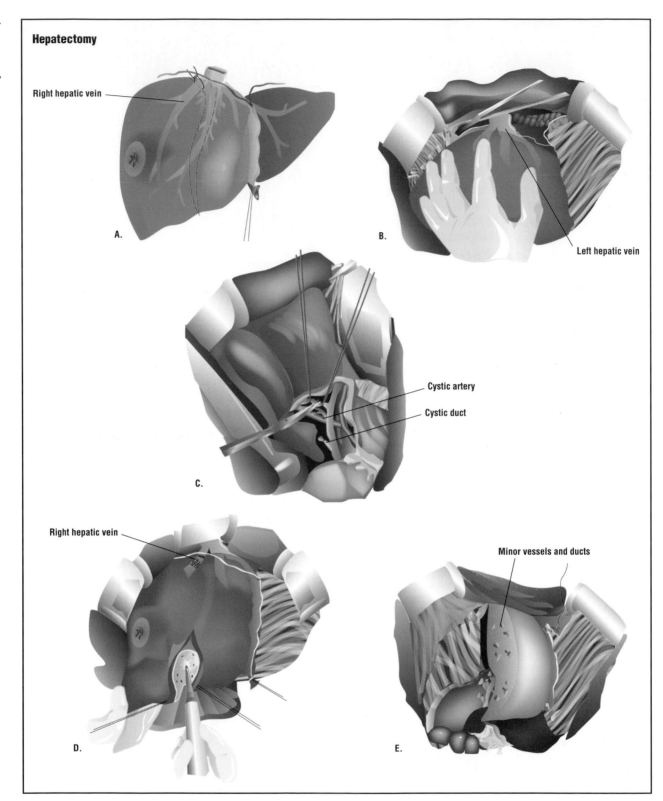

Right hepatic vein

A.

Left hepatic vein

B.

Cystic artery

Cystic duct

C.

Right hepatic vein

D.

Minor vessels and ducts

E.

To remove a portion of the liver, the surgeon enters the patient's abdomen, and frees the affected part of the liver from the connecting tissues (B). The artery to the liver and hepatic duct are disconnected from the liver (C). The diseased part of the liver is cut away, and a cauterizing tool is used to stop the bleeding as the surgeon progresses (D). *(Illustration by GGS Inc.)*

heating pad and wrappings around the arms and legs to reduce losses in body temperature during the surgery. The patient's abdomen is opened by an incision across the upper abdomen and a midline-extension incision up to the xiphoid (the cartilage located at the bottom middle of the rib cage). The main steps of a partial hepatectomy then proceed as follows:

• Freeing the liver. The first task of the surgeon is to free the liver by cutting the long fibers that wrap it.

• Removal of segments. Once the surgeon has freed the liver, the removal of segments can start. The surgeon must avoid rupturing important blood vessels to avoid a hemorrage. Two different techniques can be used. The first has the surgeon make a superficial burn with an electric lancet on the surface of the liver to mark the junction between the sections marked for removal and the rest of the liver. He/she cuts out the section, and then tears towards the hepatic parenchyma. It is the difference in resistance between the parenchyma and the vessels that allows the surgeon to identify the presence of a vessel. At this point, he/she isolates the vessel by removing the surrounding connective tissue, and then clamps it. The surgeon can then cut the vessel, without any danger to the patient. The second technique involves identifying the large vessels feeding the segments to be removed. The surgeon operates first at the level of the veins to free and then clamp the vessels required. Finally, the surgeon can make incisions without worrying about cutting little vessels.

Diagnosis/Preparation

A diagnosis of liver cancer requiring an hepatectomy is obtained with the following procedures:

• physical examination

• blood tests

• computed tomagraphy (CT) scan

• ultrasound test

• magnetic resonance imaging (MRI)

• angiograms

• biopsy

To prepare a patient for a hepactectomy, clean towels are laid across the patient's face, along the sides, and across the knees. The anterior portion of the chest, the abdomen, and the lower extremities down to the knees are scrubbed with betadine for 10 minutes. In the event of a patient being allergic to iodine, hibiscrub may be used as an alternative. On completion of the scrub, two sterile towels are used to pat the area dry. The area is then painted with iodine in alcohol, and draping proceeds with side drapes, arm board drapes, top and bot-

tom drapes, and a large steridrape. Three suction devices, one diathermy pencil, and one forceps are placed conveniently around the field.

Aftercare

After an hepatectomy, the healing process takes time; the amount of time required to recover varies from patient to patient. Patients are often uncomfortable for the first few days following surgery and they are usually prescribed pain medication. The treating physician or nurse is available to discuss **pain management**. Patients usually feel very tired or weak for a while. Also, patients may have diarrhea and a feeling of fullness in the abdomen. The health care team closely monitors the patient for bleeding, infection, liver failure, or other problems requiring immediate medical attention.

After a total hepatectomy followed by a liver transplant, the patient usually stays in the hospital for several weeks. During that time, the health care team constantly monitors how well the patient is accepting the donated liver. The patient is prescribed drugs to prevent the body from rejecting the transplant, which may cause puffiness in the face, high blood pressure, or an increase in body hair.

Risks

Patients with chronic hepatitis and cirrhosis are at high risk when an hepatectomy is performed.

There are always risks with any surgery, but a hepatectomy that removes 25–60% of the liver carries more than the average risk. Pain, bleeding, infection, and/or injury to other areas in the abdomen, as well as death, are potential risks. Other risks include postoperative fevers, pneumonia, and urinary tract infection. Patients who undergo any type of abdominal surgery are also at risk to form blood clots in their legs. These blood clots can break free and move through the heart to the lungs. In the lungs, the blood clot may cause a serious problem called pulmonary embolism, a condition usually treated with blood-thinning medication. But in some cases, embolisms can cause death. There are special devices used to keep blood flowing through the legs during surgery to try to prevent clot formation.

There are also risks that are specific only to liver surgery. During the preoperative evaluation, the treatment team tries to evaluate the patient's liver so that they can decide what piece can safely be removed. Removal of a portion of the liver may cause the remaining liver to work poorly for a short period of time. The remaining part of the liver will begin to grow back within a few weeks and will improve. However, a patient may develop liver failure.

Normal results

The results of a hepactetomy are considered normal when liver function resumes following a partial hepatectomy, or when the transplant liver starts functioning in the case of a total hepatectomy.

Morbidity and mortality rates

Liver cancer may be cured by hepatectomy, although surgery is the treatment of choice for only a small fraction of patients with localized disease. Prognosis depends on the extent of the cancer and of liver function impairment. According to the NCI, five-year survival rates are very low in the United States, usually less than 10%. Non-Hispanic white men and women have the lowest incidence of and mortality rates for primary liver cancer. Rates in the black and Hispanic populations are roughly twice as high as the rates in whites. The highest incidence rate is in Vietnamese men (41.8 per 100,000), probably reflecting risks associated with the high prevalence of viral hepatitis infections in their homeland. Other Asian-American groups also have liver cancer incidence and mortality rates several times higher than the white population.

Alternatives

There are no alternatives because hepatectomies are performed when liver cancer does not respond to other treatments.

Resources

BOOKS

Blumgart, L. H. *Surgery of the Liver and Biliary Tract.* New York: Churchill Livingstone, 1994.

Carr, B. I. *Hepatocellular Cancer: Diagnosis and Treatment (Current Clinical Oncology).* Totowa, NJ: Humana Press, 2003.

KEY TERMS

Biopsy—The removal of cells or tissues for examination under a microscope.

Cirrhosis—A type of chronic, progressive liver disease in which liver cells are replaced by scar tissue.

Computed tomagraphy (CT) scan—A series of detailed images of areas inside the body taken at various angles; the images are created on a computer linked to an x-ray machine.

Hepatitis—Disease of the liver causing inflammation. Symptoms include an enlarged liver, fever, nausea, vomiting, abdominal pain, and dark urine.

Hepatocellular carcinoma—The most common type of liver tumor.

Hepatocytes—Liver cells.

Hepatoma—A liver tumor.

Magnetic resonance imaging (MRI)—An imaging technique in which a magnet linked to a computer produces images of areas inside the body.

Parenchyma—The essential elements of an organ, used in anatomical nomenclature as a general term to designate the functional elements of an organ, as distinguished from its framework.

Resectable—Part or all of an organ that can be removed by surgery.

Dionigi, R. and J. Madariaga. *New Technologies for Liver Resections.* Basel: S. Karger Publishing, 1997.

Okita, K. *Progress in Hepatocellular Carcinoma Treatment.* New York: Springer Verlag, 2000.

PERIODICALS

Ganti, A. L., A. Sardi, and J. Gordon. "Laparoscopic Treatment of Large True Cysts of the Liver and Spleen Is Ineffective." *American Surgeon,* 68 (November 2002): 1012–1017.

Hemming, A. W., D. R. Nelson, and A. I. Reed. "Liver Transplantation for Hepatocellular Carcinoma." *Minerva Chirurgica,* 57 (October 2002): 575–585.

Joshi, R. M., P. K. Wagle, A. Darbari, D. G. Chhabra, P. S. Patnaik, and M. P. Katrak. "Hepatic Resection for Benign Liver Pathology—Report of Two Cases." *Indian Journal of Gastroenterology,* 21 (July–August 2003): 157–159.

Kammula, U. S., J. F. Buell, D. M. Labow, S. Rosen, J. M. Millis, and M. C. Posner. "Surgical Management of Benign Tumors of the Liver." *International Journal of Gastrointestinal Cancer,* 30 (2000): 141–146.

Matot, I., O. Scheinin, A. Eid, and O. Jurim. "Epidural Anesthesia and Analgesia in Liver Resection." *Anesthesia and Analgesia,* 95 (November 2002): 1179–1181.

Zhou, G., W. Cai, H. Li, Y, Zhu, and J. J. Fung. "Experiences Relating to Management of Biliary Tract Complications Following Liver Transplantation in 96 Cases." *Chinese Medical Journal,* 115 (October 2002): 1533–1537.

ORGANIZATIONS

American College of Surgeons. 633 N. Saint Clair St., Chicago, IL 60611-3211. (312) 202-5000. <www.facs.org>.

National Cancer Institute. Suite 3036A, 6116 Executive Boulevard, MSC8322, Bethesda, MD 20892-8322. (800) 422-6237. <www.cancer.gov/>.

OTHER

Cancer Information Service [cited July 6, 2003]. <http://cis. nci.nih.gov/>.

Liver Cancer Homepage [cited July 6, 2003]. <http://www. nci.nih.gov/cancerinfo/types/liver>.

Monique Laberge, PhD

Hernia repair, femoral *see* **Femoral hernia repair**

Hernia repair, incisional *see* **Incisional hernia repair**

Hernia repair, inguinal *see* **Inguinal hernia repair**

Hernia repair, umbilical *see* **Umbilical hernia repair**

Heterotopic transplant *see* **Liver transplantation**

Hip osteotomy

Definition

A hip osteotomy is a surgical procedure in which the bones of the hip joint are cut, reoriented, and fixed in a new position. Healthy cartilage is placed in the weight-bearing area of the joint, followed by reconstruction of the joint in a more normal position.

Purpose

To understand hip surgery, it is helpful to have a brief description of the structure of the human hip. The femur, or thigh bone, is connected to the knee at its lower end and forms part of the hip joint at its upper end. The femur ends in a ball-shaped piece of bone called the femoral head. The short, slanted segment of the femur

that lies between the femoral head and the long vertical femoral shaft is called the neck of the femur. In a normal hip, the femoral head fits snugly into a socket called the acetabulum. The hip joint thus consists of two parts, the pelvic socket or acetabulum, and the femoral head.

The hip is susceptible to damage from a number of diseases and disorders, including arthritis, traumatic injury, avascular necrosis, cerebral palsy, or Legg-Calve-Perthes (LCP) disease in young patients. The hip socket may be too shallow, too large, or too small, or the femoral head may lose its proper round contour. Problems related to the shape of the bones in the hip joint are usually referred to as hip dysplasia. **Hip replacement** surgery is often the preferred treatment for disorders of the hip in older patients. Adolescents and young adults, however, are rarely considered for this type of surgery due to their active lifestyle; they have few good options for alleviating their pain and improving joint function if they are stricken by a hip disorder. Osteotomies are performed in these patients, using the patient's own tissue in order to restore joint function in the hip and eliminate pain. An osteotomy corrects a hip deformity by cutting and repositioning the bone, most commonly in patients with misalignment of certain joints or mild osteoarthritis. The procedure is also useful for people with osteoarthritis in only one hip who are too young for a total joint replacement.

Demographics

The incidence of hip dysplasia is four per 1,000 live births in the general world population, although it occurs much more frequently in Lapps and Native Americans. In addition, the condition tends to run in families and is more common among girls and firstborns. Acetabular dysplasia patients are usually in their late teens to early thirties, with the female: male ratio in the United States being 5:1.

Description

A hip osteotomy is performed under general anesthesia. Once the patient has been anesthetized, the surgeon makes an incision to expose the hip joint. The surgeon then proceeds to cut away portions of damaged bone and tissue to change the way they fit together in the hip joint. This part of the procedure may involve removing bone from the femoral head or from the acetabulum, allowing the bone to be moved slightly within the joint. By changing the position of these bones, the surgeon tries to shift the brunt of the patient's weight from damaged joint surfaces to healthier cartilage. He or she then inserts a metal plate or pin to keep the bone in its new place and closes the incision.

There are different hip osteotomy procedures, depending on the type of bone correction required. Two common procedures are:

- Varus rotational osteotomy (VRO), also called a varus derotational osteotomy (VDO). In some patients, the femoral neck is too straight and is not angled far enough toward the acetabulum. This condition is called femoral neck valgus or just plain valgus. The VRO procedure corrects the shape of the femoral neck. In other patients, the femoral neck is not straight enough, in which case the condition is referred to as a femoral neck varus.

- Pelvic osteotomy. Many hip disorders are caused by a deformed acetabulum that cannot accommodate the femoral head. In this procedure, the surgeon redirects the acetabular cartilage or augments a deficient acetabulum with bone taken from outside the joint.

Diagnosis/Preparation

A **physical examination** performed by a pediatrician or an orthopaedic surgeon is the best method for diagnosing developmental dysplasia of the hip. Other aids to diagnosis include ultrasound examination of the hips during the first six months of life. An ultrasound study is better than an x ray for evaluating hip dysplasia in an infant because much of the hip is made of cartilage at this age and does not show up clearly on x rays. Ultrasound imaging can accurately determine the location of the femoral head in the acetabulum, as well as the depth of the baby's hip socket. An x-ray examination of the pelvis can be performed after six months of age when the child's bones are better developed. Diagnosis in adults also relies on x ray studies.

To prepare for a hip osteotomy, the patient should come to the clinic or hospital one to seven days prior to surgery. The physician will review the proposed surgery with the patient and answer any questions. He or she will also review the patient's medical evaluation, laboratory test results, and x-ray findings, and schedule any other tests that are required. Patients are instructed not to eat or drink anything after midnight the night before surgery to prevent nausea and vomiting during the operation.

Aftercare

Immediately following a hip osteotomy, patients are taken to the **recovery room** where they are kept for one to two hours. The patient's blood pressure, circulation, respiration, temperature, and wound drainage are carefully monitored. **Antibiotics** and fluids are given through the IV line that was placed in the arm vein during surgery. After a few days the IV is disconnected; if antibiotics are still needed, they are given by mouth for a few more days. If the patient feels some discomfort, pain medication is given every three to four hours as needed.

Patients usually remain in the hospital for several days after a hip osteotomy. Most VRO patients also require a body cast that includes the legs, which is known as a spica cast. Because of the extent of the surgery that must be done and healing that must occur to restore the pelvis to full strength, the patient's hip may be kept from bearing the full weight of the upper body for about eight to 10 weeks. A second operation may be performed after the patient's pelvis has healed to remove some of the hardware that the surgeon had inserted. Full recovery following an osteotomy usually takes longer than with a total hip replacement; it may be about four to six months before the patient can walk without assistive devices.

Risks

Although complications following hip osteotomy are rare, there is a small chance of infection or blood clot formation. There is also a very low risk of the bone not healing properly, surgical damage to a nerve or artery, or poor skin healing.

Normal results

Full recovery from an osteotomy takes six to 12 months. Most patients, however, have good outcomes following the procedure.

Alternatives

One alternative is to postpone surgery, if the patient's pain can be sufficiently controlled with medication to allow reasonable comfort, and if the patient is willing to accept a lower range of motion in the affected hip.

Surgical alternatives to a hip osteotomy include:

• Total hip replacement. Total hip replacement is an operation designed to replace the entire damaged hip joint. Various prosthetic designs and types of procedures are available. The procedure involves surgical removal of the damaged parts of the hip joint and replacing them with artificial components made from ceramic or metal alloys. The bearing surface is usually made from a durable type of polyethylene, but other materials including ceramics, newer plastics, or metals may be used.

• Arthrodesis. This procedure is rarely performed as of 2003, but is considered particularly effective for younger patients who are short in stature and otherwise healthy. Arthrodesis relieves pain by fusing the femoral head to the acetabulum. It has none of the limitations that a joint replacement or other procedure imposes on the patient's activity level. An arthrodesis is especially suited for patients with strong backs and no other symptoms. The procedure generally requires internal fixation with a plate and screws. The patient may be immobilized in a cast while healing takes place. An arthrodesis can be converted to a total hip replacement at a later date.

• Pseudarthrosis. This procedure is also called a Girdlestone operation. A pseudarthrosis involves removing the femoral head without replacing it with an artificial part. It is performed in patients with hip infections and those whose bones cannot tolerate a reconstructive procedure. Pseudarthrosis leaves the patient with one leg shorter and usually less stable than the other. After this procedure, the patient almost always needs at least one crutch, especially for long-distance walking.

See also Hip arthroscopic surgery; Hip replacement; Hip revision surgery.

Resources

BOOKS

Callaghan, J. J., A. G. Rosenberg, and A. E. Rubash, eds. *The Adult Hip*, 2 vols. Philadelphia, PA: Lippincott Williams & Wilkins Publishers, 1998.

Klapper. R., and L. Huey. *Heal Your Hips: How to Prevent Hip Surgery—and What to Do If You Need It*. New York: John Wiley & Sons, 1999.

MacNicaol, M. F., ed. *Color Atlas and Text of Osteotomy of the Hip*. St. Louis, MO: Mosby, 1996.

> ## KEY TERMS
>
> **Acetabular dysplasia**—A type of arthritis resulting in a shallow hip socket.
>
> **Acetabulum**—The hollow, cuplike portion of the pelvis into which the femoral head is fitted to make the hip joint.
>
> **Arthrodesis**—Surgical fusion of the femoral head to the acetabulum.
>
> **Avascular necrosis**—Destruction of cartilage tissue due to impaired blood supply.
>
> **Femoral head**—The upper end of the femur.
>
> **Hip dysplasia**—Abnormal development of the hip joint.
>
> **Legg-Calve-Perthes disease (LCP)**—A disorder in which the femoral head deteriorates within the hip joint as a result of insufficient blood supply.
>
> **Osteotomy**—The surgical cutting of any bone.
>
> **Valgus**—A deformity in which a body part is angled away from the midline of the body.
>
> **Varus**—A deformity in which a body part is angled toward the midline of the body.

PERIODICALS

Devane, P. A., R. Coup, and J. G. Horne. "Proximal Femoral Osteotomy for the Treatment of Hip Arthritis in Young Adults." *ANZ Journal of Surgery* 72 (March 2002): 196-199.

Ganz, R., and M. Leunig. "Osteotomy and the Dysplastic Hip: The Bernese Experience." *Orthopedics* 25 (September 2002): 945-946.

Ito, H., A. Minami, H. Tanino, and T. Matsuno. "Fixation with Poly-L-Lactic Acid Screws in Hip Osteotomy: 68 Hips Followed for 18-46 Months." *Acta Orthopaedica Scandinavica* 73 (January 2002): 60-64.

Millis, M. B., and Y. J. Kim. "Rationale of Osteotomy and Related Procedures for Hip Preservation: A Review." *Clinical Orthopaedics and Related Research* 405 (December 2002): 108-121.

ORGANIZATIONS

American Academy of Orthopaedic Surgeons (AAOS). 6300 North River Road, Rosemont, Illinois 60018-4262. (847) 823-7186. <www.aaos.org>

Arthritis Foundation. P.O. Box 7669, Atlanta, GA 30357-0669. (800) 283-7800. <www.arthritis.org>.

OTHER

AAOS. *Legg-Calve-Perthes Disease.*<orthoinfo.aaos.org/fact/thr_report.cfm?Thread_ID=159&topcategory=About%20Orthopaedics>.

Arthritis Foundation. *Types of Surgery.* <www.arthritis.org/conditions/surgerycenter/types.asp>.

MedlinePlus. *Developmental Dysplasia of the Hip.* <www.nlm. nih.gov/medlineplus/ency/article/000971.htm >.

Monique Laberge, Ph. D.

Hip prosthesis surgery *see* **Hip revision surgery**

Hip replacement

Definition

Hip replacement is a procedure in which the surgeon removes damaged or diseased parts of the patient's hip joint and replaces them with new artificial parts. The operation itself is called hip **arthroplasty**. Arthroplasty comes from two Greek words, *arthros* or joint and *plassein*, "to form or shape." It is a type of surgery done to replace or reconstruct a joint. The artificial joint itself is called a prosthesis. Hip prostheses may be made of metal, ceramic, plastic, or various combinations of these materials.

Purpose

Hip arthroplasty has two primary purposes: pain relief and improved functioning of the hip joint.

Pain relief

Because total hip replacement (THR) is considered major surgery, with all the usual risks involved, it is usually not considered as a treatment option until the patient's pain cannot be managed any longer by more conservative nonsurgical treatment. These alternatives are described below.

Joint pain interferes with a person's quality of life in many ways. If the pain in the hip area is chronic, affecting the person even when he or she is resting, it can lead to depression and other emotional disturbances. Severe chronic pain also strains a person's relationships with family members, employer, and workplace colleagues; it is now recognized to be as the most common underlying cause of suicide in the United States.

In most cases, however, pain in the hip joint is a gradual development. Typically, the patient finds that their hip begins to ache when they are exercising vigorously, walking, or standing for a long time. They may cut back on athletic activities only to find that they are starting to limp when they walk and that sitting down is also becoming uncomfortable. Many patients then begin to have trouble driving, sitting through a concert or movie, or working at a desk without pain. It is usually at this point, when a person's ability to live independently is threatened, that he or she considers hip replacement surgery.

Joint function

Restoration of joint function is the other major purpose of hip replacement surgery. The hip joint is one of the most active joints in the human body, designed for many different types of movement. It consists of the head (top) of the femur (thighbone), which is shaped like a ball; and a part of the pelvic bone called the acetabulum, which looks like a hollow or socket. In a healthy hip joint, a layer of cartilage lies between the head of the femur and the acetabulum. The cartilage keeps the bony surfaces from grinding against each other, and allows the head of the femur to rotate or swivel in different directions inside the socket formed by the acetabulum. It is this range of motion, as well as the hip's ability to support the weight of the upper body, that is gradually lost when the hip joint deteriorates. The prostheses that are used in hip replacement surgery are intended to restore as much of the functioning of to the hip joint as possible. The level of function in the hip after the surgery depends in part on the reason for the damage to the joint.

Disorders and conditions that may lead to the need for hip replacement surgery include:

- Osteoarthritis (OA). Osteoarthritis is a disorder in which the cartilage in the joints of the body gradually breaks down, allowing the surfaces of the bones to rub directly and wear against each other. Eventually the patient experiences swelling, pain, inflammation, and increasing loss of mobility. OA most often affects appears most often in adults over age 45, and is thought to result from a combination of wear and tear on the joint, lifestyle, and genetic factors. As of 2003, OA is the most common cause of joint damage requiring hip replacement.

- Rheumatoid arthritis (RA). Rheumatoid arthritis is a disease that begins earlier in life than OA and affects the whole body. Women are three times as likely as men to develop RA. Its symptoms are caused by the immune system's attacks on the body's own cells and tissues. Patients with RA often suffer intense pain even when they are not putting weight on the affected joints. One man described his pain as " … like a hot poker that's stuck from this hip right through to the other one."

- Trauma. Damage to the hip joint from a fall, automobile accident, or workplace or athletic injury may trigger the process of cartilage breakdown in the hip joint.

- Avascular necrosis. Avascular necrosis, which is also called osteonecrosis, is a disorder caused by the loss of

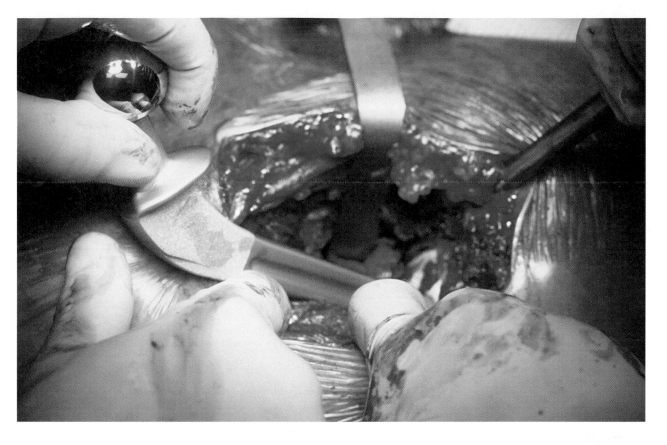

Surgeons using bone cement in the femur before inserting the prosthesis. *(Custom Medical Stock Photo. Reproduced by permission.)*

blood supply to bone tissue. Bone starved for blood supply becomes weak and eventually collapses. The most common reasons for loss of blood supply include trauma, the use of steroid medications, certain blood disorders, and alcoholism. Avascular necrosis often affects the top of the femur that forms part of the hip joint. It develops most frequently in adults between the ages of 30 and 50.

• Ankylosing spondylitis (AS). Ankylosing spondylitis is a less common form of arthritis that primarily affects the bones in the spine and pelvis. These bones gradually fuse together when the body replaces inflamed tendons or ligaments with new bone instead of elastic connective tissue. AS typically develops in the patient's late teens or early twenties, with three times as many men affected as women.

Demographics

Between 200,000 and 300,000 hip replacement operations are performed in the United States each year, most of them in patients over the age of 60. According to the American Academy of Orthopaedic Surgeons (AAOS), only 5–10% of total hip replacements as of 2002 were in patients younger than 50. There are two reasons for this concentration in older adults. Arthritis and other degenerative joint disorders are the most common health problems requiring hip replacement, and they become more severe as people grow older. The second reason is the limited life expectancy of the prostheses used in hip replacements. Because THR is a complex procedure and requires a long period of recovery after surgery, doctors generally advise patients to put off the operation as long as possible so that they will not need to undergo a second operation later to insert a new prosthesis.

This demographic picture is changing rapidly, however, because of advances in designing hip prostheses, as well as changes in older Americans' rising expectations of quality of life. Many people are less willing to tolerate years of pain or limited activity in order to postpone surgery. In addition, hip prostheses are lasting longer than those used in the 1960s; one study found that 65% of the prostheses in patients who had had THR before the age of 50 were still intact and functioning well 25 years after the surgery. A larger number of hip replacements are now being done in younger patients, and the operation itself is being performed more often. One expert estimates that the annual number of hip replacements in the United States will rise to 600,000 by 2015.

Description

Hip replacement surgery is a relatively recent procedure that had to wait for the invention of plastics and other synthetic materials to make reliable prostheses that could withstand years of wear. The first successful total hip replacement was performed in 1962 by Sir John Charnley (1911–1982), a British orthopedic surgeon who designed a device that is still known as a Charnley prosthesis. Charnley used a stainless steel ball mounted on a stem that was inserted into the patient's thighbone to replace the femoral head. A high-density polyethylene socket was fitted into the acetabular side of the joint. Both parts of the Charnley prosthesis were secured to their respective sides of the joint with an acrylic polymer cement. More recent developments include the use of cobalt chrome alloys or ceramic materials in place of stainless steel, as well as methods for holding the prosthesis in place without cement.

As of 2003, there are three major types of hip replacement surgery performed in the United States: a standard procedure for hip replacement; a newer technique known as minimally invasive surgery (MIS), pioneered in Chicago in February 2001; and revision surgery, which is done to replace a loosened or damaged prosthesis.

Standard hip replacement surgery

A standard hip replacement operation takes 1-1/2–3 hours. The patient may be given a choice of general, spinal, or epidural anesthesia. An epidural anesthesia, which is injected into the space around the spinal cord to block sensation in the lower body, causes less blood loss and also lowers the risk of blood clots or breathing problems after surgery. After the patient is anesthetized, the surgeon makes an incision 8–12 in (20–30 cm) long down the side of the patient's upper thigh. The surgeon may then choose to enter the joint itself from the side, back, or front. The back approach is the most common. The ligaments and muscles under the skin are then separated.

Once inside the joint, the surgeon separates the head of the femur from the acetabulum and removes the head with a saw. The surgeon uses a power drill and a special reamer to remove the cartilage from the acetabulum and shape it to accept the acetabular part of the prosthesis. This part of the new prosthesis is a curved piece of metal lined with plastic or ceramic.

After selecting the correct size for the patient, the surgeon inserts the acetabular component. If the new joint is to be cemented, the surgeon will attach the component to the bone with a type of epoxy. Otherwise the metal plate will be held in place by screws or by the tightness of the fit itself.

To replace the femoral head, the surgeon first drills a hollow inside the thighbone to accept a stem for the femoral component. The stem may be cemented in place or held in place by the tightness of the fit. A metal or ceramic ball to replace the head of the femur is then attached to the stem.

After the prosthesis is in place, an x ray is taken to verify that it is correctly positioned. The incision is then washed with saline solution as a safeguard against infection. The sutures used to close the deeper layers of tissue are made of a material that the body eventually absorbs, while the uppermost layer of skin is closed with metal surgical staples. The staples are removed 10–14 days after surgery.

Finally, a large triangular pillow known as a Charnley pillow is placed between the patient's ankles to prevent dislocation of the hip during the first few days after surgery.

Minimally invasive hip replacement surgery

Minimally invasive surgery (MIS) is a new technique of hip replacement introduced in 2001. Instead of making one long incision, the surgeon uses two 2-inch (5 cm) incisions or one 3.5-1/2-inch (9 cm) incision. Using newly designed smaller implements, the surgeon removes the damaged bone and inserts the parts of the new prosthesis. MIS hip replacement takes only an hour and a half; there is less bleeding and the patient can leave the hospital the next day. As of 2002, however, obese patients or those with very weak bones are not considered for MIS.

Revision surgery

Revision surgery is most commonly performed to replace a prosthesis that no longer fits or functions well because the bone in which it is implanted has deteriorated with age or disease. Revision surgery is a much more complicated process than first-time hip replacement; it sometimes requires a specialized prosthesis as well as bone grafts from the patient's pelvis, and its results are not usually as good. On the other hand, some patients have had as many as three revision operations with satisfactory results.

Diagnosis/Preparation

Because pain in the hip joint is usually a gradual development, its cause has been diagnosed in most cases by the time the patient is ready to consider hip replacement surgery. The doctor will have taken a careful med-

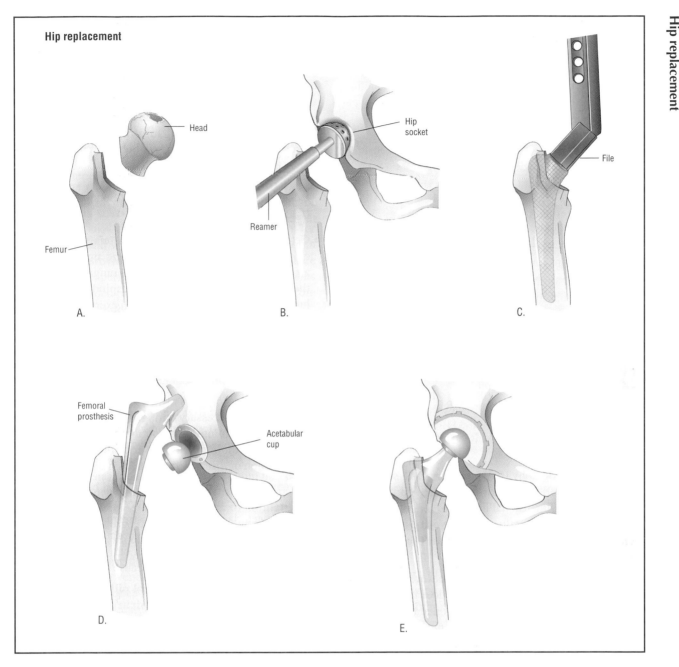

Hip replacement

In a hip replacement, the upper leg bone, or femur, is separated from the hip socket, and the damaged head is removed (A). A reamer is used to prepare the socket for the prosthesis (B). A file is used to create a tunnel in the femur for the prosthesis (C). The hip and socket prostheses are cemented in place (D), and finally connected (E). *(Illustration by Argosy.)*

ical and employment history in order to determine the most likely cause of the pain and whether the patient's job may be a factor. The doctor will also ask about a family history of osteoarthritis as well as other disorders known to run in families. The patient will be asked about injuries, falls, or other accidents that may have affected the hip joint; and about his or her use of alcohol and prescription medications—particularly steroids, which can cause avascular necrosis.

The patient will then be given a complete **physical examination** to evaluate his or her fitness for surgery. Certain disorders, including Parkinson's disease; dementia and other conditions of altered mental status; kidney disease; advanced osteoporosis; disorders associated with muscle weakness; diabetes; and an unstable cardiovascular system are generally considered contraindications to hip replacement surgery. People with weakened immune systems may also be advised against surgery. In

Risks

Hip replacement surgery involves both short- and long-term risks.

Short-term risks

The most common risks associated with hip replacement are as follows:

- Dislocation of the new prosthesis. Dislocation is most likely to occur in the first 10–12 weeks after surgery. It is a risk because the ball and socket in the prosthesis are smaller than the parts of the natural joint, and can move out of place if the patient places the hip in certain positions. The three major rules for avoiding dislocation are: Do not cross the legs when lying, sitting, or standing; never lean forward past a 90-degree angle at the waist; do not roll the legs inward toward each other— keep the feet pointed forward or turned slightly outward.

- Deep vein thrombosis (DVT). There is some risk (about 1.5% in the United States) of a clot developing in the deep vein of the leg after hip replacement surgery because the blood supply to the leg is cut off by a tourniquet during the operation. The blood-thinning medications and TED stockings used after surgery are intended to minimize the risk of DVT.

- Infection. The risk of infection is minimized by storing autologous blood for transfusion and administering intravenous **antibiotics** after surgery. Infections occur in fewer than 1% of hip replacement operations.

- Injury to the nerves that govern sensation in the leg. This problem usually resolves over time.

Long-term risks

The long-term risks of hip replacement surgery include:

- Inflammation related to wear and tear on the prosthesis. Tiny particles of debris from the prosthesis can cause inflammation in the hip joint and lead eventually to dissolution and loss of bone. This condition is known as osteolysis.

- Heterotopic bone. Heterotopic bone is bone that develops in the space between the femur and the pelvis after hip replacement surgery. It can cause stiffness and pain, and may have to be removed surgically. The cause is not completely understood as of 2002 but is thought to be a reaction to the trauma of the operation. In the United States, patients are usually given indomethacin (Indocin) to prevent this process; in Germany, surgeons are using postoperative radiation treatments together with Indocin.

- Changed length of leg. Some patients find that the operated leg remains slightly longer than the other leg even after recovery. This problem does not interfere with mobility and can usually be helped by an orthotic shoe insert.

- Loosening or damage to the prosthesis itself. This development is treated with revision surgery.

Normal results

Normal results are relief of chronic pain, greater ease of movement, and much improved quality of life. Specific areas of improvement depend on a number of factors, including the patient's age, weight, and previous level of activity; the disease or disorder that caused the pain; the type of prosthesis; and the patient's attitude toward recovery. In general, total hip replacement is considered one of the most successful procedures in modern surgery.

It is difficult to estimate the "normal" lifespan of a hip prosthesis. The figure quoted by many surgeons—10 to 15 years—is based on statistics from the early 1990s. It is too soon to tell how much longer the newer prostheses will last. In addition, as hip replacements become more common, the increased size of the worldwide patient database will allow for more accurate predictions. As of 2002, it is known that younger patients and obese patients wear out hip prostheses more rapidly.

Morbidity and mortality rates

Information about mortality and complication rates following THR is limited because the procedure is considered elective. In addition, different states and countries use different sets of measurements in evaluating THR outcomes. One Norwegian study found that patients who had THR between 1987 and 1999 had a lower long-term mortality rate than the age- and gender-matched Norwegian population. A Canadian study found a 1.6% mortality rate within 30 days of surgery for THR patients between 1981

KEY TERMS

Acetabulum—The socket-shaped part of the pelvis that forms part of the hip joint.

Analgesic—A medication given to relieve pain.

Ankylosing spondylitis—A form of inflammatory arthritis in which the bones in the spine and pelvis gradually fuse when inflamed connective tissue is replaced by bone.

Arthrodesis—A surgical procedure sometimes used to treat younger patients with hip problems, in which the head of the femur is fused directly to the acetabulum.

Arthroplasty—The medical term for surgical replacement of a joint. Arthroplasty can refer to knee as well as hip replacement.

Autologous blood—The patient's own blood, drawn and set aside before surgery for use during surgery in case a transfusion is needed.

Avascular necrosis—A disorder in which bone tissue dies and collapses following the temporary or permanent loss of its blood supply. It is also known as osteonecrosis.

Cartilage—A whitish elastic connective tissue that allows the bones forming the hip joint to move smoothly against each other.

Cortisone—A steroid compound used to treat autoimmune diseases and inflammatory conditions. It is sometimes injected into a joint to relieve the pain of arthritis.

Deep venous thrombosis (DVT)—The formation of a blood clot in the deep vein of the leg. It is considered a serious complication of hip replacement surgery.

Epidural—A method of administering anesthesia by injecting it into the lower spine in the space around the spinal cord. Epidural anesthesia blocks sensation in the parts of the body below the level of the injection.

Femur—The medical name for the thighbone.

Heterotopic bone—Bone that develops as an excess growth around the hip joint following surgery.

Nonsteroidal anti-inflammatory drugs (NSAIDs)—A term used for a group of analgesics that also reduce inflammation when used over a period of time. NSAIDs are often given to patients with osteoarthritis.

Orthopedics (sometimes spelled orthopaedics)—The branch of surgery that treats deformities or disorders affecting the musculoskeletal system.

Osteolysis—Dissolution and loss of bone resulting from inflammation caused by particles of debris from athe prosthesis.

Osteotomy—A surgical alternative to a hip prosthesis, in which the surgeon cuts through the pelvis or femur in order to realign the hip.

Prosthesis (plural, prostheses)—An artificial device that substitutes for or supplements a missing or damaged body part. Prostheses may be either external or implanted inside the body.

Tourniquet—A tube or pressure cuff that is tightened around a limb in order to compress a vein to stop bleeding.

---

and 1999. A 2002 report from the Mayo Clinic found that the overall frequency of serious complications (heart attack, pulmonary embolism, deep vein thrombosis, or death) within 30 days of THR was 2.2%, the risk being higher in patients over 70. The most important factor affecting morbidity and mortality rates in the United States, according to a 2002 Harvard study, is the volume of THRs performed at a given hospital or by a specific surgeon; the higher the volume, the better the outcomes.

Alternatives

Nonsurgical alternatives

The most common conservative alternatives to hip replacement surgery are assistive devices (canes or walkers) to reduce stress on the affected hip; exercise regimens to maintain joint flexibility; dietary changes, particularly if the patient is overweight; and **analgesics**, or painkilling medications. Most patients who try medication begin with an over-the-counter NSAID such as ibuprofen (Advil). If the pain cannot be controlled by nonprescription analgesics, the doctor may give the patient cortisone injections, which relieve the pain of arthritis by reducing inflammation. Unfortunately, the relief provided by cortisone tends to diminish with each injection; moreover, the drug can produce serious side effects.

Complementary and alternative (CAM) approaches

Complementary and alternative forms of therapy cannot be used as substitutes for hip replacement surgery, but they are helpful in managing pain before and after the operation, and in speeding physical recovery. Many patients also find that CAM therapies help them maintain a positive mental attitude in coping with the emotional stress of surgery and physical therapy. CAM therapies that have been shown to relieve the pain of rheumatoid and osteoarthritis include acupuncture, music therapy, naturopathic treatment, homeopathy, Ayurvedic medicine, and certain herbal preparations. Chronic pain from other disorders affecting the hip has been successfully treated with biofeedback, relaxation techniques, chiropractic manipulation, and mindfulness meditation.

Some types of movement therapy are recommended in order to postpone the need for hip surgery. Yoga, tai chi, qigong, and dance therapy help to maintain strength and flexibility in the hip joint, and to slow down the deterioration of cartilage and muscle tissue. Exercise in general has been shown to reduce a person's risk of developing osteoporosis.

Alternative surgical procedures

Other surgical options include:

• Osteotomy. An osteotomy is a procedure in which the surgeon cuts the thigh bone or pelvis in order to realign the hip. It is done more frequently in Europe than in the United States, but it has the advantage of not requiring artificial materials.

• Arthrodesis. This type of operation is rarely performed except in younger patients with injury to one hip. In this procedure, the head of the femur is fused to the acetabulum with a plate and screws. The major advantage of arthrodesis is that it places fewer restrictions on the patient's activity level than a hip replacement.

• Pseudarthrosis. In this procedure the head of the femur is removed without any replacement, resulting in a shorter leg on the affected side. It is usually performed when the patient's bones are too weak for implanting a prosthesis or when the hip joint is badly infected. This procedure is sometimes called a Girdlestone operation, after the surgeon who first used it in the 1940s.

Resources

BOOKS

Pelletier, Kenneth R., MD. *The Best Alternative Medicine*, Part II, "CAM Therapies for Specific Conditions." New York: Simon & Schuster, 2002.

Silber, Irwin. *A Patient's Guide to Knee and Hip Replacement: Everything You Need to Know.* New York: Simon & Schuster, 1999.

Trahair, Richard. *All About Hip Replacement: A Patient's Guide.* Melbourne, Oxford, and New York: Oxford University Press, 1998.

PERIODICALS

"Arthritis—Hip Replacement." *Harvard Health Letter* 27 (February 2002): i4.

Chapman, K., Z. Mustafa, B. Dowling, et al. "Finer Linkage Mapping of Primary Hip Osteoarthritis Susceptibility on Chromosome 11q in a Cohort of Affected Female Sibling Pairs." *Arthritis and Rheumatism* 46 (July 2002): 1780–1783.

Daitz, Ben. "In Pain Clinic, Fruit, Candy and Relief." *New York Times*, December 3, 2002.

Drake, C., M. Ace, and G. E. Maale. "Revision Total Hip Arthroplasty." *AORN Journal* 76 (September 2002): 414–417, 419–427.

"Hip Replacement Surgery Viable Option for Younger Patients, Thanks to New Prostheses." *Immunotherapy Weekly* (March 13, 2002): 10.

Hungerford, D. S. "Osteonecrosis: Avoiding Total Hip Arthroplasty." *Journal of Arthroplasty* 17 (June 2002) (4 Supplement 1): 121–124.

Joshi, A. B., L. Marcovic, K. Hardinge, and J. C. Murphy. " Total Hip Arthroplasty in Ankylosing Spondylitis: An Analysis of 181 Hips." *Journal of Arthroplasty* 17 (June 2002): 427–433.

Laupacis, A., R. Bourne, C. Rorabeck, et al. "Comparison of Total Hip Arthroplasty Performed With and Without Cement: A Randomized Trial." *Journal of Bone and Joint Surgery, American Volume* 84-A (October 2002): 1823–1828.

Lie, S. A., L. B. Engesaeter, L. I. Havelin, et al. "Early Postoperative Mortality After 67,548 Total Hip Replacements: Causes of Death and Thromboprophylaxis in 68 Hospitals in Norway from 1987 to 1999." *Acta Orthopaedica Scandinavica* 73 (August 2002): 392–399.

Mantilla, C. B., T. T. Horlocker, D. R. Schroeder, et al. "Frequency of Myocardial Infarction, Pulmonary Embolism, Deep Venous Thrombosis, and Death Following Primary Hip or Knee Arthroplasty." *Anesthesiology* 96 (May 2002): 1140–1146.

Solomon, D. H., E. Losina, J. A. Baron, et al. "Contribution of Hospital Characteristics to the Volume-Outcome Relationship: Dislocation and Infection Following Total Hip Replacement Surgery." *Arthritis and Rheumatism* 46 (September 2002): 2436–2444.

White, R. H. and M. C. Henderson. "Risk Factors for Venous Thromboembolism After Total Hip and Knee Replacement Surgery." *Current Opinion in Pulmonary Medicine* 8 (September 2002): 365–371.

ORGANIZATIONS

American Academy of Orthopaedic Surgeons (AAOS). 6300 North River Road, Rosemont, IL 60018. (847) 823-7186 or (800) 346-AAOS. <http://www.aaos.org>.

American Physical Therapy Association (APTA). 1111 North Fairfax Street, Alexandria, VA 22314. (703)684-APTA or (800) 999-2782. <http://www.apta.org>.

National Center for Complementary and Alternative Medicine (NCCAM) Clearinghouse. P.O. Box 7923, Gaithersburg, MD 20898. (888) 644-6226. TTY: (866) 464-3615. Fax: (866) 464-3616. <http://www.nccam.nih.gov.>.

National Institute of Arthritis and Musculoskeletal and Skin Diseases (NIAMS) Information Clearinghouse. National Institutes of Health, 1 AMS Circle, Bethesda, MD 20892. (301) 495-4484. TTY: (301) 565-2966. <http://www.niams.nih.gov>.

Rush Arthritis and Orthopedics Institute. 1725 West Harrison Street, Suite 1055, Chicago, IL 60612. (312) 563-2420. <www.rush.edu>.

OTHER

Hip Universe. June 15, 2003 [cited July 1, 2003]. <http://www.hipuniverse.homestead.com>.

Questions and Answers About Hip Replacement. Bethesda, MD: National Institutes of Health, 2001. NIH Publication No. 01-4907.

Rebecca Frey, Ph.D.

Hip revision surgery

Definition

Hip revision surgery, which is also known as revision total hip **arthroplasty**, is a procedure in which the surgeon removes a previously implanted artificial hip joint, or prosthesis, and replaces it with a new prosthesis. Hip revision surgery may also involve the use of bone grafts. The bone graft may be an autograft, which means that the bone is taken from another site in the patient's own body; or an allograft, which means that the bone tissue comes from another donor.

Purpose

Hip revision surgery has three major purposes: relieving pain in the affected hip; restoring the patient's mobility; and removing a loose or damaged prosthesis before irreversible harm is done to the joint. Hip prostheses that contain parts made of polyethylene typically become loose because wear and tear on the prosthesis gradually produces tiny particles from the plastic that irritate the soft tissue around the prosthesis. The inflamed tissue begins to dissolve the underlying bone in a process known as osteolysis. Eventually, the soft tissue expands around the prosthesis to the point at which the prosthesis loses contact with the bone.

In general, a surgeon will consider revision surgery for pain relief only when more conservative measures, such as medication and changes in the patient's lifestyle, have not helped. In some cases, revision surgery is performed when x-ray studies show loosening of the prosthesis, wearing of the surfaces of the hip joint, or loss of bone tissue even though the patient may not have experienced any discomfort. In most cases, however, increasing pain in the affected hip is one of the first indications that revision surgery is necessary.

Other less common reasons for hip revision surgery include fracture of the hip, the presence of infection, or dislocation of the prosthesis. In these cases the prosthesis must be removed in order to prevent long-term damage to the hip itself.

Demographics

The demographics of hip revision surgery are likely to change significantly over the next few decades as the proportion of people over 65 in the world's population continues to increase. As of 2003, however, demographic information about this procedure is difficult to evaluate. This difficulty is due in part to the fact that total **hip replacement** (THR) itself is a relatively new procedure dating back only to the early 1960s. Since the design of hip prostheses and the materials used in their manufacture have changed over the last forty years, it is difficult to predict whether prostheses implanted in 2003 will last longer than those used in the past, and if so, whether improved durability will affect the need for revision surgery. On the other hand, more THRs are being performed in younger patients who are more likely to wear out their hip prostheses relatively quickly because they are more active and living longer than the previous generation of THR recipients. In addition, recent improvements in surgical technique as well as in prosthesis design have made hip revision surgery a less risky procedure than it was even a decade ago. One Scottish surgeon has reported performing as many as four hip revisions on selected patients, with highly successful outcomes. According to one estimate, 32,000 revision total hip arthroplasties were performed in the United States in 2000.

While information on the epidemiology of both THR and hip revision surgery is limited, one study of **Medicare** patients in the United States who had had either THR or revision hip surgery between 1995 and 1996 was published in January 2003. The authors found that three to six times as many THRs were performed as revision surgeries. Women had higher rates of both procedures than men, and Caucasians had higher rates than African Americans. Other researchers have reported that one reason for the lower rate of hip replacement and revision procedures among African Americans is the difference in social networks. African Americans are less likely than Caucasians to know someone who has had hip surgery, and they are therefore less likely to consider it as a treatment option.

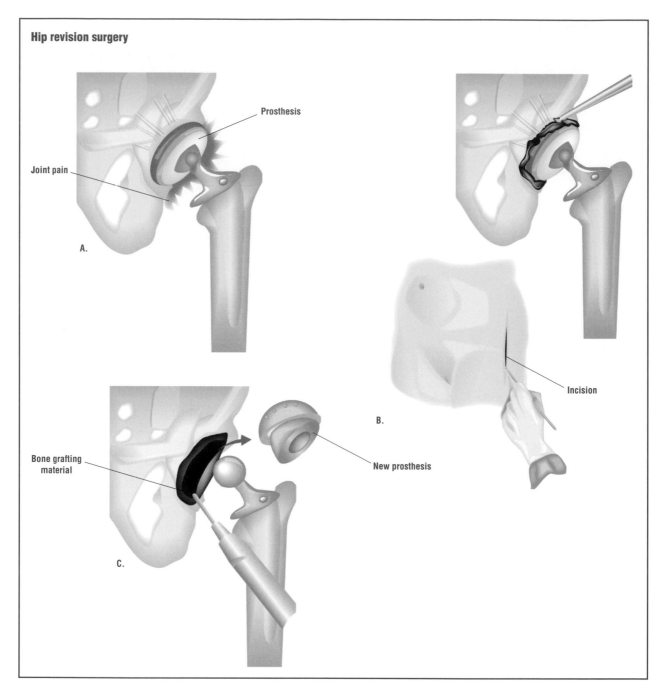

Hip revision surgery

Degeneration of the joint around the prosthesis causes pain for some patients who have undergone hip replacement (A). To repair it, an incision is made in the hip and the old prosthesis is removed (B). Bone grafts may be planted in the hip, and a new prosthesis is attached (C). *(Illustration by GGS Inc.)*

Description

Hip revision surgery is hard to describe in general terms because the procedure depends on a set of factors unique to each patient. These factors include the condition of the patient's hip and leg bones; the type of prosthesis originally used; whether the original prosthesis was cemented or held in place without cement; and the patient's age and overall health. Unlike standard THR, however, hip revision surgery is a much longer and more complicated procedure. It is not unusual for a hip revision operation to take five to eight hours.

The most critical factor affecting the length of the operation and some of the specific steps in hip revision surgery is the condition of the bone tissue in the femur.

As of 2003, defects in the bone are classified in four stages as follows:

• Type I. Minimal bone defects.

• Type II. Most of the damage lies at the metaphysis (the flared end of the femur), with minimal damage to the shaft of the bone.

• Type III. All of the damage lies at the metaphysis.

• Type IV. There is extensive bone loss in the femoral shaft as well as at the metaphysis.

The first stage in all hip revision surgery is the removal of the old prosthesis. The part attached to the acetabulum is removed first. The hip socket is cleaned and filled with morselized bone, which is bone in particle form. The new shell and liner are then pressed into the acetabulum.

Revision of the femoral component is the most complicated part of hip revision surgery. If the first prosthesis was held in place by pressure rather than cement, the surgeon usually cuts the top of the femur into several pieces to remove the implant. This cutting apart of the bone is known as osteotomy. The segments of bone are cleaned and the new femoral implant is pressed or cemented in place. If the patient's bone has been classified as Type IV, bone grafts may be added to strengthen the femur. These grafts consist of morselized bone from a donor (allograft bone) that is packed into the empty canal inside the femur. This technique is called impaction grafting. The segments of the femur are then reassembled around the new implant and bone grafts, and held in place with surgical wire.

A newer technique that was originally designed to help surgeons remove old cement from prostheses that were cemented in place can sometimes be used instead of osteotomy. This method involves the use of a ballistic chisel powered by controlled bursts of pressurized nitrogen. The ballistic chisel is used most often to break up pieces of cement from a cemented prosthesis, but it can also be used to loosen a prosthesis that was held in place only by tightness of fit. In addition to avoiding the need for an osteotomy, the ballistic chisel takes much less time. The surgeon uses an arthroscope in order to view the progress of the chisel while he or she is working inside the femur itself.

After all the cement has been removed from the inner canal of the femur, the surgeon washes out the canal with saline solution, inserts morselized bone if necessary, and implants the new femoral component of the prosthesis. After both parts of the prosthesis have been checked for correct positioning, the head of the femoral component is fitted into the new acetabular component and the incision is closed.

WHO PERFORMS THE PROCEDURE AND WHERE IS IT PERFORMED?

Hip revision surgery is performed by an orthopedic surgeon, who is an MD and who has received advanced training in surgical treatment of disorders of the musculoskeletal system. As of 2002, qualification for this specialty in the United States requires a minimum of five years of training after medical school. Most orthopedic surgeons who perform joint replacements and revision surgery have had additional specialized training in these specific procedures. It is a good idea to find out how many hip revisions the surgeon performs each year; those who perform 200 or more have had more opportunities to refine their technique.

In many cases, hip revision surgery is done by the surgeon who performed the first replacement operation. Some surgeons, however, refer patients to colleagues who specialize in hip revision procedures.

Hip revision surgery can be performed in a general hospital with a department of **orthopedic surgery**, but is also performed in specialized clinics or institutes for joint disorders.

Diagnosis/Preparation

Diagnosis

In most cases, increasing pain, greater difficulty in placing weight on the hip, and loss of mobility in the hip joint are early indications that revision surgery is necessary. The location of the pain may point to the part of the prosthesis that has been affected by osteolysis. The pain is felt in both the hip area and the thigh when both parts of the prosthesis have become loose; if only the femoral component has been affected, the patient usually feels pain only in the thigh. As was mentioned earlier, however, some patients do not experience any discomfort even though their prosthesis is loosening or wearing against surrounding structures. In addition, a minority of patients who have had THR have always had pain from their artificial joints, and these patients may not consider their discomfort new or significant.

In general, diagnostic imaging that shows bone loss, loosening of the prosthesis, or wearing away of the joint tissues is an essential aspect of hip revision surgery—many orthopedic surgeons will not consider the procedure unless the x-ray studies reveal one or more of these signs. X-ray studies are also used to diagnose fractures of the hip or dislocated prostheses. In some cases, the doctor may order a computed tomography (CT) scan to confirm the extent and location of suspected osteolysis; recent research indicates that **CT scans** can detect bone loss around a hip prosthesis at earlier stages than radiography.

Infections related to a hip prosthesis are a potentially serious matter. Estimated rates of infection following THR range between one in 300 operations and one in 100. Infections can develop at any time following THR, ranging from the immediate postoperative period to 10 or more years later. The symptoms of superficial infections include swelling, pain, and redness in the skin around the incision, but are usually treatable with **antibiotics**. With deep infections, antibiotics may not work and the new joint is likely to require revision surgery. One American specialist has said that the chances of salvaging an infected prosthesis are only 50/50.

Preoperative preparation

Certain health conditions or disorders are considered contraindications for hip revision surgery. These include:

- a current hip infection
- dementia or other severe mental disorder
- severe vascular disease
- poor condition of the skin covering the hip
- extreme obesity
- paralysis of the quadriceps muscles
- terminal illness

Patients who are considered appropriate candidates for hip revision surgery are asked to come to the hospital about a week before the operation. X rays and other diagnostic images of the hip are reviewed in order to select the new prosthesis. This review is called templating because the diagnostic images serve as a template for the new implant. The surgeon will also decide whether special procedures or instruments will be needed to remove the old prosthesis.

Aftercare

Aftercare for hip revision surgery is essentially the same as for hip replacement surgery. The major difference is that some patients with very weak bones are asked to use canes or walkers all the time following revision surgery rather than trying to walk without assistive devices.

Risks

Risk factors

Factors that lower a patient's chances for a good outcome from hip revision surgery include the following:

- Sex. Men are more likely to have poor outcomes from revision surgery than women, other factors being equal.
- Age. Older patients, particularly those over 75, are more likely to have complications following revision surgery.
- Race. African Americans have a higher rate of complications than Caucasian or Asian Americans.
- Socioeconomic status (SES). Patients with lower incomes do not do as well as patients in higher income brackets.
- Presence of other chronic diseases or disorders.
- Obesity. Many surgeons will not perform hip revision surgery on patients weighing 300 pounds or more.
- Genetic factors. Recent British research indicates that patients who carry an inflammation control gene known as TNF-238A are twice as likely to require replacement of a hip prosthesis as those who lack this gene.

Specific risks of hip revision surgery

Risks following hip revision surgery are similar to those following hip replacement surgery, including deep venous thrombosis and infection. The length of the patient's leg, however, is more likely to be affected following revision surgery. Dislocation is considerably more common because the tissues surrounding the bone are weaker as well as the bone itself usually being more fragile. One group of researchers found that the long-term rate of dislocation following revision surgery may be as high as 7.4%.

676

KEY TERMS

Acetabulum—The socket-shaped part of the pelvis that forms part of the hip joint.

Allograft—A graft of bone or other tissue taken from a donor.

Analgesic—A medication given to relieve pain.

Arthroscope—An instrument that contains a miniature camera and light source mounted on a flexible tube. It allows a surgeon to see the inside of a joint or bone during surgery.

Autograft—A graft of bone or other tissue taken from the body of the patient undergoing surgery.

Femur—The medical name for the thighbone. The femur is the largest bone in the human body.

Impaction grafting—The use of crushed bone from a donor to fill in the central canal of the femur during hip revision surgery.

Metaphysis—The widened end of the shaft of a long tubular bone such as the femur.

Orthopedics (sometimes spelled orthopaedics)—The branch of surgery that treats deformities or disorders affecting the musculoskeletal system.

Osteolysis—Dissolution and loss of bone resulting from inflammation caused by particles of polyethylene debris from a prosthesis.

Osteotomy—The cutting apart of a bone or removal of bone by cutting. An osteotomy is often necessary during hip revision surgery in order to remove the femoral part of the old prosthesis from the femur.

Prosthesis (plural, prostheses)—An artificial device that substitutes for or supplements a missing or damaged body part. Prostheses may be either external or implanted inside the body.

Quadriceps muscles—A set of four muscles on each leg located at the front of the thigh. The quadriceps straighten the knee and are used every time a person takes a step.

Templating—A term that refers to the surgeon's use of x-ray images of an old prosthesis as a template or pattern guide for a new implant.

Normal results

In general, hip revision surgery has less favorable outcomes than first-time replacement surgery. The greater length and complexity of the procedure often require a longer hospital stay as well as a longer period of **recovery at home**. The range of motion in the new joint is usually smaller than in the first prosthesis, and the patient may experience greater long-term discomfort. In addition, the new prosthesis is not expected to last as long. The life expectancy of implants used in first-time hip replacement surgery is usually given as 10–15 years, whereas revision implants may need to be removed after eight to 10 years.

Morbidity and mortality rates

There are relatively few analyses of mortality and morbidity following hip revision surgery in comparison to studies of complications following THR. One study published in 2003 reported the following figures for complications following hip revision surgeries (after 90 days) performed in the United States:

• mortality: 2.6%

• pulmonary embolism: 0.8%

• wound infection: 0.95%

• hospital readmission: 10.0%

• dislocation of prosthesis: 8.4%

Alternatives

Nonsurgical alternatives

In some cases medications can be used to control the patient's pain, or the patient may prefer to use assistive devices rather than undergo revision surgery. If infection is present, however, surgery is necessary in order to remove the old prosthesis and any areas of surrounding bone that may be infected.

Alternative and complementary treatments

Alternative and complementary approaches that have been shown to control discomfort after hip revision surgery include mindfulness meditation, biofeedback, acupuncture, and relaxation techniques. Music therapy, humor therapy, and aromatherapy are helpful to some patients in maintaining a positive mental attitude and relieving emotional stress before surgery or during recovery at home.

See also Hip replacement surgery.

Resources

BOOKS

Pelletier, Kenneth R., MD. "CAM Therapies for Specific Conditions." In *The Best Alternative Medicine*, Part II. New York: Simon & Schuster, 2002.

Silber, Irwin. *A Patient's Guide to Knee and Hip Replacement: Everything You Need to Know.* New York: Simon & Schuster, 1999.

Trahair, Richard. *All About Hip Replacement: A Patient's Guide.* Melbourne, Oxford, and New York: Oxford University Press, 1998.

PERIODICALS

Alberton, G. M., W. A. High, and B. F. Morrey. "Dislocation After Revision Total Hip Arthroplasty: An Analysis of Risk Factors and Treatment Options." *Journal of Bone and Joint Surgery, American Volume* 84-A (October 2002): 1788–1792.

Blake, V. A., J. P. Allegrante, L. Robbins, et al. "Racial Differences in Social Network Experience and Perceptions of Benefit of Arthritis Treatments Among New York City Medicare Beneficiaries with Self-Reported Hip and Knee Pain." *Arthritis and Rheumatism* 47 (August 15, 2002): 366–371.

Drake, C., M. Ace, and G. E. Maale. "Revision Total Hip Arthroplasty." *AORN Journal* 76 (September 2002): 414–417, 419–427.

Mahomed, N. N., J. A. Barrett, J. N. Katz, et al. "Rates and Outcomes of Primary and Revision Total Hip Replacement in the United States Medicare Population." *Journal of Bone and Joint Surgery, American Volume* 85-A (January 2003): 27–32.

Nelissen, R. G., E. R. Valstar, R. G. Poll, et al. "Factors Associated with Excessive Migration in Bone Impaction Hip Revision Surgery: A Radiostereometric Analysis Study." *Journal of Arthroplasty* 17 (October 2002): 826–833.

Puri, L., R. L. Wixson, S. H. Stern, et al. "Use of Helical Computed Tomography for the Assessment of Acetabular Osteolysis After Total Hip Arthroplasty." *Journal of Bone and Joint Surgery, American Volume* 84-A (April 2002): 609–614.

ORGANIZATIONS

American Academy of Orthopaedic Surgeons (AAOS). 6300 North River Road, Rosemont, IL 60018. (847) 823-7186 or (800) 346-AAOS. <http://www.aaos.org>.

American Physical Therapy Association (APTA). 1111 North Fairfax Street, Alexandria, VA 22314. (703)684-APTA or (800) 999-2782. <http://www.apta.org>.

National Center for Complementary and Alternative Medicine (NCCAM) Clearinghouse. P.O. Box 7923, Gaithersburg, MD 20898. (888) 644-6226. TTY: (866) 464-3615. Fax: (866) 464-3616. <http://www.nccam.nih.gov.>.

National Institute of Arthritis and Musculoskeletal and Skin Diseases (NIAMS) Information Clearinghouse. National Institutes of Health, 1 AMS Circle, Bethesda, MD 20892. (301) 495-4484. TTY: (301) 565-2966. <http://www.niams.nih.gov>.

Rush Arthritis and Orthopedics Institute. 1725 West Harrison Street, Suite 1055, Chicago, IL 60612. (312) 563-2420. <http://www.rush.edu>.

OTHER

Hip Universe. June 15, 2003 [cited July 1, 2003]. <http://www.hipuniverse.homestead.com>.

Questions and Answers About Hip Replacement. Bethesda, MD: National Institutes of Health, 2001. NIH Publication No. 01-4907.

Rebecca Frey, Ph.D.

Histocompatibility testing *see* **Human leukocyte antigen test**

HLA test *see* **Human leukocyte antigen test**

HMOs *see* **Managed care plans**

Home care

Definition

Home care is a form of health care service provided where a patient lives. Patients can receive home care services whether they live in their own homes, with or without family members, or in an assisted living facility. The purpose of home care is to promote, maintain, or restore a patient's health and reduce the effects of disease or disability.

Description

The goal of home care is to provide for the needs of the patient to allow the patient to remain living at home, regardless of age or disability. After surgery, a patient may require home care services that may range from such homemaking services as cooking or cleaning to skilled medical care. Some patients require home health aides or personal care attendants to help them with activities of daily living (ADL).

Medical, dental, and nursing care may all be delivered in patients' homes, which allows them to feel more comfortable and less anxious. Therapists from speech-language pathology, physical therapy, and respiratory therapy departments often make regular home visits, depending on a patient's specific needs. General nursing care is provided by both registered and licensed practical nurses; however, there are also nurses who are clinical specialists in psychiatry, obstetrics, and cardiology who may provide care when necessary. Home health aides provide what is called custodial care in domestic settings; their duties are similar to those of nurses' aides in the hospital. Professionals who deliver care to patients in their homes are employed either by independent for-profit home-care agencies, hospital agencies, or hospital departments. Personal care attendants can also be hired privately by patients; however, not only is it more difficult to evaluate an employee's specific background and credentials when he or she is not associated with a certified agency or hospital, but medical insurance may not cover the expense of an employee who does not come from an approved source.

Home care nurses provide care for patients of every age, economic class, and level of disability. Some nurses provide specialized hospice, mental health, or pediatric care. Home care nursing often involves more than biomedically based care, depending on a patient's religious or spiritual background.

Viewpoints

Most patients are more comfortable in their own homes, rather than in a hospital setting. Depending on the patient's living status and relationships with others in the home, however, the home is not always the best place for caregiving. Consequently, home care continues to grow in popularity. Hospital stays have been shortened considerably, starting in the 1980s with the advent of the diagnosis-related group (DRG) reimbursement system as part of a continuing effort to reduce health care costs. But as a result, many patients come home "quicker and sicker," and in need of some form of care or help that family or friends may not be able to offer. Community-based health care services are expanding, giving patients more options for assistance at home.

History

It is helpful to have some basic information about the evolution of home care in order to understand the public's demand for quality health care, cost containment, and the benefits of advances in both medical and communication technologies. Members of Roman Catholic religious orders in Europe first delivered home care in the late seventeenth century. Today, there are many home care agencies and visiting nurse associations (VNAs) that continue to deliver a wide range of home care services to meet the specific needs of patients throughout the United States and Canada.

Social factors have historically influenced home care delivery, and continue to do so today. Before the 1960s, home care was a community-based delivery system that provided care to patients whether they could pay for the services or not. Agencies relied on charitable contributions from private citizens or charitable organizations, as well as some limited government funding. Life expectancy of the United States population began to rise as advances in medical science saved patients who might have died in years past. As a result, more and more elderly or disabled people required medical care in their homes as well as in institutions. In response, the federal government put **Medicare** and **Medicaid** programs into

place in 1965 to help fund and regulate health care delivery for this population.

Funding and regulation

Government involvement resulted in regulations that changed the focus of home care from a nursing care delivery service to care delivery under the direction of a physician. Home care delivery is paid for either by the government through Medicare and/or Medicaid; by private insurance or health maintenance organizations (HMOs); by patients themselves; or by certain non-profit community, charitable disease advocacy organizations (e.g., ACS), or faith-based organizations.

Home care delivery services provided by Medicare-certified agencies are tightly regulated. For example, a patient must be homebound in order to receive Medicare-reimbursed home care services. The homebound requirement—one of many—means that the patient must be physically unable to leave home (other than for infrequent trips to the doctor or hospital), thereby restricting the number of persons eligible for home care services. Private insurance companies and HMOs also have certain criteria for the number of visits that will be covered for specific conditions and services. Restrictions on the payment source, the physician's orders, and the patient's specific needs determine the length and scope of services.

Assessment and implementation

Since home care nursing services are provided on a part-time basis, patients, family members, or other caregivers are encouraged and taught to do as much of the care as possible. This approach goes beyond payment boundaries; it extends to the amount of responsibility the patient and his or her family or caregivers are willing or able to assume in order to reach expected outcomes. Nurses who have received special training as case managers visit the patient's home and draw up a plan of care based on assessing the patient, listing the diagnoses, planning the care delivery, implementing specific interventions, and evaluating outcomes or the efficacy of the implementation phase. Planning the care delivery includes assessing the care resources within the circle of the patient's caregivers.

At the time of the initial assessment, the visiting nurse, who is working under a physician's orders, enlists professionals in other disciplines who might be involved in achieving expected outcomes, whether those outcomes include helping the patient return to a certain level of health and independence or maintaining the existing level of health and mobility. The nurse provides instruction to the patient and caregiver(s) regarding the patient's particular disease(s) or condition(s) in order to help the patient achieve an agreed-upon level of independence. Home care nurses are committed to helping patients make good decisions about their care by providing them with reliable information about their conditions. Since home care relies heavily on a holistic approach, care delivery includes teaching coping mechanisms and promoting a positive attitude to motivate patients to help themselves to the extent that they are able. Unless the patient is paying for home care services out-of-pocket and has unlimited resources or a specific private **long-term care insurance** policy, home care services are scheduled to end at some point. Therefore, the goal of most home care delivery is to move both the patient and the caregivers toward becoming as independent as possible during that time.

Professional implications

Home care delivery is influenced by a number of variables. Political, social, and economic factors place significant constraints on care delivery. Differences among nurses, including their level of education, years of work experience, type of work experience, and level of cultural competence (cross-cultural sensitivity) all influence care delivery to some extent.

Some of the professional issues confronting home care nurses include:

• legal issues

• ethical concerns

• safety issues

• nursing skills and professional education

Legal issues

The legal considerations connected with delivering care in a patient's private residence are similar to those of care delivered in health care facilities, but have additional aspects. For example, what would a home care nurse do if she or he had heard the patient repeatedly express the desire not to be resuscitated in case of a heart attack or other catastrophic event, and during a home visit, the nurse finds the patient unresponsive and cannot find the orders not to resuscitate in the patient's chart? What happens if the patient falls during home care delivery? While processes, protocols, and standards of practice cannot be written to address every situation that may arise in a domestic setting, timely communication and strong policy are essential to keep both patients and home care staff free of legal liability.

Ethical concerns

Ethical implications are closely tied to legal implications in home care—as in the case of missing do-not-re-suscitate (**DNR**) orders. For example, what measures are appropriate if a home care nurse finds a severe diabetic and recovered alcoholic washing down a candy bar with a glass of bourbon? The patient is in his or her own residence and has the legal right to do as he or she chooses. Or, what about the family member who has a bad fall while the nurse is in the home providing care? Should the nurse care for that family member as well? What is the nurse's responsibility to the patient when he or she notices that a family member is taking money from an unsuspecting patient? Complex ethical issues are not always addressed in policy statements. Ongoing communication between the home care agency and the nurse in the field is essential to address problematic situations.

Safety issues

Safety issues in home care require attention and vigilance. The home care nurse does not have security officers readily available if a family member becomes violent either toward the health care worker or the patient. Sometimes, home care staff is required to visit patients in high-crime areas or after dark. All agencies should have some type of supervisory personnel available 24 hours a day, seven days a week, so that field staff can reach them with any concerns. Also, clear policy statements that cover issues of personal safety must be documented and communicated regularly and effectively.

Technological advances

With advances in technology and the increased effort to control cost, home care delivery services are using "telecare," which uses communications technology to transmit medical information between the patient and the health care provider. Providing care to patients without being in their immediate presence is a relatively new form of home nursing, and is not without its problems. While some uncertainty exists regarding legal responsibilities and the potential for liability, much has been done to make telecare an effective way to hold costs down for some patients. Home care nurses who are required to make telecare visits should know what regulations exist in the particular state before providing care. The chief problem lies in diagnosing and prescribing over the phone. Technological advances have enabled patients to access telecare through the Internet using personal computers or using televisions. With the most recent advances in telecare, the following services may now be offered:

• instant access to patient records

• prescriptions for treatment

• assessment of possible dangers to the patient

• evaluation of the patient's treatment and medication

• follow-up care

KEY TERMS

Activities of daily living (ADLs)—The activities performed during the course of a normal day such as eating, bathing, dressing, toileting, etc.

Home health aide—An employee of a home care agency who provides the same services to a patient in the home as nurses aides perform in hospitals and nursing homes.

Licensed practical nurse (LPN)—A person who is licensed to provide basic nursing care under the supervision of a physician or a registered nurse.

Medicaid—The federally funded program in the United States for state-operated programs that provide medical assistance to permanently disabled patients and to low-income people.

Medicare—The federally-funded national health insurance program in the United States for all people over the age of 65.

Personal care attendant—An employee hired ei-

ther through a health care facility, home care agency, or private agency to assist a patient in performing ADLs.

Psychiatric nursing—The nursing specialty concerned with the prevention and treatment of mental disorders and their consequences.

Registered nurse—A graduate nurse who has passed a state nursing board examination and been registered and licensed to practice nursing.

Respiratory therapy—The department of any health care facility or agency that provides treatment to patients to maintain or improve their breathing function.

Speech-language pathology—Formerly known as speech therapy, it includes the study and treatment of human communication—its development and disorders.

Resources

BOOKS

Abrams, William B., Mark H Beers, and Robert Berkow, eds. *The Merck Manual of Geriatrics,* 3rd edition. Whitehouse Station, NJ: Merck & Co., Inc., 2000.

Eaton, Shirley. *Handbook for Personal Caregivers of the Elderly.* Bloomington, IN: 1stBooks Library, 2002.

Rice, Robyn. *Home Care Nursing Practice: Concepts and Application,* 3rd edition. Philadelphia: Mosby, 2001.

PERIODICALS

Goulet, C., et al. "A Randomized Clinical Trial of Care for Women with Preterm Labor: Home Management Versus Hospital Management." *CMAJ* 164, no. 7 (April 3, 2001): 985–991.

Hoenig, Helen, Donald H. Taylor, Jr, and Frank A. Sloan. "Does Assistive Technology Substitute for Personal Assistance among the Disabled Elderly?" *American Journal of Public Health* 93, no. 2 (February 2003): 330–337.

Jenkens, R.L., and P. White. "Telehealth Advancing Nursing Practice." *Nursing Outlook* 49, no. 2 (March–April 2001): 100–105.

Rhinehart, E. "Infection Control in Home Care." *Emerging Infectious Diseases* 7, no. 2 (March–April 2001): 208–212.

Spratt, G., and Petty, T.L. "Partnering for Optimal Respiratory Home Care: Physicians Working with Respiratory Therapists to Optimally Meet Respiratory Home Care Needs." *Respiratory Care,* 46, no. 5 (May 2001): 475–488.

ORGANIZATIONS

Centers for Medicare & Medicaid Services. 7500 Security Boulevard, Baltimore, MD 21244-1850. (410) 786-3000. (877) 267-2323. <http://www.medicare.gov>.

e-Healthcare Solutions Inc. 953 Route 202 North, Branchburg, NJ 08876. (908) 203-1350. Fax: (908) 203-1307. <info@e-healthcaresolutions.com>. <http://www.digitalhealthcare.com>.

Hospice Foundation of America. 2001 S. Street NW, Suite 300, Washington, DC 20009. (800) 854-3402. (202) 638-5419l. Fax: (202) 638-5312; E-mail: <jon@hospicefoundation.org>. <http://www.hospicefoundation.org>.

Joint Commission on Accreditation of Health Care Organizations. One Renaissance Blvd., Oakbrook Terrace, IL 60181. (630) 792-5000. <http://www.jcaho.org>.

National Association for Home Care & Hospice. 228 7th Street, SE, Washington, DC 20003. (202) 547-7424. Fax: (202) 547-3540.

U.S. Department of Health and Human Services. 200 Independence Avenue, S.W., Washington, DC 20201. (202) 619-0257. (877) 696-6775. <http://www.hcfa.gov>.

Visiting Nurse Associations of America. 11 Beacon Street, Suite 910, Boston, MA 02108. (888) 866-8773. (617) 523-4042. Fax: (617) 227-4843. <vnaa@vnaa.org>. <http://www.vnaa.org>.

OTHER

Coates, Karen J. "Senior Class." *Nurseweek* May 2002 [cited March 1, 2003]. <http://www.nurseweek.com/news/features/02-05/senior.asp>.

Susan Joanne Cadwallader
Crystal H. Kaczkowski, MSc

Homocysteine test *see* **Cardiac marker tests**

Hospices

Definition

The term hospice refers to an approach to end-of-life care as well as to a type of facility for supportive care of terminally ill patients. Hospice programs provide palliative (care that relieves discomfort but does not improve the patient's condition or cure the disease) patient-centered care, and other services. The goal of hospice care, whether delivered in the patient's home or in a health-care facility, is the provision of humane and compassionate medical, emotional, and spiritual care to the dying.

Description

Early history

The English word "hospice" is derived from the Latin *hospitium*, which originally referred to the guesthouse of a monastery or convent. The first hospices date back to the Middle Ages, when members of religious orders frequently took in dying people and nursed them during their last illness. Other hospices were built along the routes to major pilgrimage shrines in medieval Europe, such as Rome, Compostela, and Canterbury. Pilgrims who died during their journey were cared for in these hospices. The modern hospice movement, however, may be said to have begun in the United Kingdom during the middle of the nineteenth century. In Dublin, the Roman Catholic Sisters of Charity undertook to provide a clean, supportive environment for care for the terminally ill. Their approach spread throughout England and as far as Asia, Australia, and Africa; but until the early 1970s, it had not been accepted on any wide scale in the United States.

Two physicians, Drs. Cicely Saunders and Elisabeth Kübler-Ross, are credited with introducing the hospice concept in the United States. Dame Saunders had originally trained as a nurse in England and afterward attended medical school. She founded St. Christopher's Hospice just outside of London in 1962. St. Christopher's pioneered an interdisciplinary team approach to the care of the dying. This approach made great strides in **pain management** and symptom control. Dr. Saunders also developed the basic tenets of hospice philosophy. These include:

- acceptance of death as the natural conclusion of life
- delivery of care by a highly trained, interdisciplinary team of health professionals who communicate among themselves regularly
- an emphasis on effective pain management and comprehensive **home care** services
- counseling for the patient and bereavement counseling for the family after the patient's death

- ongoing research and education as essential features of hospice programs

During this same period, Dr. Kübler-Ross, a psychiatrist working in Illinois, published results from her ground-breaking studies of dying patients. Her books about the psychological stages of response to catastrophe and her lectures to health professionals helped to pave the way for the development and acceptance of hospice programs in the United States. The merit of the five stages of acceptance that Dr. Kübler-Ross outlines is that they are not limited to use in counseling the dying. Many patients who become disabled—especially those whose disability and physical impairment are sudden occurrences—go through the same stages of "grieving" for the loss of their previous physical health or quality of life. Paraplegics, quadriplegics, amputees, and patients with brain-stem injuries all progress through these same stages of "acceptance"—and they are not dying.

The first hospice programs in North America opened during the 1970s. In New Haven, Connecticut, the Yale University School of Medicine started a hospice home care program in 1974, adding inpatient facilities in 1979. In 1976, another hospice/home-care program, the Hospice of Marin, began in northern California. After a slow start, interest in and enthusiasm for the hospice concept grew. Health professionals as well as the public at large embraced the idea of death with dignity. The notion of quality care at the end of life combined with grief counseling and bereavement care (counseling and support for families and friends of dying persons) gained widespread acceptance. The hospice movement also benefited from government efforts to contain health-care costs when reimbursement for inpatient **hospital services** was sharply reduced. Home-based hospice care is a cost-effective alternative to end-of-life care in a hospital or skilled nursing facility.

Acceptance by mainstream medical professionals

The hospice approach emphasizes caring instead of curing, and some health professionals initially found that this orientation was inconsistent with their previous education, experiences, beliefs, and traditions. Moreover, the involvement of complementary and alternative medicine practitioners was sometimes unsettling for health professionals unaccustomed to interacting with these persons. As a result of this early period of tension, the Academy of Hospice Physicians was established in 1988 to bring together doctors from a variety of specialties to awaken interest in hospice care among their colleagues and answer their concerns.

In the 1990s, the Academy changed its name to the American Academy of Hospice and Palliative Medicine, or AAHPM. Its present purposes include the recognition of palliative care and the management of terminal illness as a distinctive medical discipline; the accreditation of training programs in hospice care; and the support of further research in the field. Most members of the AAHPM believe that more work needs to be done to encourage primary care practitioners and other physicians to refer patients to hospices. A study published in 2003 found that a significant minority of family practitioners and internists have problems interacting with hospices and hospice staff.

Models of hospice care

Hospital- and home-based hospice care

According to the National Hospice and Palliative Care Organization (NHPCO), there are 3,139 hospice programs operating in the United States as of 2003, including Puerto Rico and Guam. In 1999, hospice programs in the United States cared for over 600,000 people, or 29% of those who died that year. The Centers for Disease Control and Prevention (CDC) National Center for Health Statistics gives the following figures for combined home health and hospice care for 2000, the latest year for which data are available: number of home health and hospice care agencies, 11,400; number of patients served by these agencies, 1.5 million.

There are several successful hospice models as of 2003. At present, over 90% of hospice care is delivered in patients' homes, although the hospice programs that direct the care may be based in medical facilities. Home health agency programs care for patients at home, while hospital-based programs may devote a special wing, unit, or floor to hospice patients. Freestanding independent for-profit hospices devoted exclusively to care of the terminally ill also exist. Most hospice programs offer a combination of services, both inpatient and home-care programs, allowing patients and families to make use of either or both as needed.

One limitation of present hospice models is that most require physicians to estimate that the patient is not likely to live longer than six months. This requirement is related to criteria for **Medicare** eligibility. Unfortunately, it means that terminal patients with uncertain prognoses are often excluded from hospice care, as well as homeless and isolated patients. In addition, pressures to contain health care costs have continued to shorten the length of patients' stays in hospices. The shortened time span in turn has made it more difficult for pastoral and psychological counselors to help patients and their families deal effectively with the complex issues of terminal illness.

Another present issue for hospice care in the United States and Western Europe is the need for greater understanding of concepts of death in Eastern cultures. For example, the Chinese notion of a "good death" differs from Western perspectives in several significant ways. As more people from non-Western cultures emigrate to North America and eventually seek hospice care, their concepts of **death and dying** will need to be incorporated in hospice care programs.

Specialized hospices

The first hospices in the United States and the United Kingdom were established to meet the needs of adult patients; in the early 1970s, only four hospice programs in the United States accepted children. In 1977, a dying eight-year-old boy was denied admission to a hospice because of his age. This incident prompted the foundation of hospices just for children as well as the admission of children to other hospices. As of 2003, almost all hospices in the United States and Canada will accept children as patients.

In 1995, the National Prison Hospice Association (NPHA) was founded to meet the needs of prison inmates with terminal illness. Prisoners are much more resistant than most people to accept the fact that they are dying because death in prison feels like the ultimate defeat. Many are also very suspicious of medical care given within the prison, and are afraid to appear weak and vulnerable in the eyes of other inmates. A surprisingly high number refuse to take pain medications for this reason. The NPHA trains medical professionals and volunteers to understand the special needs of terminally ill prison inmates and their families.

Hospices in the United States and Canada accept patients from all religious backgrounds and faith traditions. Hospices that are related to a specific religion or spiritual tradition, however, often offer special facilities or programs to meet the needs of patients from that tradition. For example, there are Jewish hospices that observe the dietary regulations, Sabbath rituals, and other parts of Halakhah (Jewish religious law). Hospices related to the various branches of Christianity have a priest or pastor on call for prayer, administration of the sacraments, and similar religious observances. The Zen Hospice Project sponsors programs reflecting the Buddhist tradition of compassionate service and maintains a 24-bed unit within the Laguna Honda Hospice in California.

Aspects of hospice care

General environment

The goal of freestanding hospices and even hospital-based programs is the creation and maintenance of warm, comfortable, home-like environments. Rather than the direct overhead lights found in hospitals, these hospices use floor and table lamps along with natural light to convey a sense of brightness and uplift. Some hospices offer music or art programs and fill patient rooms with original artwork and fresh flowers.

Pain management and psychospiritual support

Along with acceptance of death as a natural part of the life cycle, health professionals who refer patients to or work in hospice programs must become especially well informed about pain management and symptom control. This knowledge is necessary because about 80% of hospice patients are dying of end-stage cancer. In traditional medical settings, pain medication is often administered when the patient requests it. Hospice care approaches pain control quite differently. By administering pain medication regularly, before it is needed, hospice caregivers hope to prevent pain from recurring. Since addiction and other long-term consequences of narcotic **analgesics** are not a concern for the terminally ill, hospice caregivers focus on relieving pain as completely and effectively as possible. Hospice patients often have **patient-controlled analgesia** (PCA) pumps that allow them to control their pain medication.

Symptom relief often requires more than simply using narcotic analgesia. Hospices consider the patient and family as the unit of care; "family" is broadly defined as embracing all persons who are close to the patient as well as blood relatives. Seeking to relieve physical, psychological, emotional, and spiritual discomfort, hospice teams rely on members of the clergy, pastoral counselors, social workers, psychiatrists, massage therapists, and trained volunteers to comfort patients and family members, in addition to the solace offered by nurses and physicians.

Since the patient and his or her family members are considered the unit of care, hospice programs continue to support families and loved ones after the patient's death. Grief and bereavement counseling as well as support groups offer opportunities to express and resolve emotional concerns and share them with others.

Complementary and alternative therapies

In addition to mainstream medicine, many hospices offer patients and families the opportunity to use complementary and alternative approaches to control symptoms and improve well being. Acupuncture, music therapy, pet therapy, bodywork, massage therapy, aromatherapy, Reiki (energy healing), Native American ceremonies, herbal treatments, and other non-Western practices may be used to calm and soothe patients and their families. A 2002 study of complementary and alternative therapies

---

KEY TERMS

Analgesic—A type of medication given to relieve pain.

Hospice—An approach for providing compassionate, palliative care to terminally ill patients and counseling or assistance for their families. The term may also refer to a hospital unit or freestanding facility devoted to the care of terminally ill patients.

Palliative—A type of care that is intended to relieve pain and suffering, but not to cure.

Patient-controlled analgesia (PCA)—An approach to pain management that allows the patient to control the timing of intravenous doses of analgesic drugs.

---

within hospice programs found that patients who received these treatments reported greater overall satisfaction with hospice care than those who did not.

Resources

BOOKS

Kübler-Ross, Elisabeth. *On Death and Dying.* New York: Macmillan, 1969.

Pelletier, Kenneth R., MD. *The Best Alternative Medicine,* Part I, Chapter 11, "Spirituality and Healing." New York: Simon & Schuster, 2002.

Rabow, Michael W., MD, Steven Z. Pantilat, MD, and Robert V. Brody, MD. "Care at the End of Life." In *Current Medical Diagnosis & Treatment 2001,* edited by Lawrence M. Tierney, Jr., MD, et al. New York: Lange Medical Books/McGraw-Hill, 2001.

Sheehan, Denise C., and Walter B. Forman. *Hospice and Palliative Care.* Boston, MA: Jones and Bartlett Publishers, 1996.

PERIODICALS

Demmer, C. and J. Sauer. "Assessing Complementary Therapy Services in a Hospice Program." *American Journal of Hospice and Palliative Care* 19 (September-October 2002): 306–314.

Mak, M. H. "Awareness of Dying: An Experience of Chinese Patients with Terminal Cancer." *Omega (Westport)* 43 (2001): 259–279.

Ogle, K., B. Mavis, and T. Wang. "Hospice and Primary Care Physicians: Attitudes, Knowledge, and Barriers." *American Journal of Hospice and Palliative Care* 20 (January-February 2003): 41–51.

Thomson, J. E. and M. R. Jordan. "Depth Oriented Brief Therapy: An Ideal Technique as Hospice Lengths-of-Stay Continue to Shorten." *Journal of Pastoral Care and Counseling* 56 (Fall 2002): 221–225.

ORGANIZATIONS

American Academy of Hospice and Palliative Medicine (AAHPM). 4700 West Lake Avenue, Glenview, IL 60025-1485. (847) 375-4712. <http://www.aahpm.org>.

Children's Hospice International (CHI). 901 North Pitt Street, Suite 230, Alexandria, VA 22314. (703) 684-0330 or (800) 2-4-CHILD. <http://www.chionline.org>.

Hospice Foundation of America. 2001 S Street NW, Suite 300, Washington, DC 20009. (800) 854-3402. <http://www.hospicefoundation.org>.

National Hospice and Palliative Care Organization (NHPCO). 1700 Diagonal Road, Suite 625, Alexandria, VA 22314. (703) 837-1500 or (800) 658-8898 (Helpline). <http://www.nhpco.org>.

National Institute for Jewish Hospice (NIJH). Cedars-Sinai Medical Center, 444 South San Vincente Blvd., Suite 601, Los Angeles, CA 90048. (800) 446-4448. <http://www.jewishla.org>.

National Prison Hospice Association (NPHA). P. O. Box 3769, Boulder, CO 80307-3769. (303) 544-5923. <http://www.npha.org>.

Zen Hospice Project. 273 Page Street, San Francisco, CA 94102. (415) 863-2910. <http://www.zenhospice.org>.

Barbara Wexler
Rebecca Frey, Ph.D.

Hospital-acquired infections

Definition

A hospital-acquired infection, also called a nosocomial infection, is an infection that first appears between 48 hours and four days after a patient is admitted to a hospital or other health-care facility.

Description

About 5–10% of patients admitted to acute care hospitals and long-term care facilities in the United States develop a hospital-acquired, or nosocomial, infection, with an annual total of more than one million people. Hospital-acquired infections are usually related to a procedure or treatment used to diagnose or treat the patient's initial illness or injury. The Centers for Disease Control (CDC) of the U.S. Department of Health and Human Services has shown that about 36% of these infections are preventable through the adherence to strict guidelines by health care workers when caring for patients. What can make these infections so troublesome is that they occur in people whose health is already compromised by the condition for which they were first hospitalized.

Hospital-acquired infections can be caused by bacteria, viruses, fungi, or parasites. These microorganisms may already be present in the patient's body or may come from the environment, contaminated hospital equipment, health care workers, or other patients. Depending on the causal agents involved, an infection may start in any part of the body. A localized infection is limited to a specific part of the body and has local symptoms. For example, if a surgical wound in the abdomen becomes infected, the area around the wound becomes red, hot, and painful. A generalized infection is one that enters the bloodstream and causes systemic symptoms such as fever, chills, low blood pressure, or mental confusion. This can lead to sepsis, a serious, rapidly progressive multi-organ infection, sometimes called blood poisoning, that can result in death.

Hospital-acquired infections may develop from the performance of surgical procedures; from the insertion of catheters (tubes) into the urinary tract, nose, mouth, or blood vessels; or from material from the nose or mouth that is aspirated (inhaled) into the lungs. The most common types of hospital-acquired infections are urinary tract infections (UTIs), ventilator-associated pneumonia, and surgical wound infections. The University of Michigan Health System reports that the most common sources of infection in their hospital are urinary catheters, central venous (in the vein) catheters, and endotrachial tubes (tubes going through the mouth into the stomach). Catheters going into the body allow bacteria to walk along the outside of the tube into the body where they find their way into the bloodstream. A study in the journal *Infection Control and Hospital Epidemiology* shows that about 24% of patients with catheters will develop catheter related infections, of which 5.2% will become bloodstream infections. Death has been shown to occur in 4–20% of catheter-related infections.

Causes

All hospitalized patients are at risk of acquiring an infection from their treatment or surgery. Some patients are at greater risk than others, especially young children, the elderly, and persons with compromised immune systems. The National Nosocomial Infection Surveillance System database compiled by the CDC shows that the overall infection rate among children in intensive care is 6.1%, with the primary causes being venous catheters and ventilator-associated pneumonia. The risk factors for hospital-acquired infections in children include parenteral nutrition (tube or intravenous feeding), the use of **antibiotics** for more than 10 days, use of invasive devices, poor postoperative status, and immune system dysfunction. Other risk factors that increase the opportunity for hospitalized adults and children to acquire infections are:

- a prolonged hospital stay
- severity of underlying illness
- compromised nutritional or immune status
- use of indwelling catheters
- failure of health care workers to wash their hands between patients or before procedures
- prevalence of antibiotic-resistant bacteria from the overuse of antibiotics

Any type of invasive (enters the body) procedure can expose a patient to the possibility of infection. Some common procedures that increase the risk of hospital-acquired infections include:

- urinary bladder catheterization
- respiratory procedures such as intubation or **mechanical ventilation**
- surgery and the dressing or drainage of surgical wounds
- gastric drainage tubes into the stomach through the nose or mouth
- intravenous (IV) procedures for delivery of medication, **transfusion**, or nutrition

Urinary tract infection (UTI) is the most common type of hospital-acquired infection and has been shown to occur after urinary catheterization. Catheterization is the placement of a catheter through the urethra into the urinary bladder to empty urine from the bladder; or to deliver medication, relieve pressure, or measure urine in the bladder; or for other medical reasons. Normally, a healthy urinary bladder is sterile, with no harmful bacteria or other microorganisms present. Although bacteria may be in or around the urethra, they normally cannot enter the bladder. A catheter, however, can pick up bacteria from the urethra and give them an easy route into the bladder, causing infection. Bacteria from the intestinal tract are the most common type to cause UTIs. Patients with poorly functioning immune systems or who are taking antibiotics are also at increased risk for UTI caused by a fungus called *Candida*. The prolonged use of antibiotics, which may reduce the effectiveness of the patient's own immune system, has been shown to create favorable conditions for the growth of this fungal organism.

Pneumonia is the second most common type of hospital-acquired infection. Bacteria and other microorganisms are easily introduced into the throat by treatment procedures performed to treat respiratory illnesses. Patients with chronic obstructive lung disease, for example, are especially susceptible to infection because of frequent and prolonged antibiotic therapy and long-term mechanical ventilation used in their treatment. The infecting microorganisms can come from contaminated equipment or the hands of health care workers as procedures are conducted such as respiratory intubation, suctioning of material from the throat and mouth, and mechanical ventilation. Once introduced through the nose and mouth, microorganisms quickly colonize the throat area. This means that they grow and form a colony, but have not yet caused an infection. Once the throat is colonized, it is easy for a patient to aspirate the microorganisms into the lungs, where infection develops that leads to pneumonia.

Invasive surgical procedures increase a patient's risk of getting an infection by giving bacteria a route into normally sterile areas of the body. An infection can be acquired from contaminated surgical equipment or from the hands of health care workers. Following surgery, the surgical wound can become infected from contaminated dressings or the hands of health-care workers who change the dressing. Other wounds can also become easily infected, such as those caused by trauma, burns, or pressure sores that result from prolonged bed rest or wheel chair use.

Many hospitalized patients need continuous medications, transfusions, or nutrients delivered into their bloodstream. An intravenous (IV) catheter is placed in a vein and the medications, blood components, or liquid nutritionals are infused into the vein. Bacteria from the surroundings, contaminated equipment, or health care workers' hands can enter the body at the site of catheter insertion. A local infection may develop in the skin around the catheter. The bacteria can also enter the blood through the vein and cause a generalized infection. The longer a catheter is in place, the greater the risk of infection.

Other hospital procedures that may put patients at risk for nosocomial infection are gastrointestinal procedures, obstetric procedures, and **kidney dialysis**.

Symptoms

Fever is often the first sign of infection. Other symptoms and signs of infection are rapid breathing, mental confusion, low blood pressure, reduced urine output, and a high white blood cell count. Patients with a UTI may have pain when urinating and blood in the urine. Symptoms of pneumonia may include difficulty breathing and inability to cough. A localized infection begins with swelling, redness, and tenderness on the skin or around a surgical wound or other open wound, which can progress rapidly to the destruction of deeper layers of muscle tissue, and eventually sepsis.

Diagnosis

An infection is suspected any time a hospitalized patient develops a fever that cannot be explained by the underlying illness. Some patients, especially the elderly, may not develop a fever. In these patients, the first signs of infection may be rapid breathing or mental confusion.

Diagnosis of a hospital-acquired infection is determined by:

- evaluation of symptoms and signs of infection

- examination of wounds and catheter entry sites for redness, swelling, or the presence of pus or an abscess

- a complete **physical examination** and review of underlying illness

- laboratory tests, including **complete blood count** (CBC) especially to look for an increase in infection-fighting white cells; **urinalysis**, looking for white cells or evidence of blood in the urinary tract; cultures of the infected area, blood, sputum, urine, or other body fluids or tissue to find the causative organism

- chest x ray may be done when pneumonia is suspected to look for the presence of white blood cells and other inflammatory substances in lung tissue

- review of all procedures performed that might have led to infection

Treatment

Cultures of blood, urine, sputum, other body fluids, or tissue are especially important in order to identify the bacteria, fungi, virus, or other microorganism causing the infection. Once the organism has been identified, it will be tested again for sensitivity to a range of antibiotics so that the patient can be treated quickly and effectively with an appropriate medicine to which the causative organism will respond. While waiting for these test results, treatment may begin with common broad-spectrum antibiotics such as penicillin, **cephalosporins**, **tetracyclines**, or erythromycin. More and more often, some types of bacteria are becoming resistant to these standard antibiotic treatments, especially when patients with chronic illnesses are frequently given antibiotic therapy for long periods of time. When this happens, a different, more powerful, and more specific antibiotic must be used to which the specific organism has been shown to respond. Two strong antibiotics that have been effective against resistant bacteria are vancomycin and imipenem, although some bacteria are developing resistance to these antibiotics as well. The prolonged use of antibiotics is also known to reduce the effectiveness of the patient's own immune system, sometimes becoming a factor in the development of infection.

Fungal infections are treated with antifungal medications. Examples of these are amphotericin B, nystatin, ketoconazole, itraconazole, and fluconazole.

Viruses do not respond to antibiotics. A number of antiviral drugs have been developed that slow the growth or reproduction of viruses, such as acyclovir, ganciclovir, foscarnet, and amantadine.

Prevention

Hospitals take a variety of steps to prevent nosocomial infections, including:

- Adopt an infection control program such as the one sponsored by the U.S. Centers for Disease Control (CDC), which includes quality control of procedures known to lead to infection, and a monitoring program to track infection rates to see if they go up or down.

- Employ an infection control practitioner for every 200 beds.

- Identify high-risk procedures and other possible sources of infection.

- Strict adherence to hand-washing rules by health care workers and visitors to avoid passing infectious microorganisms to or between hospitalized patients.

- Strict attention to aseptic (sterile) technique in the performance of procedures, including use of sterile gowns, gloves, masks, and barriers.

- Sterilization of all reusable equipment such as ventilators, humidifiers, and any devices that come in contact with the respiratory tract.

- Frequent changing of dressings for wounds and use of antibacterial ointments under dressings.

- Remove nasogastric (nose to stomach) and endotracheal (mouth to stomach) tubes as soon as possible.

- Use of an antibacterial-coated venous catheter that destroys bacteria before they can get into the blood stream.

- Prevent contact between respiratory secretions and health care providers by using barriers and masks as needed.

- Use of silver alloy-coated urinary catheters that destroy bacteria before they can migrate up into the bladder.

- Limitations on the use and duration of high-risk procedures such as urinary catheterization.

- Isolation of patients with known infections.

- Sterilization of medical instruments and equipment to prevent contamination.

- Reductions in the general use of antibiotics to encourage better immune response in patients and reduce the cultivation of resistant bacteria.

Resources
BOOKS
Andreoli, T. E., J. C. Bennet, C. C. Carpenter, and F. Plum. *Cecil Essentials of Medicine.* Philadelphia: W.B. Saunders Co., 1997.
Schaffer, S. D., et al. *Infection Prevention and Safe Practice.* New York: Mosby-Year Book, 1996.

ORGANIZATIONS

U.S. Center for Disease Control and Prevention (CDC). 1600 Clifton Road, Atlanta, GA 30333. 404-639-3311. <http://www.cdc.gov/health/disease.htm>.

OTHER

"Safer Hospital Stay, and Reducing Hospital-Born Infections." *Health Scout News,* 2003 [cited July 7, 2003]. <http://www.healthscout.com>.

Toni Rizzo
L. Lee Culvert

Hospital services

Definition

Hospital services is a term that refers to medical and surgical services and the supporting laboratories, equipment and personnel that make up the medical and surgical mission of a hospital or hospital system.

Purpose

Hospital services make up the core of a hospital's offerings. They are often shaped by the needs or wishes of its major users to make the hospital a one-stop or core institution of its local community or medical network. Hospitals are institutions comprising basic services and personnel—usually departments of medicine and surgery—that administer clinical and other services for specific diseases and conditions, as well as emergency services. Hospital services cover a range of medical offerings from basic health care necessities or training and research for major medical school centers to services designed by an industry-owned network of such institutions as health maintenance organizations (HMOs). The mix of services that a hospital may offer depends almost entirely upon its basic mission(s) or objective(s).

There are three basic types of hospitals in the United States: proprietary (for-profit) hospitals; nonprofit hospitals; and charity- or government-supported hospitals. The services within these institutions vary considerably, but are usually organized around the basic mission(s) or objective (s) of the institution:

• Proprietary hospitals. For-profit hospitals include both general and specialized hospitals, usually as part of a healthcare network like Humana or HCA, which may be corporately owned. The main objective of proprietary hospitals is to make a profit from the services provided.

• Teaching or community hospitals. These are hospitals that serve several purposes: they provide patients for the training or research of interns and residents; they also offer services to patients who are unable to pay for services, while attempting to maintain profitability. Nonprofit centers like the University of California at San Francisco (UCSF) or the Mayo Clinics combine service, teaching, and profitability without being owned by a corporation or private owner.

• Government-supported hospitals. This group includes tax-supported hospitals for counties, communities and cities with voluntary hospitals (community or charity hospitals) run by a board of citizen administrators who serve without pay. The main objective of this type of hospital is to provide health care for a community or geographic region.

Demographics

The total number of hospitals in the United States, including military and prison hospitals, is over 6,500. Of this total, approximately 3,000 are non-government-related nonprofit hospitals; almost 800 are investor-owned; and 1,156 are government (state, county, or local) hospitals.

Description

Over the past two decades, hospital services in the United States have declined markedly as a percentage of health care costs, from 43.5% in 1980 to 32.8% in 2000. This decline was due to shortened lengths of hospital stay, the move from inpatient to outpatient facilities for surgery, and a wave of hospital mergers in the 1990s that consolidated services and staff. Since 2001, however, spending on hospital care in the United States has been growing faster than other sectors of the economy as a result of increasing demand for hospital services. Forty percent of the rise in spending on hospital care is due to escalating costs for hospital services attributed to population growth, the aging of the general population, and growing discontent with the limitations imposed by managed care. In addition, new medical technologies have allowed hospitals to provide life-saving diagnostic and therapeutic alternatives that were unavailable in the 1990s.

At the same time that the use of hospital services is increasing nationwide, government support of hospital services with **Medicaid** and **Medicare** has been decreasing, putting pressure upon hospitals to treat the uninsured and make up for $21.6 billion in uncompensated care (year 2002). This trend has put pressure on for-profit, not-for-profit and teaching hospitals to provide a broader range of community services or such "low-end" services as mental health care, preventive health services, and general pediatric care. In addition, very recent changes in Federal laws governing the entry of hospitals into new markets—Certificate of Need laws—allow health care providers to offer new hospital services, resulting in the growth of ambulatory surgical centers, special tertiary surgery centers and specialty hospitals that treat a single major disease category. These legislative changes encourage the offering of "high-end" services that are increasingly demanded by consumers.

Hospital services define the core features of a hospital's organization. The range of services may be limited in such specialty hospitals as cardiovascular centers or cancer treatment centers, or very broad to meet the needs of the community or patient base, as in full service health maintenance organizations (HMOs), rural charity centers, urban health centers, or medical research centers. Hospital services are usually the most general in large urban areas or underserved rural areas, broadly encompassing many services ordinarily offered by other medical providers. The basic services that hospitals offer include:

- short-term hospitalization
- emergency room services
- general and specialty surgical services
- x ray/radiology services
- laboratory services
- blood services

HMO hospitals add a number of special and auxiliary services to the basic list, including:

- pediatric specialty care
- greater access to surgical specialists
- physical therapy and rehabilitation services
- prescription services
- home nursing services
- nutritional counseling
- mental health care
- family support services
- genetic counseling and testing
- social work or case management services
- financial services

Hospitals funded by state, regional, or local government, as well as charity hospitals and hospitals within research and teaching centers, are pressed by community needs to provide for the uninsured or underinsured with more basic services:

- primary care services
- mental health and drug treatment
- infectious disease clinics
- hospice care
- dental services
- translation and interpreter services

Diagnosis/Preparation

Most hospitals have extensive surgical services that include preoperative testing, which may include x-rays, **CT scans**, ultrasonography, blood tests, **urinalysis**, and/or an EKG. Medication counseling is offered for current patient prescriptions and how they should be taken during and after surgery. **Informed consent** forms are made available to patients, as well as patient advocate services for questions and assistance in understanding the consent form and similar documents. An anesthesiologist or an assistant discuss with the patient the patient's history of allergies, previous reactions to anesthesia and special precautions that will be taken. Intravenous medications are usually begun in the patient's room before surgery to relax the patient, with general anesthesia administered in the **operating room**.

Aftercare

According to the National Center for Health Statistics of the Centers for Disease Control and Prevention (CDC), 40 million inpatient surgical procedures were performed in the United States in 2000, followed closely by 31.5 million outpatient surgeries. The procedures that were performed most frequently included:

- digestive system: 12 million procedures
- musculoskeletal system: 7.4 million procedures
- cardiovascular system: 6.8 million procedures
- eye: 5.4 million procedures

Inpatient aftercare

After inpatient surgery, most patients are taken to a **recovery room** and monitored by nursing staff until they regain full consciousness. If there are complications or if the patient develops respiratory or cardiac problems, he or she is transferred to a surgical **intensive care unit** equipped to deal with acute needs. Intensive care units (ICU) are highly advanced facilities in which patients are monitored by special equipment that measures their heart rate, breathing, blood pressure, and blood oxygen level. Some patients require a respirator to breathe for them and additional intravenous lines to deliver medication and fluids. Once stabilized, patients are transferred to their hospital room.

After returning to the room, the patient is encouraged to sit up, start walking, and do as much as possible to return to a normal level of activity. Special diets may be provided, as well as pain-killing medications and **antibiotics** if needed. A respiratory therapist will usually visit the patient with breathing equipment intended to help the patient's lung function return to normal. A physical therapist may introduce the patient to an **exercise** program or to skills needed to manage with temporary or permanent physical limitations.

Discharge personnel help the patient plan to go home. Some hospitals follow up with an outpatient nurse or social worker service. Pharmaceutical services may be offered to fill take-home prescriptions without the requirement of visiting an outside pharmacy. Medical equipment, like wheelchairs or crutches and other durable equipment, may be provided by the hospital and then purchased by the patient for use at home.

Outpatient aftercare

Outpatient or ambulatory surgery services make up almost half of all surgeries in the United States as a result of advances in surgical equipment and technique that allow for laser treatments and other minimally invasive procedures. Outpatient procedures require comparatively little aftercare for the patient due to both the nature of the surgical procedure and the advantages of being able to use regional or local anesthesia. Aftercare in hospital outpatient clinics, **ambulatory surgery centers**, or office-based practices requires that patients recover from anesthetics in the facility. After the anesthetic has worn off, the patient is briefly monitored for complications and released to go home. Many surgical procedures now allow patients to go home after a short recovery period on the same day as the surgery, and benefit from minimal pain and a speedier recovery.

Morbidity and mortality rates

According to a health consumer organization, 98,000 people die each year in America's hospitals as a result of **medical errors**. In recent years, many hospitals have introduced special safeguards to cut down on the number of mistakes in medication and surgical services. Two new practices have been adopted by quality hospitals. Computerized order entries for medications cut down drastically on the number of misread prescriptions. The other innovation reduces the number of medical errors in intensive care units by using specially trained physicians—intensivists—in the unit. Hospitals that have introduced these patient safety features can be found on the Internet at conssumer health sites.

Proprietary hospitals generally offer more services and "high end" care than government or community hospitals, with teaching hospitals offering the most highly developed new procedures and techniques along with services for the poor and special populations. For-profit hospitals, however, do not have lower rates of morbidity or mortality in their delivery of hospital services. One study in 2000 published by General Internal Medicine found that patients at for-profit hospitals suffered two to four times more complications from surgery as well as delays in diagnosing and treating illness than did patients in nonprofit hospitals. Previous research has shown that death rates are 25% higher in proprietary hospitals than in teaching hospitals, and 6–7% higher in proprietary hospitals than in nonprofit institutions.

Resources

PERIODICALS

Birkmeyer, J. D., E. V. Finlayson, and C. M. Birkmeyer. "Volume Standards for High-Risk Surgical Procedures: Potential Benefits of the Leapfrog Initiative." *Surgery* 130 (September 2001): 415-422.

Relman, Arnold, MD. "Dr. Business." *The American Prospect* 8 (September 1, 1997).

ORGANIZATIONS

Accreditation Association for Ambulatory Health Care (AAAHC). 3201 Old Glenview Road, Suite 300, Wilmette, IL 60091-2992. (847) 853-6060. <www.aahc.org>.

American Hospital Association. One North Franklin, Chicago, IL 60606-3421. (312) 422-3000. <www.hospitalconnect.com>.

Joint Commission on Accreditation of Healthcare Organizations (JCAHO). One Renaissance Blvd., Oakbrook Ter-

KEY TERMS

Auxiliary hospital services—A term used broadly to designate such nonmedical services as financial services, birthing classes, support groups, etc. that are instituted in response to consumer demand.

Health maintenance organization (HMO)—A broad term that covers a variety of prepaid systems providing health care within a certain geographic area to all persons covered by the HMO's contract.

Intensivist—A physician who specializes in caring for patients in intensive care units.

Nonprofit hospitals—Hospitals that combine a teaching function with providing for uninsured within large, complex networks technically designated as nonprofit institutions. While the institution may be nonprofit, however, its services are allowed to make a profit.

Proprietary hospitals—Hospitals owned by private entities, mostly corporations, that are intended to make a profit as well as provide medical services. Most hospitals in health maintenance organizations and health networks are proprietary institutions.

Teaching hospitals—Hospitals whose primary mission is training medical personnel in collaboration with (or ownership by) a medical school or research center.

race, IL 60181. (630) 792-5000 or (630) 792-5085. <www.jcaho.org/>.

OTHER

Employee Benefits Research Institute (EBRI). *The Role of the Health Care Sector in the U.S. Economy.* <www.ebri.org/press/>.

HealthPages.com. *All Hospitals Are Not Created Equal.* <www.healthpages.com>.

HealthScope.com. *Hospitals.* <www.healthscope.com>.

Nancy McKenzie, PhD

Human leukocyte antigen test

Definition

The human leukocyte antigen (HLA) test, also known as HLA typing or tissue typing, identifies antigens on the white blood cells (WBCs) that determine tissue compatibility for organ transplantation (that is, histocompatibility testing). There are six loci on chromosome 6, where the genes that produce HLA antigens are inherited: HLA-A, HLA-B, HLA-C, HLA-DR, HLA-DQ, and HLA-DP.

Unlike most blood group antigens, which are inherited as products of two alleles (types of gene that occupy the same site on a chromosome), many different alleles can be inherited at each of the HLA loci. These are defined by antibodies (antisera) that recognize specific HLA antigens, or by DNA probes that recognize the HLA allele. Using specific antibodies, 26 HLA-A alleles, 59 HLA-B alleles, 10 HLA-C alleles, 26 HLA-D alleles, 22 HLA-DR alleles, nine HLA-DQ alleles, and six HLA-DP alleles can be recognized. This high degree of genetic variability (polymorphism) makes finding compatible organs more difficult than finding compatible blood for **transfusion**.

Purpose

HLA typing, along with ABO (blood type) grouping, is used to provide evidence of tissue compatibility. The HLA antigens expressed on the surface of the lymphocytes of the recipient are matched against those from various donors. Human leukocyte antigen typing is performed for kidney, bone marrow, liver, pancreas, and heart transplants. The probability that a transplant will be successful increases with the number of identical HLA antigens.

Graft rejection occurs when the immune cells (T-lymphocytes) of the recipient recognize specific HLA antigens on the donor's organ as foreign. The T-lymphocytes initiate a cellular immune response that result in graft rejection. Alternatively, T-lymphocytes present in the grafted tissue may recognize the host tissues as foreign and produce a cell-mediated immune response against the recipient. This is called graft versus host disease (GVHD), and it can lead to life-threatening systemic damage in the recipient. Human leukocyte antigen testing is performed to reduce the probability of both rejection and GVHD.

Typing is also used along with blood typing and DNA tests to determine the parentage (that is, for paternity testing). The HLA antigens of the mother, child, and alleged father can be compared. When an HLA antigen of the child cannot be attributed to the mother or the alleged father, then the latter is excluded as the father of the child.

A third use of HLA testing called linkage analysis is based on the region where the HLA loci are positioned, the major histocompatibility complex (MHC), which contains many other genes located very close to the HLA

Hydrocelectomy

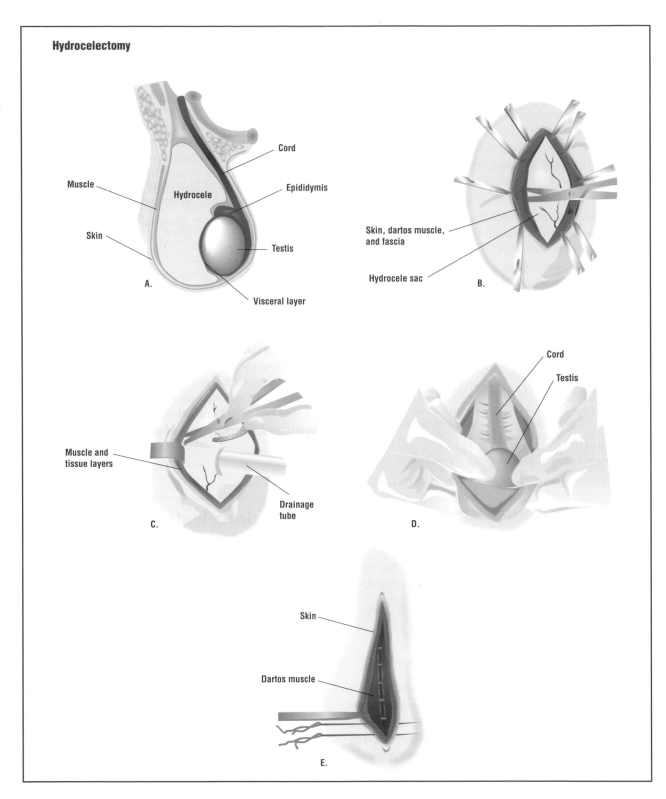

A hydrocele is a pocket of fluid inside a man's testicle (A). To remove it, the surgeon cuts through the skin and tissue layers (B), then drains the hydrocele with a tube (C). The hydrocele is opened completely (D), and skin and tissue layers are stitched (E). *(Illustration by GGS Inc.)*

Description

A hydrocele usually appears as a soft swelling in the membrane surrounding the testes. It is not usually painful and does not damage the testes. It typically occurs on one side only; only 7–10% occur on both sides of the scrotum. Inflammation is not usually present, although if the hydrocele occurs in conjunction with epididymitis (inflammation of the epididymis), the testes may be inflamed and painful. The main symptom of a hydrocele that occurs without epididymitis is scrotal swelling. As the hydrocele fills with fluid and grows, the scrotum itself gets larger. Some men may have pain or discomfort from the increased size of the scrotal mass. Hydroceles are usually congenital, found in a large percentage (80% or more) of male children and in 1% of adult males over 40.

The most common congenital hydrocele is caused by a failure of a portion of the testicular membrane (processus vaginalis, a membrane that descends with the testicles in the fetus) to close normally. This failure to close allows peritoneal (abdominal) fluid to flow into the scrotum. Although surgery is the usual treatment, it is not performed until the child is at least two years of age, giving the processus vaginalis sufficient time to close by itself. More than 80% of newborn boys are reported to have a patent (open) processus vaginalis, but it closes spontaneously in the majority of children before they are 12 months old. The processus is not expected to close spontaneously in children over 18 months.

In adults, hydroceles develop slowly, usually as a result either of a defect in the tunica vaginalis that causes overproduction of fluid, or as a result of blocked lymphatic flow that may be related to an obstruction in the spermatic cord. Hydroceles may also develop as a result of inflammation or infection of the epididymis; trauma to the scrotal area; or in association with cancerous tumors in the groin area. A hydrocele can occur at the same time as an inguinal hernia.

Hydroceles can be treated with aspiration or surgery. To aspirate the collected fluid, the doctor inserts a needle into the scrotum and directs it toward the hydrocele. Suction is applied to remove (aspirate) as much fluid as possible. While aspiration is usually successful, it is a temporary correction with a high potential for recurrence of the hydrocele. Aspiration may have longer-term success when certain medications are injected during the procedure (sclerotherapy). There is a higher risk of infection with aspiration than with surgery.

Generally, surgical repair of a hydrocele will eliminate the hydrocele and prevent recurrence. In adults, surgery is used to remove large or painful hydroceles. It is the preferred method of treatment for children over

---

WHO PERFORMS THE PROCEDURE AND WHERE IS IT PERFORMED?

A hydrocelectomy is performed in a hospital operating room or a one-day surgery center by a general surgeon or urologist.

---

two years of age. It is also standard practice to remove hydroceles that reoccur after aspiration.

Patients are given general anesthesia for hydrocele repair surgery. A hydrocelectomy is typically performed on an outpatient basis with no special precautions required. The extent of the surgery depends on whether other problems are present. If the hydrocele is uncomplicated, the doctor makes an incision directly into the scrotum. After the canal between the abdominal cavity and the scrotum is repaired, the hydrocele sac is removed, fluid is removed from the scrotum, and the incision is closed with sutures. If there are complications, such as the presence of an inguinal hernia, an incision is made in the groin area. This approach allows the doctor to repair the hernia or other complicating factors at the same time as correcting the hydrocele. Some surgeons use a minimally invasive laparoscopic approach to repair a hydrocele. The operation is performed through a tiny incision using a lighted, camera-tipped, tube-like instrument (laparoscope) that allows the passage of instruments for the repair while displaying images of the procedure on a monitor in the **operating room**.

Diagnosis

Diagnosis will begin with taking a careful history, including sexual history, recent injury, or illnesses, and observing signs and symptoms. Hydroceles can sometimes be diagnosed in the doctor's office by visual examination and palpation (touch). Hydroceles are distinguished from other testicular problems by transillumination (shining a light source through the hydrocele so that the tissue lights up) and ultrasound examinations of the area around the groin and scrotum.

Preparation

The patient will be given standard pre-operative blood and urine tests at some time prior to surgery. Before the operation, the physician or nurse will explain the procedure, the type of anesthesia to be used, and, in some cases, the need for a temporary drain to be inserted. The drain will be placed during surgery to reduce the chances of post-operative infection and fluid accumulation.

QUESTIONS TO ASK THE DOCTOR

- Why is this surgery necessary?
- How will it improve my condition (my child's condition)?
- Is surgery the only option for correction of this problem?
- How many times have you performed this surgery? What are the usual results?
- How will I (my child) feel after the surgery?
- How soon can I (my child) resume normal activities?

Aftercare

Immediately following surgery, the patient will be taken to a recovery area and checked for any undue bleeding from the incision. Body temperature and blood pressure will be monitored. Patients will usually go home the same day for a brief recovery period at home. Follow-up appointments are usually scheduled for several weeks after surgery so that the doctor can check the incision for healing and to be sure there is no infection. The patient may notice swelling for several months after the procedure; however, prolonged swelling, fever, or redness in the incision area should be reported to the surgeon immediately.

Risks

Hydrocelectomy is considered a safe surgery, with only a 2% risk of infection or complications. Injury to spermatic vessels can occur, however, and affect the man's fertility. As with all surgical procedures, reactions to anesthesia, bleeding from the surgical incision, and internal bleeding can also occur.

Normal results

Surgery usually corrects the hydrocele and the underlying defect completely; recurrence is rare. The long-term outlook is excellent. There may be swelling of the scrotum for up to a month. The adult patient is able to resume most activities within seven to 10 days, although heavy lifting and sexual activities may be delayed for up to six weeks. Children will be able to resume normal activities in four to seven days.

Morbidity and mortality rates

Chronic infection after surgical repair can increase morbidity. There are no instances reported of death following a hydrocele repair.

KEY TERMS

Aspiration—The process of removing fluids or gases from the body by suction.

Epididymis—A coiled segment of spermatic duct within the scrotum, attached to the back of the testis.

Epididymitis—Inflammation of the epididymis.

Inguinal hernia—An opening, weakness, or bulge in the lining tissue of the abdominal wall in the groin area, with protrusion of the large intestine.

Hydrocele—An accumulation of fluid in the membrane that surrounds the testes.

Scrotum—A pouch of skin containing the testes, epididymis, and portions of the spermatic cords.

Testis (plural, testes)—The male sex gland, held within the scrotum.

Transillumination—A technique in which the doctor shines a strong light through body tissues in order to examine an organ or structure.

Tunica vaginalis—A sac-like membrane covering the outer surface of the testes.

Alternatives

A hydrocele is most often a congenital defect that is commonly corrected surgically. There are no recommended alternatives and no known measures to prevent the occurrence of congenital hydroceles.

Resources

BOOKS

"Disorders of the Scrotum." Section 17, Chapter 219 in *The Merck Manual of Diagnosis and Therapy*, edited by Mark H. Beers, MD, and Robert Berkow, MD. Whitehouse Station, NJ: Merck Research Laboratories, 1999.

Sabiston, D. C., and H. K. Lyrly. *Essentials of Surgery.* Philadelphia, PA: W. B. Saunders Co., 1994.

Way, Lawrence W., MD. *Current Surgical Diagnosis and Treatment*, 10th ed. Stamford, CT: Appleton & Lange, 1994.

PERIODICALS

Chalasani, V., and H. H. Woo. "Why Not Use a Small Incision to Treat Large Hydroceles?" *ANZ Journal of Surgery* 72 (August 2002): 594-595.

Fearne, C. H., M. Abela, and D. Aquilina. "Scrotal Approach for Inguinal Hernia and Hydrocele Repair in Boys." *European Journal of Pediatric Surgery* 12 (April 2002): 116-117.

ORGANIZATIONS

National Kidney and Urologic Diseases Information Clearinghouse. 31 Center Drive, MSC 2560, Building 31, Room

9A-04, Bethesda, MD 20892-2560. (800) 891-5390. <www.niddk.nih.gov>.

OTHER

Dolan, James P., MD. *Hydrocele Repair.* <www.kernanhospital. com>.

Men's Health Topics. *Hydrocele.* <www.uro.com/hydrocele. htm>.

L. Lee Culvert

Hypophysectomy

Definition

Hypophysectomy, or hypophysis, is the surgical removal of the pituitary gland.

Purpose

The pituitary gland is a small, oval-shaped endocrine gland about the size of a pea located in the center of the brain above the back of the nose. Its major role is to produce hormones that regulate growth and metabolism in the body. Removing this important gland is a drastic step that is usually taken in the case of cancers or tumors that resist other forms of treatment, especially craniopharyngioma tumors. Hypophysectomy may also be performed to treat Cushing's syndrome, a hormonal disorder caused by prolonged exposure of the body's tissues to high levels of the hormone cortisol, in most cases associated with benign tumors called pituitary adenomas. The goal of the surgery is to remove the tumor and try to partially preserve the gland.

Demographics

Craniopharyngiomas account for less than 5% of all brain tumors. Half of all craniopharyngiomas occur in children, with symptoms most often appearing between the ages of five and ten. Cushing's syndrome is relatively rare in the United States, most commonly affecting adults aged 20–50. An estimated 10–15 of every million people are affected each year. However, the Pituitary Network Association reports that one out of every five people worldwide has a pituitary tumor. The earliest study was performed in 1936, by Dr. R. T. Costello of the Mayo Foundation who found pituitary tumors in 22.4% of his studied population with statistics not having changed significantly since that time.

Description

There are several surgical approaches to the pituitary. The surgeon chooses the best one for the specific procedure. The pituitary lies directly behind the nose, and access through the nose or the sinuses is often the best approach. A **craniotomy** (opening the skull) and lifting the frontal lobe of the brain will expose the delicate neck of the pituitary gland. This approach works best if tumors have extended above the pituitary fossa (the cavity in which the gland lies).

Surgical methods using new technology have made other approaches possible. Stereotaxis is a three-dimensional aiming technique using x rays or scans for guidance. Instruments can be placed in the brain with pinpoint accuracy through tiny holes in the skull. These instruments can then manipulate brain tissue, either to destroy it or remove it. Stereotaxis is also used to direct radiation with similar precision using a gamma knife. Access to some brain lesions can be gained through the blood vessels using tiny tubes and wires guided by x rays.

Diagnosis/Preparation

A patient best prepares for a hypophysectomy by keeping as healthy and relaxed as possible. Informed surgical consent is always required.

The patient is first seen for evaluation of pituitary functions by the treatment team. An MRI scan of the pituitary gland is performed and the patient is seen by a neurosurgeon in an outpatient clinic or at the hospital to assess whether hypophysectomy is suitable.

The patient checks into the hospital the day before surgery and undergoes blood tests, chest x rays, or an electrocardiogram to assess anesthesia fitness. Four to five sticks are attached on buttons on the forehead and marked for a special MRI scan. These buttons and scan help the neurosurgeon to accurately remove the pituitary tumor using sophisticated visualization computers. The patient is visited by the anesthesiologist (the physician who puts the patient to sleep for the operation) and he is asked to fast (nothing to eat or drink) from midnight before the day of surgery. If the hypophysectomy is performed through the nose, the patient is advised to practice breathing through the mouth as the nose will be packed after the surgery.

Aftercare

The operation takes about one to two hours, following which the patient is taken to the recovery area for about two hours before returning to the neurosurgical ward. The following postoperative measures are the normally taken:

• The patient's nose is packed to stop bleeding.

• There may be a dressing on a site of incision in the abdominal wall or thigh if a graft was necessary.

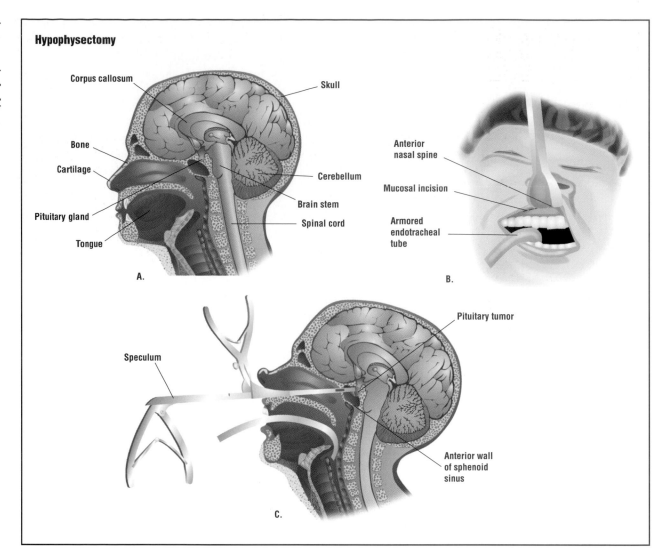

Hypophysectomy

Corpus callosum

Skull

Bone

Cartilage

Cerebellum

Brain stem

Pituitary gland

Spinal cord

Tongue

A.

Anterior nasal spine

Mucosal incision

Armored endotracheal tube

B.

Speculum

Pituitary tumor

Anterior wall of sphenoid sinus

C.

Hypophysectomy is a procedure to access and remove the pituitary gland (A). To access it, an incision is made beneath the patient's upper lip to enter the nasal cavity (B). A speculum is inserted, and special forceps are used to remove the pituitary tumor (C). *(Illustration by GGS Inc.)*

- A drip is attached to the hand and foot and other lines are attached to monitor the heart and breathing.

- A urinary catheter is placed to monitor fluid output.

- The patient has an oxygen mask.

Once in the ward, the patient is allowed to eat and drink the same night, after he or she has recovered from the anesthesia. If fluid intake and output are in balance, the drip and urinary catheter are removed the next morning. The nurses continue to monitor the amount of fluid taken and the amount of urine passed by the patient for a few days. The blood is usually tested the day following surgery. The nasal pack stays for about four days. Once the nasal pack is removed, patients commonly experience moisture coming through the nose and blood-stained mucus occurs frequently. If all is well, patients are usually discharged the following day. There are no sutures to be removed. The sutures in the nose are degradable and the graft site is usually glued together. Patients are advised not to blow their nose or insert anything in the nose.

Risks

The risks associated with hypophysectomy are numerous. Procedures are painstakingly selected to minimize risk and maximize benefit. A special risk associated with surgery on the pituitary is the risk of destroying the entire gland and leaving the entire endocrine system without regulation. Historically, this was the purpose of hypophysectomy, when the procedure was performed to

698

suppress hormone production. After the procedure, the endocrinologist, a physician specializing in the study and care of the endocrine system, would provide the patient with all the hormones needed. Patients with no pituitary function did and still do quite well because of the available hormone replacements.

Other specific risks include;

- Hypopituitarism. Following surgery, if the pituitary gland has normal activity, it may become underactive and the patient may require hormone replacement therapy. Diabetes insipidus (DI) (excessive thirst and excessive urine) is not uncommon in the first few days following surgery. The vast majority of cases clear but a small number of individuals need hormone replacement.

- Cerebrospinal fluid (CSF) leakage. CSF leakage from the nose can occur following hypophysectomy. If it happens during surgery, the surgeon will repair the leak immediately. If it occurs after the nasal pack is removed, it may require diversion of the CSF away from the site of surgery or repair.

- Infection. Infection of the pituitary gland is a serious risk as it may result in abscess formation or meningitis. The risk is very small and the vast majority of cases are treatable by **antibiotics**. Patients are usually given antibiotics during surgery and until the nasal pack is removed.

- Bleeding. Nasal bleeding or bleeding in the cavity of the tumor after removal may occur. If the latter occurs it may lead to deterioration of vision as the visual nerves are very close to the pituitary region.

- Nasal septal perforation. This may also occur during surgery, although it is very uncommon.

- Visual impairment. A very rare occurrence, but still a risk.

- Incomplete **tumor removal**. Tumors may not be completely removed, due to their attachment to vital structures.

Normal results

In the past, complete removal of the pituitary was the goal for cancer treatment. Nowadays, removal of tumors with preservation of the gland is the goal of the surgery.

Morbidity and mortality rates

A follow-up study performed at the Massachusetts General Hospital and involving 349 patients who underwent surgery for pituitary adenomas between 1978 and 1985 documented 39 deaths over the 13 year follow-up. The primary cause of death was cardiovascular (27.5%) followed by non-pituitary cancer (20%) and pituitary-related deaths (20%). When compared to the population at large, the primary cause of death was also cardiovascular (40%), followed by cancers (at 24%).

Alternatives

Surgery is a common treatment for pituitary tumors. For patients in whom hypophysectomy has failed or who are not suitable candidates for surgery, radiotherapy is another possible treatment. Radiation therapy uses high-energy x rays to kill cancer cells and shrink tumors. Radiation to the pituitary gland is given over a six-week period, with improvement occurring in 40–50% of adults and up to 80% of children. It may take several months or years before patients feel better from radiation treatment

Hypophysectomy

KEY TERMS

Adenoma—A benign tumor in which cells form recognizable glandular structures.

Cerebrospinal fluid (CSF)—A clear, colorless fluid that contains small quantities of glucose and protein. CSF fills the ventricles of the brain and the central canal of the spinal cord.

Craniotomy—A surgical incision into the skull.

Cushing's disease—A disease in which too many hormones called glucocorticoids are released into the blood. This causes fat to build up in the face, back, and chest, and the arms and legs to become very thin. Other symptoms include excessive blood sugar levels, weak muscles and bones, a flushed face, and high blood pressure.

Electrocardiogram—A recording of the electrical activity of the heart on a moving strip of paper.

Endocrine system—Group of glands and parts of glands that control metabolic activity. The pituitary, thyroid, adrenals, ovaries, and testes are all part of the endocrine system.

Hormone—A chemical made in one place that has effects in distant places in the body. Hormone production is usually triggered by the pituitary gland.

Hypopituitarism—A medical condition where the pituitary gland produces lower than normal levels of its hormones.

Magnetic resonance imaging (MRI)—A special imaging technique used to visualize internal structures of the body, particularly the soft tissues.

Metabolism—The sum of all the physical and chemical processes required to maintain life and also the transformation by which energy is made available for the uses of the body.

Pituitary gland—A small, oval-shaped endocrine gland situated at the base of the brain in the fossa (depression) of the sphenoid bone. Its overall role is to regulate growth and metabolism. The gland is divided into the posterior and anterior pituitary, each responsible for the production of its own unique hormones.

Pituitary tumors—Tumors found in the pituitary gland. Most pituitary tumors are benign, meaning that they grow very slowly and do not spread to other parts of the body.

alone. However, the combination of radiation and the drug mitotane (Lysodren) has been shown to help speed recovery. Mitotane suppresses cortisol production and lowers plasma and urine hormone levels. Treatment with mitotane alone can be successful in 30–40% of patients. Other drugs used alone or in combination to control the production of excess cortisol are aminoglutethimide, metyrapone, trilostane, and ketoconazole.

Resources

BOOKS

Biller, Beverly M. K. and Gilbert H. Daniels. "Neuroendocrine Regulation and Diseases of the Anterior Pituitary and Hypothalamus." In *Harrison's Principles of Internal Medicine,* edited by Anthony S. Fauci, et al. New York: McGraw-Hill, 1997.

Jameson, J. Larry. "Anterior Pituitary." In *Cecil Textbook of Medicine,* edited by J. Claude Bennett and Fred Plum. Philadelphia: W. B. Saunders, 1996.

Youmans, Julian R. "Hypophysectomy." In *Neurological Surgery.* Philadelphia: W. B. Saunders, 1990.

PERIODICALS

Buchinsky, F. J., T. A. Gennarelli, S. E. Strome, D. G. Deschler, and R. E. Hayden. "Sphenoid Sinus Mucocele: A Rare Complication of Transsphenoidal Hypophysectomy." *Ear Nose Throat Journal* 80 (December 2001): 886–888.

Davis, K. T., I. McDuffie, L. A. Mawhinney, and S. A. Murray. "Hypophysectomy Results in a Loss of Connexin Gap Junction Protein from the Adrenal Cortex." *Endocrine Research* 26 (November 2000): 561–570.

Dizon, M. N. and D. L. Vesely. "Gonadotropin-secreting Pituitary Tumor Associated with Hypersecretion of Testosterone and Hypogonadism After Hypophysectomy." *Endocrinology Practice* 3 (May-June 2002): 225–231.

Nakagawa, T., M. Asada, T. Takashima, and K. Tomiyama. "Sellar Reconstruction After Endoscopic Transnasal Hypophysectomy." *Laryngoscope* 11 (November 2001): 2077–2081.

Volz, J., U. Heinrich, and S. Volz-Koster. "Conception and Spontaneous Delivery After Total Hypophysectomy." *Fertility and Sterility* 77 (March 2002): 624–625.

ORGANIZATIONS

American Association of Clinical Endocrinologists (AACE). 1000 Riverside Ave., Suite 205, Jacksonville, FL 32204. (904) 353-7878. <http://www.aace.com/>.

American Association of Endocrine Surgeons (AAES). Metro-Health Medical Center, H920, 2500 MetroHealth Drive, Cleveland, OH 44109-1908. (216) 778-4753. <http://www.endocrinesurgeons.org/gt;.

OTHER

"Hypophysectomy." University of Dundee. Tayside University Hospitals. 2000 [cited June 24, 2003]. <http://www.dundee.ac.uk/medicine/tayendoweb/images/hypophysectomy.htm>

J. Ricker Polsdorfer, MD
Monique Laberge, Ph.D.

Hypospadias repair

Definition

Hypospadias repair refers to a group of surgical approaches used to correct or reconstruct parts of the external genitalia and urinary tract related to a displaced meatus, or opening of the urethra. The urethra is the passageway that carries urine from the bladder to the outside of the body. Hypospadias is the medical term for a birth defect in which the urethra opens on the underside of the penis (in boys) or into the vagina (in girls). The word hypospadias comes from two Greek words that mean underneath and rip or tear, because severe forms of hypospadias in boys look like large tears in the skin of the penis.

Hypospadias is one of the most common congenital abnormalities in males. It was described in the first and second centuries A.D. by Celsus, a Roman historian of medicine, and Galen, a Greek physician. The first attempt to correct hypospadias by surgery was made in 1874 by Duplay, a French surgeon; as of 2003, more than 200 different procedures for the condition have been reported in the medical literature.

Hypospadias repair is, however, controversial because it is genital surgery. Some people regard it as unnecessary interference with a child's body and a traumatic experience with psychological consequences extending into adult life. Others maintain that boys with untreated hypospadias are far more likely than those who have had surgery to develop fears about intimate relationships and sexuality. There is little information about the emotional aftereffects of hypospadias repair on girls.

Purpose

Although there are several different surgical procedures used at present to correct hypospadias depending on its severity, all have the following purposes:

• To permit emptying of the bladder standing up. The abnormal location of the urethral meatus on the underside of the penis forces many boys to void urine sitting down, which leads to anxiety about using public restrooms or otherwise being seen undressed by other males.

• To correct a condition associated with hypospadias known as chordee. Chordee, which comes from the French cordée, which means tied or corded, is a condition in which the penis bends downward during an erection. This curving or bending makes it difficult to have normal sexual intercourse as an adult.

• To prevent urinary tract infections (UTIs). It is common in hypospadias for the urethral meatus to be stenotic, or abnormally narrowed. A stenotic urethra increases the risk of frequent UTIs.

• To lower the risk of developing testicular cancer. Hypospadias has been identified as a risk factor for developing testicular cancer after adolescence.

• To confirm the boy's sexual identity by improving the outward appearance of the penis. The external genitals of babies with severe hypospadias may look ambiguous at birth, causing stress for the parents about their child's gender identity.

Demographics

Hypospadias is much more common in males than in females. In Canada and the United States, the incidence of hypospadias in boys is estimated to be 1:250 or 1:300 live births. In girls, the condition is very rare, estimated at 1:500,000 live births. One troubling phenomenon is the reported doubling of cases of hypospadias in both Europe and North America since the 1970s without any obvious explanation. According to a recent press release from the U.S. Centers for Disease Control and Prevention (CDC), data from two surveillance systems monitoring birth defects in the United States show that the rate of hypospadias rose from 36 per 10,000 male births in 1968 to 80 per 10,000 male births in 1993. In addition to the increase in the number of cases reported, the proportion of severe cases has also risen, which means that the numerical increase cannot be explained as the result of better reporting.

The severity of hypospadias is defined according to the distance of the urethral opening from its normal location at the tip of the penis. In mild hypospadias, which is sometimes called coronal/glandular hypospadias, the urethral opening is located on the shaft of the penis just below the glans. In mild to moderate hypospadias, the opening is located further down the shaft of the penis toward the scrotum. In severe hypospadias, which is also called penoscrotal hypospadias, the urethral opening is located on the scrotum. About 80–85% of hypospadias are classified as mild; 10–15% as mild to moderate; and 3–6% as severe.

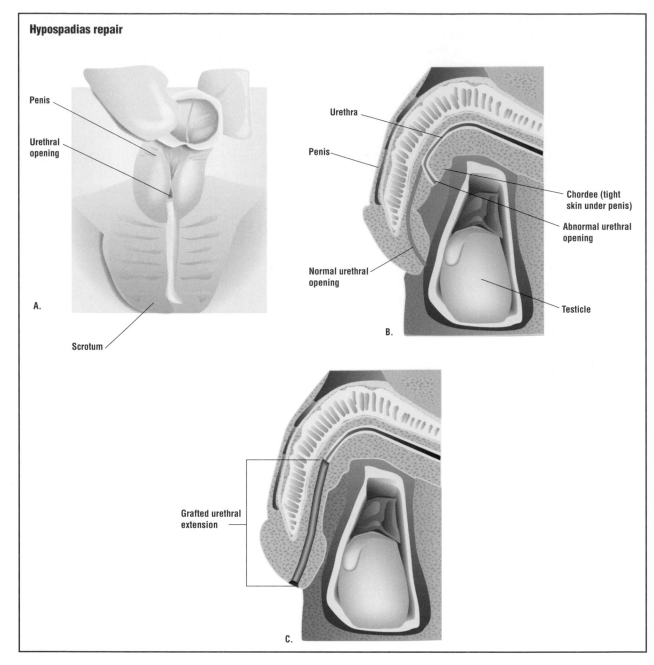

Hypospadias repair

A.

Penis

Urethral opening

Scrotum

B.

Urethra

Penis

Normal urethral opening

Chordee (tight skin under penis)

Abnormal urethral opening

Testicle

C.

Grafted urethral extension

In hypospadias, the urethral opening is at the base of the penis, instead of the tip (A). Tissue grafts are used to create an extension for the urethra (C) and alleviate the tight skin, or chordee, on the underside of the penis. *(Illustration by GGS Inc.)*

Although the causes of hypospadias are not yet fully understood, the condition is thought to be the end result of a combination of factors. The following have been associated with an increased risk of hypospadias:

• Genetic inheritance. Hypospadias is known to run in families; a boy with hypospadias has a 28% chance of having a male relative with the condition.

• Genetic disorders. Hypospadias is found in boys with a deletion on human chromosome 4p, also known as

Wolf-Hirschhorn syndrome; and in persons with a variety of intersex conditions related to chromosomal abnormalities. Several different genetic mutations responsible for a deficiency in 5-alpha reductase, an enzyme needed to convert testosterone to a stronger androgen needed for urethral development, have been found in boys with hypospadias.

• Low birth weight. Several studies in the United Kingdom as well as in the United States have shown that male infants with hypospadias weigh less and are smaller at birth than controls. It is thought that these low measurements are markers of fetal androgen dysfunction.

- Drugs taken by the mother during pregnancy. Diethylstilbestrol (DES), a synthetic hormone that was prescribed for many women between 1938 and 1971 to prevent miscarriage, has been associated with an increased risk of stenosis of the urethral meatus as well as hypospadias in the sons of women who took the medication. Boys born to mothers addicted to cocaine also have an abnormally high rate of hypospadias.

- Environmental contamination. One proposal for explaining the rising rate of hypospadias and other birth defects in males is the so-called endocrine disruptor hypothesis. Many pesticides, fungicides, and other environmental pollutants contain estrogenic or anti-androgenic substances that interfere with the normal androgen pathways in embryonic tissue development—in birds and other animals as well as in humans.

- Assisted reproduction. A study done in Baltimore of children who were conceived through in vitro fertilization (IVF) between 1988 and 1992 found that the incidence of hypospadias among the males was five times that of male infants in a control group.

With regard to ethnic and racial differences in the American population, the CDC reports that Caucasians have the highest rates of hypospadias, Hispanics have the lowest, and African Americans have intermediate rates. Other studies have found that hypospadias is more common in males of Jewish or Italian descent than in other ethnic groups.

Description

Correction of hypospadias in boys

The specific surgical procedure used depends on the severity of the hypospadias. The objectives of surgery always include widening the urethral meatus; correcting chordee, if present; reconstructing the missing part of the urethra; and making the external genitalia look as normal as possible. Most repair procedures take between one-and-a-half and three hours, and are performed under general anesthesia. Mild hypospadias can be corrected in a one-step procedure known as a meatal advancement and glanduloplasty, or MAGPI. In a MAGPI procedure, the opening of the urethra is moved forward and the head of the penis is reshaped. More severe hypospadias can also be corrected in one operation, which involves degloving the penis (separating the skin from the shaft) in order to cut the bands of tissue that cause chordee, and constructing a new urethra that will reach to the tip of the penis. The spe-

cific technique of reconstruction is usually decided in the **operating room**, when the surgeon can determine how much tissue will be needed to make the new urethra. In some cases, tissue must be taken from the inner arm or the lining of the mouth. In a few cases, the repair may require two or three stages spaced several months apart.

There is some remaining disagreement among professionals regarding the best age for hypospadias repair in boys. Most surgeons think the surgery should be done between 12 and 18 months of age, on the ground that gender identity is not fully established prior to toilet training and the child is less likely to remember the operation. Some doctors, however, prefer to wait until the child is about three years old, particularly if the repair involves extensive reconstruction of the urethra.

Recent advances in hypospadias repair include the use of tissue glues and other new surgical adhesives that speed healing and reduce the risk of fistula formation. In addition, various synthetic materials are being tested for their suitability in constructing artificial urethras, which would reduce the risk of complications related to **skin grafting**.

Correction of hypospadias in girls

The most common surgical technique for correcting hypospadias in girls is construction of a new urethra that opens to the outside of the body rather than emptying into the vagina. Tissue is taken from the front wall of the vagina for this purpose.

Diagnosis/Preparation

Diagnosis

The diagnosis of hypospadias in boys is often made at the time of delivery during the newborn examination. The condition may also be diagnosed before birth by ultrasound; according to a group of Israeli researchers, ultrasound images of severe hypospadias resemble the outline of a tulip flower. Ultrasound is also used prior to surgical repair to check for other abnormalities, as about 18% of boys with hypospadias also have cryptorchidism (undescended testicles), inguinal hernia, or defects of the upper urinary tract.

Hypospadias in girls may not be discovered for several months after birth because of the difficulty of examining the vagina in newborn females.

Preparation

Male infants with hypospadias should not be circumcised as the foreskin may be needed for tissue grafting during repair of the hypospadias.

Some surgeons prescribe small doses of male hormones to be given to the child in advance to increase the size of the penis and improve blood supply to the area. The child may also be given a mild sedative immediately before surgery to minimize memories of the procedure.

Aftercare

Short-term aftercare

Many anesthesiologists provide a penile nerve block to minimize the child's postoperative discomfort. Dressings are left in place for about four days. The surgeon places a stent, which is a short plastic tube held in place with temporary stitches, or a catheter to keep the urethra open. The patient is usually given a course of **antibiotics** to reduce the risk of infection until the dressings and the stent or catheter are removed, usually 10–14 days after surgery.

The child should be encouraged to drink plenty of fluids after returning home in order to maintain an adequate urinary output. Periodic follow-up tests of adequate urinary flow are typically scheduled for three weeks, three months, and 12 months after surgery.

Long-term aftercare

Boys who have had any type of hypospadias repair should be followed through adolescence to exclude the possibility of chronic inflammation or scarring of the urethra. In some cases, psychological counseling may also be necessary.

Risks

In addition to the risks of bleeding and infection that are common to all operations under general anesthesia, there are some risks specific to hypospadias repair:

- Wound dehiscence. Dehiscence means that the incision splits apart or reopens. It is treated by a follow-up operation.
- Bladder spasms. These are a reaction to the presence of a urinary catheter, and are treated by giving medications to relax the bladder muscles.
- Fistula formation. A fistula is an abnormal opening that forms between the reconstructed urethra and the skin. Most fistulae that form after hypospadias surgery close by themselves within a few months. The remainder can be closed surgically.
- Recurrent chordee. This complication requires another operation to remove excess fibrous tissue.
- Urethral stenosis. Narrowing of the urethral opening after surgery is treated by dilating the meatus with urethral probes.

Normal results

Hypospadias repair in both boys and girls has a high rate of long-term success. In almost all cases, the affected children are able to have normal sexual intercourse as adults, and almost all are able to have children.

Morbidity and mortality rates

Surgical repair of hypospadias has a fairly high short-term complication rate:

- leakage of urine from the area around the urethral meatus: 3–9%
- formation of a fistula: 0.6–23% for one-stage procedures; 2–37% for two-stage procedures
- urethral stenosis: 8.5%
- persistent chordee: less than 1%

KEY TERMS

Androgen—Any substance that promotes the development of masculine characteristics in a person. Testosterone is one type of androgen; others are produced in the adrenal glands located above the kidneys.

Chordee—A condition associated with hypospadias in which the penis bends downward during erections.

Circumcision—The removal of the foreskin of the penis.

Cryptorchidism—A developmental disorder in which one or both testes fail to descend from the abdomen into the scrotum before birth. It is the most common structural abnormality in the male genital tract.

Degloving—Separating the skin of the penis from the shaft temporarily in order to correct chordee.

Dehiscence—A separation or splitting apart. In hypospadias repair, dehiscence refers to the reopening of the tip of the penis or the coming apart of the entire repair.

Fistula (plural, fistulae)—An abnormal passage between two internal organs or between an internal organ and the surface of the body. The formation of fistulae is one of the possible complications of hypospadias repair.

Glans—The cap-shaped structure at the end of the penis.

Hernia—The protrusion of a loop or piece of tissue through an incision or abnormal opening in other tissues.

Inguinal—Referring to the groin area.

Meatus—The medical term for the opening of the urethra.

Stenotic—Abnormally narrowed. The urethral meatus is often stenotic in patients with uncorrected hypospadias.

Stent—A thin plastic tube inserted temporarily to hold the urethra open following hypospadias repair.

Testosterone—The major male sex hormone, produced in the testes.

Urethra—The canal or passageway that carries urine from the bladder to the outside of the body.

Urology—The branch of medicine that deals with disorders of the urinary tract in both males and females, and with the genital organs in males.

Alternatives

There are no medical treatments for hypospadias as of 2003. The only alternative to surgery in childhood is postponement until the child is old enough to decide for himself (or herself) about genital surgery.

See also Orchiectomy.

Resources

BOOKS

"Congenital Anomalies: Chromosomal Abnormalities." Section 19, Chapter 261 in *The Merck Manual of Diagnosis and Therapy*, edited by Mark H. Beers, MD, and Robert Berkow, MD. Whitehouse Station, NJ: Merck Research Laboratories, 1999.

"Congenital Anomalies: Renal and Genitourinary Defects." Section 19, Chapter 261 in *The Merck Manual of Diagnosis and Therapy*, edited by Mark H. Beers, MD, and Robert Berkow, MD. Whitehouse Station, NJ: Merck Research Laboratories, 1999.

"Drugs in Pregnancy." Section 18, Chapter 249 in *The Merck Manual of Diagnosis and Therapy*, edited by Mark H. Beers, MD, and Robert Berkow, MD. Whitehouse Station, NJ: Merck Research Laboratories, 1999.

"Infertility: Sperm Disorders." Section 18, Chapter 245 in *The Merck Manual of Diagnosis and Therapy*, edited by Mark H. Beers, MD, and Robert Berkow, MD. Whitehouse Station, NJ: Merck Research Laboratories, 1999.

PERIODICALS

Baskin, Laurence S. "Hypospadias, Anatomy, Embryology, and Reconstructive Techniques." *Brazilian Journal of Urology* 26 (November-December 2000): 621–629.

Fredell, L., et al. "Complex Segregation Analysis of Hypospadias." *Human Genetics* 111 (September 2002): 231–234.

Greenfield, S. P. "Two-Stage Repair for Proximal Hypospadias: A Reappraisal." *Current Urology Reports* 4 (April 2003): 151–155.

Hendren, W. H. "Construction of a Female Urethra Using the Vaginal Wall and a Buttock Flap: Experience with 40 Cases." *Journal of Pediatric Surgery* 33 (February 1998): 180–187.

Hughes, I. A., et al. "Reduced Birth Weight in Boys with Hypospadias: An Index of Androgen Dysfunction?" *Archives of Disease in Childhood: Fetal and Neonatal Edition* 87 (September 2002): F150–F151.

Klip, H., et al. "Hypospadias in Sons of Women Exposed to Diethylstilbestrol in Utero: A Cohort Study." *Lancet* 359 (March 30, 2002): 1102–1107.

Meizner, I., et al. "The 'Tulip Sign': A Sonographic Clue for In-Utero Diagnosis of Severe Hypospadias." *Ultrasound in Obstetrics and Gynecology* 19 (March 2002): 250–253.

ORGANIZATIONS

American Academy of Pediatrics (AAP). 141 Northwest Point Boulevard, Elk Grove Village, IL 60007. (847) 434-4000. <http://www.aap.org>.

American Board of Urology (ABU). 2216 Ivy Road, Suite 210, Charlottesville, VA 22903. (434) 979-0059. <http://www.abu.org>.

American Urological Association (AUA). 1120 North Charles Street, Baltimore, MD 21201. (410) 727-1100. <http://www.auanet.org>.

Society for Pediatric Urology (SPU). C/o HealthInfo, 870 East Higgins Road, Suite 142, Schaumburg, IL 60173. <http://www.spuonline.org>.

OTHER

Centers for Disease Control Press Release. *Hypospadias Trends in Two U.S. Surveillance Systems* [cited April 24, 2003]. <http://www.cdc.gov/od/oc/media/pressrel/hypospad.htm>.

Gatti, John M., Andrew Kirsch, and Howard M. Snyder III. "Hypospadias." *eMedicine.* January 31, 2003 [cited April 25, 2003]. <http://www.emedicine.com/PED/topic1136.htm>.

Santanelli, Fabio and Francesca R. Grippaudo. "Urogenital Reconstruction, Penile Hypospadias." *eMedicine.* November 6, 2002 [cited April 24, 2003]. <http://www.emedicine.com/plastic/topic495.htm>.

Silver, Richard I. "Recent Research Topics in Hypospadias." *Society for Pediatric Urology Newsletter* 1 (October 1999). <http://www.kids-urology.com/HypospadiasResearch.html>.

Rebecca Frey, Ph.D.

Hysterectomy

Definition

Hysterectomy is the surgical removal of all or part of the uterus. In a total hysterectomy, the uterus and cervix are removed. In some cases, the fallopian tubes and ovaries are removed along with the uterus, which is a hysterectomy with bilateral **salpingo-oophorectomy**. In a subtotal hysterectomy, only the uterus is removed. In a radical hysterectomy, the uterus, cervix, ovaries, oviducts, lymph nodes, and lymph channels are removed. The type of hysterectomy performed depends on the reason for the procedure. In all cases, menstruation permanently stops and a woman loses the ability to bear children.

Purpose

The most frequent reason for hysterectomy in American women is to remove fibroid tumors, accounting for 30% of these surgeries. Fibroid tumors are non-cancerous (benign) growths in the uterus that can cause pelvic, low back pain, and heavy or lengthy menstrual periods. They occur in 30–40% of women over age 40, and are three times more likely to be present in African-American women than in Caucasian women. Fibroids do not need to be removed unless they are causing symptoms that interfere with a woman's normal activities.

Treatment of endometriosis is the reason for 20% of hysterectomies. The endometrium is the lining of the uterus. Endometriosis occurs when the cells from the endometrium begin growing outside the uterus. The outlying endometrial cells respond to the hormones that control the menstrual cycle, bleeding each month the way the lining of the uterus does. This causes irritation of the surrounding tissue, leading to pain and scarring.

Twenty percent of hysterectomies are done because of heavy or abnormal vaginal bleeding that cannot be linked to any specific cause and cannot be controlled by other means. Another 20% are performed to treat prolapsed uterus, pelvic inflammatory disease, or endometrial hyperplasia, a potentially pre-cancerous condition.

About 10% of hysterectomies are performed to treat cancer of the cervix, ovaries, or uterus. Women with cancer in one or more of these organs almost always have the organ(s) removed as part of their cancer treatment.

Demographics

Hysterectomy is the second most common operation performed on women in the United States. About 556,000 of these surgeries are done annually. By age 60, approximately one out of every three American women will have had a hysterectomy. It is estimated that 30% of hysterectomies are unnecessary.

The frequency with which hysterectomies are performed in the United States has been questioned in recent years. It has been suggested that a large number of hysterectomies are performed unnecessarily. The United States has the highest rate of hysterectomies of any country in the world. Also, the frequency of this surgery varies across different regions of the United States. Rates are highest in the South and Midwest, and are higher for African-American women. In recent years, although the number of hysterectomies performed has declined, the number of hysterectomies performed on younger women aged 30s and 40s is increasing, and 55% of all hysterectomies are performed on women ages 35–49.

Hysterectomy (abdominal)

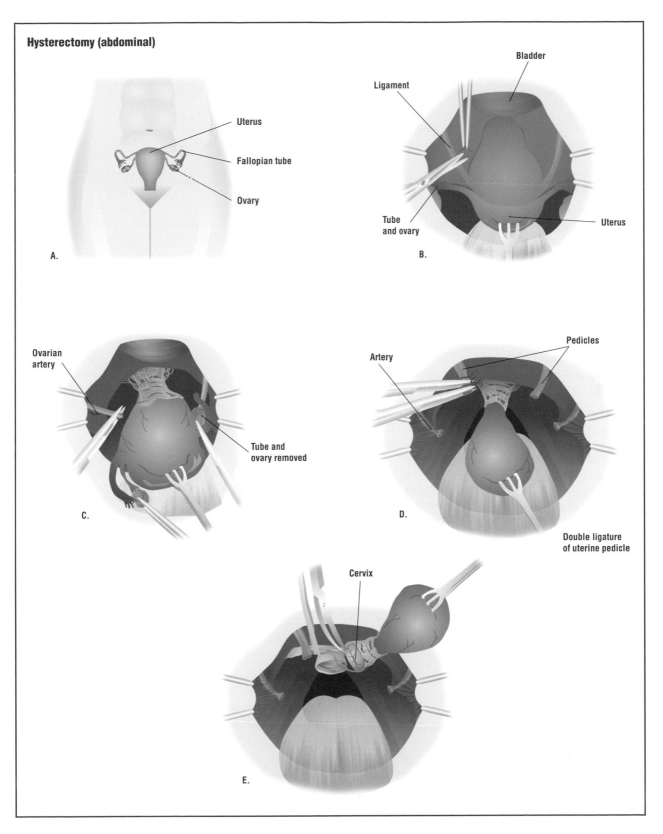

In a hysterectomy, the reproductive organs are accessed through a lower abdominal incision or laparoscopically (A). Ligaments and supporting structures called pedicles connecting the uterus to surrounding organs are severed (B). Arteries to the uterus are severed (C). The uterus, fallopian tubes, and ovaries are removed (D and E). *(Illustration by GGS Inc.)*

Description

A hysterectomy is classified according to what structures are removed during the procedure and what method is used to remove them.

Total hysterectomy

A total hysterectomy, sometimes called a simple hysterectomy, removes the entire uterus and the cervix. The ovaries are not removed and continue to secrete hormones. Total hysterectomies are usually performed in the case of uterine and cervical cancer. This is the most common kind of hysterectomy.

In addition to a total hysterectomy, a procedure called a bilateral salpingo-oophorectomy is sometimes performed. This surgery removes the ovaries and the fallopian tubes. Removal of the ovaries eliminates the main source of the hormone estrogen, so menopause occurs immediately. Removal of the ovaries and fallopian tubes is performed in about one-third of hysterectomy operations, often to reduce the risk of ovarian cancer.

Subtotal hysterectomy

If the reason for the hysterectomy is to remove uterine fibroids, treat abnormal bleeding, or relieve pelvic pain, it may be possible to remove only the uterus and leave the cervix. This procedure is called a subtotal hysterectomy (or partial hysterectomy), and removes the least amount of tissue. The opening to the cervix is left in place. Some women believe that leaving the cervix intact aids in their achieving sexual satisfaction. This procedure, which used to be rare, is now performed more frequently.

Subtotal hysterectomy is easier to perform than a total hysterectomy, but leaves a woman at risk for cervical cancer. She will still need to get yearly Pap smears.

Radical hysterectomy

Radical hysterectomies are performed on women with cervical cancer or endometrial cancer that has spread to the cervix. A radical hysterectomy removes the uterus, cervix, above part of the vagina, ovaries, fallopian tubes, lymph nodes, lymph channels, and tissue in the pelvic cavity that surrounds the cervix. This type of hysterectomy removes the most tissue and requires the longest hospital stay and a longer recovery period.

Methods of hysterectomy

There are two ways that hysterectomies can be performed. The choice of method depends on the type of hysterectomy, the doctor's experience, and the reason for the hysterectomy.

ABDOMINAL HYSTERECTOMY. About 75% of hysterectomies performed in the United States are abdominal hysterectomies. The surgeon makes a 4–6-in (10–15-cm) incision either horizontally across the pubic hair line from hip bone to hip bone or vertically from navel to pubic bone. Horizontal incisions leave a less noticeable scar, but vertical incisions give the surgeon a better view of the abdominal cavity. The blood vessels, fallopian tubes, and ligaments are cut away from the uterus, which is lifted out.

Abdominal hysterectomies take from one to three hours. The hospital stay is three to five days, and it takes four to eight weeks to return to normal activities.

The advantages of an abdominal hysterectomy are that the uterus can be removed even if a woman has internal scarring (adhesions) from previous surgery or her fibroids are large. The surgeon has a good view of the abdominal cavity and more room to work. Also, surgeons tend to have the most experience with this type of hysterectomy. The abdominal incision is more painful than with vaginal hysterectomy, and the recovery period is longer.

VAGINAL HYSTERECTOMY. With a vaginal hysterectomy, the surgeon makes an incision near the top of the vagina. The surgeon then reaches through this incision to cut and tie off the ligaments, blood vessels, and fallopian tubes. Once the uterus is cut free, it is removed through the vagina. The operation takes one to two hours. The hospital stay is usually one to three days, and the return to normal activities takes about four weeks.

The advantages of this procedure are that it leaves no visible scar and is less painful. The disadvantage is that it is more difficult for the surgeon to see the uterus and surrounding tissue. This makes complications more common. Large fibroids cannot be removed using this technique. It is very difficult to remove the ovaries during a vaginal hysterectomy, so this approach may not be possible if the ovaries are involved.

Vaginal hysterectomy can also be performed using a laparoscopic technique. With this surgery, a tube containing a tiny camera is inserted through an incision in the navel. This allows the surgeon to see the uterus on a video monitor. The surgeon then inserts two slender instruments through small incisions in the abdomen and uses them to cut and tie off the blood vessels, fallopian tubes, and ligaments. When the uterus is detached, it is removed though a small incision at the top of the vagina.

This technique, called laparoscopic-assisted vaginal hysterectomy, allows surgeons to perform a vaginal hysterectomy that might otherwise be too difficult. The hospital stay is usually only one day. Recovery time is about two weeks. The disadvantage is that this operation is relatively new and requires great skill by the surgeon.

Any vaginal hysterectomy may have to be converted to an abdominal hysterectomy during surgery if complications develop.

Diagnosis/Preparation

Before surgery the doctor will order blood and urine tests. The woman may also meet with the anesthesiologist to evaluate any special conditions that might affect the administration of anesthesia. On the evening before the operation, the woman should eat a light dinner and then have nothing to eat or drink after midnight.

Aftercare

After surgery, a woman will feel some degree of discomfort; this is generally greatest in abdominal hysterectomies because of the incision. Hospital stays vary from about two days (laparoscopic-assisted vaginal hysterectomy) to five or six days (abdominal hysterectomy with bilateral salpingo-oophorectomy). During the hospital stay, the doctor will probably order more blood tests.

Return to normal activities such as driving and working takes anywhere from two to eight weeks, again depending on the type of surgery. Some women have emotional changes following a hysterectomy. Women who have had their ovaries removed will probably start hormone replacement therapy.

Risks

Hysterectomy is a relatively safe operation, although like all major surgery it carries risks. These include unanticipated reaction to anesthesia, internal bleeding, blood clots, damage to other organs such as the bladder, and post-surgery infection.

Other complications sometimes reported after a hysterectomy include changes in sex drive, weight gain, constipation, and pelvic pain. Hot flashes and other symptoms of menopause can occur if the ovaries are removed. Women who have both ovaries removed and who do not take estrogen replacement therapy run an in-

QUESTIONS TO ASK THE DOCTOR

- Why is a hysterectomy recommended for my particular condition?
- What type of hysterectomy will be performed?
- What alternatives to hysterectomy are available to me?
- Will I have to start hormone replacement therapy?

creased risk for heart disease and osteoporosis (a condition that causes bones to be brittle). Women with a history of psychological and emotional problems before the hysterectomy are likely to experience psychological difficulties after the operation.

As in all major surgery, the health of the patient affects the risk of the operation. Women who have chronic heart or lung diseases, diabetes, or iron-deficiency anemia may not be good candidates for this operation. Heavy smoking, obesity, use of steroid drugs, and use of illicit drugs add to the surgical risk.

Normal results

Although there is some concern that hysterectomies may be performed unnecessarily, there are many conditions for which the operation improves a woman's quality of life. In the Maine Woman's Health Study, 71% of women who had hysterectomies to correct moderate or severe painful symptoms reported feeling better mentally, physically, and sexually after the operation.

Morbidity and mortality rates

The rate of complications differs by the type of hysterectomy performed. Abdominal hysterectomy is associated with a higher rate of complications (9.3%), while the overall complication rate for vaginal hysterectomy is 5.3%, and 3.6% for laparoscopic vaginal hysterectomy. The risk of death from hysterectomy is about one in every 1,000 women. The rates of some of the more commonly reported complications are:

- excessive bleeding (hemorrhaging): 1.8–3.4%
- fever or infection: 0.8–4.0%
- accidental injury to another organ or structure: 1.5–1.8%

Alternatives

Women for whom a hysterectomy is recommended should discuss possible alternatives with their doctor and consider getting a **second opinion**, since this is major surgery with life-changing implications. Whether an alternative is appropriate for any individual woman is a decision she and her doctor should make together. Some alternative procedures to hysterectomy include:

- Embolization. During uterine artery embolization, interventional radiologists put a catheter into the artery that leads to the uterus and inject polyvinyl alcohol particles right where the artery leads to the blood vessels that nourish the fibroids. By killing off those blood vessels, the fibroids have no more blood supply, and they die off. Severe cramping and pain after the procedure is common, but serious complications are less than 5% and the procedure may protect fertility.

- **Myomectomy**. A myomectomy is a surgery used to remove fibroids, thus avoiding a hysterectomy. Hysteroscopic myomectomy, in which a surgical hysteroscope (telescope) is inserted into the uterus through the vagina, can be done on an outpatient basis. If there are large fibroids, however, an abdominal incision is required. Patients typically are hospitalized for two to three days after the procedure and require up to six weeks recovery. Laparoscopic myomectomies are also being done more often. They only require three small incisions in the abdomen, and have much shorter hospitalization and recovery times. Once the fibroids have been removed, the surgeon must repair the wall of the uterus to eliminate future bleeding or infection.

- Endometrial ablation. In this surgical procedure, recommended for women with small fibroids, the entire lining of the uterus is removed. After undergoing endometrial ablation, patients are no longer fertile. The uterine cavity is filled with fluid and a hysteroscope is inserted to provide a clear view of the uterus. Then, the lining of the uterus is destroyed using a laser beam or electric voltage. The procedure is typically done under anesthesia, although women can go home the same day as the surgery. Another newer procedure involves using a balloon, which is filled with superheated liquid and inflated until it fills the uterus. The liquid kills the lining, and after eight minutes the balloon is removed.

- Endometrial resection. The uterine lining is destroyed during this procedure using an electrosurgical wire loop (similar to endometrial ablation).

Resources

PERIODICALS

Kovac, S. Robert. "Hysterectomy Outcomes in Patients with Similar Indications." *Obstetrics & Gynecology* 95, no. 6 (June 2000): 787–93.

ORGANIZATIONS

American Cancer Society. 1599 Clifton Rd., NE, Atlanta, GA 30329-4251. (800) 227-2345. <http://www.cancer.org>.
American College of Obstetricians and Gynecologists. 409 12th St., SW, P.O. Box 96920, Washington, DC 20090-6920. <http://www.acog.org>.
National Cancer Institute. Building 31, Room 10A31, 31 Center Drive, MSC 2580, Bethesda, MD 20892-2580. (800) 422-6237. <http://www.nci.nih.gov>.

OTHER

Bachmann, Gloria. "Hysterectomy." *eMedicine*. May 3, 2002 [cited March 13, 2003]. <http://www.emedicine.com/med/topic3315.htm>.
Bren, Linda. "Alternatives to Hysterectomy: New Technologies, More Options." *Food and Drug Administration*. October 29, 2001 [cited March 13, 2003]. <http://www.fda.gov/fdac/features/2001/601_tech.html>.

Debra Gordon
Stephanie Dionne Sherk

Hysteroscopy

Definition

Hysteroscopy enables a physician to look through the vagina and neck of the uterus (cervix) to inspect the cavity of the uterus with an instrument called a hysteroscope. Hysteroscopy is used as both a diagnostic and a treatment tool.

Purpose

Diagnostic hysteroscopy can be used to help determine the cause of infertility, dysfunctional uterine bleeding, and repeated miscarriages. It can also help locate polyps and fibroids, as well as intrauterine devices (IUDs).

The procedure is also used to investigate and treat gynecological conditions, often done instead of or in addition to performing a dilation and curettage (D&C). A D&C is a surgical procedure that expands the cervical canal (dilation) so that the lining of the uterus can be scraped (curettage). A D&C can be used to take a sample of the lining of the uterus for analysis. However, hysteroscopy has advantages over a D&C because the doctor can take tissue samples of specific areas and view any fibroids, polyps, or structural abnormalities. In addition, small fibroids and polyps may be removed via the hysteroscope (in combination with other instruments that are inserted through canals in the hysteroscope), thus avoiding more invasive and complicated open surgery. This approach is also used to remove IUDs that have become embedded in the wall of the uterus.

Demographics

There is no research available to indicate that hysteroscopy is performed more or less frequently on any subset of the female population.

Description

The hysteroscope is an extremely thin telescope-like instrument that looks like a lighted tube. The modern hysteroscope is so thin that it can fit through the cervix with only minimal or no dilation.

Before inserting the hysteroscope, the doctor administers an anesthetic. Once it has taken effect, the doctor dilates the cervix slightly, and then inserts the hysteroscope through the cervix to reveal the inside of the uterus. Ordinarily, the walls of the uterus are touching each other. In order to get a better view, the uterus may be inflated with carbon dioxide gas or fluid. Hysteroscopy takes approximately 30 minutes.

Treatment involving the use of hysteroscopy is usually performed as a short-stay hospital procedure with regional or general anesthesia. Tiny **surgical instruments** may be inserted through the hysteroscope to remove polyps or fibroids. A small sample of tissue lining the uterus is often removed for examination, especially if the patient has experienced any abnormal bleeding.

Diagnosis/Preparation

If the procedure is performed under general anesthesia, the patient should have nothing to eat or drink after

midnight the night before the procedure. Routine lab tests may be ordered if the procedure is performed in a hospital. Occasionally, a mild sedative is administered to help the patient relax. The patient is asked to empty her bladder. She is then placed in position (usually in a special chair that tilts back) and the vagina is cleansed. Usually, a local anesthetic is administered around the cervix, although a regional anesthetic that blocks nerves connected to the pelvic region or a general anesthetic may be required for some patients.

Aftercare

It is normal to experience light bleeding for one to two days after surgical hysteroscopy. Mild cramping or pain is common after operative hysteroscopy, but usually diminishes within eight hours. If carbon dioxide gas was used, the resulting discomfort usually subsides within 24 hours.

Risks

Diagnostic hysteroscopy rarely causes complications. The primary risk is infection. Prolonged bleeding may follow a surgical hysteroscopy to remove a growth. Another complication is perforation of the uterus, bowel, or bladder, caused by over-forceful advancement of the hysteroscope. An infrequent but dangerous complication is increased fluid absorption from the uterus into the bloodstream. Keeping track of the amount of fluid used during the procedure can minimize this complication. Surgery under general anesthesia poses the additional risks typically associated with this type of anesthesia.

The procedure is not performed on women with acute pelvic inflammatory disease (PID) due to the potential of exacerbating the condition. Hysteroscopy should be scheduled after menstrual bleeding has ended and before ovulation to avoid a potential interruption of a new pregnancy.

Patients should notify their health care provider if, after the hysteroscopy, they develop any of the following symptoms:

- abnormal discharge
- heavy bleeding
- fever over 101°F (38.3°C)
- severe lower abdominal pain

Normal results

Normal hysteroscopy reveals a healthy uterus with no fibroids or other growths. Abnormal results include uterine fibroids, polyps, or a septum (an extra fold of tissue down the center of the uterus). Sometimes, precancerous or malignant growths are discovered.

Morbidity and mortality rates

The rate of complications during diagnostic hysteroscopy is very low, about 0.01%. Surgical hysteroscopy is associated with a higher number of complications. Perforation of the uterus occurs in 0.8% of procedures and excess bleeding in 1.2–3.5% of cases. Death as a result of hysteroscopy occurs at a rate of 2.4 per 100,000 procedures performed.

Alternatives

A laparoscope (an instrument with a video camera inserted through the abdominal wall) may be used to visualize the outside of the uterus or perform a surgical procedure on the pelvic organs. **Laparoscopy** and hys-

teroscopy are sometimes performed simultaneously to maximize their diagnostic capabilities.

Resources

BOOKS
Pagana, Kathleen D., and Timothy J. Pagana. *Diagnostic Testing and Nursing Implications.* 5th edition. St. Louis: Mosby, 1999.

PERIODICALS
Murdoch, J. A., and T. J. Gan. "Anesthesia for Hysteroscopy." *Anesthesiology Clinics of North America* 19, no. 1 (March 2001): 125–40.

Neuwirth, R. S. "Special Article: Hysteroscopy and Gynecology: Past, Present, and Future." *Journal of American Association of Gynecology Laparoscopy* 8, no. 2 (May 2001): 193–8.

ORGANIZATIONS
American College of Obstetricians and Gynecologists. 409 12th St., S.W., P.O. Box 96920, Washington, DC 20090-6920. <http://www.acog.org/>.

OTHER
Gordon, A. G. "Complications of Hysteroscopy." *Practical Training and Research in Gynecologic Endoscopy.* February 17, 2003 [cited March 13, 2003]. <http://www.gfmer.ch/Books/Endoscopy_book/Ch24_Complications_hyster.html>.

Maggie Boleyn, RN, BSN
Stephanie Dionne Sherk

Ibuprophen *see* **Nonsteroidal anti-inflammatory drugs**

ICU *see* **Intensive care unit**

ICU equipment *see* **Intensive care unit equipment**

Ileal conduit surgery

Definition

There are many surgical techniques for urinary diversion surgery. They fall into two categories: continent diversion and conduit diversion. In continent diversion, also known as continent catheterizable stomal reservoir, a separate rectal reservoir for urine is created, which allows evacuation from the body. In conduit diversion, or orthotopic urethral anastomotic procedure, an intestinal stoma or conduit for release of urine is created in the abdominal wall so that a catheter or ostomy can be attached for the release of urine. An ileal conduit is a small urine reservoir that is surgically created from a small segment of bowel. Both techniques are forms of reconstructive surgery to replace the bladder or bypass obstructions or disease in the bladder so that urine can pass out of the body. Both procedures have been used for years and should be considered for all appropriate patients. Ileal conduit surgery, the easiest of the reconstructive surgeries, is the gold standard by which other surgical techniques, both continent and conduit, have been compared as the techniques have advanced over the decades.

Purpose

The bladder creates a reservoir for the liquid wastes created by the kidneys as a result of the ability of these organs to filter and retain glucose, salts, and minerals that the body needs. When the bladder must be removed; or becomes diseased, injured, obstructed, or develops leak points; the release of urinary wastes from the kidneys becomes impaired, endangering the kidneys with an overburden of poisons. Reasons for disabling the urinary bladder are: cancer of the bladder; neurogenic sources of bladder dysfunction; bladder sphincter detrusor overactivity that causes continual urge incontinence; chronic inflammatory diseases of the bladder; tuberculosis; and schistosomiasis, which is an infestation of the bladder by parasites, mostly occurring Africa and Asia. Radical **cystectomy**, removal of the bladder, is the predominant treatment for cancer of the bladder, with radiation and chemotherapy as other alternatives. In both cases, urinary diversion is often necessitated, either due to the whole or partial removal of the bladder or to damage done by radiation to the bladder.

Demographics

Urinary diversion has a long history and, over the last two decades, has developed new techniques for urinary tract reconstruction to preserve renal function and to increase the quality of life. A number of difficulties had to be solved for such progress to take place. Clean intermittent catherization by the patient became possible in the 1980s, and many patients with loss of bladder function were able to continue to have urine release through the use of catheters. However, it soon became clear that catherization left a residue that cumulatively, and over time, increased the risk of infection, which subsequently decreased kidney function through reflux, or backup, of urine into the kidneys. A new way had to be found. With the advent of surgical anatomosis (the grafting of vascularizing tissue for the repair and expansion of organ function) as well as with the ability to include a flap-type of valve to prevent backup, bladder reconstructive surgery that allowed for protection of the kidneys became possible.

Description

Ileal conduit surgery consists of open abdominal surgery that proceeds in the following three stages:

- Isolating the ileum, which is the last section of small bowel. The segment used is about 5.9–7.8 in (15–20 cm) in length.

- The segment is then anastomosized, or grafted, to the ureters with absorbable sutures.

- A stoma, or opening in skin, is created on the right side of the abdomen.

- The other end of the bowel segment is attached to the stoma, which drains into a ostomy bag.

Stents are used to bypass the surgical site and divert urine externally, ensuring that the anastomotic site has adequate healing time. Continent surgeries are more extensive than the ileal conduit surgery and are not described here. Both types of surgery require an extensive hospitalization with careful monitoring of the patient for infections, removal of stents placed in the bowel during surgery, and removal of catheters.

Diagnosis/Preparation

Ileal conduit surgery is recommended depending on what conditions are being treated; whether the urinary diversion is immediately necessary; for the relief of pain or discomfort; or for relatively healthy individuals or individuals with terminal illness. Three major decisions that must be made by the physician and patient include:

- The type of surgery to restore bladder function: either by sending urine through the ureters to a new repository fashioned in the rectum, or by creating a conduit for the removal of the urine out through the stomach wall and into a permanent storage pouch, or ostomy outside the body.

- The type of material out of which to fashion the reservoir or conduit.

- Where to place the stoma outlet for patient use.

Recent research has shown there is little difference in infection rates or in renal deterioration between the conduit surgical techniques and the continent techniques. The patient's preference becomes important as to which type of surgery and resulting procedures for urination

they want. Of course, some patients, unable to conduct catheterization due to debilitating diseases like multiple sclerosis or neurological injuries, should be encouraged to have the reservoir or continent procedures.

Materials for fashioning continent channels have included sections of the appendix, stomach, ileum and cecum of the intestines, and for the reservoir, sigmoid and ureter tissues, usually with an anti-refluxing mechanism to maximize continence. A segment of the ileum is often preferred, unless the tissue has received radiation. In this case, other tissue must be used. Ileum is preferred because the ileal tissue of the intestines accommodates larger urine volume at lower pressure.

Many urinary diversion procedures are performed in conjunction with surgery for recurrent cancer or complications of pelvic radiation. Fistula development and repeated repair as well as ureteral obstruction also are reasons to have the surgery. If the surgery is considered because of cancer, the physician and the patient need to discuss how appropriate the surgery is for cure or for relieving pain. Highly relevant are the patient's age, medical condition, and ability to comprehend both the procedure and the patient's role in the changed state that will result with the surgery. In general, ileal conduit surgery is easier, faster, and has fewer complications than continent reservoir surgery.

In addition to these considerations, great emphasis must be put on preparing the patient psychologically, and physicians must make themselves available for counseling and questions before proceeding with patient evaluation for the procedures. The renal system must be assessed using pylography, which is the visualization of the renal pelvis of the kidneys to determine the health of each renal system. Patients with renal disease or abnormalities are not good candidates for urinary diversion. Bowel preparation and prophylactic **antibiotics** are necessary to avoid infection with the surgery. Bowel preparation includes injecting a clear-liquid diet preoperatively for two days, followed by using a cleansing enema or enemas until the bowel runs clear. The importance of these preparations must be explained to the patient: leaking from the bowel during surgery can be life threatening. For ileal conduits, the placement of the stoma must be decided. This is accomplished after the physician evaluates the patient's abdomen in both a sitting and standing position, to avoid placing the stoma in a fatty fold of the abdomen. The input from a stomal therapist is important for this preparation with the patient.

Aftercare

Ureteral stents are generally removed one week after surgery. A urine culture is taken from each stent.

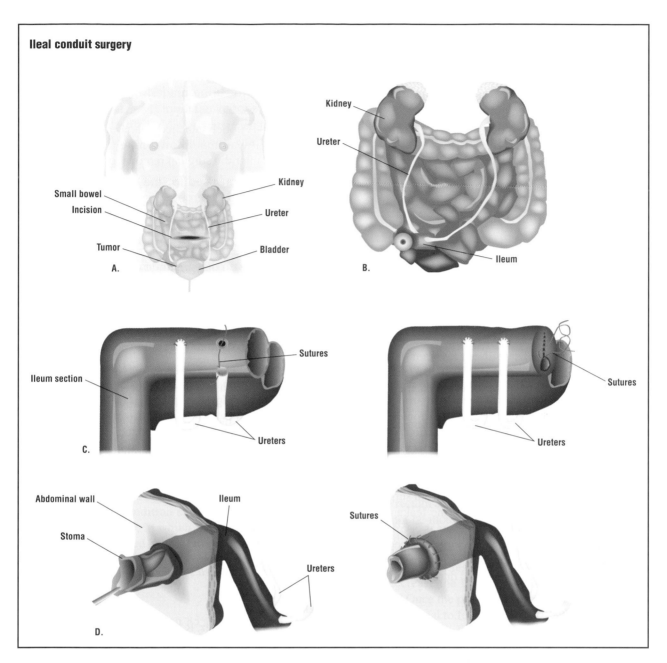

Ileal conduit surgery

In a cystectomy with ileal conduit, an incision is made in the patient's lower abdomen (A). The ureters are disconnected from the bladder, which is then removed (B). They are then attached to a section of ileum (small intestine) that has been removed and refashioned for that purpose (C). A stoma, or hole in the abdominal wall, is created at the site to allow drainage of the urine (D). *(Illustration by GGS Inc.)*

Radiologic contrast studies are carried out to ensure against ureteral anastomotic leakage or obstruction. On the seventh postoperative day, a contrast study is performed to ensure pouch integrity. Thereafter, ureteral stents may be removed, again with radiologic control. When it has been determined that the ureteral anastomoses and pouch are intact, the suction drain is removed. The patient is shown how to support the operative site when sleeping and with breathing and coughing. Fluids and electrolytes are infused intravenously until the patient can take liquids by mouth. The patient is usually able to get up in eight to 24 hours and leave the hospital in about a week.

Patients are taught how to care for the ostomy, and family members are educated as well. Appropriate supplies and a schedule of how to change the pouch are discussed, along with skin care techniques for the area sur-

Ileoanal anastomosis

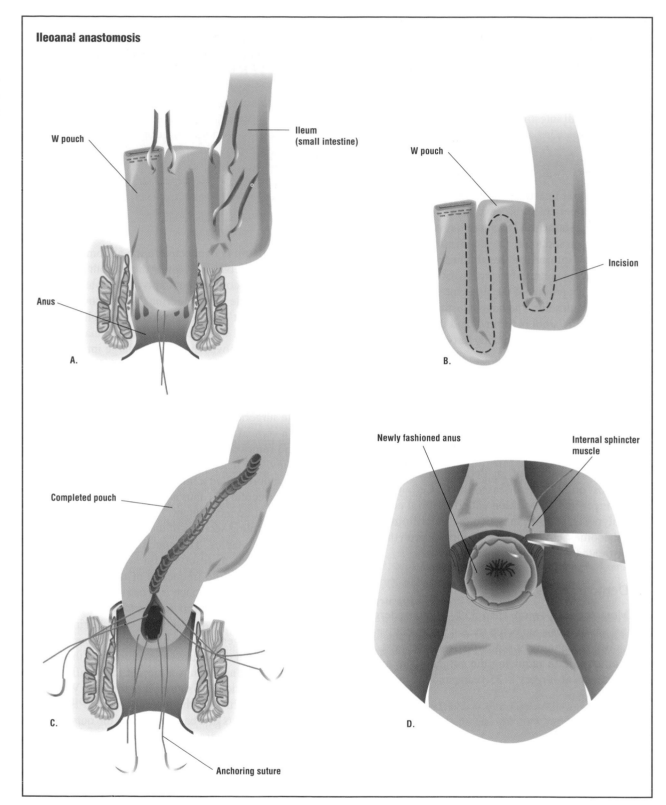

W pouch

Ileum
(small intestine)

Anus

A.

W pouch

Incision

B.

Completed pouch

C.

Anchoring suture

Newly fashioned anus

Internal sphincter
muscle

D.

In an ileoanal anastomosis, a pouch is used to create a large section of bowel whose function replaces that of the large intestine, or colon. In this operation, the ileum (part of the small intestine) is shaped into a W-shaped pouch (A). An incision is made (B) to open up the shape and create the larger pouch, which is left open at one end and brought through the rectal area (C). The bottom of the pouch acts as a new rectum, and a new anus is fashioned (D). *(Illustration by GGS Inc.)*

runs from the small intestine through the ileal pouch and anal canal to the outside of the body. In some instances, the surgeon may decide to combine the two surgeries into one operation without creating a temporary ileostomy.

Diagnosis/Preparation

Because an ileoanal anastomosis is a procedure that is done after a patient has failed to respond to other therapies, the patient's condition has been diagnosed by the time the doctor suggests this surgery.

The patient meets with the operating physician prior to surgery to discuss the details of the surgery and receive instructions on pre- and post-operative care. Immediately before the operation, an intravenous (IV) line is placed in the patient's arm to administer fluid and medications, and the patient is given a bowel preparation to cleanse the bowel for surgery. The location of the stoma is marked on the skin so that it is placed away from bones, abdominal folds, and scars.

Aftercare

Following surgery, the staff will instruct the patient in the care of the stoma, placement of the ileostomy bag, and necessary changes regarding diet and lifestyle. Visits with an enterostomal therapist (ET) or a support group for individuals with ostomies may be recommended to help the patient adjust to living with a stoma. After the anastomosis has healed, which usually takes about two to three months, the ileostomy can then be closed. A dietician may suggest permanent changes in the patient's diet to minimize gas and diarrhea.

Risks

Risks associated with any surgery that involves opening the abdomen include excessive bleeding, infection, and complications due to general anesthesia. Specific complications following an ileoanal anastomosis include leakage of stool, anal stenosis (narrowing of the anus), pouchitis (inflammation of the ileal pouch), and pouch failure. Patients who have received a temporary ileostomy may experience obstruction (blockage) of the stoma, stomal prolapse (protrusion of the ileum through the stoma), or a rash or skin irritation around the stoma.

Normal results

After ileoanal anastomosis, patients will usually experience between four and nine bowel movements during the day and one at night; this frequency generally decreases over time. Because of the nature of the surgery, persons with an ileoanal anastomosis retain the ability to control their bowel movements. They can refrain from defecating

---

QUESTIONS TO ASK THE DOCTOR

- Why are you recommending an ileoanal anastomosis?
- What type of pouch will be created?
- Will an ileostomy be created? When will it be reversed?
- Are there any nonsurgical alternatives to this procedure?
- When will I be able to resume my normal diet and activities?

---

for extended periods of time, an advantage not afforded by a conventional ileostomy. One study found that 97% of patients were satisfied with the results of the surgery and would recommend it to others with similar disorders.

Morbidity and mortality rates

The overall rate of complications associated with ileoanal anastomosis is approximately 10%. Between 10% and 15% of patients will experience at least one episode of pouchitis, and 10–20% will develop postsurgical pelvic or wound infections. The rate of anastomosis failure requiring the creation of a permanent ileostomy is approximately 5–10%.

Alternatives

An ileostomy is a surgical alternative for patients who are not good candidates for an ileoanal anastomosis. If the patient wishes to retain continence, the surgeon may perform a continent ileostomy. Portions of the small intestine are used to form a pouch and valve; these are then directly attached to the abdominal wall skin to form a stoma. Waste collects inside the internal pouch and is expelled by insertion of a soft, flexible tube through the stoma several times a day.

Resources

BOOKS

Pemberton, John H., and Sidney F. Phillips. "Ileostomy and Its Alternatives." In *Sleisenger and Fordtran's Gastrointestinal and Liver Disease*, 7th ed. Philadelphia: Elsevier Science, 2002.

PERIODICALS

Becker, James M. "Surgical Therapy for Ulcerative Colitis and Crohn's Disease." *Gastroenterology Clinics of North America* 28 (June 1, 1999): 371-90.

KEY TERMS

Anastomosis (plural, anastomoses)—A surgically created joining or opening between two organs or body spaces that are normally separate.

Colon—The portion of the large intestine where stool is formed.

Continent—Able to hold the contents of the bladder or bowel until one can use a bathroom. A continent surgical procedure is one that allows the patient to keep waste products inside the body rather than collecting them in an external bag attached to a stoma.

Enterostomal therapist—A health care provider who specializes in the care of patients with enterostomies (e.g., ileostomies or colostomies).

Ostomy—The surgical creation of an opening from an internal structure to the outside of the body.

Polyp—Any mass of tissue that grows out of a mucous membrane in the digestive tract, uterus, or elsewhere in the body.

Stoma (plural, stomata)—A surgically created opening in the abdominal wall to allow digestive wastes to pass to the outside of the body.

ORGANIZATIONS

Crohn's and Colitis Foundation of America. 386 Park Ave. S., 17th Floor, New York, NY 10016. (800) 932-2423. <www.ccfa.org>.

United Ostomy Association, Inc. 19772 MacArthur Blvd., Suite 200, Irvine, CA 92612-2405. (800) 826-0826. <www.uoa.org>.

OTHER

Hurst, Roger D. "Surgical Treatment of Ulcerative Colitis." *Crohn's and Colitis Foundation of America.* [cited May 1, 2003]. <www.ccfa.org/medcentral/library/surgery/ucsurg. htm>.

Stephanie Dionne Sherk

Ileoanal reservoir surgery

Definition

Ileoanal reservoir surgery or **ileoanal anastomosis** is a two-stage restorative procedure that removes a part of the colon and uses the ileum (a section of the small intestine) to form a new reservoir for waste that can be expelled through the anus. This surgery is one of several continent surgeries that rely upon a newly created pouch to replace the resected colon and retain the patient's sphincter for natural defecation. Ileoanal reservoir surgery is also called a J-pouch, endorectal pullthrough, or pelvic pouch procedure.

Purpose

A number of diseases require removal of the entire colon or parts of the colon. Proctolectomies (removal of the entire colon) are often performed to treat colon cancer. Another surgical option is the creation of an ileoanal pouch to serve as an internal waste reservoir—an alternative to the use of an external ostomy pouch. An ileoanal reservoir procedure is performed primarily on patients with ulcerative colitis, inflammatory bowel disease (IBD), familial polyposis, or familial adenomatous polyposis (FAP), which is a relatively rare cancer that covers the colon with 100 or more polyps. FAP is caused by a gene mutation on the long arm of human chromosome 5. Ileoanal reservoir surgery is recommended only in those patients who have not previously lost their rectum or anus.

Demographics

The prevalence of familial adenomatous polyposis (FAP) in the United States is two to three cases per 100,000 persons. It develops before age 40 and accounts for about 0.5% of colorectal cancers; this figure is declining, however, as more at-risk families are undergoing detection and prophylactic colon surgery. The annual incidence of ulcerative colitis is 10.4–12 cases per 100,000 people. The prevalence rate is 35–100 cases per 100,000. People of Jewish descent have two to four times the risk of developing ulcerative colitis than people from other ethnic backgrounds. About 20% of ulcerative colitis patients require surgery of the colon.

Description

Conventional ileoanal reservoir surgery is an open procedure that is done in two stages. In the first stage, the surgeon removes the diseased colon and creates a pouch. The second stage is performed three months later, when the temporary drainage conduit is closed and the newly created reservoir allows the patient to defecate in the normal fashion. Both surgeries can also be done together, bypassing the creation of a temporary **ileostomy**.

Some surgeons use a laparoscopic approach to ileoanal surgery. This technique involves the insertion of scaled-down **surgical instruments** and a scope that allows the surgeon to see inside the abdomen through several relatively small incisions (3.5 inches [9 cm] or about compared to 6.3 inches [16 cm] or for an open procedure) in the abdominal wall. Studies indicate that there are few differences in the rates of mortality or complications between laparoscopic surgery and conventional open surgery. Because the incisions are smaller, patients typically require less pain medication with laparoscopic surgery.

Ileoanal surgery includes the following steps:

• The surgeon isolates the ileum or small segment of bowel.

• The segment is then attached to the anus with absorbable sutures.

• A pouch is created out of the small bowel above the anus.

• If the surgeon is performing the procedure in two stages, he or she creates a temporary ileostomy. An ileostomy is a tubular bowel segment attached to a stoma at the abdomen that drains into a bag outside the abdomen.

• In the second-stage operation, the surgeon uses an open abdominal procedure to close the temporary pouch.

The surgeon will insert stents to bypass the surgical site and divert urinary and digestive wastes to the outside of the body, thus allowing the new connection between the ileum and the anus to heal properly.

Diagnosis/Preparation

The diagnosis of FAP is usually made after symptoms caused by polyps in the colon, such as rectal bleeding, diarrhea, and abdominal pain, have led to a **physical examination**, the taking of a family history, and in some cases a genetic test. Ulcerative colitis or inflammatory bowel disease patients have usually been treated with medical alternatives before they decide to have surgery. All patients who are candidates for an ileoanal procedure will have an evaluation of the upper gastrointestinal tract, an x ray of the small bowel, and a **colonoscopy**

with a pathology review. Most patients will also be given a **sigmoidoscopy** and a digital rectal examination.

The surgeon will need to perform an ileostomy in about 5–10% of cases because the patient's rectal muscles are not strong enough for an anastomosis. This possibility is discussed with the patient, as well as the fact that complications in surgery may lead to an ostomy procedure. The placement of a stoma must be decided in the event that an ileostomy is necessary. The physician evaluates the patient's abdomen while the patient is sitting and then standing, in order to avoid placing the stoma inside a fatty fold of the abdomen. A stomal therapist is often called in to prepare the patient for the possibility that an appliance will be needed. In addition to the medical and surgical considerations of the procedure, the patient requires psychological preparation regarding the changes in function and appearance that accompany this surgery.

Prior to surgery, the patient must undergo a bowel preparation, which includes a clear-liquid diet for two days before the procedure. In addition to drinking nothing but clear fluids, the patient must have a cleansing enema until the bowel runs clear. The importance of a thorough bowel preparation must be explained to the patient, because leakage from the bowel during surgery can be life-threatening.

Aftercare

Open ileaoanal reservoir surgery is a lengthy procedure (as long as five hours) with a slow recovery rate (approximately six weeks) and a relatively long stay in the hospital (about 10 days). The catheters and stents that were used are removed several days after surgery. The patient will be introduced to a special diet in the hospital, and the diet will be altered if needed in response to changes in the chemistry of the colon. The patient's stools are measured, and he or she is monitored for dehydration. In addition, the patient will have the op-

KEY TERMS

Anastomosis—A surgically created joining or opening between two organs or body spaces that are normally separate.

Colon—The portion of the large intestine where stool is formed.

Continent—Ability to hold the contents of the bladder or bowel until one can use a bathroom. A continent surgical procedure is one that allows the patient to keep waste products inside the body rather than collecting them in an external bag attached to a stoma.

Ileoanal anastomosis—A reservoir for fecal waste surgically created out of the small intestine. It retains the sphincter function of the anus and allows the patient to defecate in the normal fashion.

Ileum—The third and lowest portion of the small intestine, extending from the jejunum to the beginning of the large intestine.

Polyp—Any mass of tissue that grows out of a mucous membrane in the digestive tract, uterus, or elsewhere in the body.

Sphincter—A circular band of muscle fibers that constricts or closes a passageway in the body.

Stent—A thin rodlike or tubelike device made of wire mesh, inserted into a blood vessel or a section of the digestive tract to keep the structure open.

Stoma (plural, stomata)—A surgically created opening in the abdominal wall to allow digestive wastes to pass to the outside of the body.

portunity to discuss his or her concerns about care of the new reservoir and frequency of defecation with staff members before leaving the hospital.

Results

For carefully selected patients this procedure, developed over 30 years, is the preferred form of radical colon surgery when the patient's sphincter and rectum are still intact. The advantage of the ileoanal reservoir surgery is that the patient has an internal pouch for the collection of waste material and can pass this waste normally through the anus. Bowel movements may be more fluid, however, and more frequent with the new reservoir. In a small percentage of cases, the surgeon may eventually need to perform an ileostomy due to complications. In one quality of life study for patients who have undergone ileoanal reservoir surgery, researchers found only slight differences in their general health and level of daily activity compared with subjects recruited from the general population.

Morbidity/mortality

Morbidity rates with this procedure have decreased over time due to improvements in technique. The most common complication is inflammation of the pouch, which occurs in as many as 40% of patients. This complication can be treated with medication. Other complications include severe scarring around the incision, and some risk of injury to the nerves that control erection and bladder function. In one major study of 379 patients, researchers at the University of Cincinnati reported that 79 patients had pouch infections (24.3%) and another 20 patients required further surgery for obstructions of the small bowel (6.2%).

Alternatives

The major surgical alternative to an ileoanal reservoir procedure is an ileostomy. In an ileostomy, the patient's fecal matter drains into a plastic bag attached to a stoma on the outside of the patient's abdomen or into a pouch attached to the abdominal wall to be withdrawn through a plastic tube.

Resources

BOOKS

Pemberton, John H., and Sidney F. Phillips. "Ileostomy and Its Alternatives" In *Sleisenger and Fordtran's Gastrointestinal and Liver Disease*, 7th ed. Philadelphia: Elsevier Science, 2002.

"Tumors of the Gastrointestinal Tract: Large-Bowel Tumors." In *The Merck Manual of Diagnosis and Therapy*, edited by Mark H. Beers, MD, and Robert Berkow, MD. Whitehouse Station, NJ: Merck Research Laboratories, 1999.

PERIODICALS

Allison, Stephen, and Marvin L. Corman. "Intestinal Stomas in Crohn's Disease." *Surgical Clinics of North America* 81, no. 1 (February 1, 2001): 185-95.

Blumberg, D., and D. E. Beck. "Surgery for Ulcerative Colitis." *Gastroenterology Clinics of North America* 31 (March 2002): 219-235.

Pasupathy, S., K. W. Eu, Y. H. Ho, and F. Seow-Choen. "A Comparison Between Open Versus Laparoscopic Assisted Colonic Pouches for Rectal Cancer." *Techniques in Coloproctology* 5 (April 2001): 19-22.

Robb, B., et al. "Quality of Life in Patients Undergoing Ileal Pouch-Anal Anastomosis at the University of Cincinnati." *American Journal of Surgery* 183 (April 2002): 353-360.

ORGANIZATIONS

American Gastroenterological Association, American Digestive Health Foundation. 7910 Woodmont Aveenue, 7th Floor, Bethesda, MD 20814. (301) 654-2055. <www.gasto.org.>

American Society of Colon and Rectal Surgeons. 85 W. Algonquin Rd., Suite 550, Arlington Heights, IL 60005. <fascrs.org,>

National Digestive Diseases Information Clearinghouse. 2 Information Way, Bethesda, MD 20892-3570. <www.niddk.nih.gov.>

United Ostomy Association, Inc. (UOA). 19772 MacArthur Blvd., Suite 200, Irvine, CA 92612-2405. (800) 826-0826. <www.uoa.org.>

OTHER

MDconsult.com. *Inflammatory Bowel Disease (Crohn's Disease and Ulcerative Colitis)*. <www.MDconsult.com.>

Nancy McKenzie, PhD

Ileorectal anastomosis *see* **Ileoanal anastomosis**

Ileostomy

Definition

An ileostomy is a surgical procedure in which the small intestine is attached to the abdominal wall in order to bypass the large intestine; digestive waste then exits the body through an artificial opening called a stoma (from the Greek word for "mouth").

Purpose

In general, an ostomy is the surgical creation of an opening from an internal structure to the outside of the body. An ileostomy, therefore, creates a temporary or permanent opening between the ileum (the portion of the small intestine that empties to the large intestine) and the abdominal wall. The colon and/or rectum may be removed or bypassed. A temporary ileostomy may be recommended for patients undergoing bowel surgery (e.g., removal of a segment of bowel), to provide the intestines with sufficient time to heal without the stress of normal digestion.

Chronic ulcerative colitis is an example of a medical condition that is treated with the removal of the large in-

---

WHO PERFORMS THE PROCEDURE AND WHERE IS IT PERFORMED?

Ileostomies are usually performed in a hospital **operating room**. The surgery may be performed by a general surgeon, a colorectal surgeon (a medical doctor who focuses on diseases of the colon, rectum, and anus), or gastrointestinal surgeon (a medical doctor who focuses on diseases of the gastrointestinal system).

---

testine. Ulcerative colitis occurs when the body's immune system attacks the cells in the lining of the large intestine, resulting in inflammation and tissue damage. Patients with ulcerative colitis often experience pain, frequent bowel movements, bloody stools, and loss of appetite. An ileostomy is a treatment option for patients who do not respond to medical or dietary therapies for ulcerative colitis.

Other conditions that may be treated with an ileostomy include:

• bowel obstructions

• cancer of the colon and/or rectum

• Crohn's disease (chronic inflammation of the intestines)

• congenital bowel defects

• uncontrolled bleeding from the large intestine

• injury to the intestinal tract

Demographics

The United Ostomy Association estimates that approximately 75,000 ostomy surgeries are performed each year in the United States, and that 750,000 Americans have an ostomy. Ulcerative colitis and Crohn's disease affect approximately one million Americans. There is a greater incidence of the diseases among Caucasians under the age of 30 or between the ages of 50 and 70.

Description

For some patients, an ileostomy is preceded by removal of the colon (colonectomy) or the colon and rectum (protocolectomy). After the patient is placed under general anesthesia, an incision approximately 8 in (20 cm) long is made down the patient's midline, through the abdominal skin, muscle, and other subcutaneous tissues. Once the abdominal cavity has been opened, the colon and rectum are isolated and removed. The anal canal is stitched closed.

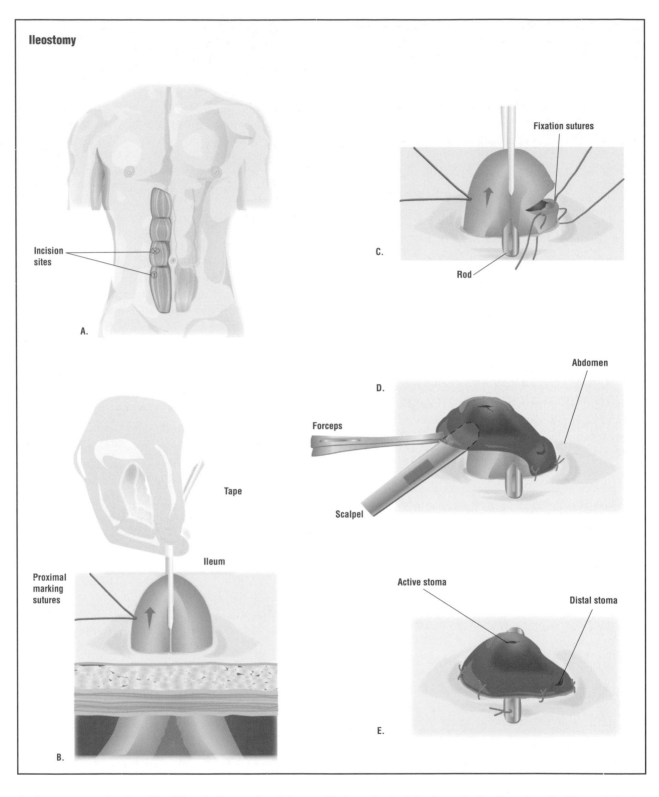

Ileostomy

An ileostomy can be placed in different sites on the abdomen (A). Once the incision is made, the ileum is pulled through the incision (B), and a rod is placed under the loop. The loop is cut open, one side is stitched to the abdomen (C). The portion of intestine is flipped open to expose the interior surface (D), and the opposite side is stitched in place (E). *(Illustration by GGS Inc.)*

Other patients undergoing ileostomy will have only a temporary bypass of the colon and rectum; examples are patients undergoing **small bowel resection** or the creation of an **ileoanal anastomosis**. An ileoanal anastomosis is a procedure in which the surgeon forms a pouch out of tissue from the ileum and connects it directly to the anal canal.

There are two basic types of permanent ileostomy: conventional and continent. A conventional ileostomy, also called a Brooke ileostomy, involves a separate, smaller incision through the abdominal wall skin (usually on the lower right side) to which the cut end of the ileum is sutured. The ileum may protrude from the skin, often as far as 2 in (5 cm). Patients with this type of stoma are considered fecal-incontinent, meaning they can no longer control the emptying of wastes from the body. After a conventional ileostomy, the patient is fitted with a plastic bag worn over the stoma and attached to the abdominal skin with adhesive. The ileostomy bag collects waste as it exits from the body.

An alternative to conventional ileostomy is the continent ileostomy. Also called a Kock ileostomy, this procedure allows a patient to control when waste exits the stoma. Portions of the small intestine are used to form a pouch and valve; these are directly attached to the abdominal wall skin to form a stoma. Waste collects internally in the pouch and is expelled by insertion of a soft, flexible tube through the stoma several times a day.

Diagnosis/Preparation

The patient meets with the operating physician prior to surgery to discuss the details of the surgery and receive instructions on pre- and post-operative care. Directly preceding surgery, an intravenous (IV) line is placed to administer fluid and medications, and the patient is given a bowel prep to cleanse the bowel and prepare it for surgery. The location where the stoma will be placed is marked, away from bones, abdominal folds, and scars.

Aftercare

Following surgery, the patient is instructed in the care of the stoma, placement of the ileostomy bag, and necessary changes to diet and lifestyle. Because the large intestine (a site of fluid absorption) is no longer a part of the patient's digestive system, fecal matter exiting the stoma has a high water content. The patient must therefore be diligent about his or her fluid intake to minimize the risk of dehydration. Visits with an enterostomal therapist (ET) or a support group for individuals with ostomies may be recommended to help the patient adjust to living with a stoma. Once the ileostomy has healed, a normal diet can usually be resumed, and the patient can return to normal activities.

QUESTIONS TO ASK THE DOCTOR

- Why is an ileostomy being recommended?
- What type of ileostomy would work best for me?
- What are the risks and complications associated with the recommended procedure?
- Are any nonsurgical treatment alternatives available?
- How soon after surgery may I resume my normal diet and activities?

Risks

Risks associated with the ileostomy procedure include excessive bleeding, infection, and complications due to general anesthesia. After surgery, some patients experience stomal obstruction (blockage), inflammation of the ileum, stomal prolapse (protrusion of the ileum through the stoma), or irritation of the skin around the stoma.

Normal results

The physical quality of life of most patients is not affected by an ileostomy, and with proper care most patients can avoid major medical complications. Patients with a permanent ileostomy, however, may suffer emotional aftereffects and benefit from psychotherapy.

Morbidity and mortality rates

Among patients who have undergone a Brooke ileostomy, medical literature reports a 19–70% risk of complications. Small bowel obstruction occurs in 15% of patients; 30% have problems with the stoma; 20–25% require further surgery to repair the stoma; and 30% experience postsurgical infections. The rate of complications is also high among patients who have had a continent ileostomy (15–60%). The most common complications associated with this procedure are small bowel obstruction (7%), wound complications (35%), and failure to restore continence (50%). The mortality rate of both procedures is less than 1%.

Alternatives

Patients with mild to moderate ulcerative colitis may be able to manage their disease with medications. Medications that are given to treat ulcerative colitis in-

---

Anastomosis—A surgically created joining or opening between two organs or body spaces that are normally separate.

Colon—The portion of the large intestine where stool is formed.

Enterostomal therapist—A health care provider who specializes in the care of individuals with enterostomies (e.g. ileostomies or colostomies).

Rectum—The portion of the large intestine where stool is stored until exiting the body through the anal canal.

Stoma (plural, stomata)—A surgically created opening in the abdominal wall to allow digestive wastes to pass to the outside of the body.

clude enemas containing hydrocortisone or mesalamine; oral sulfasalazine or olsalazine; oral **corticosteroids**; or cyclosporine and other drugs that affect the immune system.

A surgical alternative to ileostomy is the ileal pouch-anal anastomosis, or ileoanal anastomosis. This procedure, used more frequently than permanent ileostomy in the treatment of ulcerative colitis, is similar to a continent ileostomy in that an ileal pouch is formed. The pouch, however, is not attached to a stoma but to the anal canal. This procedure allows the patient to retain fecal continence. An ileoanal anastomosis usually requires the placement of a temporary ileostomy for two to three months to give the connected tissues time to heal.

Resources

BOOKS

"Inflammatory Bowel Diseases: Ulcerative Colitis." In *The Merck Manual of Diagnosis and Therapy*, edited by Mark H. Beers, MD, and Robert Berkow, MD. Whitehouse Station, NJ: Merck Research Laboratories, 1999.

Pemberton, John H., and Sidney F. Phillips. "Ileostomy and Its Alternatives" (Chapter 105). In *Sleisenger and Fordtran's Gastrointestinal and Liver Disease*, 7th ed. Philadelphia: Elsevier Science, 2002.

Rolandelli, Rolando H., and Joel J. Roslyn. "Colon and Rectum," (Chapter 46), In *Sabiston Textbook of Surgery*. Philadelphia: W. B. Saunders Company, 2001.

PERIODICALS

Allison, Stephen, and Marvin L. Corman. "Intestinal Stomas in Crohn's Disease." *Surgical Clinics of North America* 81, no. 1 (February 1, 2001): 185-95.

ORGANIZATIONS

Crohn's and Colitis Foundation of America. 386 Park Ave. S., 17th Floor, New York, NY 10016. (800) 932-2423. <www.ccfa.org>.

United Ostomy Association, Inc. 19772 MacArthur Blvd., Suite 200, Irvine, CA 92612-2405. (800) 826-0826. <www.uoa.org>.

OTHER

Hurst, Roger D. "Surgical Treatment of Ulcerative Colitis." [cited May 1, 2003]. <www.ccfa.org/medcentral/library/surgery/ucsurg.htm>.

Stephanie Dionne Sherk

Immunoassay tests

Definition

Immunoassays are chemical tests used to detect or quantify a specific substance, the analyte, in a blood or body fluid sample, using an immunological reaction. Immunoassays are highly sensitive and specific. Their high specificity results from the use of antibodies and purified antigens as reagents. An antibody is a protein (immunoglobulin) produced by B-lymphocytes (immune cells) in response to stimulation by an antigen. Immunoassays measure the formation of antibody-antigen complexes and detect them via an indicator reaction. High sensitivity is achieved by using an indicator system (e.g., enzyme label) that results in amplification of the measured product.

Immunoassays may be qualitative (positive or negative) or quantitative (amount measured). An example of a qualitative assay is an immunoassay test for pregnancy. Pregnancy tests detect the presence of human chorionic gonadotropin (hCG) in urine or serum. Highly purified antibodies can detect pregnancy within two days of fertilization. Quantitative immunoassays are performed by measuring the signal produced by the indicator reaction. This same test for pregnancy can be made into a quantitative assay of hCG by measuring the concentration of product formed.

Purpose

The purpose of an immunoassay is to measure (or, in a qualitative assay, to detect) an analyte. Immunoassay is the method of choice for measuring analytes normally present at very low concentrations that cannot be determined accurately by other less expensive tests. Common uses include measurement of drugs, hormones, specific proteins, tumor markers, and markers of cardiac injury. Qualitative immunoassays are often used to detect antigens on infectious agents and antibodies that the body produces to fight them. For example, immunoassays are used to detect antigens on *Hemophilus, Cryptococcus,* and *Streptococcus* organisms in the cerebrospinal fluid (CSF) of meningitis patients. They are also used to detect antigens associated with organisms that are difficult to culture, such as hepatitis B virus and *Chlamydia trichomatis.* Immunoassays for antibodies produced in viral hepatitis, HIV, and Lyme disease are commonly used to identify patients with these diseases.

Description

There are several different methods used in immunoassay tests.

• Immunoprecipitation. The simplest immunoassay method measures the quantity of precipitate, which forms after the reagent antibody (precipitin) has incubated with the sample and reacted with its respective antigen to form an insoluble aggregate. Immunoprecipitation reactions may be qualitative or quantitative.

• Particle immunoassays. By linking several antibodies to the particle, the particle is able to bind many antigen molecules simultaneously. This greatly accelerates the speed of the visible reaction. This allows rapid and sensitive detection of antibodies that are markers of such diseases, as infectious mononucleosis and rheumatoid arthritis.

• Immunonephelometry. The immediate union of antibody and antigen forms immune complexes that are too small to precipitate. However, these complexes will scatter incident light and can be measured using an instrument called a nephelometer. The antigen concentration can be determined within minutes of the reaction.

• Radioimmunoassay (RIA) is a method employing radioactive isotopes to label either the antigen or antibody. This isotope emits gamma raysare, which are usually measured following removal of unbound (free) radiolabel. The major advantages of RIA, compared with other immunoassays, are higher sensitivity, easy signal detection, and well-established, rapid assays. The major disadvantages are the health and safety risks posed by the use of radiation and the time and expense associated with maintaining a licensed radiation safety and disposal program. For this reason, RIA has been largely replaced in routine clinical laboratory practice by enzyme immunoassay.

• Enzyme (EIA) immunoassay was developed as an alternative to radioimmunoassay (RIA). These methods use an enzyme to label either the antibody or antigen. The sensitivity of EIA approaches that for RIA, without the danger posed by radioactive isotopes. One of the most widely used EIA methods for detection of infectious diseases is the enzyme-linked immunosorbent assay (ELISA).

• Fluorescent immunoassay (FIA) refers to immunoassays which utilize a fluorescent label or an enzyme label which acts on the substrate to form a fluorescent product. Fluorescent measurements are inherently more sensitive than colorimetric (spectrophotometric) measurements. Therefore, FIA methods have greater analytical sensitivity than EIA methods, which employ absorbance (optical density) measurement.

• Chemiluminescent immunoassays utilize a chemiluminescent label. Chemiluminescent molecules produce light when they are excited by chemical energy. These emissions are measured by a light detector.

Precautions

Blood samples are collected by vein puncture with a needle. It is not necessary to restrict fluids or food prior to collection. Blood should be collected in tubes containing no additive. Risks of vein puncture include bruising of the skin or bleeding into the skin. Random urine samples are acceptable for drug assays; however, 24-hour urine samples are preferred for hormones and other substances which show diurnal or pulse variation.

Special safety precautions must be observed when performing RIA methods. Radioactive isotopes are used by RIA tests to label antigens or antibodies. Pregnant females should not work in an area where RIA tests are being performed. Personnel handling isotope reagents must wear badges which monitor their exposure to radiation. Special sinks and waste disposal containers are required for disposal of radioactive waste. The amount of radioisotope discarded must be documented for both liquid and solid waste. Leakage or spills of radioactive reagents must be measured for radioactivity; the amount of radiation and containment and disposal processes must be documented.

Normal results

Immunoassays which are qualitative are reported as positive or negative. Quantitative immunoassays are reported in mass units, along with reference intervals (normal ranges) for the test. Normal ranges may be age- and gender-dependent. Positive immunoassay test results for HIV and drugs of abuse generally require confirmatory testing.

Although immunoassays are both highly sensitive and specific, false positive and negative results may occur. False-negative results may be caused by improper

KEY TERMS

Antibody—A protein produced by B-lymphocytes in response to stimulation by an antigen.

Antigen—Any substance which induces an immune response.

Human chorionic gonadotropin (hCG)—A hormone that is measured to detect early pregnancy.

Immunoassay—A method that measures antibody-antigen complexes formed by reacting purified antibody or antigen with the sample.

Nephelometry—A method for measuring the light scattering properties of a sample.

Radioimmunoassay—A method that uses a radioisotope label in an immunoassay.

sample storage or treatment, reagent deterioration, or improper washing technique. False-positive results are sometimes seen in persons who have certain antibodies, especially to mouse immunoglobulins (immune cells) that may be used in the test. False-positive results have been reported for samples containing small fibrin strands that adhere to the solid phase matrix. False-positives may also be caused by substances in the blood or urine that cross-react or bind to the antibody used in the test.

Preparation

Generally, no special instructions need be given to patients for immunoassay testing. Some assays require a timed specimen collection, while others may have special dietary restrictions.

Aftercare

When blood testing is used for the immunoassay, the vein puncture site will require a bandage or light dressing to accomplish blood clotting.

Risks

Immunoassay is an *in vitro* procedure, and is therefore not associated with complications. When blood is collected, slight bleeding into the skin and subsequent bruising may occur. The patient may become lightheaded or queasy from the sight of blood.

Resources

BOOKS

Bishop, M. L., J. L. Duben-Engelkirk, and E. P. Fody. *Clinical Chemistry Principles, Procedures, Correlations.* 4th ed. Lippincott, Williams, and Wilkins, 2001.

Burtis, C. A., and E. R. Ashwood, eds. *Tietz Fundamentals of Clinical Chemistry.* 5th ed. Philadelphia: W.B. Saunders, 2001.

Henry, J. B., ed. *Clinical Diagnosis and Management by Laboratory Methods.* 20th ed. Philadelphia: W. B. Saunders, 2001.

Wallach, Jacques. *Interpretation of Diagnostic Tests.* 7th ed. Philadelphia: Lippincott Williams & Wilkens, 2000.

Wild, D., ed. *Immunoassay Handbook.* 2nd ed. London: Nature Publishing Group, 2000.

Robert Harr
Paul Johnson
Mark A. Best

Immunologic therapies

Definition

Immunologic therapy is an approach to the treatment of disease that uses medicines for stimulating the body's natural immune response.

Purpose

Immunologic therapy is used to improve the immune system's natural ability to fight such diseases as cancer, hepatitis, and AIDS. These drugs may also be used to help the body recover from immunosuppression resulting from such treatments as chemotherapy or radiation therapy.

Description

Most drugs in this category are synthetic versions of substances produced naturally in the body. In their natural forms, these substances help defend the body against disease. For example, aldesleukin (Proleukin) is an artificial form of interleukin-2, which helps white blood cells work. Aldesleukin is administered to patients with kidney cancers and skin cancers that have spread to other parts of the body. Filgrastim (Neupogen) and sargramostim (Leukine) are versions of natural substances called colony stimulating factors, which encourage the bone marrow to make new white blood cells. Another type of drug, epoetin (Epogen, Procrit), is a synthetic version of human erythropoietin, which stimulates the bone marrow to make new red blood cells. Thrombopoietin stimulates the production of platelets, which are disk-shaped bodies in the blood that are important in clotting. Interferons are substances that the body produces naturally, using cells in the immune system to fight infections and tumors. Synthetic interferons carry such brand names as Alferon, Roferon or Intron A. Some of the interferons that are currently in use as medications are recombinant interferon alfa-2a, recombinant interferon alfa-2b, interferon alfa-n1, and interferon alfa-n3. Alfa interferons are used to treat hairy cell leukemia, malignant melanoma, and Kaposi's sarcoma, which is a type of cancer associated with HIV infection. In addition, interferons are also used to treat such other conditions as laryngeal papillomatosis, genital warts, and certain types of hepatitis.

Recommended dosage

The recommended dosage depends on the type of immunologic therapy. For some medicines, the physician will decide the dosage for each patient, taking into account a patient's weight and whether he or she is taking other medicines. Some drugs used in immunologic therapy are given only in a hospital under a physician's supervision. Patients who are taking drugs that can be used at home should consult the physician who prescribed the medicine or the pharmacist who filled the prescription for the correct dosage.

Most of these drugs come in an injectable form, which is generally administered by a cancer care provider.

Precautions

Aldesleukin

This drug may temporarily increase the patient's risk of getting infections. It may also lower the number of platelets in the blood, and thus interfere with the blood's ability to clot. Taking the following precautions may reduce the chance of such complications:

- Avoid people with infectious diseases whenever possible.

- Be alert to such signs of infection as fever, chills, sore throat, pain in the lower back or side, cough, hoarseness, or painful or difficult urination. If any of these symptoms occur, the patient should call their physician immediately.

- Be alert to such signs of bleeding problems as black or tarry stools; tiny red spots on the skin; blood in the urine or stools; or any other unusual bleeding or bruising.

- Take care to avoid cuts or other injuries, particularly when using knives, razors, nail clippers, and other sharp objects. The patient should consult his or her dentist for the best ways to clean the teeth and mouth without injuring the gums. In addition, patients should not have any dental work done without checking with their primary physician.

- Wash hands frequently, and avoiding touching the eyes or inside of the nose unless the hands have just been washed.

Aldesleukin may make some disorders worse, including chickenpox, shingles (herpes zoster), liver disease, lung disease, heart disease, underactive thyroid, psoriasis, immune system problems and mental problems. The medicine may also increase the risk of seizures (convulsions) in people with epilepsy or other seizure disorders. In addition, the drug's effects may be intensified in people with kidney disease, because their kidneys are slow to clear the medicine from their bodies.

Colony stimulating factors

Certain drugs used in treating cancer reduce the body's ability to fight infections. Although colony stimulating factors help restore the body's natural defenses, the process takes time. Getting prompt treatment for infections is important, even while the patient is taking these medications. Patients taking colony stimulating factors should call their physician at the first sign of illness or infection, including a sore throat, fever, or chills.

People with certain medical conditions may have problems if they take colony stimulating factors. Patients with kidney disease, liver disease, or conditions related to inflammation or immune system disorders may find that colony stimulating factors make their disorder worse. People with heart disease may be more likely to experience such side effects as water retention and irregular heart rhythm while taking these drugs. Patients with lung disease may increase their risk of shortness of breath. People with any of these medical conditions should consult their personal physician before using colony stimulating factors.

Epoetin

Epoetin is a medicine that may cause seizures (convulsions), especially in people with epilepsy or other seizure disorders. No one who takes epoetin should drive, operate heavy machinery, or do anything that would be dangerous to themselves or others in the event of a seizure.

Epoetin helps the body make new red blood cells, but it is not effective unless there are adequate stores of iron in the body. The patient's physician may recommend taking iron supplements or certain vitamins that help to maintain the body's iron supply. It is necessary to follow the physician's advice in this instance, as with any dietary supplements that should come only from a physician.

Studies of laboratory animals indicate that epoetin taken during pregnancy causes birth defects in these species, including damage to the bones and spine. The drug, however, has not been reported to cause problems in human babies whose mothers took it during pregnancy. Nevertheless, women who are or may become pregnant should check with their physicians for the most up-to-date information on the safety of taking this medicine during pregnancy.

People with certain medical conditions may have problems if they take epoetin. For example, there appears to be a greater risk of side effects in people with high blood pressure, disorders of the heart or blood vessels, or a history of blood clots. In addition, epoetin may not work properly in people who have bone disorders or sickle cell anemia.

Interferons

Interferons may intensify the effects of alcohol and other drugs that slow down the central nervous system, including antihistamines, over-the-counter cold medicines, allergy medications, sleep aids, anticonvulsants, tranquilizers, some pain relievers, and **muscle relaxants**. Interferons may also intensify the effects of anesthetics, including the local anesthetics used for dental procedures. Patients taking interferons should consult their physicians before taking any of the medications listed above.

Some people experience dizziness, unusual fatigue, or drowsiness while taking these drugs. Because of these possible problems, anyone who takes these drugs should not drive, use heavy machinery, or do anything else that requires full alertness until they have determined how the drugs affect them.

Interferons often cause flu-like symptoms, including fever and chills. The physician who prescribes this medicine may recommend taking **acetaminophen** (Tylenol) before—and sometimes after—each dose to keep the fever from getting too high. If the physician recommends taking acetaminophen, the patient should follow his or her instructions carefully.

Like aldesleukin, interferons may temporarily increase the risk of getting infections and lower the number of platelets in the blood, which may lead to clotting problems. Patients should observe the precautions listed above for reducing the risk of infection and bleeding for aldesleukin.

People who have certain medical conditions may have problems if they take interferons. For example, the drugs may worsen some medical conditions, including heart disease, kidney disease, liver disease, lung disease, diabetes, bleeding problems, and certain psychiatric disorders. In people who have overactive immune systems, these drugs can even increase the activity of the immune system. People who have shingles or chickenpox, or who have recently been exposed to chickenpox, may increase their risk of developing severe problems in other parts of the body if they take interferons. People with a history of seizures or associated mental disorders may be at risk if they take interferon.

Elderly people appear to be at increased risk of side effects from taking interferons.

Interferons may cause changes in the menstrual cycles of teenagers. Young women should discuss this possibility with their physicians. These drugs are not known to cause fetal death, birth defects, or other problems in humans when taken during pregnancy. Women who are pregnant or who may become pregnant should ask their physicians for the latest information on the safety of taking these drugs during pregnancy.

Women who are breastfeeding their babies may need to stop while taking this medicine. It is not yet known whether interferons pass into breast milk; however, because of the chance of serious side effects that might affect the baby, women should not breastfeed while taking interferon. Patients should consult their physician for more specific advice.

General precautions for all types of immunologic therapy

Regular appointments with the doctor are necessary during immunologic therapy treatment. These checkups give the physician a chance to make sure the medicine is working and to monitor the patient for unwanted side effects.

Anyone who has had unusual reactions to the drugs used in immunologic therapy should inform the doctor before resuming the drugs. Any allergies to foods, dyes, preservatives, or other substances should also be reported.

Side effects

Aldesleukin

Aldesleukin may cause serious side effects. It is ordinarily given only in a hospital, where medical professionals can watch for early signs of problems. Medical tests may be performed to check for unwanted side effects. In general, anyone who has breathing problems, fever or chills while being given aldesleukin should consult their doctor at once.

Other side effects should be brought to a physician's attention as soon as possible:

• dizziness
• drowsiness
• confusion
• agitation

- depression
- nausea and vomiting
- diarrhea
- sores in the mouth and on the lips
- tingling of hands or feet
- decrease in urination
- unexplained weight gain of five or more pounds (2 or more kilograms)

Some side effects of aldesleukin are usually temporary and do not need medical attention unless they are bothersome. These include dry skin, itchy or burning rash or redness followed by peeling, loss of appetite, and a general feeling of illness or discomfort.

Colony stimulating factors

Patients sometimes experience mild pain in the lower back or hips in the first few days of treatment with colony stimulating factors. This side effect is not a cause for concern, and usually goes away within a few days. If the pain is intense or causes discomfort, the physician may prescribe a painkiller.

Other possible side effects include headache, joint or muscle pain, and skin rash or itching. These side effects tend to disappear as the body adjusts to the medicine, and do not need medical treatment. If they continue, or if they interfere with normal activities, the patient should consult their physician.

Epoetin

Epoetin may cause such flu-like symptoms as muscle aches, bone pain, fever, chills, shivering, and sweating within a few hours after it is taken. These symptoms usually go away within 12 hours. If they persist or are severe, the patient should call their doctor. Other possible side effects of epoetin that do not need medical attention are diarrhea, nausea or vomiting, and fatigue or weakness.

Other side effects, however, should be brought to a physician's attention as soon as possible. These include headache; vision problems; a rise in blood pressure; fast heartbeat; weight gain; or swelling of the face, fingers, lower legs, ankles, or feet. Anyone who has chest pain or seizures after taking epoetin should seek professional emergency medical attention immediately.

Interferons

Interferons may cause temporary hair loss (alopecia). Although this side effect may be upsetting because it affects the patient's appearance, it is not a sign that something is seriously wrong. The hair should grow back normally after treatment ends.

As the body adjusts to these medications, the patient may experience other side effects that usually go away during treatment. These include flu-like symptoms, alterations in the sense of taste, loss of appetite (anorexia), nausea and vomiting, skin rashes, and unusual fatigue. The patient should consult a doctor if these problems persist or if they interfere with normal life.

Other side effects are more serious and should be brought to a physician's attention as soon as possible:

- confusion
- difficulty thinking or concentrating
- nervousness
- depression
- sleep problems
- numbness or tingling in the fingers, toes, and face

General precautions regarding side effects for all types of immunologic therapy

Other side effects are possible with any type of immunologic therapy. Anyone who has unusual symptoms during or after treatment with these drugs should contact the physician immediately.

Interactions

Anyone who has immunologic therapy should give their physician a list of all other medications that they take, including over-the-counter and herbal preparations. Some combinations of drugs may increase or decrease the effects of one or both drugs, or increase the likelihood of side effects.

Alternatives

Immunoprevention

Immunoprevention is a form of treatment that has been proposed as a form of cancer therapy. There are two types of immunoprevention, active and passive. Treatment that involves such immune molecules as cytokines, which are prepared synthetically, or other immune molecules that are not produced by patients themselves are called passive immunotherapy. By contrast, vaccines are a form of active immune therapy because they elicit an immune response from the patient's body. Cancer vaccines may be made of whole tumor cells or from substances or fragments from the tumor known as antigens.

Adoptive immunotherapy

Adoptive immunotherapy involves stimulating T lymphocytes by exposing them to tumor antigens. These modified cells are grown in the laboratory and then in-

KEY TERMS

Bone marrow—Soft tissue that fills the hollow centers of bones. Blood cells and platelets (disk-shaped bodies in the blood that are important in clotting) are produced in the bone marrow.

Chemotherapy—Treatment of an illness with chemical agents. The term is usually used to describe the treatment of cancer with drugs.

Hepatitis—Inflammation of the liver caused by a virus, chemical, or drug.

Immune response—The body's natural protective reaction against disease and infection.

Immune system—The system that protects the body against disease and infection through immune responses.

Inflammation—Pain, redness, swelling, and heat that usually develop in response to injury or illness.

Seizure—A sudden attack, spasm, or convulsion.

Shingles—A disease caused the Herpes zoster virus—the same virus that causes chickenpox. Symptoms of shingles include pain and blisters along one nerve, usually on the face, chest, stomach, or back.

Sickle cell anemia—An inherited disorder in which red blood cells contain an abnormal form of hemoglobin, a protein that carries oxygen.

Wilson, Billie Ann, RN, PhD, Carolyn L. Stang, PharmD, and Margaret T. Shannon, RN, PhD. *Nurses Drug Guide 2000.* Stamford, CT: Appleton and Lange, 1999.

PERIODICALS

"Immunoprevention of Cancer: Is the Time Ripe?" *Cancer Research* 60 (May 15, 2000): 2571-2575.

Rosenberg, S. A. "Progress in the Development of Immunotherapy for the Treatment of Patients with Cancer." *Journal of Internal Medicine* 250 (December 2001): 462-475.

Rosenberg, S. A. "Progress in Human Tumor Immunology and Immunotherapy." *Nature* 411 (May 17, 2001): 380-385.

ORGANIZATIONS

American Society of Health-System Pharmacists (ASHP). 7272 Wisconsin Avenue, Bethesda, MD 20814. (301) 657-3000. <www.ashp.org>.

National Cancer Institute (NCI). NCI Public Inquiries Office, Suite 3036A, 6116 Executive Boulevard, MSC8332, Bethesda, MD 20892-8322. (800) 4-CANCER or (800) 332-8615 (TTY). <www.nci.nih.gov>.

United States Food and Drug Administration (FDA). 5600 Fishers Lane, Rockville, MD 20857-0001. (888) INFO-FDA. <www.fda.gov>.

OTHER

National Cancer Institute (NCI). *Treating Cancer with Vaccine Therapy.* <www.cancertrials.nci.nih.gov/news/features/vaccine/html/page05.htm>.

Nancy Ross-Flanigan
Samuel Uretsky, PharmD
Kausalya Santhanam, Ph.D.

jected into patients. Since the cells taken from a different person for this purpose are often rejected, patients serve both as donor and recipient of their own T cells. Adoptive immunotherapy is particularly effective in patients who have received massive doses of radiation and chemotherapy. In such patients, therapy results in immunosuppression (weakened immune systems), making them vulnerable to viral infections. For example, CMV-specific T cells can reduce the risk of cytomegalovirus (CMV) infection in organ transplant patients.

Resources

BOOKS

"Factors Affecting Drug Response: Drug Interactions." In *The Merck Manual of Diagnosis and Therapy*, edited by Mark H. Beers, MD, and Robert Berkow, MD. Whitehouse Station, NJ: Merck Research Laboratories, 1999.

Reiger, Paula T. *Biotherapy: A Comprehensive Overview.* Sudbury: Jones and Bartlett, Inc. 2000.

Stern, Peter L., P. C. Beverley, and M. Carroll. *Cancer Vaccines and Immunotherapy.* New York: Cambridge University Press, 2000.

Immunosuppressant drugs

Definition

Immunosuppressant drugs, which are also called anti-rejection drugs, are used to prevent the body from rejecting a transplanted organ.

Purpose

When an organ, such as a liver, heart or kidney, is transplanted from one person (the donor) into another (the recipient), the immune system of the recipient triggers the same response against the new organ that it would have against any foreign material, setting off a chain of events that can damage the transplanted organ. This process is called rejection. It can occur rapidly (acute rejection), or over a long period of time (chronic rejection). Rejection can occur despite close matching of the donated organ and the transplant patient. Immunosuppressant drugs greatly decrease the risks of rejection, protecting the new organ and preserving its function. These drugs act by blocking the recipient's immune system so that it is less likely to react against the transplanted organ. A wide variety of drugs are available to achieve this aim but work in different ways to reduce the risk of rejection.

In addition to being used to prevent organ rejection, immunosuppressant drugs are also used to treat such severe skin disorders as psoriasis and such other diseases as rheumatoid arthritis, Crohn's disease (chronic inflammation of the digestive tract), and patchy hair loss (alopecia areata). Some of these conditions are termed "autoimmune" diseases, indicating that the immune system is reacting against the body itself.

Description

Immunosuppressant drugs can be classified according to their specific molecular mode of action. The four main categories of immunosuppressant drugs currently used in treating patients with transplanted organs are the following:

- Cyclosporins (Neoral, Sandimmune, SangCya). These drugs act by inhibiting T-cell activation, thus preventing T-cells from attacking the transplanted organ.

- Azathioprines (Imuran). These drugs disrupt the synthesis of DNA and RNA as well as the process of cell division.

- Monoclonal antibodies, including basiliximab (Simulect), daclizumab (Zenpax), and muromonab (Orthoclone OKT3). These drugs act by inhibiting the binding of interleukin-2, which in turn slows down the production of T-cells in the patient's immune system.

- Such **corticosteroids** as prednisolone (Deltasone, Orasone). These drugs suppress the inflammation associated with transplant rejection.

Most patients are prescribed a combination of drugs after their transplant, one from each of the above main groups; for example, they may be given a combination of cyclosporin, azathioprine, and prednisolone. Over a period of time, the doses of each drug and the number of drugs taken may be reduced as the risks of rejection decrease. Most transplant patients, however, will need to take at least one immunosuppressive medication for the rest of their lives.

Immunosuppressants can also be classified according to the specific organ that is transplanted:

- Basiliximab (Simulect) is also used in combination with such other drugs as cyclosporin and corticosteroids in kidney transplants.

- Daclizumab (Zenapax) is also used in combination with such other drugs as cyclosporin and corticosteroids in kidney transplants.

- Muromonab CD3 (Orthoclone OKT3) is used along with cyclosporin in kidney, liver and heart transplants.

- Tacrolimus (Prograf) is used in liver and kidney transplants. It is under study for bone marrow, heart, pancreas, pancreatic island cell, and small bowel transplantation

Some immunosuppressants are also used to treat a variety of autoimmune diseases:

- Azathioprine (Imuran) is used not only to prevent organ rejection in kidney transplants, but also in treatment of rheumatoid arthritis. It has been used to treat chronic ulcerative colitis, although it has proved to be of limited value for this use.

- Cyclosporin (Sandimmune, Neoral) is used in heart, liver, kidney, pancreas, bone marrow, and heart/lung transplantation. The Neoral form of cyclosporin has been used to treat psoriasis and rheumatoid arthritis. The drug has also been used to treat many other conditions, including multiple sclerosis, diabetes, and myasthenia gravis.

- Glatiramer acetate (Copaxone) is used in the treatment of relapsing-remitting multiple sclerosis. In one study, glatiramer reduced the frequency of multiple sclerosis attacks by 75% over a two-year period.

- Mycopehnolate (CellCept) is used along with cyclosporin in kidney, liver, and heart transplants. It has also been used to prevent the kidney problems associated with lupus erythematosus.

- Sirolimus (Rapamune) is used in combination with other drugs, including cyclosporin and corticosteroids, in kidney transplants. The drug is also used to treat patients with psoriasis.

Recommended dosage

Immunosuppressant drugs are available only with a physician's prescription. They come in tablet, capsule, liquid, and injectable forms. The recommended dosage depends on the type and form of immunosuppressant drug and the purpose for which it is being used. Doses may be different for different patients. The prescribing physician or the pharmacist who filled the prescription will advise the patient on the correct dosage.

Patients who are taking immunosuppressant drugs should take them *exactly as directed*. They should never take smaller, larger, or more frequent doses of these medications. In addition, immunosuppressant drugs should never be taken for a longer period of time than directed. The physician will decide exactly how much of the medicine each patient needs. Blood tests are usually necessary to monitor the action of these drugs.

Patients should always consult the prescribing physician before they stop taking an immunosuppressant drug.

Precautions

Patients who are taking immunosuppressant drugs should see their doctor on a regular basis. Periodic checkups will allow the physician to make sure the drug is working as it should and to monitor the patient for unwanted side effects. These drugs are very powerful and can cause such serious side effects as high blood pressure, kidney problems and liver disorders. Some side effects may not show up until years after the medicine was used. Anyone who has been advised to take immunosuppressant drugs should thoroughly discuss the risks and benefits of these medications with the prescribing physician.

Immunosuppressant drugs lower a person's resistance to infection and can make infections harder to treat. The drugs can also increase the chance of uncontrolled bleeding. Anyone who has a serious infection or injury while taking immunosuppressant drugs should get prompt medical attention and should make sure that the treating physician knows that he or she is taking an immunosuppressant medication. The prescribing physician should be immediately informed if such signs of infection as fever or chills; cough or hoarseness; pain in the lower back or side; painful or difficult urination; bruising or bleeding; blood in the urine; bloody or black, tarry stools occur. Other ways of preventing infection and injury include washing the hands frequently, avoiding sports in which injuries may occur, and being careful when using knives, razors, fingernail clippers, or other sharp objects. Avoiding contact with people who have infections is also important.

In addition, people who are taking or have been taking immunosuppressant drugs should not have such immunizations as smallpox vaccinations without consulting their physician. Because their resistance to infection has been lowered, people taking these drugs might get the disease that the vaccine is designed to prevent. People taking immunosuppressant drugs should avoid contact with anyone who has had a recent dose of oral polio vaccine, as there is a chance that the virus used to make the vaccine could be passed on to them.

Immunosuppressant drugs may cause the gums to become tender and swollen or to bleed. If this happens, a physician or dentist should be notified. Regular brushing, flossing, cleaning, and gum massage may help prevent this problem. A dentist can provide advice on how to clean the teeth and mouth without causing injury.

Special conditions

People who have certain diseases or disorders, or who are taking certain other medicines may have problems if they take immunosuppressant drugs. Before taking these drugs, patients should inform the prescribing physician about any of the following conditions:

ALLERGIES. Anyone who has had unusual reactions to immunosuppressant drugs in the past should let his or her physician know before taking the drugs again. The physician should also be told about any allergies to foods, dyes, preservatives, or other substances.

PREGNANCY. Azathioprine has been considered a cause of birth defects. The British National Formulary, however, states: "Transplant patients immunosuppressed with azathioprine should not discontinue it on becoming pregnant; there is no evidence that azathioprine is teratogenic. There is less experience of ciclosporin in pregnancy but it does not appear to be any more harmful than azathioprine. The use of these drugs during pregnancy needs to be supervised in specialist units. Any risk to the offspring of azathioprine-treated men is small." Nonetheless, patients who are taking any immunosuppressive drug should consult with their physician before conceiving a child, and they should notify the doctor at once when there is any indication of pregnancy.

Basiliximab should not be used during pregnancy. The manufacturer recommends using adequate contraception during use of this drug, and for eight weeks following the final dose.

The manufacturers warn against the use of tacrolimus and mycophenolate during pregnancy, on the basis of findings from animal studies. They recommend using adequate contraception while taking these drugs, and for six weeks after the last dose.

The safety of corticosteroids during pregnancy has not been absolutely determined. There is some evidence that use of these drugs during pregnancy may affect the baby's growth; however, this result is not certain, and may vary with the medication used. Patients taking any steroid drug should consult with their physician before starting a family, and should notify the doctor at once if they think they are pregnant.

Most of these medicines have not been studied in humans during pregnancy. Women who are pregnant or who may become pregnant and who need to take immunosuppressants should consult their physicians.

LACTATION. Immunosuppressant drugs pass into breast milk and may cause problems in nursing babies

KEY TERMS

Antibody—A protein produced by the immune system in response to the presence in the body of an antigen.

Antigen—Any substance or organism that is foreign to the body. Examples of antigens include bacteria, bacterial toxins, viruses, or other cells or proteins.

Autoimmune disease—A disease in which the immune system is overactive and produces antibodies that attack the body's own tissues.

Corticosteroids—A class of drugs that are synthetic versions of the cortisone produced by the body. They rank among the most powerful anti-inflammatory agents.

Cortisone—A glucocorticoid compound produced by the adrenal cortex in response to stress. Cortisone is a steroid with anti-inflammatory and immunosuppressive properties.

Inflammation—A process occurring in body tissues, characterized by increased circulation and the accumulation of white blood cells. Inflamma-

tion also occurs in such disorders as arthritis and causes harmful effects.

Immune system—The network of organs, cells, and molecules that work together to defend the body from such foreign substances and organisms causing infection and disease as bacteria, viruses, fungi, and parasites.

Immunosuppresive cytotoxic drugs—A class of drugs that function by destroying cells and suppressing the immune response.

Lymphocyte—A type of white blood cell involved in the immune response. The two main groups of lymphocytes are the B cells, which carry antibody molecules on their surface; and T cells, which destroy antigens.

Psoriasis—A skin disease characterized by itchy, scaly, red patches on the skin.

T cells—Any of several lymphocytes that have specific antigen receptors, and are involved in cell-mediated immunity and the destruction of antigen-bearing cells.

whose mothers take it. Breastfeeding is not recommended for women taking immunosuppressants.

OTHER MEDICAL CONDITIONS. People with any of the following conditions may have problems if they take immunosuppressant drugs:

• People who have shingles (herpes zoster) or chickenpox, or who have recently been exposed to chickenpox, may develop severe disease in other parts of their bodies when they take these medicines.

• Immunosuppressants may produce more intense side effects in people with kidney disease or liver disease, because their bodies are slow to get rid of the medicine.

• Oral forms of immunosuppressants may be less effective in people with intestinal problems, because the medicine cannot be absorbed into the body.

Before using immunosuppressants, people with these or other medical problems should make sure their physicians are aware of their conditions.

Side effects

Increased risk of infection is a common side effect of all immunosuppressant drugs. The immune system protects the body from infections; when the immune system is suppressed, infections are more likely. Taking

such **antibiotics** as co-trimoxazole prevents some of these infections. Immunosuppressant drugs are also associated with a slightly increased risk of cancer because the immune system plays a role in protecting the body against some forms of cancer. For example, the long-term use of immunosuppressant drugs carries an increased risk of developing skin cancer as a result of the combination of the drugs and exposure to sunlight.

Other side effects of immunosuppressant drugs are minor and usually go away as the body adjusts to the medicine. These include loss of appetite, nausea or vomiting, increased hair growth, and trembling or shaking of the hands. Medical attention is not necessary unless these side effects continue or cause problems.

The treating physician should be notified immediately if any of the following side effects occur:

• unusual tiredness or weakness

• fever or chills

• frequent need to urinate

Interactions

Immunosuppressant drugs may interact with other medicines. When interactions occur, the effects of one or both drugs may change or the risk of side effects may be greater. Other drugs may also have adverse effects on immunosuppressant therapy. It is particularly important for patients taking cyclosporin or tacrolimus to be careful about the possibility of drug interactions. Other examples of problematic interactions are:

• The effects of azathioprine may be greater in people who take allopurinol, a medicine used to treat gout.

• A number of drugs, including female hormones (estrogens), male hormones (androgens), the antifungal drug ketoconazole (Nizoral), the ulcer drug cimetidine (Tagamet), and the **erythromycins** (used to treat infections), may intensify the effects of cyclosporine.

• When sirolimus is taken at the same time as cyclosporin, the blood levels of sirolimus may be increased to a level that produces severe side effects. Although these two drugs are usually used together, the dose of sirolimus should be taken four hours after the dose of cyclosporin.

• Tacrolimus is eliminated through the kidneys. When this drug is used with other medications that may harm the kidneys, such as cyclosporin, the antibiotics gentamicin and amikacin, or the antifungal drug amphotericin B, the blood levels of tacrolimus may rise. Careful kidney monitoring is essential when tacrolimus is given with any drug that might cause kidney damage.

• The risk of cancer or infection may be greater when immunosuppressant drugs are combined with certain other drugs that also lower the body's ability to fight disease and infection. These drugs include corticosteroids, especially prednisone; the anticancer drugs chlorambucil (Leukeran), cyclophosphamide (Cytoxan), and mercaptopurine (Purinethol); and the monoclonal antibody muromonab-CD3 (Orthoclone), which is also used to prevent transplanted organ rejection.

Not every drug that may interact with immunosuppressant drugs is listed here. Anyone who takes immunosuppressant drugs should give their doctor a list of all other medicines that he or she is taking and should ask whether there are any potential interactions that might interfere with treatment.

Resources

BOOKS

Abbas, A. K., and A. H. Lichtman. *Basic Immunology: Functions and Disorders of the Immune System.* Philadelphia: W. B. Saunders Co., 2001.

Sompayrac, L. M. *How the Immune System Works.* Boston: Blackwell Science, 1999.

Travers, P. *Immunobiology: The Immune System in Health and Disease,* 5th ed. New York: Garland Publishers, 2001.

ORGANIZATIONS

American Association of Immunologists (AAI). 9650 Rockville Pike, Bethesda, MD 20814. (301) 634-7178. <www.12.17.12.70/aai/default/asp>.

American Society of Health-System Pharmacists (ASHP). 7272 Wisconsin Avenue, Bethesda, MD 20814. (301) 657-3000. <www.ashp.org>.

British National Formulary. <www.bnf.vhn.net/bnf/documents/bnf.2.html#BNFID_35091>.

National Cancer Institute (NCI). NCI Public Inquiries Office, Suite 3036A, 6116 Executive Boulevard, MSC8332, Bethesda, MD 20892-8322. (800) 4-CANCER or (800) 332-8615 (TTY). <www.nci.nih.gov>.

United States Food and Drug Administration (FDA). 5600 Fishers Lane, Rockville, MD 20857-0001. (888) INFO-FDA. <www.fda.gov>.

Nancy Ross-Flanigan
Samuel Uretsky, PharmD

Implantable cardioverter-defibrillator

Definition

The implantable cardioverter-defibrillator (ICD) is a surgically implanted electronic device that directs an electric charge directly into the heart to treat life-threatening arrhythmias.

Purpose

The implantable cardioverter-defibrillator is used to detect and stop life-threatening arrhythmias and restore a productive heartbeat that is able to provide adequate cardiac output to sustain life. The exact indications for the implantation of the device are controversial, but patients suffering from ventricular fibrillation (unproductive heartbeat), ventricular tachycardia (abnormally fast heartbeat), long QT syndrome (an inherited heart disease), or others at risk for sudden cardiac death are potential candidates for this device. A study by the National Institute for Heart, Lung, and Blood of the National Institutes of Health showed a significant increase in survival for patients suffering from ventricular arrhythmias when ICD implant is compared to medication. Several follow-up studies indicate that this may be due to the marked increase in survival for the sickest patients, generally defined as those having a heart weakened to less than 50% of normal, as measured by the ability of the left side of the heart to pump blood. Overall, studies have documented a very low mortality rate of 1–2% an-

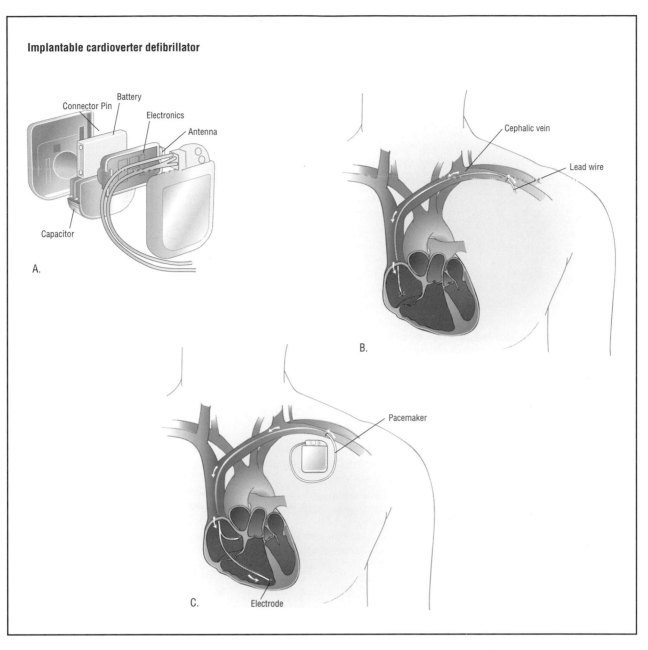

Implantable cardioverter defibrillator

To place an implantable cardioverter defibrillator, a lead wire is inserted into the cephalic vein of the shoulder and fed into the heart chambers (B). An electrode is implanted in the heart muscle of the lower chamber, and the device is attached (C). *(Illustration by Argosy.)*

nually for persons implanted with the device, compared to approximately 15–25% for patients on drug therapy.

Demographics

ICD implant is limited to patients that face the risk of sudden cardiac death from sustained ventricular arrhythmia, including ventricular tachycardia and ventricular fibrillation. Less than 1% of the more than 100,000 device implants done in the United States are performed on pediatric patients. Reduction in the risk of sudden cardiac death improves to less than 2% for both populations.

Diagnosis

Patients experiencing syncope (fainting) will be monitored with a **cardiac monitor** for arrhythmias. Following unsuccessful medical treatment for sustained ventricular arrhythmias, ICD implant will be indicated.

Description

Similar in structure to a pacemaker, an ICD has three main components: a generator, leads, and an electrode. The generator is encased in a small rectangular container, usually about 2 in (5 cm) wide and around 3 oz (85 g) in weight. Even smaller generators have been developed, measuring 1 in (2.5 cm) in diameter and weighing about 0.5 oz (14 g). The generator is powered by lithium batteries and is responsible for generating the electric shock. The generator is controlled by a computer chip that can be programmed to follow specific steps according to the input gathered from the heart. The programming is initially set and can be changed using a wand programmer, a device that communicates by radio waves through the chest of the patient after implantation. One or two leads, or wires, are attached to the generator. These wires are generally made of platinum with an insulating coating of either silicone or polyurethane. The leads carry the electric shock from the generator. At the tip of each lead is a tiny device called an electrode that delivers the necessary electrical shock to the heart. Thus, the electric shock is created by the generator, carried by the leads, and delivered by the electrodes to the heart. The decision of where to put the leads depends on the needs of the patient, but they can be located in the left ventricle, the left atrium, or both.

According to the American College of Cardiology, more than 100,000 persons worldwide currently have an ICD. The battery-powered device rescues the patient from a life-threatening arrhythmia by performing a number of functions in order to reestablish normal heart rhythm, which varies with the particular problem of the patient. Specifically, if encountered with ventricular tachycardia, many devices will begin treatment with a pacing regimen. If the tachycardia is not too fast, the ICD can deliver several pacing signals in a row. When those signals stop, the heart may go back to a normal rhythm. If the pacing treatment is not successful, many devices will move onto **cardioversion**. With cardioversion, a mild shock is sent to the heart to stop the fast heartbeat. If the problem detected is ventricular fibrillation, a stronger shock called a **defibrillation** is sent. This stronger shock can stop the fast rhythm and help the heartbeat return to normal. Finally, many ICDs can also detect heartbeats that are too slow; they can act like a pacemaker and bring the heart rate up to normal. ICDs that defibrillate both the ventricles and the atria have also been developed. Such devices not only provide dual-chamber pacing but also can distinguish ventricular from atrial fibrillation. Patients that experience both atrial and ventricle fibrillations, or atrial fibrillation alone, that would not be controlled with a single-chamber device are candidates for this kind of ICD.

Operation

ICD insertion is considered minor surgery, and can be performed in either an **operating room** or an electrophysiology laboratory. The insertion site in the chest will be cleaned, shaved, and numbed with local anesthetic. Generally, left-handed persons have ICDs implanted on the right side, and visa versa, to speed return to normal activities. Two small cuts (incisions) are made, one in the chest wall and one in a vein just under the collarbone. The wires of the ICD are passed through the vein and attached to the inner surface of the heart. The other ends of the wires are connected to the main box of the ICD, which is inserted into the tissue under the collarbone and above the breast. Once the ICD is implanted, the physician will test it several times before the anesthesia wears off by causing the heart to fibrillate and making sure the ICD responds properly. The doctor then closes the incision with sutures (stitches), staples, or surgical glue. The entire procedure takes about an hour.

Immediately following the procedure, a **chest x ray** will be taken to confirm the proper placement of the wires in the heart. The ICD's programming may be adjusted by passing the programming wand over the chest. After the initial operation, the physician may induce ventricular fibrillation or ventricular tachycardia one more time prior to the patient's discharge, although recent studies suggest that this final test is not generally necessary.

A short stay in the hospital is usually required following ICD insertion, but this varies with the patient's age and condition. If there are no complications, complete recovery from the procedure will take about four weeks. During that time, the wires will firmly take hold where they were placed. In the meantime, the patient should avoid heavy lifting or vigorous movements of the arm on the side of the ICD, or else the wires may become dislodged.

After implantation, the cardioverter-defibrillator is programmed to respond to rhythms above the patient's **exercise** heart rate. Once the device is in place, many tests will be conducted to ensure that the device is sensing and defibrillating properly. About 50% of patients with ICDs require a combination of drug therapy and the ICD.

Morbidity and mortality rates

Perioperative mortality demonstrates a 0.4–1.8% risk of death for primary non-thoracotomy implants. The ICD showed improved survival compared to medical therapy, improving by 38% at one year. There is a 96% survival rate at four years for those implanted with ICD. Less then 2% of patients require termination of the device, with a return to only medical therapy.

Normal results

Ventricular tachycardia can be successfully relieved by pacing in 96% of instances with the addition of defibrillation converting 98% of patients to a productive rhythm that is able to sustain cardiac output. Ventricular fibrillation is successfully converted in 98.6–98.8% of all cases. Atrial fibrillation and rapid ventricular response leads to erroneous fibrillation in as many as 11% of patients.

Risks

Environmental conditions that can affect the functioning of the ICD after installation include:

- strong electromagnetic fields such as those used in arc-welding

- contact sports

- shooting a rifle from the shoulder nearest the installation site

- cell phones used on that side of the body

- magnetic mattress pads such as those believed to treat arthritis

- some medical tests such as **magnetic resonance imaging** (MRI)

Environmental conditions often erroneously thought to affect ICDs include:

- microwave ovens (the waves only affect old, unshielded **pacemakers** and do not affect ICDs)

- airport security (although metal detector alarms could be set off, so patients should carry a card stating they have an ICD implanted)

- anti-theft devices in stores (although patients should avoid standing near the devices for prolonged periods)

Patients should also be instructed to memorize the manufacturer and make of their ICD. Although manufacturing defects and recalls are rare, they do occur and a patient should be prepared for that possibility.

Aftercare

In general, if the condition of the patient's heart, drug intake, and metabolic condition remain the same, the ICD requires only periodic checking every two months or so for battery strength and function. This is done by placing a special device over the ICD that allows signals to be sent over the telephone to the doctor, a process called trans-telephonic monitoring.

If changes in medications or physical condition occur, the doctor can adjust the ICD settings using a programmer, which involves placing the wand above the pacemaker and remotely changing the internal settings. One relatively common problem is the so-called "ICD storm," in which the machine inappropriately interprets an arrhythmia and gives a series of shocks. Reprogramming can sometimes help alleviate that problem.

When the periodic testing indicates that the battery is getting low, an elective ICD replacement operation is

KEY TERMS

Arrhythmia—A variation of the normal rhythm of the heartbeat.

Cardioverter—A device to apply electric shock to the chest to convert an abnormal heartbeat into a normal heartbeat.

Defibrillation—An electronic process that helps reestablish a normal heart rhythm.

Ventricles—The two large lower chambers of the heart that pump blood to the lungs and the rest of the human body.

Ventricular fibrillation—An arrhythmia in which the heart beats very fast, but blood is not pumped out to the body, which can become fatal if not corrected.

Ventricular tachycardia—An arrhythmia in which the heart rate is more than 100 beats per minute.

scheduled. The entire signal generator is replaced because the batteries are sealed within the case. The leads can often be left in place and reattached to the new generator. Batteries usually last from four to eight years.

Alternatives

Patients are treated with medical therapy to reduce the chance of arrhythmia. This alternative has been shown to have a higher rate of sudden death when compared to ICD over the initial three years of treatment, but has not been compared at five years. If the site of ventricular tachycardia generation can be mapped by electrophysiology studies, the aberrant cells can be removed or destroyed. Less then 5% of patients suffer peri-operative mortality with this cell removal.

Resources

BOOKS

Gersh, Bernard J., ed. *Mayo Clinic Heart Book.* New York: William Morrow and Company, Inc., 2000.

PERIODICALS

Gregoratos, Gabriel, et al. "ACC/AHA Guidelines for Implantation of Cardiac Pacemakers and Antiarrhythmia Devices." *Journal of the American College of Cardiologists* 31, no. 5 (April 1998): 1175–1209.

Moss, A. "Implantable Cardioverter-Defibrillator Therapy: The Sickest Patients Benefit Most." *Circulation* 101 (April 2000): 1638–1640.

Sears, Samuel F. Jr., et al. "Fear of Exertion Following ICD Storm: Considering ICD Shock and Learning History."

Journal of Cardiopulmonary Rehabilitation 21 (January/February 2001): 47.

ORGANIZATIONS

American Heart Association. National Center. 7272 Greenville Avenue, Dallas, TX, 75231-4596. (214) 373-6300. <http://www.americanheart.org>.

North American Society of Pacing and Electrophysiology. 6 Strathmore Road, Natick, MA, 01760-2499. (508) 647-0100. <http://www.naspe.org/index.html>.

OTHER

"Implantable Cardioverter-Defibrillator." *American Academy of Family Physicians.* May 7, 2001. <http://www.family-doctor.org/handouts/270.html>.

"Implantable Cardioverter-Defibrillators (ICDs)" *North American Society of Pacing and Electrophysiology.* 2000. <http://www.naspe.org/your_heart/treatments/icds.html>.

Michelle L. Johnson, MS, JD
Allison J. Spiwak, MSBME

In vitro fertilization

Definition

In vitro fertilization (IVF) is a procedure in which eggs (ova) from a woman's ovary are removed, they are fertilized with sperm in a laboratory procedure, and then the fertilized egg (embryo) is returned to the woman's uterus.

Purpose

IVF is one of several assisted reproductive techniques (ART) used to help infertile couples to conceive a child. If after one year of having sexual intercourse without the use of birth control a woman is unable to get pregnant, infertility is suspected. Some of the reasons for infertility are damaged or blocked fallopian tubes, hormonal imbalance, or endometriosis in the woman. In the man, low sperm count or poor quality sperm can cause infertility.

IVF is one of several possible methods to increase the chances for an infertile couple to become pregnant. Its use depends on the reason for infertility. IVF may be an option if there is a blockage in the fallopian tube or endometriosis in the woman, or low sperm count or poor quality sperm in the man. There are other possible treatments for these conditions, such as surgery for blocked tubes or endometriosis, which may be attempted before IVF.

IVF will not work for a woman who is incapable of ovulating or with a man who is not able to produce at least a few healthy sperm.

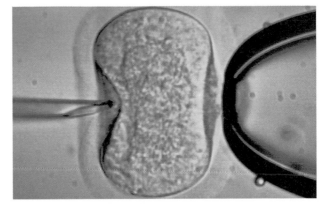

A microscopic image of a needle (left) injecting sperm cells directly into a human egg (center). The broad object at right is a pipette used to hold the ovum steady. *(Phototake NYC. Reproduced by permission.)*

Demographics

IVF has been used successfully since 1978, when the first child to be conceived by this method was born in England. Over the past 20 years, thousands of couples have used this method of ART or similar procedures to conceive.

Description

In vitro fertilization is a procedure in which the joining of egg and sperm takes place outside of a woman's body. A woman may be given fertility drugs before this procedure so that several eggs mature in the ovaries at the same time. The mature eggs (ova) are removed from the woman's ovaries using a long, thin needle. The physician has access to the ovaries using one of two possible procedures. One involves inserting the needle through the vagina (transvaginally); the physician guides the needle to the location in the ovaries with the help of an ultrasound machine. In the other procedure, called **laparoscopy**, a small thin tube with a viewing lens is inserted through an incision in the navel. This allows the physician to see on a video monitor inside the uterus to locate the ovaries.

Once the eggs are removed, they are mixed with sperm in a laboratory dish or test tube. (This is the origin of the term "test tube baby.") The eggs are monitored for several days. Once there is evidence that fertilization has occurred and the cells have begun to divide, they are then returned to the woman's uterus.

In the procedure to remove eggs, a sufficient number may be gathered to be frozen and saved (either fertilized or unfertilized) for additional IVF attempts.

Diagnosis/Preparation

Once a woman is determined to be a good candidate for *in vitro* fertilization, she will generally be given fertility drugs to stimulate ovulation and the development of multiple eggs. These drugs may include gonado-tropin-releasing hormone agonists (GnRHa), Pergonal, Clomid, or human chorionic gonadotropin (hcg). The maturation of the eggs is then monitored with ultrasound tests and frequent blood tests. If enough eggs mature, a physician will perform the procedure to remove them. The woman may be given a sedative prior to the procedure. A local anesthetic agent may also be used to reduce discomfort during the procedure.

The screening procedures and treatments for infertility can become a long, expensive, and, sometimes, disappointing process. Each IVF attempt takes at least an entire menstrual cycle and can cost $5,000–10,000, which may or may not be covered by health insurance. The anxiety of dealing with infertility can challenge both individuals and their relationship. The added stress and expense of multiple clinic visits, testing, treatments, and surgical procedures can become overwhelming. Couples may want to receive counseling and support through the process.

Aftercare

After the IVF procedure is performed, the woman can resume normal activities. A pregnancy test can be done approximately 12–14 days after the procedure to determine if it was successful.

Risks

The risks associated with in vitro fertilization include the possibility of multiple pregnancy (since several embryos may be implanted) and ectopic pregnancy (an embryo that implants in the fallopian tube or in the abdominal cavity outside the uterus). There is a slight risk of ovarian rupture, bleeding, infections, and complications of anesthesia. If the procedure is successful and pregnan-

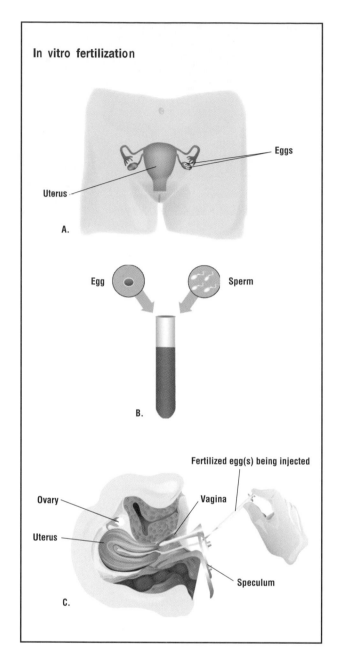

In vitro fertilization

Eggs

Uterus

A.

Egg

Sperm

B.

Fertilized egg(s) being injected

Ovary

Vagina

Uterus

Speculum

C.

For *in vitro* fertilization, hormones are administered to the patient, and then eggs are harvested from her ovaries (A). The eggs are fertilized by sperm donated by the father (B). Once the cells begin to divide, one or more embryos are placed into the woman's uterus to develop (C). *(Illustration by GGS Inc.)*

cy is achieved, the pregnancy carries the same risks as any pregnancy achieved without assisted technology.

Normal results

Success rates vary widely among clinics and among physicians performing the procedure. A couple has about a 10% chance of becoming pregnant each time the pro-

cedure is performed. Therefore, the procedure may have to be repeated more than once to achieve pregnancy.

Abnormal results include ectopic or multiple pregnancy that may abort spontaneously or that may require termination if the health of the mother is at risk.

Morbidity and mortality rates

The most common cause of morbidity is ecotopic pregnancy. Pain is associated with most components of the procedure. Mortality as a result of IVF is extremely rare.

Alternatives

Other types of assisted reproductive technologies might be used to achieve pregnancy. A procedure called intracytoplasmic sperm injection (ICSI) utilizes a manipulation technique that must be performed using a microscope to inject a single sperm into each egg. The fertilized eggs can then be returned to the uterus, as in IVF. In gamete intrafallopian tube transfer (GIFT), the eggs and sperm are mixed in a narrow tube, and then deposited in the fallopian tube, where fertilization normally takes place. Another variation on IVF is zygote intrafallopian tube transfer (ZIFT). As in IVF, the fertilization of the eggs occurs in a laboratory dish. And, similar to GIFT, the embryos are placed in the fallopian tube, rather than in the uterus as with IVF.

Resources

BOOKS

Boggs, William M., and Rosella D. Smith. *The Journey to Fertility: A Couple's Guide to In Vitro Fertilization*. Timonium, MD: Wilrose Books, 2001.

DeJonge, Christopher J. *Assisted Reproductive Technologies: Current Accomplishments and New Horizons*. Oxford: Cambridge University Press, 2002.

Elder, Kay, and Brian Dale. *In Vitro Fertilization, 2nd edition*. Oxford: Cambridge University Press, 2000.

Trounson, Alan O., and David K. Gaardner. *Handbook of In Vitro Fertilization, 2nd edition*. Boca Raton, FL: CRC Press, 1999.

PERIODICALS

Aboulghar, M. A., R. T. Mansour, G. I. Serour, H. G. Al-Inany, and M. M. Aboulghar. "The Outcome of In Vitro Fertilization in Advanced Endometriosis with Previous Surgery: A Case-controlled Study." *American Journal of Obstetrics and Gynecology* 188, no. 2 (2003): 371–375.

Kolibianakis, E. M., et al. "Outcome for Donors and Recipients in Two Egg-sharing Policies." *Fertility and Sterility* 79, no. 1 (2003): 69–73.

Puskar, J. M. "Prenatal Adoption: The Vatican's Proposal to the *In Vitro* Fertilization Disposition Dilemma." *New York University Law School Journal of Human Rights* 14, no. 3 (1998): 757–793.

KEY TERMS

Endometriosis—An inflammation of the endometrium, the mucous lining of the uterus.

Fallopian tubes—In a woman's reproductive system, a pair of narrow tubes (one for each ovary) that carries eggs from the ovary to the uterus.

Gamete intrafallopian tube transfer (GIFT)—A process where eggs are taken from a woman's ovaries, mixed with sperm, and then deposited into the woman's fallopian tube.

Intracytoplasmic sperm injection (ICSI)—A process used to inject a single sperm into each egg before fertilized eggs are put back into a woman's body; the procedure may be used if the male has a low sperm count.

Zygote intrafallopian tube transfer (ZIFT)—The woman's eggs are fertilized in a laboratory dish and then placed in her fallopian tube.

Squires, J., A. Carter, and P. Kaplan. "Developmental Monitoring of Children Conceived by Intracytoplasmic Sperm Injection and *In Vitro* Fertilization." *Fertility and Sterility* 79, no. 2 (2003): 453–454.

ORGANIZATIONS

American Board of Obstetrics and Gynecology. 2915 Vine Street, Suite 300, Dallas, TX 75204. (214) 871-1619; Fax: (214) 871-1943. info@abog.org. <http://www.abog.org>.

American College of Obstetricians and Gynecologists. 409 12th St., SW, P.O. Box 96920, Washington, DC 20090-6920. <http://www.acog.org>.

American Infertility Association. 666 Fifth Avenue, Suite 278, New York, NY 10103. (718) 621-5083. E-mail: <info@americaninfertility.org>. <http://www.americaninfertility.org>.

American Society for Reproductive Medicine. 1209 Montgomery Highway, Birmingham, AL 35216-2809. (205) 978-5000. <http://www.asrm.com>.

International Council on Infertility Information Dissemination, Inc. P.O. Box 6836, Arlington, VA 22206. (703) 379-9178. <http://www.inciid.org>.

OTHER

American Society for Reproductive Medicine. [cited March 1, 2003]. <http://www.asrm.org/Patients/FactSheets/invitro.html>.

Columbia University College of Physicians and Surgeons. [cited March 2, 2003]. <http://www.columbia.edu/cu/news/01/09/in_vitro_prayer.html>.

Encyclopedia.Com. [cited March 2, 2003]. <http://www.encyclopedia.com/html/i1/invitro.asp>.

International Council on Infertility Information Dissemination. <http://www.inciid.org/ivf.html>.

L. Fleming Fallon Jr., MD, DrPH

Incision care

Definition

Incision care refers to a series of procedures and precautions related to closing a wound or surgical incision; protecting the cut or injured tissues from contamination or infection; and caring properly for the new skin that forms during the healing process. Incision care begins in the hospital or outpatient clinic and is continued by the patient during **recovery at home**.

Purpose

There are several reasons for caring properly for an incision or wound. These include:

• lowering the risk of postoperative complications, particularly infection

• avoiding unnecessary pain or discomfort

• minimizing scarring

• preventing blood loss

Description

Types of wound or incision closure

Proper care of an incision begins with knowing what material or technique the surgeon used to close the cut. There are four major types of closure used in Canada and the United States as of 2003.

SURGICAL SUTURES. Sutures, or stitches, are the oldest method still in use to close an incision. The surgeon uses a sterilized thread, which may be made of natural materials (silk or catgut) or synthetic fibers, to stitch the edges of the cut together with a special curved needle. There are two major types of sutures, absorbable and nonabsorbable. Absorbable sutures are gradually broken down in the body, usually within two months. Absorbable sutures do not have to be removed. They are used most commonly to close the deeper layers of tissue in a large incision or in such areas as the mouth. Nonabsorbable sutures are not broken down in the body and must be removed after the incision has healed. They are used most often to close the outer layers of skin or superficial cuts.

Sutures have several disadvantages. Because they are made of materials that are foreign to the body, they must be carefully sterilized and the skin around the incision cleansed with Betadine or a similar antiseptic to minimize the risk of infection. Suturing also requires more time than newer methods of closure. If the patient is not under general anesthesia, the surgeon must first apply or inject a local anesthetic before suturing. Lastly, there is a higher risk of scarring with sutures, particularly if the surgeon puts too much tension on the thread while stitching or selects thread that is too thick for the specific procedure.

SURGICAL STAPLES. Surgical staples are a newer method of incision closure. Staples are typically made of stainless steel or titanium. They are used most commonly to close lacerations on the scalp or to close the outer layers of skin in orthopedic procedures. They cannot be used on the face, hand, or other areas of the body where tendons and nerves lie close to the surface. Staples are usually removed seven to 10 days after surgery.

Staples are less likely to cause infections than sutures, and they also take less time to use. They can, however, leave noticeable scars if the edges of the wound or incision have not been properly aligned. In addition, staples require a special instrument for removal.

STERI-STRIPS. Steri-strips are pieces of adhesive material that can be used in some surgical procedures to help the edges of an incision grow together. They have several advantages, including low rates of infection, speed of application, no need for local anesthesia, and no need for special removal. Steri-strips begin to curl and peel away from the body, usually within five to seven days after surgery. They should be pulled off after two weeks if they have not already fallen off. Steri-strips, however, have two disadvantages: they are not as precise as sutures in bringing the edges of an incision into alignment; and they cannot be used on areas of the body that are hairy or that secrete moisture, such as the palms of the hands or the armpits.

LIQUID TISSUE GLUES. Tissue glues are the newest type of incision closure. They are applied to the edges of the incision and form a bond that holds the tissues together until new tissue is formed. The tissue glues most commonly used as of 2003 belong to a group of chemicals known as cyanoacrylates. In addition to speed of use and a low infection rate, tissue glues are gradually absorbed by the body. They are less likely to cause scarring, which makes them a good choice for facial surgery and other cosmetic procedures. They are also often used to close lacerations or incisions in children, who find them less frightening or painful than sutures or staples. Like Steri-strips, however, tissue glues cannot be used on areas of high moisture. They are also ineffective for use on the knee or elbow joints.

Dressings and drainage devices

After the incision is closed, it is covered with a dressing of some sort to keep it dry and clean, and prevent infection. Most dressings consist of gauze pads held in place by strips of adhesive tape or ACE bandages. An antibiotic ointment may also be applied to the gauze. A newer type of dressing, called OpSite, is a thin transparent membrane made of polyurethane coated with adhesive. It keeps disease organisms out of the wound while holding a layer of moisture close to the skin. This moist environment keeps scabs from forming and speeds up healing of the incision. OpSite can also be used to hold catheters or drainage tubes in place. It cannot, however, be used for severe (third-degree) burns or deep incisions.

Some surgical procedures, such as a mastectomy or removal of a ruptured appendix, require the surgeon to insert a drainage device to remove blood, pus, or other tissue fluids from the area of the incision. It is important to prevent these fluids from collecting under the incision because they encourage the growth of disease organisms. The drain may be left in place after the patient leaves the hospital. If so, the patient will need to check and empty the drain daily in addition to general incision care.

Home care of incisions

Guidelines for home care of an incision vary somewhat depending on the material that was used for closure, the location and size of the incision, and the nature of the operation. The following section is a general description of the major aspects of incision care.

Patients should ask their doctor for specific information about caring for their incision:

- the type of closure used

- whether another appointment will be needed to remove any sutures or staples

- the length of time that the incision should be kept covered, and the type of dressing that should be used

- whether the incision must be kept dry, and for how long

- any specific signs or symptoms that should be reported to the doctor

Most hospitals and surgery clinics provide patients with written handouts or checklists about incision care; however, it is always helpful to go over the information in the handout with the doctor or nurse, and to ask any further questions that may arise.

BATHING AND SHOWERING. Incisions should be kept dry for several days after surgery, with the exception of incisions closed with tissue glue. Incisions closed with nonabsorbable sutures or staples must be kept dry until the doctor removes the sutures or staples, usually about seven to 10 days after surgery. Incisions closed with Steri-strips should be kept dry for about four to five days. If the incision gets wet accidentally, it must be dried at once. Patients with incisions on the face, hands, or arms may be able to take showers or tub baths as long as they are able to hold the affected area outside the water. Patients with incisions in other parts of the body can usually take sponge baths.

It is usually safe to allow incisions closed with tissue glue to get wet during showering or bathing. The patient should, however, dry the area around the incision carefully after washing.

PHYSICAL ACTIVITY AND EXERCISE. Patients should avoid any activity that is likely to pull on the edges of the incision or put pressure on it. Walking and other light activities are encouraged, as they help to restore normal energy levels and digestive functions. Patients should not, however, participate in sports, engage in sexual activity, or lift heavy objects until they have had a postoperative checkup.

MEDICATIONS. Patients are asked to avoid **aspirin** or over-the-counter medications containing aspirin for a week to 10 days after surgery, because aspirin interferes with blood clotting and makes it easier for bruises to form in the skin near the incision. The doctor will usually prescribe codeine or another non-aspirin medication for pain control.

Patients with medications prescribed for other conditions or disorders should ask the doctor before starting to take them again.

SUN EXPOSURE. As an incision heals, the new skin that is formed over the cut is very sensitive to sunlight and will burn more easily than normal skin. Sunburn in turn will lead to worse scarring. Patients should keep the incision area covered for three to nine months from direct sun exposure in order to prevent burning and severe scarring.

SPECIAL CONSIDERATIONS FOR FACIAL INCISIONS. Patients who have had facial surgery are usually given very detailed instructions about incision care because the skin of the face is relatively thin, and incisions in this area can be easily stretched out of alignment. In addition, patients should not apply any cosmetic creams or make-up after surgery without the surgeon's approval because of the risk of infection or allergic reaction.

GENERAL HYGIENE. Infection is the most common complication of surgical procedures. It can be serious; of the 300,000 patients whose incisions become infected each year in the United States, about 10,000 will die. It is important, therefore, to minimize the risk of an infection when caring for an incision at home.

Patients should observe the following precautions about general cleanliness and personal habits:

• wash hands carefully after using the toilet and after touching or handling trash or garbage; pets and pet equipment; dirty laundry or soiled incision dressings; and anything else that is dirty or has been used outdoor

• ask family members, close friends, and others who touch the patient to wash their hands first

• avoid contact with family members and others who are sick or recovering from a contagious illness

• stop smoking (smoking slows down the healing process)

Risks

Some patients are more likely to develop infections or to have their incision split open, which is known as dehiscence. Risk factors for infection or dehiscence include:

• obesity

• diabetes

• malnutrition

• a weakened immune system

• taking corticosteroid medications prescribed for another disorder or condition

• a history of heavy smoking

Warning signs

Patients who notice any of the following signs or symptoms should call their doctor:

• fever of 100.5°F (38°C) or higher

• severe pain in the area of the incision

• intense redness in the area of the incision

• bruising

• bleeding or increased drainage of tissue fluid

Normal results

As an incision heals, it is normal to experience some redness, swelling, itching, minor skin irritation or oozing of tissue fluid, or small lumps in the skin near the incision. At first, the skin over the incision will feel thick and hard. After a period of two to six months, the swelling and irritation will go down and the scar tissue will soften and begin to blend into the surrounding tissue.

See also Bandages and dressings; Hospital-acquired infections; Postoperative care; Wound care.

KEY TERMS

Catgut—The oldest type of absorbable suture. In spite of its name, catgut is made from collagen derived from sheep or cattle intestines. Synthetic absorbable sutures have been available since the 1980s.

Dehiscence—Separation or splitting open of the different layers of tissue in a surgical incision. Dehiscence may be partial, involving only a few layers of surface tissue; or complete, reopening all the layers of the incision.

Drainage—The withdrawal or removal of blood and other fluid matter from an incision or wound. An incision that is oozing blood or tissue fluids is said to be draining.

Dressing—A bandage, gauze pad, or other material placed over a wound or incision to cover and protect it.

Incision—The medical term for a cut made by a surgeon into a tissue or organ.

Laceration—A type of wound with rough, torn, or ragged edges.

Suture—A loop of thread, catgut, or synthetic material used to draw together and align the edges of a wound or incision. Sutures may be either absorbable or nonabsorbable.

Resources

BOOKS

Graber, Mark, MD. "General Surgery: Wound Management," In *The University of Iowa Family Practice Handbook*. 4th edition. Edited by Mark Graber, MD, and Matthew L. Lanternier, MD. St. Louis, MO: Mosby, 2001.

PERIODICALS

Farion, K., M. H. Osmond, L. Hartling, et al. "Tissue Adhesives for Traumatic Lacerations in Children and Adults." *Cochrane Database Systems Review* 2002: CD003326.

Higgins, Robert V., Wendel Naumann, and James Hall. "Abdominal Incisions and Sutures in Gynecologic Oncological Surgery." *eMedicine*. December 11, 2002 [cited February 19, 2003].

Mattick, A., G. Clegg, T. Beattie, and T. Ahmad. "A Randomised, Controlled Trial Comparing a Tissue Adhesive (2-octylcyanoacrylate) with Adhesive Strips (Steri-strips) for Paediatric Laceration Repair." *Emergency Medicine Journal* 19 (September 2002): 405–407.

Passey, Andrew. "Does the Suture Have a Future?" *Medica.de*, November 15, 2002 [cited February 19, 2003]. <http://www.11.medica.de/cgi-bin/md_medica/pub/content,lang,2/ticket,g_a_s_t/oid,7456/local_lang,2>.

Selo-Ojeme, D. O., and K. B. Lim. "Randomised Clinical Trial of Suture Compared with Adhesive Strip for Skin Closure After HRT Implant." *BJOG: An International Journal of Obstetrics and Gynaecology* 109 (October 2002): 1178–1180.

Takahashi, K., T. Muratani, M. Saito, et al. "Evaluation of the Disinfective Efficacy of Povidone-Iodine with the Use of the Transparent Film Dressing OpSite Wound." *Dermatology* 204 (2002), Supplement 1: 59–62.

Rebecca Frey, Ph.D.

Incisional hernia repair

Definition

Incisional hernia repair is a surgical procedure performed to correct an incisional hernia. An incisional hernia, also called a ventral hernia, is a bulge or protrusion that occurs near or directly along a prior abdominal surgical incision. The surgical repair procedure is also known as incisional or ventral herniorrhaphy.

Purpose

Incisional hernia repair is performed to correct a weakened area that has developed in the scarred muscle tissue around a prior abdominal surgical incision, occurring as a result of tension (pulling in opposite directions) created when the incision was closed with sutures, or by any other condition that increases abdominal pressure or interferes with proper healing.

Demographics

Because incisional hernias can occur at the site of any type of abdominal surgery previously performed on a wide range of individuals, there is no outstanding profile of an individual most likely to have an incisional hernia. Men, women, and children of all ages and ethnic backgrounds may develop an incisional hernia after abdominal surgery. Incisional hernia occurs more commonly among adults than among children.

Description

An incisional hernia can develop in the scar tissue around any surgery performed in the abdominal area, from the breastbone down to the groin. Depending upon the location of the hernia, internal organs may press through the weakened abdominal wall. The rate of incisional hernia occurrence can be as high as 13%

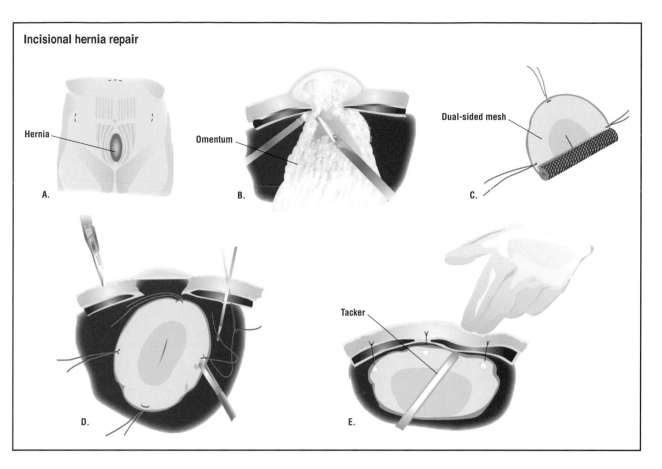

Incisional hernia repair

A. Hernia

B. Omentum

C. Dual-sided mesh

D.

E. Tacker

An incisional hernia occurs at the site of a previous incision (A). Intestinal contents break through the abdominal wall and bubble up under the skin. In a laparoscopic repair, the surgeon uses laparoscopic forceps to pull the material, omentum, from the hernia site (B). A mesh pad is inserted into the site to line the hernia site (C and D), and is tacked into place (E). *(Illustration by GGS Inc.)*

with some abdominal surgeries. These hernias may occur after large surgeries such as intestinal or vascular (heart, arteries, and veins) surgery, or after smaller surgeries such as an **appendectomy** or a **laparoscopy**, which typically requires a small incision at the navel. Incisional hernias themselves can be very small or large and complex, involving growth along the scar tissue of a large incision. They may develop months after the surgery or years after, usually because of inadequate healing or excessive pressure on an abdominal wall scar. The factors that increase the risk of incisional hernia are conditions that increase strain on the abdominal wall, such as obesity, advanced age, malnutrition, poor metabolism (digestion and assimilation of essential nutrients), pregnancy, dialysis, excess fluid retention, and either infection or hematoma (bleeding under the skin) after a prior surgery.

Tension created when sutures are used to close a surgical wound may also be responsible for developing an incisional hernia. Tension is known to influence poor healing conditions because of related swelling and wound separation. Tension and abdominal pressure are greater in people who are overweight, creating greater risk of developing incisional hernias following any abdominal surgery, including surgery for a prior inguinal (groin) hernia. People who have been treated with steroids or chemotherapy are also at greater risk for developing incisional hernias because of the affect these drugs have on the healing process.

The first symptom a person may have with an incisional hernia is pain, with or without a bulge in the abdomen at or near the site of the original surgery. Incisional hernias can increase in size and gradually produce more noticeable symptoms. Incisional hernias may or may not require surgical treatment.

The effectiveness of surgical repair of an incisional hernia depends in part on reducing or eliminating tension at the surgical wound. The tension-free method used by many medical centers and preferred by surgeons who specialize in hernia repair involves the permanent placement of surgical (prosthetic) steel or polypropylene mesh patches well beyond the edges of the weakened area of the abdominal wall. The mesh is sewn to the area, bridging the hole or weakened area beneath it. As the area heals, the mesh becomes firmly integrated into the inner abdominal wall membrane (peritoneum) that protects the organs of the abdomen. This method creates little or no tension and has a lower rate of hernia recurrence, as well as a faster recovery with less pain. Incisional hernias recur more frequently when staples are used rather than sutures to secure mesh to the abdominal wall. Autogenous tissue (skin from the patient's own body) has also been used for this type of repair.

Two surgical approaches are used to treat incisional hernias: either a laporoscopic incisional herniorrhaphy, which uses small incisions and a tube-like instrument with a camera attached to its tip; or a conventional open repair procedure, which accesses the hernia through a larger abdominal incision. Open procedures are necessary if the intestines have become trapped in the hernia (incarceration) or the trapped intestine has become twisted and its blood supply cut off (strangulation). Extremely obese patients may also require an open procedure because deeper layers of fatty tissue will have to be removed from the abdominal wall. Mesh may be used with both types of surgical access.

Minimally invasive laporoscopic surgery has been shown to have advantages over conventional open procedures, including:

- reduced hospital stays
- reduced postoperative pain
- reduced wound complications
- reduced recovery time

Surgical procedure

In both open and laparoscopic procedures, the patient lies on the operating table, either flat on the back or on the side, depending on the location of the hernia. General anesthesia is usually given, though some pa-

tients may have local or regional anesthesia, depending on the location of the hernia and complexity of the repair. A catheter may be inserted into the bladder to remove urine and decompress the bladder. If the hernia is near the stomach, a gastric (nose or mouth to stomach) tube may be inserted to decompress the stomach.

In an open procedure, an incision is made just large enough to remove fat and scar tissue from the abdominal wall near the hernia. The outside edges of the weakened hernial area are defined and excess tissue removed from within the area. Mesh is then applied so that it overlaps the weakened area by several inches (centimeters) in all directions. Non-absorbable sutures (the kind that must be removed by the doctor) are placed into the full thickness of the abdominal wall. The sutures are tied down and knotted.

In the less-invasive laparoscopic procedure, two or three small incisions will be made to access the hernia site—the laparoscope is inserted in one incision and **surgical instruments** in the others to remove tissue and place the mesh in the same fashion as in an open procedure. Significantly less abdominal wall tissue is removed in laparoscopic repair. The surgeon views the entire procedure on a video monitor to guide the placement and suturing of mesh.

Diagnosis/Preparation

Diagnosis

Reviewing the patient's symptoms and medical history are the first steps in diagnosing an incisional hernia. All prior surgeries will be discussed. The doctor will ask how much pain the patient is experiencing, when it was first noticed, and how it has progressed. The doctor will palpate (touch) the area, looking for any abnormal bulging or mass, and may ask the patient to cough or strain in order to see and feel the hernia more easily. To confirm the presence of the hernia, an ultrasound examination or other scan such as computed tomography (CT) may be performed. Scans will allow the doctor to visualize the hernia and to make sure that the bulge is not another type of abdominal mass such as a tumor or enlarged lymph gland. The doctor will be able to determine the size of the defect and whether or not surgery is an appropriate way to treat it. A referral to a surgeon will be made if the doctor believes that medical treatment will not effectively correct the incisional hernia.

Preparation

Many months before the surgery, the patient's doctor may advise weight loss to help reduce the risks of surgery and to improve the surgical results. Control of diabetes and smoking cessation are also recommended for a better surgical result. Close to the time of the scheduled surgery, the patient will have standard preoperative blood and urine tests, an electrocardiogram, and a **chest x ray** to make sure that heart and lungs and major organ systems are functioning well. A week or so before surgery, medications may be discontinued, especially **aspirin** or anticoagulant (blood-thinning) drugs. Starting the night before surgery, patients must not eat or drink anything. Once in the hospital, a tube may be placed into a vein in the arm (intravenous line) to deliver fluid and medication during surgery. The patient will be given a preoperative injection of **antibiotics** before the procedure. A sedative may be given to relax the patient.

Aftercare

Immediately after surgery, the patient will be observed in a recovery area for several hours, for monitoring of body temperature, pulse, blood pressure, and heart function, as well as observation of the surgical wound for undue bleeding or swelling. Patients will usually be discharged on the day of the surgery; only more complex hernias such as those with incarcerated or strangulated intestines will require overnight hospitalization. Some patients may have prolonged suture-site pain, which may be treated with pain medication or anti-inflammatory drugs. Antibiotics may be prescribed to help prevent postoperative infection.

Once the patient is home, the hernia repair site must be kept clean, and any sign of swelling or redness reported to the surgeon. Patients should also report a fever or any abdominal pain. Outer sutures may have to be removed by the surgeon in a follow-up visit about a week after surgery. Activities may be limited to non-strenuous movement for up to two weeks, depending on the type of surgery performed. To allow proper healing of muscle tissue, hernia repair patients should avoid heavy lifting for at least six to eight weeks after surgery, or longer as advised.

Risks

Long-term complications seldom occur after incisional hernia repair. Short-term risks are greater with obese patients or those who have had multiple earlier operations or the prior placement of mesh patches. The risk of complications has been shown to be about 13%. The risk of recurrence and repeat surgery is as high as 52%, particularly with open procedures or those using staples rather than sutures for wound closure. Some of the factors that cause incisional hernias to occur in the first place, such as obesity and nutritional disorders, will persist in certain patients and encourage the development of a second incisional hernia and repeat surgery. Each subsequent time, the surgery will become more difficult and the risk

---

QUESTIONS TO ASK THE DOCTOR

- What procedure will be performed to correct my hernia?
- What is your experience with this procedure? How often do you perform this procedure?
- Why must I have the surgery?
- What are my options if I do not have the surgery?
- How can I expect to feel after surgery?
- What are the risks involved in having this surgery?
- How quickly will I recover? When can I return to school or work?
- What are my chances of having this type of hernia again?
- What can I do to avoid getting this type of hernia again?

---

of complications greater. Postoperative infection is higher with open procedures than with laparoscopic procedures.

Postoperative complications may include:

- fluid buildup at the site of mesh placement, sometimes requiring aspiration (draining off)
- postoperative bleeding, though seldom enough to require repeat surgery
- prolonged suture pain, treated with pain medication or anti-inflammatory drugs
- intestinal injury
- nerve injury
- fever, usually related to surgical wound infection
- intra-abdominal (within the abdominal wall) abscess
- urinary retention
- respiratory distress

Normal results

Good outcomes are expected with incisional hernia repair, particularly with the laparoscopic method. Patients will usually go home the day of surgery and can expect a one- to two-week recovery period at home, and then a return to normal activities. The American College of Surgeons reports that recurrence rates after the first repair of an incisional hernia range from 25–52%. Recurrence is more frequent when conventional surgical

KEY TERMS

Autogenous tissue—Tissue or skin taken from any part of a person's body to graft onto another part of the body that needs repairing; laid on as a patch.

Herniorrhaphy—The surgical repair of any type of hernia.

Incarcerated intestine—Intestines trapped in the weakened area of the hernia that cannot slip back into the abdominal cavity.

Incisional hernia—Hernia occuring at the site of a prior surgery.

Inguinal hernia—A weak spot in the lower abdominal muscles of the groin through which body organs, usually the large intestines, can push through as a result of abdominal pressure.

Laparoscopy—The use of a camera-tipped viewing tube called a laparoscope to perform minimally invasive surgery while viewing the procedure on a video screen.

Strangulated hernia—A twisted piece of herniated intestine that can block blood flow to the intestines.

---

wound closure with standard sutures (stitches) is used. Recurrence after open procedures has been shown to be less likely when mesh is used, although complications, especially infection, have been shown to increase because of the larger abdominal incisions. Laparoscopy with mesh has shown rates of recurrence as low as 3.4%, with fewer complications as well.

Morbidity and mortality rates

Deaths are not reported resulting directly from the performance of herniorrhaphy for incisional hernia.

Alternatives

The alternatives to first-time and recurrent incisional hernia repair begin with preventive measures such as:

- Losing weight; maintaining suitable weight for age and height.
- Strengthening abdominal muscles through regular moderate **exercise** such as walking, tai chi, yoga, or stretching exercises and gentle aerobics.
- Reducing abdominal pressure by avoiding constipation and the buildup of excess body fluids, achieved by adopting a high-fiber, low-salt diet.

- Learning to lift heavy objects in a safe, low-strain way using arm and leg muscles.
- Controlling diabetes and poor metabolism with regular medical care and dietary changes as recommended.
- Eating a healthy, balanced diet of whole foods, high in essential nutrients, including whole grains, fruits and vegetables, limited meat and dairy, and eliminating prepared and refined foods.

See also Femoral hernia repair; Inguinal hernia repair.

Resources

BOOKS

Maddern, Guy J. *Hernia Repair: Open vs. Laparoscopic Approaches*. London: Churchill Livingstone, 1997.

ORGANIZATIONS

American College of Surgeons (ACS), Office of Public Information. 633 North Saint Clair Street, Chicago, IL 60611-3211. (312) 202-5000. <http://www.facs.org>.

The National Digestive Diseases Information Clearinghouse (NIDDK). 2 Information Way, Bethesda, MD 20892-3570. <http://www.niddk.nih.gov/health/digest/nddic.htm>.

OTHER

"Focus on Men's Health: Hernia." January 2003. *MedicineNet Home*.<http://www.medicinenet.com>.

Incisional and Ventral Hernias (Patient Information). Central Montgomery Medical Center, Outpatient Surgery Department. 2100 N. Broad Street, Lansdale, PA 19446. (215) 368-1122.

L. Lee Culvert

Inflatable sphincter *see* **Artificial sphincter insertion**

Informed consent

Definition

Informed consent is a legal document in all 50 states. It is an agreement for a proposed medical treatment or non-treatment, or for a proposed invasive procedure. It requires physicians to disclose the benefits, risks, and alternatives to the proposed treatment, non-treatment, or procedure. It is the method by which fully informed, rational persons may be involved in choices about their health care.

Description

Informed consent stems from the legal and ethical right an individual has to decide what is done to his or her body, and from the physician's ethical duty to make sure that individuals are involved in decisions about their own health care. The process of securing informed consent has three phases, all of which involve information exchange between doctor and patient and are part of patient education. First, in words an individual can understand, the physician must convey the details of a planned procedure or treatment, its potential benefits and serious risks, and any feasible alternatives. The patient should be presented with information on the most likely outcomes of the treatment. Second, the physician must evaluate whether or not the person has understood what has been said, must ascertain that the risks have been accepted, and that the patient is giving consent to proceed with the procedure or treatment with full knowledge and forethought. Finally, the individual must sign the consent form, which documents in generic format the major points of consideration. The only exception to this is securing informed consent during extreme emergencies.

It is critical that a patient receive enough information on which to base informed consent, and that the consent is wholly voluntary and has not been forced in any way. It is the responsibility of the physician who discusses the particulars with the patient to detail the conversation in the medical record. A physician may, at his or her discretion, appoint another member of the health care team to obtain the patient's signature on the consent form, with the assurance that the physician has satisfied the requirements of informed consent.

The law requires that a reasonable physician/patient standard be applied when determining how much information is considered adequate when discussing a procedure or treatment with the patient. There are three approaches to making this discussion: what the typical physician would say about the intervention (the reasonable physician standard); what an average patient would need to know to be an informed participant in the decision (the reasonable patient standard); and what a patient would need to know and understand to make a decision that is informed (the subjective standard).

There is a theory that the practice of acquiring informed consent is rooted in the post-World War II Nuremberg Trials. At the war crimes tribunal in 1949, 10 standards were put forth regarding physicians' requirements for experimentation on human subjects. This established a new standard of ethical medical behavior for the post-WW II human rights age, and the concept of voluntary informed consent was established. A number of rules accompanied voluntary informed consent. It could only be requested for experimentation for the gain of society, for the potential acquisition of knowledge of the pathology of disease, and for studies performed that avoided physical and mental suffering to the fullest extent possible.

Today, all of the 50 United States have legislation that delineates the required standards for informed consent. For example, the State of Washington employs the second approach outlined as the reasonable patient standard (what an average patient would need to know to be an informed participant in the decision). This approach ensures that a doctor fulfills all professional responsibilities and provides the best care possible and that patients have choices in decisions about their health care. However, the patient's competence in making a decision is considered. This points to the issue of the patient's mental capacity. Anyone suffering from an illness, anticipating surgery, or undergoing treatment for a disease is under a great deal of stress and anxiety. It may be natural for a patient to be confused or indecisive. When the attending physician has serious doubts about the patient's understanding of the intervention and its risks, the patient may be referred for a psychiatric consultation. This is strictly a precaution to ensure that the patient understands what has been explained; declining to be treated or operated on does not necessarily mean the person is incompetent. It could mean that the person is exercising the right to make his or her own health care decisions.

Although the law requires a formal presentation of the procedure or treatment to the patient, physicians do express doubt as to the wisdom of this. Some believe that informing patients of the risks of treatment might scare them into refusing it, even when the risks of non-treatment are even greater. But patients might have a different view. Without the complete story, for example, a patient might consent to beginning a particular course of chemotherapy. Convinced by the pressures from a pharmaceutical company, it is conceivable that a doctor will use an agent less effective than a newer treatment. By withholding information about treatment alternatives, the physician may be denying the patient a choice and, worse, perhaps a chance of an extended life of greater quality.

Undeniably, physicians in surgery, anesthesia, oncology, infectious disease, and other specialties are faced with issues regarding informed consent. As the federal government takes a more active role in deciding the extent to which patients must be informed of treatments, procedures, and clinical trials in which they voluntarily become enrolled, more and more health care providers must become educated in what must be conveyed to patients. This is emphasized by the report of a case in which a federal court (Hutchinson vs. United States [91 F2d 560 (9th Cir. 1990)]) ruled in favor of the physician, despite his failure to advise his asthmatic patient, for whom he had prescribed the steroid, prednisone, of the drug's well-known risk of developing aseptic necrosis (bone death), which did occur. The practitioner neglected to inform the patient that there were other drugs available with much less serious side effects that could have treated the asthma. However, a higher appellate court reversed the ruling and found the physician guilty. Apparently, the patient had used more conservative drugs in the past with good results. The court believed that if the physician had merely advised the patient of the more serious side effects of prednisone and offered the patient more conservative treatment, the physician would have avoided liability.

Nursing professionals have a greater role than they might believe in evaluating whether or not consent is informed. When a nurse witnesses the signature of a patient for a procedure, or surgery, he or she is not responsible for providing the details. Rather, the role is to be the patient's advocate, to protect the patient's dignity, to identify any fears, and to determine the patient's degree of comprehension and approval of care to be received. Each patient is an individual, and each one will have a different and unique response depending on his or her personality, level of education, emotions, and cognitive status. If a patient can restate the information that has been imparted, then that will help to confirm that he or she has received enough information and has understood it. The nurse is obligated to report any doubts about the patient's understanding regarding what has been said or any concerns about his or her capacity to make decisions.

Results

The result of informed consent is greater safety and protection for patients, physicians, and society.

See also Do not resuscitate order; Patient confidentiality; Patient rights.

Resources

BOOKS

Berg, J. W., C. W. Lidz, P. S. Appelbaum, and L. S. Parker. *Informed Consent: Legal Theory and Clinical Practice, 2nd edition.* London: Oxford University Press, 2001.

Donnelly, Mary. *Consent.* Crosses Green, Ireland: Cork University Press, 2002.

Jonsen, A. R., W. J. Winslade, and M. Siegler. *Clinical Ethics: A Practical Approach to Ethical Decisions in Clinical Medicine, 5th edition.* New York: McGraw-Hill, 2002.

Radford, Roger. *Informed Consent.* Bangor, Maine: Booklocker. com, 2002.

PERIODICALS

Hanson, L. R. "Informed Consent and the Scope of a Physician's Duty of Disclosure." *Specialty Law Digest: Health Care Law* 285 (2003): 9–34.

Karpman, A. "Informed Consent: Does the First Amendment Protect a Patient's Right to Choose Alternative Treatment?" *New York Law School Journal of Human Rights* 16, no. 3 (2000): 933–957.

Luce, J. M. "Is the Concept of Informed Consent Applicable to Clinical Research Involving Critically Ill Patients?" *Critical Care Medicine* 31, no. 3 (2003): S153–S160.

Marr, S. "Protect Your Practice: Informed Consent." *Plastic Surgical Nursing* 22, no. 4 (2002): 180–197.

Meadows, M. "Drug Research and Children." *FDA Consumer* 37, no. 1 (2003): 12–17.

ORGANIZATIONS

American Academy of Family Physicians. 11400 Tomahawk Creek Parkway, Leawood, KS 66211-2672. (913) 906-6000. fp@aafp.org. <http://www.aafp.org>.

American Bar Association. 750 N Lake Shore Drive, Chicago, IL 60611. 312-988-5000. <http://www.abanet.org/home. html>.

American College of Physicians. 190 N Independence Mall West, Philadelphia, PA 19106-1572. (800) 523-1546, x2600, or (215) 351-2600. <http://www.acponline.org>.

American Medical Association. 515 N. State Street, Chicago, IL 60610. 312) 464-5000. <http://www.ama-assn.org>.

OTHER

American Academy of Pediatrics. [cited March 23, 2003]. <http://www.aap.org/policy/00662.html>.

Food and Drug Administration. [cited March 23, 2003]. <http://www.fda.gov/opacom/morechoices/fed996.html>.

Office for Protection from Research Risks, Department of Health and Human Services. [cited March 23, 2003]. <http://ohrp.osophs.dhhs.gov/humansubjects/guidance/ ictips.htm>.

University of Washington School of Medicine. [cited March 23, 2003]. <http://eduserv.hscer.washington.edu/bioethics/ topics/consent.html>.

L. Fleming Fallon Jr., MD, DrPH

Inguinal hernia repair

Definition

Inguinal hernia repair, also known as herniorrhaphy, is the surgical correction of an inguinal hernia. An inguinal hernia is an opening, weakness, or bulge in the lining tissue (peritoneum) of the abdominal wall in the groin area between the abdomen and the thigh. The surgery may be a standard open procedure through an incision large enough

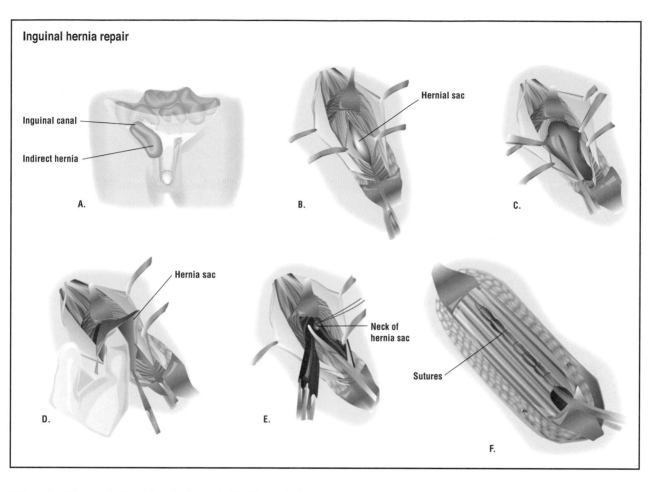

Inguinal hernia repair

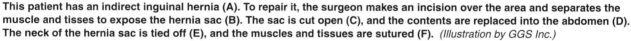

This patient has an indirect inguinal hernia (A). To repair it, the surgeon makes an incision over the area and separates the muscle and tisses to expose the hernia sac (B). The sac is cut open (C), and the contents are replaced into the abdomen (D). The neck of the hernia sac is tied off (E), and the muscles and tissues are sutured (F). *(Illustration by GGS Inc.)*

to access the hernia or a laparoscopic procedure performed through tiny incisions, using an instrument with a camera attached (laparoscope) and a video monitor to guide the repair. When the surgery involves reinforcing the weakened area with steel mesh, the repair is called hernioplasty.

Purpose

Inguinal hernia repair is performed to close or mend the weakened abdominal wall of an inquinal hernia.

Demographics

The majority of hernias occur in males. Nearly 25% of men and only 2% of women in the United States will develop inguinal hernias. Inguinal hernias occur nearly three times more often in African American adults than in Caucasians. Among children, the risk of groin hernia is greater in premature infants or those of low birth weight. Indirect inguinal hernias will occur in 10–20 children in every 1,000 live births.

Description

About 75% of all hernias are classified as inguinal hernias, which are the most common type of hernia occurring in men and women as a result of the activities of normal living and aging. Because humans stand upright, there is a greater downward force on the lower abdomen, increasing pressure on the less muscled and naturally weaker tissues of the groin area. Inguinal hernias do not include those caused by a cut (incision) in the abdominal wall (incisional hernia). According to the National Center for Health Statistics, about 700,000 inguinal hernias are repaired annually in the United States. The inguinal hernia is usually seen or felt first as a tender and sometimes painful lump in the upper groin where the inguinal canal passes through the abdominal wall. The inguinal canal is the normal route by which testes descend into the scrotum in the male fetus, which is one reason these hernias occur more frequently in men.

Hernias are divided into two categories: congenital (from birth), also called indirect hernias, and acquired, also called direct hernias. Among the 75% of hernias classified as inguinal hernias, 50% are indirect or congenital hernias, occurring when the inguinal canal entrance fails to close normally before birth. The indirect inguinal hernia pushes down from the abdomen and through the inguinal canal. This condition is found in 2% of all adult males and in 1–2% of male children. Indirect inguinal hernias can occur in women, too, when abdominal pressure pushes folds of genital tissue into the inquinal canal opening. In fact, women will more likely have an indirect inguinal hernia than direct. Direct or acquired inguinal hernias occur when part of the large intestine protrudes through a weakened area of muscles in the groin. The weakening results from a variety of factors encountered in the wear and tear of life.

Inguinal hernias may occur on one side of the groin or both sides at the same or different times, but occur most often on the right side. About 60% of hernias found in children, for example, will be on the right side, about 30% on the left, and 10% on both sides. The muscular weak spots develop because of pressure on the abdominal muscles in the groin area occurring during normal activities such as lifting, coughing, straining during urination or bowel movements, pregnancy, or excessive weight gain. Internal organs such as the intestines may then push through this weak spot, causing a bulge of tissue. A congenital indirect inguinal hernia may be diagnosed in infancy, childhood, or later in adulthood, influenced by the same causes as direct hernia. There is evidence that a tendency for inguinal hernia may be inherited.

A direct and an indirect inguinal hernia may occur at the same time; this combined hernia is called a pantaloon hernia.

A femoral hernia is another type of hernia that appears in the groin, occurring when abdominal organs and tissue press through the femoral ring (passageway where the major femoral artery and vein extend from the leg into the abdomen) into the upper thigh. About 3% of all hernias are femoral, and 84% of all femoral hernias occur in women. These are not inquinal hernias, but they can sometimes confuse the diagnosis of inguinal hernias because they curve over the inguinal area. They are more often accompanied by intestinal obstruction than inguinal hernias.

Because inguinal hernias do not heal on their own and can become larger or twisted, which may close off the intestines, the prevailing medical opinion is that hernias must be treated surgically when they cause pain or limit activity. Protruding intestines can sometimes be pushed back temporarily into the abdominal cavity, or an external support (truss) may be worn to hold the area in place until surgery can be performed. Sometimes, other medical conditions complicate the presence of a hernia by adding constant abdominal pressure. These conditions, including chronic coughing, constipation, fluid retention, or urinary obstruction, must be treated simultaneously to reduce abdominal pressure and the recurrence of hernias after repair. A relationship between smoking and hernia development has also been shown. Groin hernias occur more frequently in smokers than nonsmokers, especially in women. A hernia may become incarcerated, which means that it is trapped in place and cannot slip back into the abdomen. This causes bowel obstruction, which may require the removal of affected parts of the intestines (**bowel resection**) as well as hernia repair. If the herniated intestine becomes twisted, blood supply to the intestines may be cut off (intestinal ischemia) and the hernia is said to be strangulated, a condition causing severe pain and requiring immediate surgery.

Surgical procedures

In open inguinal hernia repair procedures, the patient is typically given a light general anesthesia of short duration. Local or regional anesthetics may be given to some patients. Open surgical repair of an indirect hernia begins with sterilizing and draping the inguinal area of the abdomen just above the thigh. An incision is made in the abdominal wall and fatty tissue removed to expose the inguinal canal and define the outer margins of the hole or weakness in the muscle. The weakened section of tissue is dissected (cut and removed) and the inguinal canal opening is sutured closed (primary closure), making sure that no abdominal organ tissue is within the sutured area. The exposed inguinal canal is examined for any other trouble spots that may need reinforcement. Closing the underlayers of tissue (subcutaneous tissue) with fine sutures and the outer skin with staples completes the procedure. A sterile dressing is then applied.

An open repair of a direct hernia begins just as the repair of an indirect hernia, with an incision made in the same location above the thigh, just large enough to allow visualization of the hernia. The surgeon will look for and palpate (touch) the bulging area of the hernia and will reduce it by placing sutures in the fat layer of the abdominal wall. The hernial sac itself will be closed, as in the repair of the indirect hernia, by using a series of sutures from one end of the weakened hernia defect to the other. The repair will be checked for sturdiness and for any tension on the new sutures. The subcutaneous tissue and skin will be closed and a sterile dressing applied.

Laparoscopic procedures are conducted using general anesthesia. The surgeon will make three tiny incisions in the abdominal wall of the groin area and inflate the abdomen with carbon dioxide to expand the surgical area. A laparoscope, which is a tube-like fiber-optic instrument with a small video camera attached to its tip, will be inserted in one incision and **surgical instruments** inserted in the other incisions. The surgeon will view the movement of the instruments on a video monitor, as the hernia is pushed back into place and the hernial sac is repaired with surgical sutures or staples. Laparoscopic surgery is believed to produce less postoperative pain and a quicker recovery time. The risk of infection is also reduced because of the small incisions required in laparoscopic surgery.

The use of surgical (prosthetic) steel mesh or polypropylene mesh in the repair of inguinal hernias has been shown to help prevent recurrent hernias. Instead of the tension that develops between sutures and the skin in a conventionally repaired area, hernioplasty using mesh patches has been shown to virtually eliminate tension. The procedure is often performed in an outpatient facility with local anesthesia and patients can walk away the same day, with little restrictions in activity. Tension-free repair is also quick and easy to perform using the laparoscopic method, although general anesthesia is usually used. In either open or laparoscopic procedures, the mesh is placed so that it overlaps the healthy skin around the hernia opening and then is sutured into place with fine silk. Rather than pulling the hole closed as in conventional repair, the mesh makes a bridge over the hole and as normal healing take place, the mesh is incorporated into normal tissue without resulting tension.

Diagnosis/Preparation

Diagnosis

Reviewing the patient's symptoms and medical history are the first steps in diagnosing a hernia. The surgeon will ask when the patient first noticed a lump or bulge in the groin area, whether or not it has grown larger, and how much pain the patient is experiencing. The doctor will palpate the area, looking for any abnormal bulging or mass, and may ask the patient to cough or strain in order to see and feel the hernia more easily. This may be all that is needed to diagnose an inguinal hernia.

To confirm the presence of the hernia, an ultrasound examination may be performed. The ultrasound scan will allow the doctor to visualize the hernia and to make sure that the bulge is not another type of abdominal mass such as a tumor or enlarged lymph gland. It is not usually possible to determine whether the hernia is direct or indirect until surgery is performed.

Preparation

Patients will have standard preoperative blood and urine tests, an electrocardiogram, and a **chest x ray** to make sure that the heart, lungs, and major organ systems are functioning well. A week or so before surgery, medications may be discontinued, especially **aspirin** or anticoagulant (blood-thinning) drugs. Starting the night before surgery, patients must not eat or drink anything. Once in the hospital, a tube may be placed into a vein in the arm (intravenous line) to deliver fluid and medication during surgery. A sedative may be given to relax the patient.

Aftercare

The hernia repair site must be kept clean and any sign of swelling or redness reported to the surgeon. Patients should also report a fever, and men should report any pain or swelling of the testicles. The surgeon may remove the outer sutures in a follow-up visit about a week after surgery. Activities may be limited to non-strenuous movement for up to two weeks, depending on the type of surgery performed and whether or not the surgery is the first hernia repair. To allow proper healing of muscle tis-

KEY TERMS

Incarcerated hernia—An inguinal hernia that is trapped in place and cannot slip back into the abdominal cavity, often causing intestinal obstruction.

Incisional hernia—Hernia occurring at the site of a prior surgery.

Inguinal hernia—A weak spot in the lower abdominal muscles of the groin through which body organs, usually the large intestines, can push through as a result of abdominal pressure.

Ischemia—The death of tissue that results from lack of blood flow and oxygen.

Laparoscopy—The use of a camera-tipped viewing tube called a laparoscope to perform minimally invasive surgery while viewing the procedure on a video screen.

Strangulated hernia—A twisted piece of herniated intestine that can block blood flow to the intestines.

sue, hernia repair patients should avoid heavy lifting for six to eight weeks after surgery. The postoperative activities of patients undergoing repeat procedures may be even more restricted.

Prevention of indirect hernias, which are congenital, is not possible. However, preventing direct hernias and reducing the risk of recurrence of direct and indirect hernias can be accomplished by:

• maintaining body weight suitable for age and height

• strengthening abdominal muscles through regular exercise

• reducing abdominal pressure by avoiding constipation and the build-up of excess body fluids, achieved by adopting a high-fiber, low-salt diet

• lifting heavy objects in a safe, low-stress way, using arm and leg muscles

Risks

Hernia surgery is considered to be a relatively safe procedure, although complication rates range from 1–26%, most in the 7–12% range. This means that about 10% of the 700,000 inguinal hernia repairs each year will have complications. Certain specialized clinics report markedly fewer complications, often related to whether open or laparoscopic technique is used. One of the greatest risks of inquinal hernia repair is that the her-

nia will recur. Unfortunately, 10–15% of hernias may develop again at the same site in adults, representing about 100,000 recurrences annually. The risk of recurrence in children is only about 1%. Recurrent hernias can present a serious problem because incarceration and strangulation are more likely and because additional surgical repair is more difficult than the first surgery. When the first hernia repair breaks down, the surgeon must work around scar tissue as well as the recurrent hernia. Incisional hernias, which are hernias that occur at the site of a prior surgery, present the same circumstance of combined scar tissue and hernia and even greater risk of recurrence. Each time a repair is performed, the surgery is less likely to be successful. Recurrence and infection rates for mesh repairs have been shown in some studies to be lower than with conventional surgeries.

Complications that can occur during surgery include injury to the spermatic cord structure; injuries to veins or arteries, causing hemorrhage; severing or entrapping nerves, which can cause paralysis; injuries to the bladder or bowel; reactions to anesthesia; and systemic complications such as cardiac arrythmias, cardiac arrest, or death. Postoperative complications include infection of the surgical incision (less in **laparoscopy**); the formation of blood clots at the site that can travel to other parts of the body; pulmonary (lung) problems; and urinary retention or urinary tract infection.

Normal results

Inguinal hernia repair is usually effective, depending on the size of the hernia, how much time has gone by between its first appearance and the corrective surgery, and the underlying condition of the patient. Most first-time hernia repair procedures will be one-day surgeries, in which the patient will go home the same day or in 24 hours. Only the most challenging cases will require an overnight stay. Recovery times will vary, depending on the type of surgery performed. Patients undergoing open surgery will experience little discomfort and will resume normal activities within one to two weeks. Laparoscopy patients will be able to enjoy normal activities within one or two days, returning to a normal work routine and lifestyle within four to seven days, with the exception of heavy lifting and contact sports.

Morbidity and mortality rates

Mortality related to inguinal hernia repair or postoperative complications is unlikely, but with advanced age or severe underlying conditions, deaths do occur. Recurrence is a notable complication and is associated with increased morbidity, with recurrence rates for indirect hernias from less than 1–7% and 4–10% for direct.

Alternatives

If a hernia is not surgically repaired, an incarcerated or strangulated hernia can result, sometimes involving life-threatening bowel obstruction or ischemia.

Resources

BOOKS

Maddern, Guy J. *Hernia Repair: Open vs. Laparoscopic approaches.* London: Churchill Livingstone, 1997.

ORGANIZATIONS

American College of Surgeons (ACS), Office of Public Information. 633 North Saint Clair Street, Chicago, IL 60611-3211. (312) 202-5000. <http://www.facs.org>.
The National Digestive Diseases Information Clearinghouse (NIDDK). 2 Information Way, Bethesda, MD 20892-3570. <http://www.niddk.nih.gov/health/digest/nddic.htm>.

OTHER

"Focus on Men's Health: Hernia." *MedicineNet Home* Jan. 2003. <http://www.medicinenet.com>.
"Inguinal Hernia." Healthwise, Inc. February 2001. <http://www.laurushealth.com/library.>.

L. Lee Culvert

Inner ear tube insertion *see* **Endolymphatic shunt**

Intensive care unit

Definition

An intensive care unit, or ICU, is a specialized section of a hospital that provides comprehensive and continuous care for persons who are critically ill and who can benefit from treatment.

Purpose

The purpose of the intensive care unit (ICU) is simple even though the practice is complex. Healthcare professionals who work in the ICU or rotate through it during their training provide around-the-clock intensive monitoring and treatment of patients seven days a week. Patients are generally admitted to an ICU if they are likely to benefit from the level of care provided. Intensive care has been shown to benefit patients who are severely ill and medically unstable—that is, they have a potentially life-threatening disease or disorder.

Although the criteria for admission to an ICU are somewhat controversial—excluding patients who are either too well or too sick to benefit from intensive care—there are four recommended priorities that intensivists (specialists in critical care medicine) use to decide this question. These priorities include:

- Critically ill patients in a medically unstable state who require an intensive level of care (monitoring and treatment).
- Patients requiring intensive monitoring who may also require emergency interventions.
- Patients who are medically unstable or critically ill and who do not have much chance for recovery due to the severity of their illness or traumatic injury.
- Patients who are generally not eligible for ICU admission because they are not expected to survive. Patients in this fourth category require the approval of the director of the ICU program before admission.

ICU care requires a multidisciplinary team that consists of but is not limited to intensivists (clinicians who specialize in critical illness care); pharmacists and nurses; respiratory care therapists; and other medical consultants from a broad range of specialties including surgery, pediatrics, and anesthesiology. The ideal ICU will have a team representing as many as 31 different health care professionals and practitioners who assist in patient evaluation and treatment. The intensivist will provide treatment management, diagnosis, interventions, and individualized care for each patient recovering from severe illness.

Demographics

A large and comprehensive study conducted in 1992 by the Society of Critical Care Medicine in collaboration with the American Hospital Association found that approximately 8% of all licensed hospital beds in the United States were designated for intensive care. The average size of an adult or pediatric ICU averaged 10–12 beds per unit. Small hospitals with fewer than 100 beds usually had one ICU, whereas larger hospitals with more than 300 beds usually had several ICUs designated for medical, surgical, and coronary patients. Smaller hospitals do not usually have a full-time board-certified specialist in critical care medicine, whereas larger medical centers generally employ certified intensivists—60% of hospitals with more than 500 beds had full-time specialist directors at the time the survey was conducted.

With regard to the nursing staff in ICUs, the proportion of nurses with specialized and advanced training in critical care medicine is higher in larger medical centers—about 16% in hospitals with 100 beds or fewer, but 21% in hospitals with more than 500 beds.

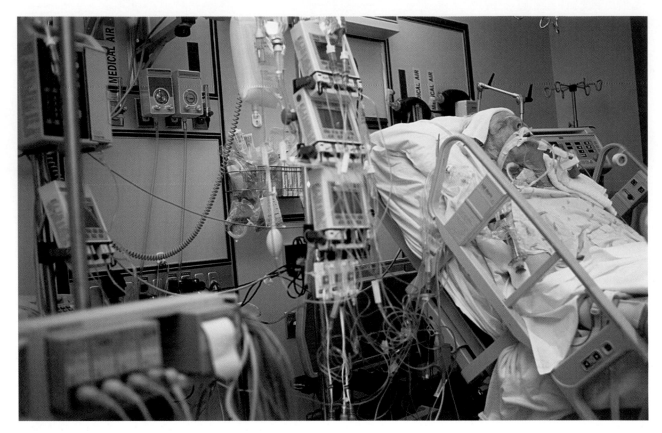

This man is recovering from quadruple bypass surgery in an intensive care unit. *(Custom Medical Stock Photo. Reproduced by permission.)*

Most pediatric ICUs have four to six beds per unit. The mortality rate in pediatric ICUs tends to increase in proportion to size, with larger units reporting more deaths (approximately 8% in the larger units). Eighty percent of pediatric ICUs have full-time medical directors.

Description

ICUs are highly regulated departments, typically limiting the number of visitors to the patient's immediate family even during visiting hours. The patient usually has several monitors attached to various parts of his or her body for real-time evaluation of medical stability. The intensivist will make periodic assessments of the patient's cardiac status, breathing rate, urinary output, and blood levels for nutritional and hormonal problems that may arise and require urgent attention or treatment. Patients who are admitted to the ICU for observation after surgery may have special requirements for monitoring. These patients may have catheters placed to detect hemodynamic (blood pressure) changes, or require **endotracheal intubation** to help their breathing, with the breathing tube connected to a mechanical ventilator.

In addition to the intensivist's role in direct patient care, he or she is usually the lead physician when multiple consultants are involved in an intensive care program. The intensivist coordinates the care provided by the consultants, which allows for an integrated treatment approach to the patient.

Nursing care has an important role in an intensive care unit. The nurse's role usually includes clinical assessment, diagnosis, and an individualized plan of expected treatment outcomes for each patient (implementation of treatment and patient evaluation of results). The ICU pharmacist evaluates all drug therapy, including dosage, route of administration, and monitoring for signs of allergic reactions. In addition to checking and supervising all levels of medication administration, the ICU pharmacist is also responsible for enteral and parenteral nutrition (tube feeding) for patients who cannot eat on their own. ICUs also have respiratory care therapists with specialized training in cardiorespiratory (heart and lung) care for critically ill patients. Respiratory therapists generally provide medications to help patients breathe as well as the care and support of mechanical ventilators. Respiratory therapists also evaluate all respiratory therapy procedures to maximize efficiency and cost-effectiveness.

Large medical centers may have more than one ICU. These specialized intensive care units typically include a CCU (coronary care unit); a pediatric ICU (PICU, dedicated to the treatment of critically ill children); a newborn ICU or NICU, for the care of premature and critically ill infants; and a surgical ICU (SICU, dedicated to the treatment of postoperative patients).

Preparation

Persons who are critically ill may be admitted to the ICU from the emergency room, a surgical ward, or from any other hospital department. ICUs are arranged around a central station so that patients can be seen either through the room windows or from a nursing station a few steps away. Patients are given 24-hour assessments by the intensivist. Preparatory orders for the ICU generally vary from patient to patient since treatment is individualized. The initial workup should be coordinated by the attending ICU staff (intensivist and ICU nurse specialist), pharmacists (for medications and IV fluid therapy), and respiratory therapists for stabilization, improvement, or continuation of cardiopulmonary care. Well-coordinated care includes prompt consultation with other specialists soon after the patient is admitted to the ICU. The patient is connected to monitors that record his or her **vital signs** (pulse, blood pressure, and breathing rate). Orders for medications, laboratory tests, or other procedures are instituted upon arrival.

In general there are eight categories of diseases and disorders that are regarded as medical justification for admission to an ICU. These categories include disorders of the cardiac, nervous, pulmonary, and endocrine (hormonal) systems, together with postsurgical crises and medication monitoring for drug ingestion or overdose. Cardiac problems can include heart attacks (myocardial infarction), shock, cardiac arrhythmias (abnormal heart rhythm), heart failure (congestive heart failure or CHF), high blood pressure, and unstable angina (chest pain). Lung disorders can include acute respiratory failure, pulmonary emboli (blood clots in the lungs), hemoptysis (coughing up blood), and respiratory failure. Neurological disorders may include acute stroke (blood clot in the brain), coma, bleeding in the brain (intracranial hemorrhage), such infections as meningitis, and traumatic brain injury (TBI). Medication monitoring is essential, including careful attention to the possibility of seizures and other drug side effects.

When patients are transferred to the ICU from another hospital department, treatment orders and planning must be reviewed and new treatment plans written for

the patient's current status. For example, a chronically ill inpatient may grow markedly worse within a few hours and may be transferred to the ICU, where the staff must reevaluate orders for his or her care.

Resources

PERIODICALS

Brilli, R. J., A. Spevetz, R. D. Branson, et al. "Critical Care Delivery in the Intensive Care Unit: Defining Clinical Roles and the Best Practice Model." *Critical Care Medicine* 29 (October 2001): 2007-2019.

Ethics Committee, Society of Critical Care Medicine. "Consensus Statement of the SCCM Ethics Committee Regarding Futile and Other Possibly Inadvisable Treatments." *Critical Care Medicine* 25 (May 1997): 887-891.

Truog, R. D., A. F. Cist, S. E. Brackett, et al. "Recommendations for End-of-Life Care in the Intensive Care Unit: The Ethics Committee of the Society of Critical Care Medicine." *Critical Care Medicine* 29 (December 2001): 2332-2348.

ORGANIZATIONS

American Hospital Association. One North Franklin, Chicago, IL 60606-3421. (312) 422-3000. <www.hospitalconnect.com>.

Joint Commission on Accreditation of Healthcare Organizations (JCAHO). One Renaissance Blvd., Oakbrook Terrace, IL 60181. (630) 792-5000 or (630) 792-5085. <www.jcaho.org/>.

Society of Critical Care Medicine (SCCM). 701 Lee Street, Suite 200, Des Plaines, IL 60016. (847) 827-6869; Fax: (847) 827-6869. <www.sccm.org>.

Laith Farid Gulli, M.D., M.S.
Bilal Nasser, M.D., M.S.
Uchechukwu Sampson, M.D., M.P.H., M.B.A.

Intensive care unit equipment

Definition

Intensive care unit (ICU) equipment includes patient monitoring, respiratory and cardiac support, **pain**

management, emergency resuscitation devices, and other life support equipment designed to care for patients who are seriously injured, have a critical or life-threatening illness, or have undergone a major surgical procedure, thereby requiring 24-hour care and monitoring.

Purpose

An ICU may be designed and equipped to provide care to patients with a range of conditions, or it may be designed and equipped to provide specialized care to patients with specific conditions. For example, a neuromedical ICU cares for patients with acute conditions involving the nervous system or patients who have just had neurosurgical procedures and require equipment for monitoring and assessing the brain and spinal cord. A neonatal ICU is designed and equipped to care for infants who are ill, born prematurely, or have a condition requiring constant monitoring. A trauma/burn ICU provides specialized injury and **wound care** for patients involved in auto accidents and patients who have gunshot injuries or burns.

Description

Intensive care unit equipment includes patient monitoring, life support and emergency resuscitation devices, and diagnostic devices.

Patient monitoring equipment

Patient monitoring equipment includes the following:

- Acute care physiologic monitoring system—comprehensive patient monitoring systems that can be configured to continuously measure and display a number of parameters via electrodes and sensors that are connected to the patient. These may include the electrical activity of the heart via an EKG, respiration rate (breathing), blood pressure, body temperature, cardiac output, and amount of oxygen and carbon dioxide in the blood. Each patient bed in an ICU has a physiologic monitor that measure these body activities. All monitors are networked to a central nurses' station.

- Pulse oximeter—monitors the arterial hemoglobin oxygen saturation (oxygen level) of the patient's blood with a sensor clipped over the finger or toe.

- Intracranial pressure monitor—measures the pressure of fluid in the brain in patients with head trauma or other conditions affecting the brain (such as tumors, edema, or hemorrhage). These devices warn of elevated pressure and record or display pressure trends. Intracranial pressure monitoring may be a capability included in a physiologic monitor.

- Apnea monitor—continuously monitors breathing via electrodes or sensors placed on the patient. An apnea monitor detects cessation of breathing in infants and adults at risk of respiratory failure, displays respiration parameters, and triggers an alarm if a certain amount of time passes without a patient's breath being detected. Apnea monitoring may be a capability included in a physiologic monitor.

Life support and emergency resuscitative equipment

Intensive care equipment for life support and emergency resuscitation includes the following:

- Ventilator (also called a respirator)—assists with or controls pulmonary ventilation in patients who cannot breathe on their own. Ventilators consist of a flexible breathing circuit, gas supply, heating/humidification mechanism, monitors, and alarms. They are microprocessor-controlled and programmable, and regulate the volume, pressure, and flow of patient respiration. Ventilator monitors and alarms may interface with a central monitoring system or information system.

- Infusion pump—device that delivers fluids intravenously or epidurally through a catheter. Infusion pumps employ automatic, programmable pumping mechanisms to deliver continuous anesthesia, drugs, and blood infusions to the patient. The pump is hung on an intravenous pole placed next to the patient's bed.

- Crash cart—also called a resuscitation or code cart. This is a portable cart containing emergency resuscitation equipment for patients who are "coding." That is, their **vital signs** are in a dangerous range. The emergency equipment includes a defibrillator, airway intubation devices, a resuscitation bag/mask, and medication box. Crash carts are strategically located in the ICU for immediate availability for when a patient experiences cardiorespiratory failure.

- Intraaortic balloon pump—a device that helps reduce the heart's workload and helps blood flow to the coronary arteries for patients with unstable angina, myocardial infarction (heart attack), or patients awaiting organ transplants. Intraaortic balloon pumps use a balloon placed in the patient's aorta. The balloon is on the end of a catheter that is connected to the pump's console, which displays heart rate, pressure, and electrocardiogram (ECG) readings. The patient's ECG is used to time the inflation and deflation of the balloon.

Diagnostic equipment

The use of diagnostic equipment is also required in the ICU. Mobile x-ray units are used for bedside radiography, particularly of the chest. Mobile x-ray units use a battery-operated generator that powers an x-ray tube. Handheld, portable clinical laboratory devices, or point-

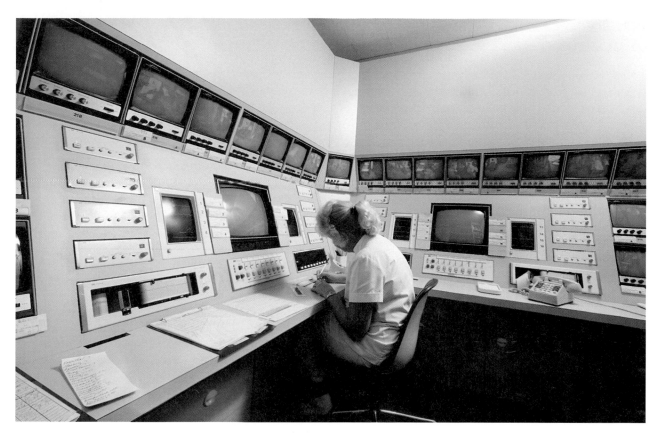

Nurse monitoring a central station for intensive care unit (ICU) equipment. *(Custom Medical Stock Photo. Reproduced by permission.)*

of-care analyzers, are used for blood analysis at the bedside. A small amount of whole blood is required, and blood chemistry parameters can be provided much faster than if samples were sent to the central laboratory.

Other ICU equipment

Disposable ICU equipment includes urinary (Foley) catheters, catheters used for arterial and central venous lines, Swan-Ganz catheters, chest and endotracheal tubes, gastrointestinal and nasogastric feeding tubes, and monitoring electrodes. Some patients may be wearing a posey vest, also called a Houdini jacket for safety; the purpose is to keep the patient stationary. Spenco boots are padded support devices made of lamb's wool to position the feet and ankles of the patient. Support hose may also be placed on the patient's legs to support the leg muscles and aid circulation.

Operation

The ICU is a demanding environment due to the critical condition of patients and the variety of equipment necessary to support and monitor patients. Therefore, when operating ICU equipment, staff should pay atten-

tion to the types of devices and the variations between different models of the same type of device so they do not make an error in operation or adjustment. Although many hospitals make an effort to standardize equipment—for example, using the same manufacturer's infusion pumps or patient monitoring systems, older devices and nonstandardized equipment may still be used, particularly when the ICU is busy. Clinical staff should be sure to check all devices and settings to ensure patient safety.

Intensive care unit patient monitoring systems are equipped with alarms that sound when the patient's vital signs deteriorate—for instance, when breathing stops, blood pressure is too high or too low, or when heart rate is too fast or too slow. Usually, all patient monitors connect to a central nurses' station for easy supervision. Staff at the ICU should ensure that all alarms are functioning properly and that the central station is staffed at all times.

For reusable patient care equipment, clinical staff make certain to properly disinfect and sterilize devices that have contact with patients. Disposable items, such as catheters and needles, should be disposed of in a properly labeled container.

KEY TERMS

Apnea—Cessation of breathing.

Arterial line—A catheter inserted into an artery and connected to a physiologic monitoring system to allow direct measurement of oxygen, carbon dioxide, and invasive blood pressure.

Catheter—A small, flexible tube used to deliver fluids or medications. A catheter may also be used to drain fluid or urine from the body.

Central venous line—A catheter inserted into a vein and connected to a physiologic monitoring system to directly measure venous blood pressure.

Chest tube—A tube inserted into the chest to drain fluid and air from around the lungs.

Critical care—The multidisciplinary health care specialty that provides care to patients with acute, life-threatening illness or injury.

Edema—An abnormal accumulation of fluids in intercellular spaces in the body; causes swelling.

Endotracheal tube—A tube inserted through the patient's nose or mouth that functions as an airway and is connected to the ventilator.

Foley catheter—A catheter inserted into the bladder to drain urine into a bag.

Gastrointestinal tube—A tube surgically inserted into the stomach for feeding a patient unable to eat by mouth.

Heart monitor leads—Sticky pads placed on the chest to monitor the electrical activity of the heart.

The pads are connected to an electrocardiogram machine.

Infectious disease team—A team of physicians who help control the hospital environment to protect patients against harmful sources of infection.

Life support—Methods of replacing or supporting a failing bodily function, such as using mechanical ventilation to support breathing. In treatable or curable conditions, life support is used temporarily to aid healing, until the body can resume normal functioning.

Nasogastric tube—A tube inserted through the nose and throat and into the stomach for direct feeding of the patient.

Sepsis—The body's response to infection. Normally, the body's own defense system fights infection, but in severe sepsis, the body "overreacts," causing widespread inflammation and blood clotting in tiny vessels throughout the body.

Swan-Ganz catheter—Also called a pulmonary artery catheter. This type of catheter is inserted into a large vessel in the neck or chest and is used to measure the amount of fluid in the heart and to determine how well the heart is functioning.

Tracheostomy tube—A breathing tube inserted in the neck, used when assisted breathing is needed for a long period of time.

Maintenance

Since ICU equipment is used continuously on critically ill patients, it is essential that equipment be properly maintained, particularly devices that are used for life support and resuscitation. Staff in the ICU should perform daily checks on equipment and inform biomedical engineering staff when equipment needs maintenance, repair, or replacement. For mechanically complex devices, service and preventive maintenance contracts are available from the manufacturer or third-party servicing companies, and should be kept current at all times.

Health care team roles

Equipment in the ICU is used by a team specialized in their use. The team usually comprises a critical care attending physician (also called an intensivist), critical care nurses, an infectious disease team, critical care respiratory ther-

apists, pharmacologists, physical therapists, and dietitians. Physicians trained in other specialties, such as anesthesiology, cardiology, radiology, surgery, neurology, pediatrics, and orthopedics, may be consulted and called to the ICU to treat patients who require their expertise. Radiologic technologists perform mobile x ray examinations (bedside radiography). Either nurses or clinical laboratory personnel perform point-of-care blood analysis. Equipment in the ICU is maintained and repaired by hospital biomedical engineering staff and/or the equipment manufacturer.

Some studies have shown that patients in the ICU following high-risk surgery are at least three times as likely to survive when cared for by "intensivists," physicians trained in critical care medicine.

Training

Manufacturers of more sophisticated ICU equipment, such as ventilators and patient monitoring devices, provide clinical training for all staff involved in ICU treatment when the device is purchased. All ICU staff must have undergone specialized training in the care of critically ill patients and must be trained to respond to life-threatening situations, since ICU patients are in critical condition and may experience respiratory or cardiac emergencies.

Resources

PERIODICALS

Savino, Joseph S., C. William Hanson III, and Timothy J. Gardner. "Cardiothoracic Intensive Care: Operation and Administration." *Seminars in Thoracic and Cardiovascular Surgery* 12 (October 2000): 362–70.

ORGANIZATIONS

American Association of Critical Care Nurses (ACCN). 101 Columbia, Aliso Viejo, CA 92656-4109. (800) 889-AACN [(800) 889-2226] or (949) 362-2000. <http://www.aacn.org>.

National Association of Neonatal Nurses. 4700 West Lake Ave., Glenview, IL 60025-1485. (847) 375-3660 or (800) 451-3795. <http://www.nann.org>.

National Heart, Lung and Blood Institute. Information Center. P.O. Box 30105, Bethesda, MD 20824-0105. (301) 251-2222. <http://www.nhlbi.nih.gov >.

National Institutes of Health, U.S. Department of Health and Human Services, 9000 Rockville Pike, Bethesda, MD 20892. (301) 496-4000. <http://www.nih.gov>.

Society of Critical Care Medicine. 701 Lee St., Suite 200, Des Plaines, IL 60016. (847) 827-6869. info@sccm.org. <http://www.sccm.org>.

OTHER

ICU Guide. 2002. <http://www.waiting.com/waitingicu.html>.

ICU-USA, Society of Critical Care Medicine, 2002 <http://www.icu-usa.com/tour/>.

"Intensive Care Units." 2003. <http://www.pulmonologychannel.com/icu/index.html>.

Pediatric Critical Care Medicine <http://pedsccm.wustl.edu/>.

Virtual Pediatric Intensive Care Unit <http://www.picu.net/>.

Jennifer E. Sisk, M.A.
Angela M. Costello

Interpositional reconstruction *see*
Arthroplasty

Intestinal anastomosis *see* **Ileoanal anastomosis**

Intestinal obstruction repair

Definition

An intestinal obstruction is a partial or complete blockage of the small or large intestine. Surgery is sometimes necessary to relieve the obstruction.

> ### WHO PERFORMS THE PROCEDURE AND WHERE IS IT PERFORMED?
>
> Ileoanal anastomoses are usually performed in a hospital **operating room**. Surgery may be performed by a general surgeon or a colorectal surgeon, a medical doctor who focuses on the surgical treatment of diseases of the colon, rectum, and anus.

Purpose

The small intestine is composed of three major sections: the duodenum just below the stomach; the jejunum, or middle portion; and the ileum, which empties into the large intestine. The large intestine is composed of the colon, where stool is formed; and the rectum, which empties to the outside of the body through the anal canal. A blockage that occurs in the small intestine is called a small bowel obstruction, and one that occurs in the colon is a colonic obstruction.

There are numerous conditions that may lead to an intestinal obstruction. The three most common causes of small bowel obstruction are adhesions, which are bands of scar tissue that form in the abdomen following injury or surgery; hernias, which develop when a portion of the intestine protrudes through a weak spot in the abdominal wall; and cancerous tumors. Adhesions account for approximately 50% of all small bowel obstructions, hernias for 15%, and tumors for 15%. Other causes include volvulus, or formation of kinks or knots in the bowel; the presence of foreign bodies in the digestive tract; intussusception, which occurs when a portion of the intestine telescopes or pulls over another portion; infection; and congenital defects. While most small bowel blockages can be treated with the administration of intravenous (IV) fluids and decompression of the bowel by the insertion of a nasogastric (NG) tube, surgical intervention is necessary in approximately 25% of patients with a partial obstruction, and 50%–65% of patients with a complete obstruction.

An obstruction of the large intestine is less common than blockages of the small intestine. Blockages of the large bowel are usually caused by colon cancer; volvulus; diverticulitis (inflammation of sac-like structures called diverticula that form in the intestines); ischemic colitis (inflammation of the colon resulting from insufficient blood flow); Crohn's disease (a disease that causes chronic inflammation of the intestines); inflammation due to radiation therapy; and the presence of foreign

QUESTIONS TO ASK THE DOCTOR

- Why are you recommending intestinal obstruction repair?
- What diagnostic tests will be performed to determine if an obstruction is present?
- Will an ileostomy or colostomy be created? Will it be temporary or permanent?
- Are any nonsurgical treatments available?
- How soon after surgery may normal diet and activities be resumed?

bodies. As in the case of small bowel obstruction, most patients with a blockage of the large intestine can be treated with IV fluids and bowel decompression.

Demographics

Approximately 300,000 intestinal obstruction repairs are performed in the United States each year. Among patients who are admitted to the hospital for severe abdominal pain, 20% have an intestinal obstruction. While bowel obstruction can affect individuals of any age, different conditions occur at higher rates in certain age groups. Children under the age of two, for example, are more likely to present with intussusceptions or congenital defects. Elderly patients, on the other hand, have a higher rate of colon cancer.

Description

After the patient has been prepared for surgery and given general anesthesia, the surgeon usually enters the abdominal cavity by way of a laparotomy, which is a large incision made through the patient's abdominal wall. This type of surgery is sometimes referred to as open surgery. An alternative to laparotomy is **laparoscopy**, a surgical procedure in which a laparoscope (a thin tube with a built-in light source) and other instruments are inserted into the abdomen through small incisions. The internal operating field is then visualized on a video monitor that is connected to the scope. In some patients, the technique may be used for abdominal exploration in place of a laparotomy. Laparoscopy is associated with faster recovery times, shorter hospital stays, and smaller surgical scars, but requires advanced training on the part of the surgeon as well as costly equipment. Moreover, it offers a more limited view of the operating field.

Treating an intestinal obstruction depends on the condition causing the blockage. Some of the more common surgical procedures used to treat bowel obstructions include:

- Lysis of adhesions. The process of removing these bands of scar tissue is called lysis. After the abdominal cavity has been opened, the surgeon locates the obstructed area and delicately dissects the adhesions from the intestine using surgical scissors and forceps.

- Hernia repair. This procedure involves an incision placed near the location of the hernia through which the hernia sac is opened. The herniated intestine is placed back in the abdominal cavity and the muscle wall is repaired.

- Resection with end-to-end anastomosis. "Resection" means to remove part or all of a tissue or structure. Resection of the small or large intestine, therefore, involves the removal of the obstructed or diseased section. Anastomosis is the connection of two cut ends of a tubular structure to form a continuous channel; the anastomosis of the intestine is most often accomplished with sutures or surgical staples.

- Resection with **ileostomy** or **colostomy**. In some patients, an anastomosis is not possible because of the extent of the diseased tissue. After the obstruction and diseased tissue is removed, an ileostomy or colostomy is created. Ileostomy is a surgical procedure in which the small intestine is attached to the abdominal wall; waste then exits the body through an artificial opening called a stoma and collects in a bag attached to the skin with adhesive. Colostomy is a similar procedure with the exception that the colon is the part of the digestive tract that is attached to the abdominal wall.

Diagnosis/Preparation

To diagnose an intestinal obstruction, the physician first gives a **physical examination** to determine the severity of the patient's condition. The abdomen is examined for evidence of scars, hernias, distension, or pain. The patient's medical history is also taken, as certain factors increase a person's risk of developing a bowel obstruction (including previous surgery, older age, and a history of constipation). A series of x rays may be taken of the abdomen, as a definitive diagnosis of obstruction can be made by x ray in 50–60% of patients. Computed tomography (CT; an imaging technique that uses x rays to produce two-dimensional cross-sections on a viewing screen) or ultrasonography (an imaging technique that uses high-frequency sounds waves to visualize structures inside the body) may also be used to diagnosis intestinal obstruction.

Unless a patient presents with symptoms that indicate immediate surgery may be necessary (high fever, severe pain, a rapid heart beat, etc.), a course of IV fluids, NG decompression, and antibiotic therapy is usually prescribed in an effort to avoid surgery.

Aftercare

After surgery, the patient's NG tube remains until bowel function returns. The patient is closely monitored for signs of infection, leakage from an anastomosis, or other complications.

Risks

Complications associated with intestinal obstruction repair include excessive bleeding; infection; formation of abscesses (pockets of pus); leakage of stool from an anastomosis; adhesion formation; paralytic ileus (temporary paralysis of the intestines); and reoccurrence of the obstruction.

Normal results

Most patients who undergo surgical repair of an intestinal obstruction have an uneventful recovery and do not experience a recurrence of the obstruction.

Morbidity and mortality rates

The mortality rate of small bowel obstruction ranges from 2% for a simple obstruction to 25% for a strangulation obstruction that compromises the blood supply and is treated after a lapse of 36 hours. Large bowel obstruction carries a mortality rate of 2% for volvulus to 40% if part of the bowel is gangrenous.

Alternatives

Such nonsurgical techniques as the administration of IV fluids and bowel decompression with a NG tube are often successful in relieving an intestinal obstruction. Patients who present with more severe symptoms that are indicative of a bowel perforation or strangulation, however, require immediate surgery.

Resources

BOOKS

Bitterman, Robert A., and Michael A. Peterson. "Large Intestine." In *Rosen's Emergency Medicine.* 5th ed. St. Louis, MO: Mosby, Inc., 2002.

Evers, B. Mark. "Small Bowel." In *Sabiston Textbook of Surgery.* Philadelphia, PA: W. B. Saunders Company, 2001.

"Mechanical Intestinal Obstruction." In *The Merck Manual of Diagnosis and Therapy,* edited by Mark H. Beers, MD, and Robert Berkow, MD. Whitehouse Station, NJ: Merck Research Laboratories, 1999.

KEY TERMS

Adhesion—A band of fibrous tissue forming an abnormal bond between two adjacent tissues or organs.

Anastomosis (plural, anastomoses)—A surgically created joining or opening between two organs or body spaces that are normally separate.

Congenital defect—A defect present at birth.

Gangrenous—Referring to tissue that is dead.

Intestinal perforation—A hole in the intestinal wall.

Intussusception—The telescoping of one part of the intestine inside an immediately adjoining part.

Lysis—The process of removing adhesions from an organ. The term comes from a Greek word that means "loosening."

Simple obstruction—A blockage in the intestine that does not affect the flow of blood to the area.

Stoma (plural, stomata)—A surgically created opening in the abdominal wall to allow digestive wastes to pass to the outside of the body.

Strangulation obstruction—A blockage in the intestine that closes off the flow of blood to the area.

Volvulus—An intestinal obstruction caused by a knotting or twisting of the bowel.

Torrey, Susan P., and Philip L. Henneman. "Small Intestine." In *Rosen's Emergency Medicine.* 5th ed. St. Louis, MO: Mosby, Inc., 2002.

PERIODICALS

Basson, Marc D. "Colonic Obstruction." *eMedicine,* September 26, 2001 [cited May 2, 2003]. <http://www.emedicine.com/med/topic415.htm>.

Khan, Ali Nawaz, and John Howat. "Small-Bowel Obstruction." *eMedicine,* April 18, 2003 [cited May 2, 2003]. <http://www.emedicine.com/radio/topic781.htm>.

ORGANIZATIONS

American Society of Colon and Rectal Surgeons. 85 W. Algonquin Rd., Suite 550, Arlington Heights, IL 60005. (847) 290-9184. <www.fascrs.org>.

United Ostomy Association, Inc. 19772 MacArthur Blvd., Suite 200, Irvine, CA 92612-2405. (800) 826-0826. <www.uoa.org>.

Stephanie Dionne Sherk

Intracranial aneurysm repair *see* **Cerebral aneurysm repair**

Intravenous rehydration

Definition

Intravenous (IV) rehydration is a treatment for fluid loss in which a sterile water solution containing small amounts of salt or sugar is injected into the patient's bloodstream.

Purpose

Rehydration is usually performed to treat the symptoms associated with dehydration, or excessive loss of body water. Fever, vomiting, and diarrhea can cause a person to become dehydrated fairly quickly. Infants and children are especially vulnerable to dehydration. Patients can become dehydrated due to an illness, surgery, metabolic disorder, hot weather, or accident. Athletes who have overexerted themselves may also require rehydration with IV fluids. An IV for rehydration can be used for several hours to several days, and is generally used if a patient is unable to keep down oral fluids due to excessive vomiting.

Description

A basic IV rehydration solution consists of sterile water with small amounts of sodium chloride (NaCl; salt) and dextrose (sugar) added. It is supplied in bottles or thick plastic bags that can hang on a pole or rolling stand mounted next to a patient's bed. Additional electrolytes (i.e., potassium, calcium, bicarbonate, phosphate, magnesium, chloride), vitamins, or drugs can be added as needed either in a separate minibag or via an injection into the intravenous line.

Diagnosis/Preparation

Signs and symptoms of dehydration include:

• extreme thirst
• sunken eyes
• reduced urine output; urine that is dark in color
• weakness and fatigue
• rapid weight loss
• dry, warm skin
• skin that is wrinkled or has little elasticity
• rapid pulse
• dry mouth
• "tearless" crying
• muscle cramps
• headache

In infants, dehydration may also be indicated by a sunken fontanelle (the soft spot on the head).

A doctor orders the IV solution and any additional nutrients or drugs to be added to it. The doctor also specifies the rate at which the IV will be infused. The intravenous solutions are prepared under the supervision of a pharmacist using sanitary techniques that prevent bacterial contamination. Just like a prescription, the IV is clearly labeled to show its contents and the amounts of any additives. A nurse will examine the patient's arm to find a suitable vein for insertion of the intravenous line. Once the vein is located, the skin around the area is cleaned and disinfected. The needle is inserted and is taped to the skin to prevent it from moving out of the vein.

Patients receiving IV therapy must be monitored to ensure that the IV solutions are providing the correct amounts of fluids and minerals needed. People with kidney and heart disease are at increased risk for overhydration, so they must be carefully monitored when receiving IV therapy.

Aftercare

Patients must be able to take (and keep down) fluids by mouth before an IV rehydration solution is discontinued. After the needle is removed, the insertion site should be inspected for any signs of bleeding or infection.

Risks

As with any invasive procedure, there is a small risk of infection or bruising at the injection site. It is possible that the IV solution may not provide all of the nutrients needed, leading to a deficiency or an imbalance. If the needle becomes dislodged, the solution may flow into tissues around the injection site rather than into the vein, resulting in swelling.

Morbidity and mortality rates

According to the United Nations Children's Fund (UNICEF), over two million children die of diarrhea-related dehydration each year. Eighty percent of these children were two years of age or younger. In the United States, an estimated 300 people (children and adults) die of dehydration annually.

Alternatives

For patients who are able to tolerate fluids by mouth, oral rehydration therapy (ORT) with oral rehydration salts (ORS) in solution is the preferred treatment alternative. Another technique in which fluid replacement is injected subcutaneously (under the skin into tissues) rather than into a vein is called hypodermoclysis. Hypodermoclysis is easier to administer than IV therapy, especially in the home setting. It may be used to treat mild to moderate dehydration in patients who are unable to take in adequate fluids by mouth and who prefer to be treated at home (geriatric or terminally ill patients).

Resources

BOOKS

Hankins, Judy, et al., eds. *Infusion Therapy in Clinical Practice*. 2nd ed. Philadelphia: WB Saunders, 2001.

Otto, Shirlie. *Pocket Guide to Intravenous Therapy*. 4th ed. St. Louis: Mosby Inc., 2001.

PERIODICALS

Suhayda, Rosemarie, and Jane C. Walton. "Preventing and Managing Dehydration." *MedSurg Nursing* 11 (December 2002): 267-278.

OTHER

Rehydration Project. P. O. Box 1, Samara, 5235, Costa Rica. (506) 656-0504. <www.rehydrate.org>.

Altha Roberts Edgren
Paula Ford-Martin

Intussusception reduction

Definition

Intussusception is a condition in which one portion of the intestine "telescopes" into or folds itself inside another portion. The term comes from two Latin words, *intus*, which means "inside" and *suscipere*, which means "to receive." The outer "receiving" portion of an intussusception is called the intussuscipiens; the part that has been received inside the intussuscipiens is called the intussusceptum. The result of an intussusception is that the bowel is obstructed and its blood supply gradually cut off. Surgery is sometimes necessary to relieve the obstruction.

Purpose

The purpose of an intussusception reduction is to prevent gangrene of the bowel, which may lead to perforation of the bowel, severe infection, and death.

The cause of intussusception is idiopathic in most children diagnosed with the condition (88–99%). Idiopathic means that the condition has developed spontaneously or that the cause is unknown. In the remaining 1–12% of child patients, certain conditions called lead points have been associated with intussusception. These lead points include cystic fibrosis; recent upper respiratory or gastrointestinal illness; congenital abnormalities of the digestive tract; benign or malignant tumors; chemotherapy; or the presence of foreign bodies.

In contrast to children, there is a lead point in 90% of adults diagnosed with intussusception.

Demographics

About 95% of all cases of intussusception occur in children. Children under two years of age are most likely to be affected by the condition; the average age at diagnosis is seven to eight months. Among children, the rate of intussusception is one to four per 1000. Conversely,

Intussusception reduction

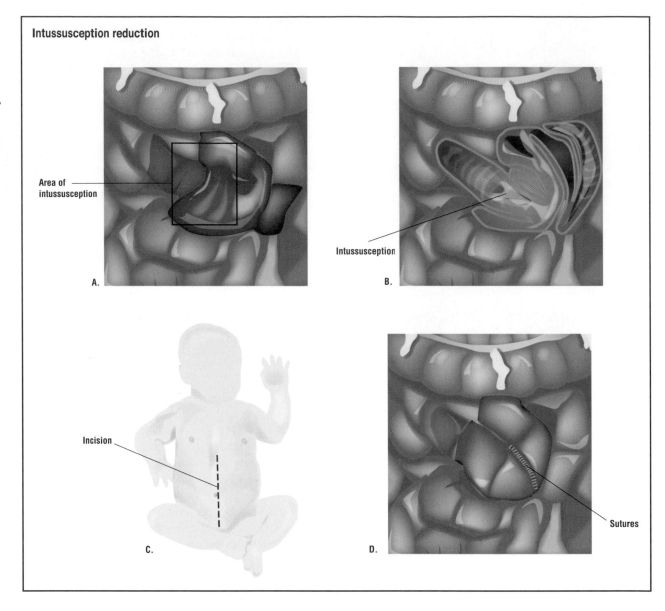

Area of
intussusception

A.

Intussusception

B.

Incision

C.

Sutures

D.

Intussusception of the bowel results in the bowel telescoping onto itself (A and B). An incision is made in the baby's abdomen to expose the bowel (C). If the surgeon cannot manipulate the bowel into a normal shape manually, the area of intussusception wil be removed and remaining bowel sutured together (D). *(Illustration by GGS Inc.)*

only two to three adults out of every 1,000,000 are diagnosed with intussusception each year. Intussusception is more likely to affect males than females in all age groups. Among children, the male: female ratio is 3:2; in persons over the age of four, the male:female ratio is 8:1.

As of 2003, racial or ethnic differences do not appear to affect the occurrence of intussusception.

Description

Surgical correction of an intussusception is done with the patient under general anesthesia. The surgeon usually enters the abdominal cavity by way of a laparo-

tomy, a large incision made through the abdominal wall. The intestines are examined until the intussusception is identified and brought through the incision for closer examination. The surgeon first attempts to reduce the intussusception by "milking" or applying gentle pressure to ease the intussusceptum out of the intussuscipiens; this technique is called manual reduction. If manual reduction is not successful, the surgeon may perform a resection of the intussusception. Resect means to remove part or all of a tissue or structure; resection of the intussusception, therefore, involves the removal of the area of the intestine that has prolapsed. The two cut ends of the intestine may then be reconnected with sutures or surgical staples; this reconnection is called an end-to-end anastomosis.

More rarely, the segment of bowel that is removed is too large to accommodate an end-to-end anastomosis. These patients may require a temporary or permanent enterostomy. In this procedure, the surgeon creates an artificial opening in the abdomen wall called a stoma, and attaches the intestine to it. Waste then exits the body through the stoma and empties into a collection bag.

An alternative to the traditional abdominal incision is **laparoscopy**, a surgical procedure in which a laparoscope (a thin, lighted tube) and other instruments are inserted into the abdomen through small incisions. The internal operating field is then visualized on a video monitor that is connected to the scope. In some patients, the surgeon may perform a laparoscopy for abdominal exploration in place of a laparotomy. Laparoscopy is associated with speedier recoveries shorter hospital stays, and smaller surgical scars; on the other hand, however, it requires costly equipment and advanced training on the surgeon's part. In addition, it offers a relatively limited view of the operating field.

Diagnosis/Preparation

The diagnosis of intussusception is usually made after a complete **physical examination**, medical history, and series of imaging studies. In children, the pediatrician may suspect the diagnosis on the basis of such symptoms as abdominal pain, fever, vomiting, and "currant jelly" stools, which consist of blood-streaked mucus and pieces of the tissue that lines the intestine. When the doctor palpates (feels) the child's abdomen, he or she will typically find a sausage-shaped mass in the right lower quadrant of the abdomen. Diagnosis of intussusception in adults, however, is much more difficult, partly because the disorder is relatively rare in the adult population.

X rays may be taken of the abdomen with the patient lying down or sitting upright. Ultrasonography (an imaging technique that uses high-frequency sounds waves to visualize structures inside the body) and computed tomography (an imaging technique that uses x rays to produce two-dimensional cross-sections on a viewing screen) are also used to diagnose intussusception. A contrast enema is a diagnostic tool that has the potential to reduce the intussusception; during this procedure, x-ray photographs are taken of the intestines after a contrast material such as barium or air is introduced through the anus.

Children diagnosed with intussusception are started on intravenous (IV) fluids and nasogastric decompression (in which a flexible tube is inserted through the nose down to the stomach) in an effort to avoid surgery. An enema may also be given to the patient, as 40–90% of cases are successfully treated by this method. If these noninvasive treatments fail, surgery becomes necessary to relieve the obstruction.

There is some controversy among doctors about the usefulness of barium enemas in reducing intussusceptions in adults. In general, enemas are less successful in adults than in children, and surgical treatment should not be delayed.

Aftercare

After surgical treatment of an intussusception, the patient is given fluids intravenously until bowel function returns; he or she may then be allowed to resume a normal diet. Follow-up care may be indicated if the intussusception occurred as a result of a specific condition (e.g., cancerous tumors).

Risks

Complications associated with intussusception reduction include reactions to general anesthesia; perfora-

KEY TERMS

Adhesion—A fibrous band of tissue that forms an abnormal connection between two adjacent organs or other structures.

Anastomosis—The connection of separate parts of a body organ or an organ system.

Benign tumor—A noncancerous growth that does not have the potential to spread to other parts of the body.

Congenital—Present at birth.

Gangrene—The death of a considerable mass of tissue, usually associated with loss of blood supply and followed by bacterial infection.

Idiopathic—Having an unknown cause or arising spontaneously. Most cases of intussusception in children are idiopathic.

Lead point—A well-defined abnormality in the area where the intussusception begins.

Malignant tumor—A cancerous growth that has the potential to spread to other parts of the body.

Stoma (plural, stomata)—A surgically created opening in the abdominal wall to allow digestive wastes to pass to the outside of the body.

Strangulation—A condition in which the blood circulation in a part of the body is shut down by pressure. Intussusception can lead to strangulation of a part of the intestine.

tion of the bowel; wound infection; urinary tract infection; excessive bleeding; and formation of adhesions (bands of scar tissue that form after surgery or injury to the abdomen).

Normal results

If intussusception is treated in a timely manner, most patients are expected to recover fully, retain normal bowel function, and have only a small chance of recurrence. The mortality rate is lowest among patients who are treated within the first 24 hours.

Morbidity and mortality rates

Intussusception recurs in approximately 1–4% of patients after surgery, compared to 5–10% after nonsurgical reduction. Adhesions form in up to 7% of patients who undergo surgical reduction. The rate of intussusception-related deaths in Western countries is less than 1%.

Alternatives

Such nonsurgical techniques as the administration of IV fluids, bowel decompression with a nasogastric tube, or a therapeutic enema are often successful in reducing intussusception. Patients whose symptoms point to bowel perforation or strangulation, however, require immediate surgery. If left untreated, gangrene of the bowel is almost always fatal.

Resources

BOOKS

"Congenital Anomalies: Gastrointestinal Defects." In *The Merck Manual of Diagnosis and Therapy*, edited by Mark H. Beers, MD, and Robert Berkow, MD. Whitehouse Station, NJ: Merck Research Laboratories, 1999.

Engum, Scott A. and Jay L. Grosfeld. "Pediatric Surgery: Intussusception." In *Sabiston Textbook of Surgery*. Philadelphia: W. B. Saunders Company, 2001.

Wyllie, Robert. "Ileus, Adhesions, Intussusception, and Closed-Loop Obstructions." In *Nelson Textbook of Pediatrics*, 16th ed. Philadelphia, PA: W. B. Saunders Company, 2000.

PERIODICALS

Chahine, A. Alfred, MD. "Intussusception." *eMedicine*, April 4, 2002 [cited May 4, 2003]. <www.emedicine.com/PED/topic1208.htm>.

Irish, Michael, MD. "Intussusception: Surgical Perspective." *eMedicine*, April 29, 2003 [cited May 4, 2003]. <www.emedicine.com/PED/topic2972.htm>.

Waseem, Muhammad and Orlando Perales. "Diagnosis: Intussusception." *Pediatrics in Review* 22, no. 4 (April 1, 2001): 135-140.

ORGANIZATIONS

American Academy of Family Physicians. PO Box 11210, Shawnee Mission, KS 66207. (800) 274-2237. <www.aafp.org>.

American Academy of Pediatrics. 141 Northwest Point Blvd., Elk Grove Village, IL 60007-1098. (847) 434-4000. <www.aap.org>.

American College of Radiology. 1891 Preston White Dr., Reston, VA 20191-4397. (800) 227-5463. <www.acr.org>.

Stephanie Dionne Sherk

Iridectomy

Definition

An iridectomy is a procedure in eye surgery in which the surgeon removes a small, full-thickness piece of the iris, which is the colored circular membrane behind the cornea of the eye. An iridectomy is also known as a corectomy. In recent years, lasers have also been used to perform iridectomies.

Purpose

Today, an iridectomy is most often performed to treat closed-angle glaucoma or melanoma of the iris. An iridectomy performed to treat glaucoma is sometimes called a peripheral iridectomy, because it removes a portion of the periphery or root of the iris.

In some cases, an iridectomy is performed prior to cataract surgery in order to make it easier to remove the lens of the eye. This procedure is referred to as a preparatory iridectomy.

Closed-angle glaucoma

Closed-angle glaucoma is a condition in which fluid pressure builds up inside the eye because the fluid, or aqueous humor, that is produced in the anterior chamber at the front of the eye cannot leave the chamber through the usual opening. This opening lies at the angle where the iris meets the cornea, which is the clear front portion of the exterior cover of the eye. In closed-angle glaucoma, the fluid is blocked because a part of the iris has moved forward and closed off the angle. As a result, fluid pressure in the eye rises rapidly, which can damage the optic nerve and lead to blindness. About 10% of all cases of glaucoma reported in the United States is closed-angle. This type of glaucoma is also called angle-closure glaucoma, acute congestive glaucoma, narrow-angle glaucoma, and pupillary block glaucoma. It usually develops in only one eye at a time.

There are two major types of closed-angle glaucoma: primary and secondary. Primary closed-angle glaucoma most commonly results from pupillary block, in which the iris closes off the angle when the pupil of the eye becomes dilated. In some cases, the blockage happens only occasionally, as when the pupil dilates in dim light, in situations of high stress or anxiety, or in response to the drops instilled by a doctor during an eye examination. This condition is referred to as intermittent, subacute, or chronic open-angle glaucoma. In other cases, the blockage is abrupt and complete, leading to an attack of acute closed-angle glaucoma. In primary glaucoma, the difference between the chronic or intermittent forms and an acute attack is usually due to small variations in the anatomical structure of the eye. These include an unusually shallow anterior chamber; a lens that is thicker than average and situated further forward in the eye; or a cornea that is smaller in diameter than average. Any of these differences can narrow the angle between

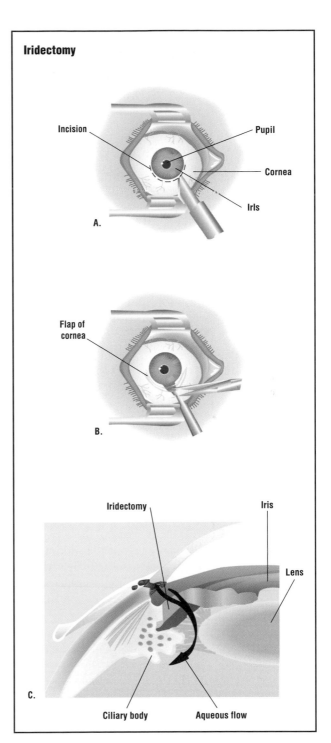

Iridectomy

A.

B.

C.

For an iridectomy, an incision is made in the cornea just below the iris (A). A piece of the iris is removed (B). This allows fluid to flow between the areas to the front and rear of the iris (C). *(Illustration by GGS Inc.)*

the iris and the cornea, which is about 45° in the normal eye. In addition, as people age, the lens tends to grow larger and thicker; this change may cause fluid pressure

WHO PERFORMS THE PROCEDURE AND WHERE IS IT PERFORMED?

Iridectomies are performed by ophthalmologists, who are physicians who have completed four to five years of specialized training in the medical and surgical treatment of eye disorders. Ophthalmology is one of 24 specialties recognized by the American Board of Medical Specialties.

Laser iridotomies or iridectomies are done as an outpatient procedure, either in the ophthalmologist's office or in an ambulatory surgery center. Surgical iridectomy is done in an operating room, either in a surgery center that specializes in ophthalmology or in a specialized eye hospital.

to build up behind the iris. Eventually, pressure from the aqueous humor may force the iris forward, blocking the drainage angle.

Secondary closed-angle glaucoma results from changes in the angle caused by disorders, medications, trauma, or surgery, rather than by the anatomy of the eye itself. In some cases, the iris is pulled up into the angle by scar tissue resulting from the abnormal formation of blood vessels in diabetes. Another common cause of secondary closed-angle glaucoma is uveitis, or inflammation of the uvea, which is the covering of the eye that includes the iris. Cases have been reported in which uveitis related to HIV infection has led to closed-angle glaucoma. Melanoma of the iris has also been associated with closed-angle glaucoma.

Any medication that causes the pupil of the eye to dilate may cause an acute attack of closed-angle glaucoma, including antihistamines and over-the-counter cold preparations. Medications that are given to treat anxiety and depression, particularly the tricyclic antidepressants and the selective serotonin reuptake inhibitors (SSRIs), may trigger the onset of closed-angle glaucoma in some patients. In other instances, anesthesia for procedures on other parts of the body produces an acute attack.

In terms of trauma, a direct blow to the eye can dislocate the lens, bringing it forward and blocking the angle; overly vigorous **exercise** may have the same effect. Lastly, certain types of eye surgery performed to treat other conditions may result in secondary closed-angle glaucoma. These procedures include implantation of an intraocular lens; cataract surgery; **scleral buckling** to treat retinal detachment; and injection of silicone oil

to replace the vitreous body in front of the retina following a vitrectomy.

Melanoma of the iris

Melanoma of the iris is a malignant tumor that develops within the pigmented cells of the iris; it is not a cancer that has developed elsewhere in the body and then spread to the eye. Melanoma of the iris can, however, enlarge and gradually destroy the patient's vision. If left untreated, it can also metastasize or spread to other organs—most commonly the liver—and eventually cause death.

Demographics

Closed-angle glaucoma affects between 350,000 and 400,000 people in the United States; in some Asian countries such as China, however, it is more common than open-angle glaucoma.

Risk factors for closed-angle glaucoma include:

- a family history of this type of glaucoma
- farsightedness
- small eyes
- age over 40
- scarring inside the eye from diabetes or uveitis
- a cataract in the lens that is growing
- Eskimo or Asian heritage (Eskimos have the highest rate of closed-angle glaucoma of any ethnic group)

Melanoma of the iris is a relatively rare form of cancer, representing only about 10% of cases of intraocular melanoma. The American Cancer Society estimates that about 220 cases of melanoma of the iris are diagnosed in the United States each year. People over 50 are the most likely to develop this form of cancer, although it can occur at any age. It appears to affect men and women equally. Melanoma of the iris is more common in Caucasians and in people with light-colored irides than in people of Asian or African descent. Suspected causes include genetic mutations and exposure to sunlight.

Description

Laser iridotomy/iridectomy

A person who is at risk for an acute episode of closed-angle glaucoma or who has already had emergency medical treatment for an attack may be treated with a **laser iridotomy** to reduce the level of fluid pressure in the affected eye. The drawback of a laser iridotomy in treating closed-angle glaucoma is that the hole may not remain open, requiring repeated iridotomies, a laser iridectomy, or a surgical iridectomy. In addition, laser iridotomies have a higher rate of success when used preventively rather than after the patient has already had an acute attack.

To perform a laser iridotomy, the ophthalmologist uses a laser, usually an argon or an Nd:YAG laser, to burn a small hole into the iris to relieve fluid pressure behind the iris. If the procedure is an iridectomy, the laser is used to remove a full-thickness section of the iris. The patient sits in a special chair with his or her chin resting on a frame or support to prevent the head from moving. The ophthalmologist numbs the eye with anesthetic eye drops. After the anesthetic has taken effect, the doctor shines the laser beam into the affected eye. The entire procedure takes between 10–30 minutes.

Conventional (surgical) iridectomy

Melanoma of the iris is usually treated by surgical iridectomy to prevent the tumor from causing secondary closed-angle glaucoma and from spreading to other parts of the body.

A surgical iridectomy is a more invasive procedure that requires an **operating room**. The patient lies on an operating table with a piece of sterile cloth placed around the eye. The procedure is usually done under general anesthesia. The surgeon uses a microscope and special miniature instruments to make an incision in the cornea and remove a section of the iris, usually at the 12 o'clock position. The incision in the cornea is self-sealing.

Diagnosis/Preparation

Closed-angle glaucoma

Closed-angle glaucoma may be diagnosed in the course of a routine eye examination or during emergency treatment for symptoms of an acute attack. A doctor who is performing a standard eye examination may notice that the patient's eye has a shallow anterior chamber or a narrow angle between the iris and the cornea. He or she may perform one or both of the following tests to evaluate the patient's risk of developing closed-angle glaucoma. One test, called tonometry, measures the amount of fluid pressure in the eye. It is a painless procedure that involves blowing a puff of pressurized air toward the patient's eye as the patient sits near a lamp and measuring the changes in the light reflections on the patient's corneas. Other methods of tonometry involve the application of a local anesthetic to the outside of the eye and touching the cornea briefly with an instrument that measures the fluid pressure directly. The second test, gonioscopy, involves the use of a special mirrored contact lens to evaluate the anatomy of the angle between the iris and the cornea. The doctor numbs the outside of the eye

with a local anesthetic and touches the outside of the cornea with the gonioscopic lens. He or she can use a slit lamp to magnify what appears on the lens. Patients with subacute, intermittent, or chronic closed-angle glaucoma can then be treated before they develop acute symptoms.

If the patient is having a sudden attack of closed-angle glaucoma, he or she will feel intense pain, and is likely to be seen on an emergency basis with the following symptoms:

- nausea and vomiting
- severe pain in or above the eye
- visual disturbances that include seeing halos around lights and hazy or foggy vision
- headache
- redness and watering in the affected eye
- a dilated pupil that does not close normally in bright light

These symptoms are produced by the sharp rise in intraocular pressure (IOP) that occurs when the angle is completely blocked. This increase can occur in a matter of hours and cause permanent loss of vision in as little as two to five days. *An acute attack of closed-angle glaucoma is a medical emergency requiring immediate treatment.* Emergency treatment includes application of eye drops to reduce the pressure in the eye quickly, other eye drops to shrink the size of the pupil, and acetazolamide or a similar medication to stop the production of aqueous humor. In severe cases, the patient may be given drugs intravenously to lower the intraocular pressure. After the pressure has been relieved with medications, the eye will require surgical treatment.

Melanoma of the iris

Melanoma of the iris is usually discovered in the course of a routine eye examination because it will be visible to the ophthalmologist as he or she looks through the pupil in the center of the iris. A melanoma on the iris

---

QUESTIONS TO ASK THE DOCTOR

- What are the alternatives to a surgical iridectomy for my condition?
- What are the risks of my having an acute attack of closed-angle glaucoma?
- What further treatment would you recommend if an iridectomy is unsuccessful?

KEY TERMS

Angle—The open point in the anterior chamber of the eye at which the iris meets the cornea. Blockage of the angle prevents fluid from leaving the anterior chamber, resulting in closed-angle glaucoma.

Aqueous humor—The watery fluid produced in the eye that ordinarily leaves the eye through the angle of the anterior chamber.

Corectomy—Another term for iridectomy.

Cornea—The transparent front portion of the exterior cover of the eye.

Enucleation—Surgical removal of the eyeball.

Glaucoma—A group of eye disorders characterized by increased fluid pressure inside the eye that eventually damages the optic nerve. As the cells in the optic nerve die, the patient gradually loses vision.

Gonioscopy—A technique for examining the angle between the iris and the cornea with the use of a special mirrored lens applied to the cornea.

Iridotomy—A procedure in which a laser is used to make a small hole in the iris to relieve fluid pressure in the eye.

Iris (plural, irides)—The circular pigmented membrane behind the cornea of the eye that gives the eye its color. The iris surrounds a central opening called the pupil.

Ocular melanoma—A malignant tumor that arises within the structures of the eye. It is the most common eye tumor in adults.

Ophthalmology—The branch of medicine that deals with the diagnosis and treatment of eye disorders.

Pupil—The opening in the center of the iris of the eye that allows light to enter the eye.

Tonometry—Measurement of the fluid pressure inside the eye.

Tunica (plural, tunicae)—The medical term for a membrane or piece of tissue that covers or lines a body part. The eyeball is surrounded by three tunicae.

Uvea—The middle of the three tunicae surrounding the eye, comprising the choroid, iris, and ciliary body. The uvea is pigmented and well supplied with blood vessels.

Uveitis—Inflammation of any part of the uvea.

Vitrectomy—Surgical removal of the vitreous body.

Vitreous body—The transparent gel that fills the inner portion of the eyeball between the lens and the retina. It is also called the vitreous humor or crystalline humor.

may look like a dark spot or ring, or it may resemble tapioca. The doctor can perform a gonioscopy, and use specialized imaging studies to rule out other possible eye disorders. An ultrasound study can be made by using a small probe placed on the eye that directs sound waves in the direction of the tumor. Another test is called fluorescein **angiography**, which involves injecting a fluorescent dye into a vein in the patient's arm. As the dye circulates throughout the body, it is carried to the blood vessels in the back of the eye. These blood vessels can be photographed through the pupil.

In a minority of patients, melanoma of the iris is discovered because the patient is experiencing eye pain resulting from a rise in IOP caused by tumor growth.

Preparation for treatment

Patients scheduled for a laser iridotomy or iridectomy are not required to fast or make other special preparations before the procedure. They may, however, be given a sedative to help them relax. Patients scheduled

for a conventional iridectomy are asked to avoid eating or drinking for about eight hours before the procedure.

Aftercare

Short-term aftercare following laser iridectomy or iridotomy is minimal. Patients are asked to make arrangements for someone to drive them home after surgery, but can usually go to work the next day and resume other activities with no restrictions. They should not need any medication stronger than **aspirin** for discomfort.

Short-term aftercare following a surgical iridectomy includes wearing a patch over the affected eye for several days and using eye drops to minimize the risk of infection. The surgeon may also prescribe medication for discomfort. It will take about six weeks for vision to return to normal. Long-term aftercare following an iridectomy for closed-angle glaucoma usually involves taking medications to help control the fluid pressure in the eye and seeing the ophthalmologist for periodic checkups.

Aftercare for melanoma of the iris includes eye checkups to be certain that the tumor has not recurred. In addition, patients are advised to reduce their exposure to sunlight and other sources of ultraviolet light.

Risks

The risks of a laser iridotomy or iridectomy include the following:

• irritation in the eye for two to three days after the procedure

• bleeding

• scarring

• failure to relieve fluid pressure in the eye

The risks of a conventional iridectomy include:

• infection

• bleeding

• scarring in the area of the incision

• failure to relieve fluid pressure

• formation of a cataract

The risks of an iridectomy for melanoma of the iris include glaucoma resulting from the formation of new blood vessels near the angle, cataract formation, and recurrence of the tumor. In the event of a recurrence, the standard treatment is enucleation, or surgical removal of the entire eye.

Normal results

Normal results for a laser-assisted or conventional iridectomy are long-term lowering of IOP and/or complete removal of a melanoma on the iris.

Morbidity and mortality rates

About 60% of patients who have had conventional iridectomies consider the operation a success; 15%, on the other hand, maintain that their vision was better before the procedure.

Fortunately for patients, melanoma of the iris is a relatively slow-growing form of cancer; it metastasizes to the liver in only 2–4% of cases. If treated promptly, it has a high survival rate of 95–97% after five years.

Alternatives

Alternatives to a conventional iridectomy for the treatment of closed-angle glaucoma include repeated laser iridotomies or the long-term use of such medications as pilocarpine. Another surgical alternative, which is most commonly done when the size of the lens is a factor in pupillary block, is removal of the lens.

Alternatives to iridectomy in the treatment of melanoma of the iris include watchful waiting, periodic eye examinations, and the use of medication to control any symptoms of closed-angle glaucoma.

See also Laser iridotomy.

Resources

BOOKS

"Angle-Closure Glaucoma." In *The Merck Manual of Diagnosis and Therapy,* edited by Mark H. Beers and Robert Berkow. Whitehouse Station, NJ: Merck Research Laboratories, 1999.

PERIODICALS

Aung, T., and P. T. Chew. "Review of Recent Advancements in the Understanding of Primary Angle-Closure Glaucoma." *Current Opinion in Ophthalmology* 13 (April 2002): 89–93.

Cardine, S., et al. "Iris Melanomas. A Retrospective Study of 11 Patients Treated by Surgical Excision." [in French] *Journal français d'ophtalmologie* 26 (January 2003): 31–37.

Chang, B. M., J. M. Liebmann, and R. Ritch. "Angle Closure in Younger Patients." *Transactions of the American Ophthalmological Society* 100 (2002): 201–212.

Goldberg, D. E., and W. R. Freeman. "Uveitic Angle Closure Glaucoma in a Patient with Inactive Cytomegalovirus Retinitis and Immune Recovery Uveitis." *Ophthalmic Surgery and Lasers* 33 (September–October 2002): 421–425.

Jackson, T. L., et al. "Pupil Block Glaucoma in Phakic and Pseudophakic Patients After Vitrectomy with Silicone Oil Inhection." *American Journal of Ophthalmology* 132 (September 2001): 414–416.

Jacobi, P. C., et al. "Primary Phacoemulsification and Intraocular Lens Implantation for Acute Angle-Closure Glaucoma." *Ophthalmology* 109 (September 2002): 1597–1603.

Jiminez-Jiminez, F. J., M. Orti-Pareja, and J. M. Zurdo. "Aggravation of Glaucoma with Fluvoxamine." *Annals of Pharmacotherapy* 35 (December 2001): 1565–1566.

Kumar, A., S. Kedar, V. K. Garodia, and R. P. Singh. "Angle Closure Glaucoma Following Pupillary Block in an Aphakin Perfluoropropane Gas-Filled Eye." *Indian Journal of Ophthalmology* 50 (September 2002): 220–221.

Lentschener, C., et al. "Acute Postoperative Glaucoma After Nonocular Surgery Remains a Diagnostic Challenge." *Anesthesia and Analgesia* 94 (April 2002): 1034–1035.

Schwartz, G. P., and L. W. Schwartz. "Acute Angle Closure Glaucoma Secondary to a Choroidal Melanoma." *CLAO Journal* 28 (April 2002): 77–79.

Shields, C. L., et al. "Factors Associated with Elevated Intraocular Pressure in Eyes with Iris Melanoma." *British Journal of Ophthalmology* 85 (June 2001): 666–669.

Shields, C. L., et al. "Iris Melanoma: Risk Factors for Metastasis in 169 Consecutive Patients." *Ophthalmology* 108 (January 2001): 172–178.

Waheed, Nadia K., and C. Stephen Foster. "Melanoma, Iris." *eMedicine* February 28, 2003 [cited April 2, 2003]. <http://www.emedicine.com/oph/topic405.htm>.

Wang, N., H. Wu, and Z. Fan. "Primary Angle Closure Glaucoma in Chinese and Western Populations." *Chinese Medical Journal* 115 (November 2002): 1706–1715.

ORGANIZATIONS

American Academy of Ophthalmology. P. O. Box 7424, San Francisco, CA 94120-7424. (415) 561-8500. <http://www.aao.org>.

Canadian Ophthalmological Society (COS). 610-1525 Carling Avenue, Ottawa ON K1Z 8R9 Canada. <http://www.eyesite.ca>.

National Eye Institute. 2020 Vision Place, Bethesda, MD 20892-3655. (301) 496-5248. <http://www.nei.nih.gov>.

Prevent Blindness America. 500 East Remington Road, Schaumburg, IL 60173. (800) 331-2020. <http://www.prevent-blindness.org>.

Wills Eye Hospital. 840 Walnut Street, Philadelphia, PA 19107. (215) 928-3000. <http://www.willseye.org>.

OTHER

National Cancer Institute (NCI) Physician Data Query (PDQ). *Intraocular (Eye) Melanoma: Treatment* January 2, 2003 [cited April 2, 2003]. <http://www.nci.nih.gov/cancerinfo/pdq/treatment/intraocularmelanoma/healthprofessional>.

National Eye Institute (NEI). *Facts About Glaucoma.* 2001. NIH Publication No. 99–651.

Prevent Blindness America. *Vision Problems in the U.S.: Prevalence of Adult Vision Impairment and Age-Related Eye Disease in America.* 2002.

Tanasescu, I., and F. Grehn. "Advantage of Surgical Iridectomy Over Nd:YAG Laser Iridotomy in Acute Primary Angle Closure Glaucoma." Presentation on September 29, 2001, at the 99th annual meeting of the Deutsche Ophthalmologische Gesellschaft. <http://www.dog.org/2001/abstract-german/Tanasescu-e.htm>.

Rebecca Frey, PhD

Iridotomy *see* **Laser iridotomy**

Islet cell transplantation

Definition

Pancreatic islet cell transplantation involves taking the cells that produce insulin from a second source such as a donor pancreas and transplanting them into a patient.

Purpose

Once transplanted, the new islet cells make and release insulin. Islet cell transplantation is primarily a treatment method for type 1 (juvenile) diabetes, but it can also be used to treat patients who have had their pan-

---

creas removed or damaged from other medical conditions or injuries.

Demographics

An estimated 120–140 million people worldwide suffer from type 1 diabetes and could benefit from this procedure. However, islet cell transplantation remains highly experimental at this time and occurs only as part of a clinical trial. The latest available data from the International Islet Transplant Registry indicate that, as of December 2000, about 500 procedures had been performed.

Description

The transplantation procedure is very straightforward, relatively noninvasive, and takes less than an hour to complete. After the patient is given light sedation, the surgeon begins by using an ultrasound to guide the placement of a small plastic tube, known as a catheter, through the upper abdomen into the liver. The liver is used as the site for transplantation because the portal vein of liver is larger and easier to access than the veins that supply the pancreas, also, it is known that islet cells that grow in the liver closely mimic normal insulin secretion.

Once the catheter is in place, the surgeon takes the cells that have been extracted from the donor pancreas and infuses them into the liver. Extraction is done as close as possible to the time of transplantation because of the fragility of the islet cells. The extraction process uses specialized enzymes to isolate the islet cells from the other cell types found in the pancreas. Only 1–2% of the pancreas is made up of islet cells, an average of two pancreases are needed for one successful transplant.

Recent study has shown that the use of perfluorocarbon in the solution that preserves the pancreas before transplant allows older organs to be used as islet cell donors. New techniques have also been developed that allow the organs to be transported before being used for transplantation. These developments are initial steps to relieving the extreme shortage of donor pancreases needed for the procedure.

During the infusion process, the cells travel through the portal vein and become lodged in the capillaries of the liver, where they remain to produce insulin as they normally would in the pancreas.

Diagnosis/Preparation

To qualify as a candidate for islet cell transplantation, the patient must suffer from type 1 (juvenile) diabetes and current insulin treatment methods must be insufficient. For example, some participants suffer from hypoglycemic unawareness, a condition where low blood sugar will cause very dangerous, unpredictable blackouts that cannot be controlled with insulin injections. The potential patient must also undergo extensive medical and psychological tests to determine their physical and mental appropriateness for enrollment in the trial. If the results of these tests support the candidacy, then sufficient donor pancreas tissue in the patient's blood type must be located. The patient is placed on an organ donor list. Waiting for more than a year is common.

In response to this long wait, research is ongoing to provide alternative sources of donor islet cells such as animal cells, a process known as a xenograft. Pigs are a particularly advantageous source of islet cells because human and pig insulin proteins differ by only one amino acid, and there is an extensive amount of fresh pancreases available from the pork industry. Other potential sources of donor islets cells include embryonic stem cells and cell lines of islet beta cells.

Prior to the transplantation, the patient must undergo a drug regime that suppresses the immune system so that the new cells will be accepted. Even though only cells are being transplanted, the amount of immunosuppression is the same as that required for a whole organ transplant. Current protocols for islet transplantation use a mixture of non-steroidal drugs, as those that include steroids have been shown to aggravate the diabetic condition of the patient and inhibit the insulin-producing function of the transplanted cells.

Future research in this area may include the use of monoclonal antibody therapy to induce tolerance in patients prior to transplantation.

Aftercare

Recovery time from the procedure itself is minimal. However, current technology requires that patients continuously remain on immunosuppressive drugs to avoid rejection of the new islet cells. Side effects from these drugs can increase the amount of time that the patient must remain hospitalized.

QUESTIONS TO ASK THE DOCTOR

- What are the chances that the procedure will allow me to no longer require insulin or is being able to reduce the amount that I use a more realistic outcome?
- Will the immunosuppression before my procedure involve the use of steroids?
- What are my risks concerning long-term use of immunosuppressive drugs?

It takes some time for the cells to attach to the liver blood vessels and begin producing insulin. Until then, numerous blood **glucose tests** are performed, and injected insulin is used to keep blood glucose levels within normal ranges.

Risks

Until recently, success rates for this procedure were not promising. With success being defined as not requiring insulin for a full year after transplantation, the success rate from 1998–2000 was only about 14% of patients transplanted. However, newer procedures have been achieving at least short-term success rates approaching 80–100%, making the possibility of widespread use of this procedure much more feasible in the near future.

Because of the newness of these procedures, the long-term success rate of these new protocols is not yet known. Graft death is significant risk even years after a successful transplant. The longest reported successful graft using the older protocols was six years. As time goes on, the ability of the graft transplanted using the new protocols and sustained by the new immunosuppressive drug mixtures will be determined.

A third important risk is the long-term use of immunosuppressive drugs by the patient. There is relatively little experience with the long-term use of these drugs, so it is difficult to predict what the exact physical effects long-term immunosuppression may have. Some of the known side effects include high blood pressure, toxicity of the kidneys, and opportunistic infections.

Alternatives

One alternative to islet cell transplantation is a transplant with a whole pancreas, a much more invasive procedure. Whole organ transplant has historically had a better success rate than islet transplantation. However,

KEY TERMS

Immunosuppression—A drug-induced state that prevents rejection of transplanted body parts.

Invasive—Used to describe a procedure that involves surgical cutting into the body.

Islet cell—The cell type within the pancreas that produces insulin.

Portal vein—The main vessel that carries blood to the liver.

Steroids—A component of commonly used immunosuppressive drugs that have negative effects on insulin production.

newer islet cell transplant protocols are approaching whole organ results, thus overcoming one of the most important differences between the two procedures.

Resources

BOOKS

Farney, Alan C., and David E. R. Sutherland. "Pancrease and Islet Transplantation." In *The Pancreas: Biology, Pathobiology, and Disease,* edited by Vay Liang W. Go, et al. New York: Raven Press, 1993.

Robertson, R. Paul. "Pancreas and Islet Transplantation." In *Endocrinology,* edited by Leslie J. DeGroot, et al. Philadelphia: W.B. Saunders Company, 2001.

PERIODICALS

"Islet Cell Transplantation for Diabetes Turns Corner." *Science Daily Magazine* (August 28, 2002).

Perry, Patrick. "Zeroing in on a Cure for Diabetes." *The Saturday Evening Post* (January/February 2002): 38–43.

ORGANIZATIONS

American Diabetes Association. 1701 North Beauregard Street, Alexandria, VA 22311. (800) 342-2383. <www.diabetes.org>.

Immune Tolerance Network (ITN). 5743 South Drexel Avenue, Suite 200, Chicago, IL 60637. (773) 834-5341. <www.immunetolerance.org>.

Michelle Johnson, MS, JD

IV rehydration *see* **Intravenous rehydration**

Joint radiography *see* **Arthrography**

Joint resection *see* **Arthroplasty**

Joint x rays *see* **Arthrography**

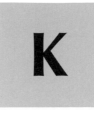

K

Keratoplasty *see* **Corneal transplantation**

Ketone test *see* **Urinalysis**

Kidney dialysis

Definition

Dialysis treatment replaces the function of the kidneys, which normally serve as the body's natural filtration system. Through the use of a blood filter and a chemical solution known as dialysate, the treatment removes waste products and excess fluids from the bloodstream, while maintaining the proper chemical balance of the blood. There are two types of dialysis treatment: hemodialysis and peritoneal dialysis.

Purpose

Dialysis is most commonly prescribed for patients with temporary or permanent kidney failure. People with end-stage renal disease (ESRD) have kidneys that are no longer capable of adequately removing fluids and wastes from their body or of maintaining the proper level of certain kidney-regulated chemicals in the bloodstream. For these individuals, dialysis is the only treatment option available outside of **kidney transplantation**. Dialysis may also be used to simulate kidney function in patients awaiting a transplant until a donor kidney becomes available. Also, dialysis may be used in the treatment of patients suffering from poisoning or overdose in order to quickly remove drugs from the bloodstream.

Demographics

As of December 31, 2000, in the United States, over 275,000 people were undergoing regular dialysis treatments to manage their ESRD. Diabetes mellitus is the leading single cause of ESRD. According to the 2002 Annual Data Report of the United States Renal Data System

(USRDS), 42% of non-Hispanic dialysis patients in the United States have ESRD caused by diabetes. People of Native American and Hispanic descent are at an elevated high risk for both kidney disease and diabetes. ESRD caused by diabetes occurred in 65% of Hispanic dialysis patients. And of those Native Americans who had been on dialysis for one year in 1999, 82% had diabetes.

Hypertension (high blood pressure) is the second leading cause of ESRD in adults, accounting for 25.5% of the patient population, followed by glomerulonephritis (8.4%). African-Americans are more likely to develop hypertension-related ESRD than whites and Hispanics.

Among children and young adults under 20 on dialysis, glomerulonephritis is the leading cause of ESRD (31%), and hereditary, cystic, and congenital diseases account for 37%. Pediatric patients typically spend less

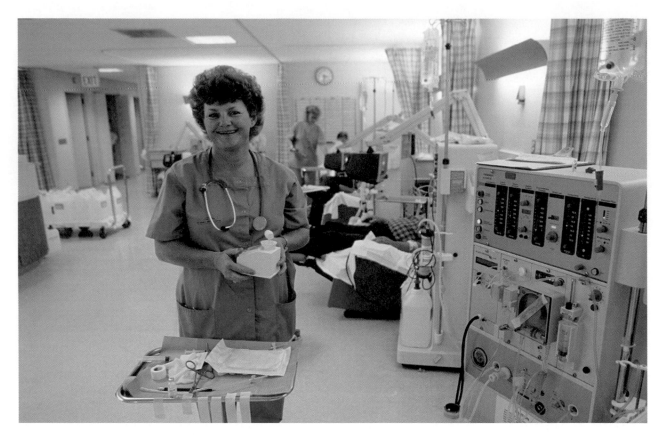

Nurse working in a kidney dialysis unit. *(Custom Medical Stock Photo. Reproduced by permission.)*

time on dialysis than adults; according to the USRDS the average waiting period for a kidney transplant for patients under age 20 is 10 months, compared to the adult wait of approximately two years.

Description

There are two types of dialysis treatment: hemodialysis and peritoneal dialysis.

Hemodialysis

Hemodialysis is the most frequently prescribed type of dialysis treatment in the United States. The treatment involves circulating the patient's blood outside of the body through an extracorporeal circuit (ECC), or dialysis circuit. Two needles are inserted into the patient's vein, or access site, and are attached to the ECC, which consists of plastic blood tubing, a filter known as a dialyzer (artificial kidney), and a dialysis machine that monitors and maintains blood flow and administers dialysate. Dialysate is a chemical bath that is used to draw waste products out of the blood.

Since the 1980s, the majority of hemodialysis treatments in the United States have been performed with hollow fiber dialyzers. A hollow fiber dialyzer is composed of thousands of tube-like hollow fiber strands encased in a clear plastic cylinder several inches in diameter. There are two compartments within the dialyzer (the blood compartment and the dialysate compartment).

The membrane that separates these two compartments is semipermeable. This means that it allows the passage of certain sized molecules across it, but prevents the passage of other, larger molecules. As blood is pushed through the blood compartment in one direction, suction or vacuum pressure pulls the dialysate through the dialysate compartment in a countercurrent, or opposite direction. These opposing pressures work to drain excess fluids out of the bloodstream and into the dialysate, a process called ultrafiltration.

A second process called diffusion moves waste products in the blood across the membrane and into the dialysate compartment, where they are carried out of the body. At the same time, electrolytes and other chemicals in the dialysate solution cross the membrane into the blood compartment. The purified, chemically balanced blood is then returned to the body.

Most hemodialysis patients require treatment three times a week, for an average of three to four hours per dialysis "run." Specific treatment schedules depend on the type of dialyzer used and the patient's current physical condition.

Blood pressure changes associated with hemodialysis may pose a risk for patients with heart problems. Peritoneal dialysis may be the preferred treatment option in these cases.

Peritoneal dialysis

In peritoneal dialysis, the patient's peritoneum, or lining of the abdomen, acts as a blood filter. A catheter is surgically inserted into the patient's abdomen. During treatment, the catheter is used to fill the abdominal cavity with dialysate. Waste products and excess fluids move from the patient's bloodstream into the dialysate solution. After a waiting period of six to 24 hours, depending on the treatment method used, the waste-filled dialysate is drained from the abdomen and replaced with clean dialysate.

There are three types of peritoneal dialysis:

• Continuous ambulatory peritoneal dialysis (CAPD). CAPD is a continuous treatment that is self-administered and requires no machine. The patient inserts fresh dialysate solution into the abdominal cavity, waits four to six hours, and removes the used solution. The solution is immediately replaced with fresh dialysate. A bag attached to the catheter is worn under clothing.

• Continuous cyclic peritoneal dialysis (CCPD). Also called automated peritoneal dialysis (APD), CCPD is an overnight treatment that uses a machine to drain and refill the abdominal cavity, CCPD takes 10 to 12 hours per session.

• Intermittent peritoneal dialysis (IPD). This hospital-based treatment is performed several times a week. A machine administers and drains the dialysate solution, and sessions can take 12 to 24 hours.

Peritoneal dialysis is often the treatment option of choice in infants and children, whose small size can make vascular (through a vein) access difficult to maintain. Peritoneal dialysis can also be done outside of a clinical setting, which is more conducive to regular school attendance.

Peritoneal dialysis is not recommended for patients with abdominal adhesions or other abdominal defects, such as a hernia, that might compromise the efficiency of the treatment. It is also not recommended for patients who suffer frequent bouts of diverticulitis, an inflammation of small pouches in the intestinal tract.

Diagnosis/Preparation

Patients are weighed immediately before and after each hemodialysis treatment to evaluate their fluid retention. Blood pressure and temperature are taken and the patient is assessed for physical changes since their last dialysis run. Regular blood tests monitor chemical and waste levels in the blood. Prior to treatment, patients are typically administered a dose of heparin, an anticoagulant that prevents blood clotting, to ensure the free flow of blood through the dialyzer and an uninterrupted dialysis run for the patient.

Aftercare

Both hemodialysis and peritoneal dialysis patients need to be vigilant about keeping their access sites and catheters clean and infection-free during and between dialysis runs.

Dialysis is just one facet of a comprehensive treatment approach for ESRD. Although dialysis treatment is very effective in removing toxins and fluids from the body, there are several functions of the kidney it cannot mimic, such as regulating high blood pressure and red blood cell production. Patients with ESRD need to watch their dietary and fluid intake carefully and take medications as prescribed to manage their disease.

Risks

Many of the risks and side effects associated with dialysis are a combined result of both the treatment and the poor physical condition of the ESRD patient. Dialysis patients should always report side effects to their healthcare provider.

Anemia

Hematocrit (Hct) levels, a measure of red blood cells, are typically low in ESRD patients. This deficiency

• When and where will my dialysis treatments be scheduled?

• How should my diet change now that I'm on dialysis?

• What kind of vascular access will I get?

• Does my new dialysis center have a dialyzer reuse program? If so, what safety checks are in place to ensure I receive a properly treated dialyzer?

• What can I do to make dialysis more effective?

• Can you refer me to any ESRD patient support groups?

• Should I change my medication routine?

KEY TERMS

Access site—The vein tapped for vascular access in hemodialysis treatments. For patients with temporary treatment needs, access to the bloodstream is gained by inserting a catheter into the subclavian vein near the patient's collarbone. Patients in long-term dialysis require stronger, more durable access sites, called fistulas or grafts, that are surgically created.

Dialysate—A chemical bath used in dialysis to draw fluids and toxins out of the bloodstream and supply electrolytes and other chemicals to the bloodstream.

Dialysis prescription—The general parameters of dialysis treatment that vary according to each patient's individual needs. Treatment length, type of dialyzer and dialysate used, and rate of ultrafiltration are all part of the dialysis prescription.

Dialyzer—An artificial kidney usually composed of hollow fiber which is used in hemodialysis to eliminate waste products from the blood and remove excess fluids from the bloodstream.

Erythropoietin—A hormone produced by the kidneys that stimulates the production of red blood cells by bone marrow.

ESRD—End-stage renal disease; chronic or permanent kidney failure.

Extracorporeal circuit (ECC)—The path the hemodialysis patient's blood takes outside of the body. It typically consists of plastic tubing, a hemodialysis machine, and a dialyzer.

Glomerulonephritis—A disease of the kidney that causes inflammation and scarring and impairs the kidney's ability to filter waste products from the blood.

Hematocrit (Hct) level—A measure of red blood cells.

Glomerulonephritis—Kidney disease caused by scarring of the glomeruli, the small blood vessels in the nephrons, or filtering centers, of the kidneys.

Peritoneum—The abdominal cavity; the peritoneum acts as a blood filter in peritoneal dialysis.

is caused by a lack of the hormone erythropoietin, which is normally produced by the kidneys. The problem is elevated in hemodialysis patients, who may incur blood loss during hemodialysis treatments. Epoetin alfa, or EPO (sold under the trade name Epogen), a hormone therapy, and intravenous or oral iron supplements are used to manage anemia in dialysis patients.

Cramps, nausea, vomiting, and headaches

Some hemodialysis patients experience cramps and flu-like symptoms during treatment. These can be caused by a number of factors, including the type of dialysate used, composition of the dialyzer membrane, water quality in the dialysis unit, and the ultrafiltration rate of the treatment. Adjustment of the dialysis prescription often helps alleviate many symptoms.

Hypotension

Because of the stress placed on the cardiovascular system with regular hemodialysis treatments, patients are at risk for hypotension, a sudden drop in blood pressure. This can often be controlled by medication and adjustment of the patient's dialysis prescription.

Infection

Both hemodialysis and peritoneal dialysis patients are at risk for infection. Hemodialysis patients should keep their access sites clean and watch for signs of redness and warmth that could indicate infection. Peritoneal dialysis patients must follow the same precautions with their catheter. Peritonitis, an infection of the peritoneum, causes flu-like symptoms and can disrupt dialysis treatments if not caught early.

Infectious diseases

Because there is a great deal of blood exposure involved in dialysis treatment, a slight risk of contracting hepatitis B and hepatitis C exists. The hepatitis B vaccination is recommended for most hemodialysis patients. As of 2001, there has only been one documented case of HIV being transmitted in a United States dialysis unit to a staff member, and no documented cases of HIV ever being transmitted between dialysis patients in the United States. The strict standards of infection control practiced in modern hemodialysis units minimizes the chance of contracting one of these diseases.

Normal results

Because dialysis is an ongoing treatment process for many patients, a baseline for normalcy can be difficult to gauge. Puffiness in the patient related to edema, or fluid retention, may be relieved after dialysis treatment. The patient's overall sense of physical well being may also be improved.

Monthly blood tests to check the levels of urea, a waste product, help to determine the adequacy of the dialysis prescription. Another test, called Kt/V (dialyzer clearance multiplied by time of treatment and divided by the total volume of water in the patient's body), is also performed to assess patient progress. A urea reduction ratio (URR) of 65% or higher, and a Kt/V of at least 1.2 are considered the benchmarks of dialysis adequacy by the Kidney Disease Outcomes Quality Initiative (K/DOQI) of the National Kidney Foundation.

Morbidity and mortality rates

The USRDS reports that mortality rates for individuals on dialysis are also significantly higher than both kidney transplant patients and the general population, and expected remaining lifetimes of chronic dialysis patients are only one-fourth to one-fifth that of the general population. The hospitalization rates for people with ESRD are four times greater than that of the general population.

Alternatives

The only alternative to dialysis for ESRD patients is a successful kidney transplant. However, demand for donor kidneys has traditionally far exceeded supply. As of March 1, 2003, there were 53,619 patients on the United Network for Organ Sharing (UNOS) waiting list for a kidney transplant, with an additional 2,405 waiting for a combination kidney and pancreas transplant. In the entire year of 2001, only 14,095 donors gave kidneys, according to UNOS.

For patients with diabetes, the number one cause of chronic kidney failure in adults, the best way to avoid ESRD and subsequent dialysis is to maintain tight control of blood glucose levels through diet, **exercise**, and medication. Controlling high blood pressure is also important.

Resources

BOOKS

Cameron, J. S. *Kidney Failure: The Facts.* New York: Oxford University Press, 1999.
National Kidney Foundation. *Dialysis Outcomes Quality Initiatives (NOQI).* Vol. 1-5. New York: National Kidney Foundation, 1997.
U.S. Renal Data System. *USRDS 2002 Annual Data Report: Atlas of End-Stage Renal Disease in the United States.* Bethesda, MD: The National Institutes of Health, National Institute of Diabetes and Digestive and Kidney Diseases, 2002.

PERIODICALS

Eknoyan G., G. J. Beck, et al. "Effect of Dialysis Dose and Membrane Flux in Maintenance Hemodialysis." *New England Journal of Medicine* 347 (December 19, 2002): 2010–2019.

ORGANIZATIONS

American Association of Kidney Patients. 3505 E. Frontage Rd., Suite 315, Tampa, FL 33607. (800) 749-2257. <http://www.aakp.org>.
American Kidney Fund (AKF). Suite 1010, 6110 Executive Boulevard, Rockville, MD 20852. (800) 638-8299. <http://www.akfinc.org>.
National Kidney Foundation. 30 East 33rd St., Suite 1100, New York, NY 10016. (800) 622-9010. <http://www.kidney.org>.
United States Renal Data System (USRDS), Coordinating Center. The University of Minnesota, 914 South 8th Street, Suite D-206, Minneapolis, MN 55404. 1-888-99USRDS. <http://www.usrds.org>.

Paula Anne Ford-Martin

Kidney function tests

Definition

Kidney function tests is a collective term for a variety of individual tests and procedures that can be done to evaluate how well the kidneys are functioning. A doctor who orders kidney function tests and uses the results to assess the functioning of the kidneys is called a nephrologist.

Purpose

The kidneys, the body's natural filtration system, perform many vital functions, including removing metabolic waste products from the bloodstream, regulating the body's water balance, and maintaining the pH (acidity/alkalinity) of the body's fluids. Approximately one and a half quarts of blood per minute are circulated through the kidneys, where waste chemicals are filtered out and eliminated from the body (along with excess water) in the form of urine. Kidney function tests help to determine if the kidneys are performing their tasks adequately.

Precautions

The doctor should take a complete history prior to conducting kidney function tests to evaluate the patient's food and drug intake. A wide variety of prescription and over-the-counter medications can affect blood and urine kidney function test results, as can some food and beverages.

Description

Many conditions can affect the ability of the kidneys to carry out their vital functions. Some conditions can lead to a rapid (acute) decline in kidney function; others lead to a gradual (chronic) decline in function. Both can result in a build-up of toxic waste substances in the blood. A number of clinical laboratory tests that measure the levels of substances normally regulated by the kidneys can help to determine the cause and extent of kidney dysfunction. Urine and blood samples are used for these tests.

The nephrologist uses these results in a number of ways. Once a diagnosis is made that kidney disease is present and what kind of kidney disease is causing the problem, the nephrologist may recommend a specific treatment. Although there is no specific drug therapy that will prevent the progression of kidney disease, the doctor will make recommendations for treatment to slow the disease as much as possible. For instance, the doctor might prescribe blood pressure medications, or treatments for patients with diabetes. If kidney disease is getting worse, the nephrologist may discuss hemodialysis (blood cleansing by removal of excess fluid, minerals, and wastes) or **kidney transplantation** (surgical procedure to implant a healthy kidney into a patient with kidney disease or kidney failure) with the patient.

Laboratory tests

There are a number of urine tests that can be used to assess kidney function. A simple, inexpensive screening test—a routine urinalysis—is often the first test conducted if kidney problems are suspected. A small, randomly collected urine sample is examined physically for things like color, odor, appearance, and concentration (specific gravity); chemically, for substances such a protein, glucose, and pH (acidity/ alkalinity); and microscopically for the presence of cellular elements (red blood cells [RBCs], white blood cells [WBCs], and epithelial cells), bacteria, crystals, and casts (structures formed by the deposit of protein, cells, and other substances in the kidneys's tubules). If results indicate a possibility of disease or impaired kidney function, one or more of the following additional tests is usually performed to pinpoint the cause and the level of decline in kidney function.

• Creatinine clearance test. This test evaluates how efficiently the kidneys clear a substance called creatinine from the blood. Creatinine, a waste product of muscle energy metabolism, is produced at a constant rate that is proportional to the individual's muscle mass. Because the body does not recycle it, all creatinine filtered by the kidneys in a given amount of time is excreted in the urine, making creatinine clearance a very specific measurement of kidney function. The test is performed on a timed urine specimen—a cumulative sample collected over a two to 24-hour period. Determination of the blood creatinine level is also required to calculate the urine clearance.

• Urea clearance test. Urea is a waste product that is created by protein metabolism and excreted in the urine. The urea clearance test requires a blood sample to measure the amount of urea in the bloodstream and two urine specimens, collected one hour apart, to determine the amount of urea that is filtered, or cleared, by the kidneys into the urine.

• Urine osmolality test. Urine osmolality is a measurement of the number of dissolved particles in urine. It is a more precise measurement than specific gravity for evaluating the ability of the kidneys to concentrate or dilute the urine. Kidneys that are functioning normally will excrete more water into the urine as fluid intake is increased, diluting the urine. If fluid intake is decreased, the kidneys excrete less water and the urine becomes more concentrated. The test may be done on a urine sample collected first thing in the morning, on multiple timed samples, or on a cumulative sample collected over a 24-hour period. The patient will typically be prescribed a high-protein diet for several days before the test and be asked to drink no fluids the night before the test.

• Urine protein test. Healthy kidneys filter all proteins from the bloodstream and then reabsorb them, allowing no protein, or only slight amounts of protein, into the urine. The persistent presence of significant amounts of protein in the urine, then, is an important indicator of kidney disease. A positive screening test for protein (included in a routine **urinalysis**) on a random urine sample is usually followed up with a test on a 24-hour urine sample that more precisely measures the quantity of protein.

There are also several blood tests that can aid in evaluating kidney function. These include:

• Blood urea nitrogen test (BUN). Urea is a byproduct of protein metabolism. Formed in the liver, this waste product is then filtered from the blood and excreted in the urine by the kidneys. The BUN test measures the amount of nitrogen contained in the urea. High BUN levels can indicate kidney dysfunction, but because BUN is also affected by protein intake and liver function, the test is usually done together with a blood creatinine, a more specific indicator of kidney function.

• Creatinine test. This test measures blood levels of creatinine, a by-product of muscle energy metabolism that, similar to urea, is filtered from the blood by the kidneys and excreted into the urine. Production of creatinine

KEY TERMS

Blood urea nitrogen (BUN)—The nitrogen portion of urea in the bloodstream. Urea is a waste product of protein metabolism in the body.

Creatinine—The metabolized by-product of creatinine, an organic compound that assists the body in producing muscle contractions. Creatinine is found in the bloodstream and in muscle tissue. It is removed from the blood by the kidneys and excreted in the urine.

Creatinine clearance rate—The clearance of creatinine from the plasma compared to its appearance in the urine. Since there is no reabsorption of creatinine, this measurement can estimate glomerular filtration rate.

Diuretic—A drug that increases the excretion of salt and water, increasing the output of urine.

Kilogram—Metric unit of weight.

Osmolality—A measurement of urine concentration that depends on the number of particles dissolved in it. Values are expressed as milliosmols per kilogram (mOsm/kg) of water.

Nephrologist—A doctor specializing in kidney disease.

Specific gravity—The ratio of the weight of a body fluid when compared with water.

Urea—A by-product of protein metabolism that is formed in the liver. Because urea contains ammonia, which is toxic to the body, it must be quickly filtered from the blood by the kidneys and excreted in the urine.

Uric acid—A product of purine breakdown that is excreted by the kidney. High levels of uric acid, caused by various diseases, can cause the formation of kidney stones.

Urine—A fluid containing water and dissolved substances excreted by the kidney.

---

depends on an person's muscle mass, which usually fluctuates very little. With normal kidney function, then, the amount of creatinine in the blood remains relatively constant and normal. For this reason, and because creatinine is affected very little by liver function, an elevated blood creatinine level is a more sensitive indicator of impaired kidney function than the BUN.

• Other blood tests. Measurement of the blood levels of other elements regulated in part by the kidneys can also be useful in evaluating kidney function. These include sodium, potassium, chloride, bicarbonate, calcium, magnesium, phosphorus, protein, uric acid, and glucose.

Results

Normal values for many tests are determined by the patient's age and gender. Reference values can also vary by laboratory, but are generally within the following ranges:

Urine tests

• Creatinine clearance. For a 24-hour urine collection, normal results are 90 mL/min–139 mL/min for adult males younger than 40, and 80–125 mL/min for adult females younger than 40. For people over 40, values decrease by 6.5 mL/min for each decade of life.

• Urine osmolality. With restricted fluid intake (concentration testing), osmolality should be greater than 800 mOsm/kg of water. With increased fluid intake (dilution testing), osmolality should be less than 100 mOSm/kg in at least one of the specimens collected. A 24-hour urine osmolality should average 300–900 mOsm/kg. A random urine osmolality should average 500–800 mOsm/kg.

• Urine protein. A 24-hour urine collection should contain no more than 150 mg of protein.

• Urine sodium. A 24-hour urine sodium should be within 75–200 mmol/day.

Blood tests

• Blood urea nitrogen (BUN) should average 8–20 mg/dL.

• Creatinine should be 0.8–1.2 mg/dL for males, and 0.6–0.9 mg/dL for females.

• Uric acid levels for males should be 3.5–7.2 mg/dL and for females 2.6–6.0 mg/dL.

Low clearance values for creatinine indicate a diminished ability of the kidneys to filter waste products from the blood and excrete them in the urine. As clearance levels decrease, blood levels of creatinine, urea, and uric acid increase. Because it can be affected by other factors, an elevated BUN, alone, is suggestive, but not diagnostic for kidney dysfunction. An abnormally elevated plasma creatinine is a more specific indicator of kidney disease than is BUN.

Low clearance values for creatinine and urea indicate a diminished ability of the kidneys to filter these waste products from the blood and to excrete them in the urine. As clearance levels decrease, blood levels of creatinine and urea nitrogen increase. Since it can be affected by other factors, an elevated BUN alone is certainly suggestive for kidney dysfunction. However, it is not diagnostic. An abnormally elevated blood creatinine, a more specific and sensitive indicator of kidney disease than the BUN, is diagnostic of impaired kidney function.

The inability of the kidneys to concentrate the urine in response to restricted fluid intake, or to dilute the urine in response to increased fluid intake during osmolality testing, may indicate decreased kidney function. Because the kidneys normally excrete almost no protein in the urine, its persistent presence, in amounts that exceed the normal 24-hour urine value, usually indicates some type of kidney disease.

Patient education

Some kidney problems are the result of another disease process, such as diabetes or hypertension. Doctors should take the time to inform patients about how their disease or its treatment will affect kidney function, as well as the different measures patients can take to help prevent these changes.

Resources

BOOKS

Brenner, Barry M. and Floyd C. Rector Jr., eds. *The Kidney, 6th Edition.* Philadelphia, PA: W. B. Saunders Company, 1999.

Burtis, Carl A. and Edward R. Ashwood. *Tietz Textbook of Clinical Chemistry.* Philadelphia, PA: W.B. Saunders Company, 1999.

Henry, J. B. *Clinical Diagnosis and Management by Laboratory Methods,* 20th ed. Philadelphia, PA: W. B. Saunders Company, 2001.

Pagana, Kathleen Deska. *Mosby's Manual of Diagnostic and Laboratory Tests.* St. Louis, MO: Mosby, Inc., 1998.

Wallach, Jacques. *Interpretation of Diagnostic Tests,* 7th ed. Philadelphia: Lippincott Williams & Wilkens, 2000.

ORGANIZATIONS

National Kidney Foundation (NKF). 30 East 33rd Street, New York, NY 10016. (800)622-9020. <http://www.kidney.org>.

National Institute of Diabetes and Digestive and Kidney Diseases (NIDDK). National Institutes of Health, Building 31, Room 9A04, 31 Center Drive, MSC 2560, Bethesda, MD 208792-2560. (301) 496-3583. <http://www.niddk.nih.gov/health/kidney/kidney.htm>.

OTHER

National Institutes of Health. [cited April 5, 2003]. <http://www.nlm.nih.gov/medlineplus/encyclopedia.html>.

National Institutes of Health. [cited June 29, 2003] <http://www.nlm.nih.gov/medlineplus/ency/article/003005.htm>.

Paula Ann Ford-Martin
Mark A. Best, M.D.

Kidney removal *see* **Nephrectomy**

Kidney transplant

Definition

Kidney transplantation is a surgical procedure to remove a healthy, functioning kidney from a living or brain-dead donor and implant it into a patient with non-functioning kidneys.

Purpose

Kidney transplantation is performed on patients with chronic kidney failure, or end-stage renal disease (ESRD). ESRD occurs when a disease, disorder, or congenital condition damages the kidneys so that they are no longer capable of adequately removing fluids and wastes from the body or of maintaining the proper level of certain kidney-regulated chemicals in the bloodstream. Without long-term dialysis or a kidney transplant, ESRD is fatal.

Demographics

Diabetes mellitus is the leading single cause of ESRD. According to the 2002 Annual Data Report of the United States Renal Data System (USRDS), 42% of non-Hispanic dialysis patients in the United States have ESRD caused by diabetes. People of Native American and Hispanic descent are at an elevated risk for both kidney disease and diabetes.

Hypertension (high blood pressure) is the second leading cause of ESRD in adults, accounting for 25.5% of the patient population, followed by glomerulonephritis (8.4%). African Americans are more likely to develop hypertension-related ESRD than Caucasians and Hispanics.

Among children and young adults under 20 on dialysis, glomerulonephritis is the leading cause of ESRD

Kidney transplantation

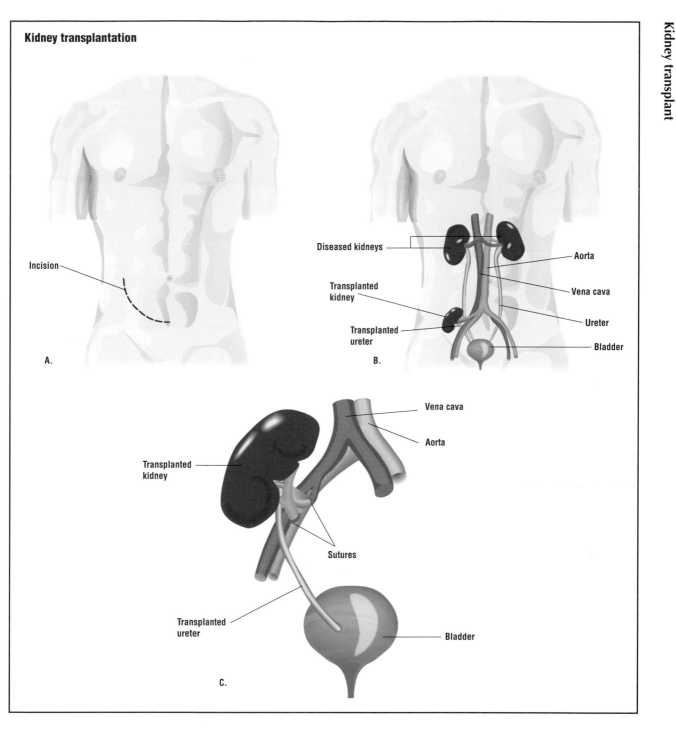

For a kidney transplant, an incision is made in the lower abdomen (A). The donor kidney is connected to the patient's blood supply lower in the abdomen than the native kidneys, which are usually left in place (B). A transplanted ureter connects the donor kidney to the patient's bladder (C). *(Illustration by GGS Inc.)*

(31%), and hereditary, cystic, and congenital diseases account for 37%. According to USRDS, the average waiting period for a kidney transplant for patients under age 20 is 10 months, compared to the adult wait of approximately two years.

Description

Kidney transplantation involves surgically attaching a functioning kidney, or graft, from a brain-dead organ donor (a cadaver transplant) or from a living donor to a patient with ESRD. Living donors may be related or unrelated to the patient, but a related donor has a better chance of having a kidney that is a stronger biological match for the patient.

Open nephrectomy

The surgical procedure to remove a kidney from a living donor is called a **nephrectomy**. In a traditional, open nephrectomy, the kidney donor is administered general anesthesia and a 6–10-in (15.2–25.4-cm) incision through several layers of muscle is made on the side or front of the abdomen. The blood vessels connecting the kidney to the donor are cut and clamped, and the ureter is also cut and clamped between the bladder and kidney. The kidney and an attached section of ureter are removed from the donor. The vessels and ureter in the donor are then tied off and the incision is sutured together again. A similar procedure is used to harvest cadaver kidneys, although both kidneys are typically removed at once, and blood and cell samples for tissue typing are also taken.

Laparoscopic nephrectomy

Laparoscopic nephrectomy is a form of minimally invasive surgery using instruments on long, narrow rods to view, cut, and remove the donor kidney. The surgeon views the kidney and surrounding tissue with a flexible videoscope. The videoscope and **surgical instruments** are maneuvered through four small incisions in the abdomen, and carbon dioxide is pumped into the abdominal cavity to inflate it for an improved visualization of the kidney. Once the kidney is freed, it is secured in a bag and pulled through a fifth incision, approximately 3 in (7.6 cm) wide, in the front of the abdominal wall below the navel. Although this surgical technique takes slightly longer than an open nephrectomy, studies have shown that it promotes a faster recovery time, shorter hospital stays, and less postoperative pain for kidney donors.

A modified laparoscopic technique called hand-assisted laparoscopic nephrectomy may also be used to remove the kidney. In the hand-assisted surgery, a small incision of 3–5 in (7.6–12.7 cm) is made in the patient's abdomen. The incision allows the surgeon to place his hand in the abdominal cavity using a special surgical glove that also maintains a seal for the inflation of the abdominal cavity with carbon dioxide. The technique gives the surgeon the benefit of using his or her hands to feel the kidney and related structures. The kidney is then removed through the incision by hand instead of with a bag.

Once removed, kidneys from live donors and cadavers are placed on ice and flushed with a cold preservative solution. The kidney can be preserved in this solution for 24–48 hours until the transplant takes place. The sooner the transplant takes place after harvesting the kidney, the better the chances are for proper functioning.

Kidney transplant

During the transplant operation, the kidney recipient is typically under general anesthesia and administered **antibiotics** to prevent possible infection. A catheter is placed in the bladder before surgery begins. An incision is made in the flank of the patient, and the surgeon implants the kidney above the pelvic bone and below the existing, non-functioning kidney by suturing the kidney artery and vein to the patient's iliac artery and vein. The ureter of the new kidney is attached directly to the kidney recipient's bladder. Once the new kidney is attached, the patient's existing, diseased kidneys may or may not be removed, depending on the circumstances surrounding the kidney failure. Barring any complications, the transplant operation takes about three to four hours.

Since 1973, **Medicare** has picked up 80% of ESRD treatment costs, including the costs of transplantation for both the kidney donor and the recipient. Medicare also covers 80% of immunosuppressive medication costs for up to three years. To qualify for Medicare ESRD benefits, a patient must be insured or eligible for benefits under Social Security, or be a spouse or child of an eligible American. Private insurance and state **Medicaid** programs often cover the remaining 20% of treatment costs.

Patients with a history of heart disease, lung disease, cancer, or hepatitis may not be suitable candidates for receiving a kidney transplant.

Diagnosis/Preparation

Patients with chronic renal disease who need a transplant and do not have a living donor registered with United Network for Organ Sharing (UNOS) to be placed on a waiting list for a cadaver kidney transplant. UNOS is a non-profit organization that is under contract with the federal government to administer the Organ Procurement and Transplant Network (OPTN) and the national Scientific Registry of Transplant Recipients (SRTR).

Kidney allocation is based on a mathematical formula that awards points for factors that can affect a successful transplant, such as time spent on the transplant list, the patient's health status, and age. The most important part of the equation is that the kidney be compatible with the patient's body. A human kidney has a set of six antigens, substances that stimulate the production of antibodies. (Antibodies then attach to cells they recognize as foreign and attack them.) Donors are tissue matched for 0–6 of the antigens, and compatibility is determined by the number and strength of those matched pairs. Blood type matching is also important. Patients with a living donor who is a close relative have the best chance of a close match.

Before being placed on the transplant list, potential kidney recipients must undergo a comprehensive physical evaluation. In addition to the compatibility testing, radiological tests, urine tests, and a psychological evaluation will be performed. A panel of reactive antibody (PRA) is performed by mixing the patient's serum (white blood cells) with serum from a panel of 60 randomly selected donors. The patient's PRA sensitivity is determined by how many of these random samples his or her serum reacts with; for example, a reaction to the antibodies of six of the samples would mean a PRA of 10%. High reactivity (also called sensitization) means that the recipient would likely reject a transplant from the donor. The more reactions, the higher the PRA and the lower the chances of an overall match from the general population. Patients with a high PRA face a much longer waiting period for a suitable kidney match.

Potential living kidney donors also undergo a complete medical history and **physical examination** to evaluate their suitability for donation. Extensive blood tests are performed on both donor and recipient. The blood samples are used to tissue type for antigen matches, and confirm that blood types are compatible. A PRA is performed to ensure that the recipient antibodies will not have a negative reaction to the donor antigens. If a reaction does occur, there are some treatment protocols that can be attempted to reduce reactivity, including immunosuppressant drugs and plasmapheresis (a blood filtration therapy).

The donor's kidney function will be evaluated with a urine test as well. In some cases, a special dye that shows up on x rays is injected into an artery, and x rays are taken to show the blood supply of the donor kidney (a procedure called an arteriogram).

Once compatibility is confirmed and the physical preparations for kidney transplantation are complete, both

QUESTIONS TO ASK THE DOCTOR

- How many kidney transplants have both you and the hospital performed?
- What are your transplant success rates? How about those of the hospital?
- Who will be on my transplant team?
- Can I get on the waiting list at more than one hospital?
- Will my transplant be performed with a laparoscopic or an open nephrectomy?
- What type of immunosuppressive drugs will I be on post-transplant?

donor and recipient may undergo a psychological or psychiatric evaluation to ensure that they are emotionally prepared for the transplant procedure and aftercare regimen.

Aftercare

A typical hospital stay for a transplant recipient is about five days. Both kidney donors and recipients will experience some discomfort in the area of the incision after surgery. Pain relievers are administered following the transplant operation. Patients may also experience numbness, caused by severed nerves, near or on the incision.

A regimen of immunosuppressive, or anti-rejection, medication is prescribed to prevent the body's immune system from rejecting the new kidney. Common immunosuppressants include cyclosporine, prednisone, tacrolimus, mycophenolate mofetil, sirolimus, baxsiliximab, daclizumab, and azathioprine. The kidney recipient will be required to take a course of **immunosuppressant drugs** for the lifespan of the new kidney. Intravenous antibodies may also be administered after **transplant surgery** and during rejection episodes.

Because the patient's immune system is suppressed, he or she is at an increased risk for infection. The incision area should be kept clean, and the transplant recipient should avoid contact with people who have colds, viruses, or similar illnesses. If the patient has pets, he or she should not handle animal waste. The transplant team will provide detailed instructions on what should be avoided post-transplant. After recovery, the patient will still have to be vigilant about exposure to viruses and other environmental dangers.

Transplant recipients may need to adjust their dietary habits. Certain immunosuppressive medications cause increased appetite or sodium and protein retention, and the patient may have to adjust his or her intake of calories, salt, and protein to compensate.

Risks

As with any surgical procedure, the kidney transplantation procedure carries some risk for both a living donor and a graft recipient. Possible complications include infection and bleeding (hemorrhage). A lymphocele, a pool of lymphatic fluid around the kidney that is generated by lymphatic vessels damaged in surgery, occurs in up to 20% of transplant patients and can obstruct urine flow and/or blood flow to the kidney if not diagnosed and drained promptly. Less common is a urine leak outside of the bladder, which occurs in approximately 3% of kidney transplants when the ureter suffers damage during the procedure. This problem is usually correctable with follow-up surgery.

A transplanted kidney may be rejected by the patient. Rejection occurs when the patient's immune system recognizes the new kidney as a foreign body and attacks the kidney. It may occur soon after transplantation, or several months or years after the procedure has taken place. Rejection episodes are not uncommon in the first weeks after transplantation surgery, and are treated with high-dose injections of immunosuppressant drugs. If a rejection episode cannot be reversed and kidney failure continues, the patient will typically go back on dialysis. Another transplant procedure can be attempted at a later date if another kidney becomes available.

The biggest risk to the recovering transplant recipient is not from the operation or the kidney itself, but from the immunosuppressive medication he or she must take. Because these drugs suppress the immune system, the patient is susceptible to infections such as cytomegalovirus (CMV) and varicella (chickenpox). Other medications that fight viral and bacterial infections can offset this risk to a degree. The immunosuppressants can also cause a host of possible side effects, from high blood pressure to osteoporosis. Prescription and dosage adjustments can lessen side effects for some patients.

Normal results

The new kidney may start functioning immediately, or may take several weeks to begin producing urine. Living donor kidneys are more likely to begin functioning earlier than cadaver kidneys, which frequently suffer some reversible damage during the kidney transplant and storage procedure. Patients may have to undergo dialysis for several weeks while their new kidney establishes an acceptable level of functioning.

Studies have shown that after they recover from surgery, kidney donors typically have no long-term complications from the loss of one kidney, and their remaining kidney will increase its functioning to compensate for the loss of the other.

Morbidity and mortality rates

Survival rates for patients undergoing kidney transplants are 95–96% one year post-transplant, and 91% three years after transplant. More than 2,900 patients on the transplant waiting list died in 2001. The success of a kidney transplant graft depends on the strength of the match between donor and recipient and the source of the kidney. According to the OPTN 2002 annual report, cadaver kidneys have a five-year survival rate of 63%, compared to a 76% survival rate for living donor kidneys. However, there have been cases of cadaver and living, related donor kidneys functioning well for over 25 years. In addition, advances in transplantation over the past decade have decreased the rate of graft failure; the USRDS reports that graft failure dropped by 23% in the years 1998–2000 compared to failures occurring between 1994 and 1997.

Alternatives

Patients who develop chronic kidney failure must either go on dialysis treatment or receive a kidney transplant to survive.

Resources

BOOKS

Cameron, J. S. *Kidney Failure: The Facts.* New York: Oxford University Press, 1999.

Finn, Robert, ed., et al. *Organ Transplants: Making the Most of Your Gift of Life.* Cambridge, MA: O'Reilly Publishing, 2000.

Mitch, William, and Saulo Klahr, eds. *Handbook of Nutrition and the Kidney, 4th edition.* Philadelphia: Lippincott, Williams, and Wilkins, 2002.

Parker, James, and Philip Parker, eds. *The 2002 Official Patient Sourcebook on Kidney Failure.* San Diego: Icon Health Publications, 2002.

University Renal Research and Education Associates (URREA); United Network for Organ Sharing (UNOS). *2002 Annual Report of the U.S. Organ Procurement and Transplantation Network and the Scientific Registry of Transplant Recipients: Transplant Data 1992–2001.* Rockville, MD: HHS/HRSA/OSP/DOT, 2003. <http://www.optn.org/data/annualReport.asp.>.

U.S. Renal Data System. *USRDS 2002 Annual Data Report.* Bethesda, MD: The National Institutes of Health, National Institute of Diabetes and Digestive and Kidney Diseases, 2003.

KEY TERMS

Arteriogram—A diagnostic test that involves viewing the arteries and/or attached organs by injecting a contrast medium, or dye, into the artery and taking an x ray.

Congenital—Present at birth.

Dialysis—A blood filtration therapy that replaces the function of the kidneys, filtering fluids, and waste products out of the bloodstream. There are two types of dialysis treatment: hemodialysis, which uses an artificial kidney, or dialyzer, as a blood filter; and peritoneal dialysis, which uses the patient's abdominal cavity (peritoneum) as a blood filter.

Glomerulonephritis—A disease of the kidney that causes inflammation and scarring and impairs the kidney's ability to filter waste products from the blood.

Iliac artery—Large blood vessel in the pelvis that leads into the leg.

Immunosuppressive medication—Drugs given to a transplant recipient to prevent his or her immune system from attacking the transplanted organ.

Rejection—The process in which the immune system attacks foreign tissue such as a transplanted organ.

Videoscope—A surgical camera.

PERIODICALS

Waller, J. R., et al. "Living Kidney Donation: A Comparison of Laparoscopic and Conventional Open Operations." *Postgraduate Medicine Journal* 78, no. 917 (March 2002): 153.

ORGANIZATIONS

American Association of Kidney Patients. 3505 E. Frontage Rd., Suite 315, Tampa, FL 33607. (800) 749-2257. info@aakp.org. <http://www.aakp.org>.

American Kidney Fund (AKF). Suite 1010, 6110 Executive Boulevard, Rockville, MD 20852. (800) 638-8299. helpline@akfinc.org. <http://www.akfinc.org>.

National Kidney Foundation. 30 East 33rd St., Suite 1100, New York, NY 10016. (800) 622-9010. <http://www.kidney.org>.

United Network for Organ Sharing (UNOS). 700 North 4th St., Richmond, VA 23219. (888) 894-6361. <http://www.transplantliving.org>.

United States Renal Data System (USRDS). USRDS Coordinating Center, 914 S. 8th St., Suite D-206, Minneapolis, MN 55404. (612) 347-7776. <http://www.usrds.org>.

OTHER

Infant Kidney Transplantation. Lucille Packard Children's Hospital. 725 Welch Road, Palo Alto, CA 94304. (650) 497-8000. <http://www.lpch.org/clinicalSpecialtiesServices/COE/Transplant/KidneyTransplant/infantAdultToinfantKidneyTransplant.html>.

A Patient's Guide to Kidney Transplant Surgery. University of Southern California Kidney Transplant Program. <http://www.kidneytransplant.org/patientguide/index.html>.

Paula Anne Ford-Martin

Knee arthroscopic surgery

Definition

Knee **arthroscopic surgery** is a procedure performed through small incisions in the skin to repair injuries to tissues such as ligaments, cartilage, or bone within the knee joint area. The surgery is conducted with the aid of an arthroscope, which is a very small instrument guided by a lighted scope attached to a television monitor. Other instruments are inserted through three incisions around the knee. Arthroscopic surgeries range from minor procedures such as flushing or smoothing out bone surfaces or tissue fragments (lavage and **debridement**) associated with osteoarthritis, to the realignment of a dislocated knee and ligament grafting surgeries. The range of surgeries represents very different procedures, risks, and aftercare requirements.

While the clear advantages of arthrocopic surgery lie in surgery with less anesthetic, less cutting, and less recovery time, this surgery nonetheless requires a very thorough examination of the causes of knee injury or pain prior to a decision for surgery.

Purpose

There are many procedures that currently fall under the general surgical category of knee arthroscopy. They fall into roughly two groups—acute injuries that destabilize the knee, and **pain management** for floating or displaced cartilage and rough bone. Acute injuries are usually the result of traumatic injury to the knee tissues such as ligaments and cartilage through accidents, sports movements, and some overuse causes. Acute injuries involve damage to the mechanical features, including ligaments and patella of the knee. These injuries can result in knee instability, severe knee dislocations, and complete lack of knee mobility. Ligament, tendon, and patella placements are key elements of the surgery. The type of treatment for

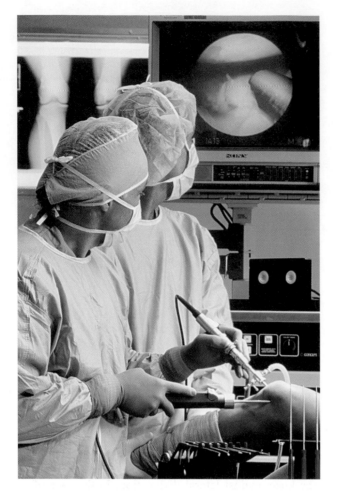

Surgeons watching a monitor showing the inside of a patient's knee during arthroscopic knee surgery. *(Custom Medical Stock Photo. Reproduced by permission.)*

acute injuries depends in large part on a strict grading system that rates the injury. For instance, grades I and II call for rest, support by crutches or leg brace, pain management, and rehabilitation. Grades III and IV indicate the need for surgery. Acute injuries to the four stabilizing ligaments of the knee joint—the anterior cruciate ligament (ACL), the posterior cruciate ligament (PCL), the medial collateral ligament (MCL), and the lateral collateral ligament (LCL)—as well as to the "tracking," or seating of the patella, can be highly debilitating.

Treatment of these acute injuries include such common surgeries as:

- Repairs of a torn ligament or reconstruction of the ligament.

- Release of a malaligned kneecap. This involves tendon surgery to release and fit the patella better into its groove.

- Grafts to ligaments to support smoother tracking of the knee with the femur.

Pain management surgeries, on the other hand, are used to relieve severe discomfort of the knee due to osteoarthritis conditions. These treatments aim at relieving pain and instability caused by more chronic, "wear and tear" kinds of conditions and involve minor and more optional surgical procedures to treat cartilage and bone surfaces. These include arthroscopic techniques to remove detached or obtruding pieces of cartilage in the joint space such as the meniscus (a fibrous cushion for the patella), to smooth aged, rough surface bone, or to remove parts of the lining of the joint that are inflamed.

Treatment distinctions between arthroscopic surgery for acute injuries and those for pain management are important and should be kept in mind. They have implications for the necessity for surgery, risks of surgery, complications, aftercare, and expectations for improvement. Arthroscopic surgery for acute injuries is less controversial because clear dysfunction and/or severe instability are measurable indications for surgery and easily identifiable. Surgery indications for pain management are largely for chronic damage and for the milder grades or stages of acute injuries (severity Grade I and II). These are controversial due to the existence of pain management and rehabilitation alternatives. Arthroscopic surgery for pain management is currently under debate.

Demographics

More than five and a half million people visit orthopedic surgeons each year because of knee problems. Over 600,000 arthroscopic surgeries are performed annually; 85% of them are for knee surgery. One very common knee injury is a torn anterior cruciate ligament (ACL) that often occurs in athletic activity. The most common source of ACL injury is skiing. Approximately 250,000 people in the United States sustain a torn or ruptured ACL each year. Research indicates that ACL injuries are on the rise in the United States due to the increase in sport activity.

The incidence of ACL injuries in women is two to eight times greater than in men. While the exact causes are not clear, differences in anatomy, strength, or conditioning are thought to play major roles. Women also seem to be more prone to patella-femoral syndrome (PFS), which is the inability of the patella to track smoothly with the femur. PFS is due primarily to development of tendons that influence the ways in which the knee tracks in movement. It can also be due to misalignments to other parts of the lower body like foot pronation. Other ligament surgeries can be caused by injury or overuse.

Knee dislocations are a focus of recent research because of their increasing frequency. Incidences range from 0.001% to 0.013% of all patients evaluated for orthopedic injuries. Many of these injuries heal without treatment and go undetected. Many people with multiple traumas in accidents have knee dislocations that go undiagnosed. Knee dislocations are of special concern, especially in traumatic injury, because their early diagnosis is required if surgery is to be effective. Knee dislocations in the morbidly obese individuals often occur spontaneously and may be associated with artery injury. This surgery involves complications related to the obesity. Finally, knee dislocations have been reported to occur in up to 6% of trampoline-associated accidents.

Description

Arthroscopic surgery for acute injuries

The knee bone sits between the femur and the tibia, attached by four ligaments that keep the knee stable as the leg moves. These ligaments can be damaged or torn through injuries and accidents. Once damaged, they do not offer stability to the knee and can cause buckling, or allow the knee to "give way." Ligaments can also "catch" and freeze the knee or make the knee track in a different direction than its leg movement, causing the knee to dislocate. Traumatic injuries such as automobile accidents may cause more than one ligament injury, necessitating multiple repairs to ligaments.

Four arthroscopic procedures relate to damage to each of the four ligaments that stabilize the knee joint movement. The four procedures are:

• Anterior cruciate ligament (ACL). A front-crossing ligament attaching the femur to the tibia through the knee; this ligament keeps the knee from hyperextension or being displaced back from the femur. The ACL is a rather large ligament that can withstand 500 lb (227 kg) of pressure. If it is torn or becomes detached, it remains that way and surgery is indicated. In the most severe cases, a graft to the ligament is necessary to reattach it to the bone. The surgery can use tissue from the patient, called an autograft, or from a cadaver, called an allograft. The patella tendon, which connects the patella to the tibia, is the most commonly used autograft. ACL reconstructive surgery involves drilling a tunnel into the tibia and the femur. The graft is then pushed through the tunnels and secured by stapling or sutures.

• Posterior cruciate ligament (PCL). A back-crossing ligament that attaches the front of the femur to back of the tibia behind the knee that keeps the knee from hyperextension or being displaced backward. PCL injuries are not as frequent as ACL injuries. These injuries are largely due to falls directly on the knee or hitting the knee on the dashboard of a car in an accident. Both displace the tibia too far back and tear the ligament. Surgery to the

PCL is rare, because the tear can usually be treated with rest and with rehabilitation. If surgery is required, it is usually to reattach the PCL to the tibia bone.

• Medial collateral ligament (MCL). This is an inside lateral ligament connecting the femur and tibia and stabilizing the knee against lateral dislocation to the left or to the right. The injury is usually due to external pressure against the inside of the knee. In the case of a grade I or II collateral ligament tear, doctors are likely to brace the knee for four to six weeks. A grade III tear may require surgery to repair ligament tear and is followed by three months of bracing. Physical therapy may be necessary before resuming full activity.

• Lateral collateral ligament (LCL). An outside lateral ligament connecting the femur and tibia and stabilizing the knee against lateral dislocation. In the case of a grade I or II collateral ligament tear, doctors are likely to brace the knee for four to six weeks. A Grade III tear may require surgery to reattach the ligament to bone. Surgery will be followed by three months of bracing. Physical therapy may be necessary before resuming full activity.

Patello-femoral syndrome (PFS)

The patella rests in a groove on the femur. Anything but a good fit can cause the patella to be unstable in its movement and very painful. Some individuals have chronic problems with the proper tracking of the patella with the femur. This may be associated with conditions related to physical features like foot pronation, or to types of body development in exercising or overuse of muscles. In the case of damage, an examination of the cartilage surrounding the patella can identify cartilage that increases friction as the patella moves. Smoothing the damaged cartilage can increase the ease of movement and eliminate pain. Finally, a tendon can occasionally make the patella track off center of the femur. By moving where the tendon is attached through lateral release surgery, the patella can be forced back into its groove.

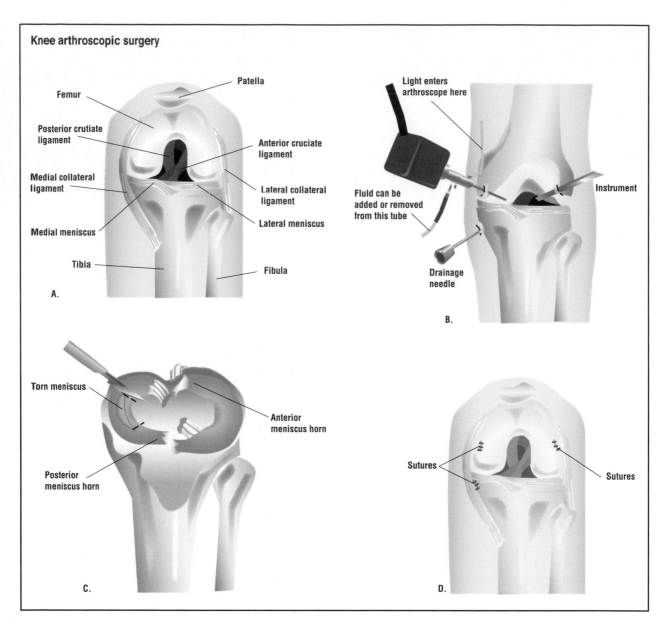

Knee arthroscopic surgery

Step A shows the anatomy of the knee from the front with the leg bent. To repair a torn meniscus, three small incisions are made into the knee to admit laparoscopic instruments (B). Fluid is injected into the joint to aid in the operation. The injury is visualized via the instruments, and the torn area is removed (C). *(Illustration by GGS Inc.)*

Pain management with lavage and debridement

In addition to the ligament and patella surgeries that are largely required for traumatic injuries, arthroscopic surgery treats the wear and tear injuries related to a torn meniscus, which is the crescent-shaped cartilage that cushions the knee, as well as injuries to the surface of bone that makes joint movement painful. These are related to osteoarthritis and rheumatoid arthritis.

In lavage and debridement, the surgeon identifies floating or displaced tissue pieces and either flushes them out with a solution applied with arthroscopy or

smoothes the surface of bone to decrease pain. These two surgical treatments are controversial because research has not indicated that alternatives to surgery are not as successful.

All of the above procedures are conducted through the visualization offered by the lighted arthroscope that allows the surgeon to follow the surgery on a television monitor. Instruments only about 0.15 in (4 mm) thick are inserted in a triangular fashion around the knee. The arthroscope goes in one incision, and instruments to cut and/or smooth and to engage in other maneuvers are put through the other incisions. In this fashion, the surgeon has magnification, perspective, and the ability to make tiny adjustments to the tissue without open surgery. The triangular approach is highly effective and safe.

Diagnosis/Preparation

Disease and injury can damage joints, ligaments, cartilage, and bone surfaces. Because the knee carries most of the weight of the body, this damage occurs almost inevitably as people age, due to sports injuries and through accidents.

The diagnosis of knee injuries or damage includes a medical history, **physical examination**, x rays, and the additional, more detailed imaging techniques with MRI or CT scan. Severe or chronic pain and/or knee instability initially brings the patient to an orthopedic physician. From there, the decision is made for surgery or for rehabilitation. Factors that influence the decision for surgery are the likelihood for repair and recovery of function, the patient's health and age, and, most importantly, the willingness of the patient to consider changes in lifestyle, especially as this relates to sport activity. Arthroscopic viewing is the most accurate tool for diagnosis, as well as for some repairs. The surgeon may provide only a provisional diagnosis until the actual surgery but will apprise the patient of the most likely course the surgery will take.

Arthroscopic surgery can be performed under local, regional, or general anesthetic. The type used depends largely upon the severity of damage, the level of pain after surgery, patient wishes, and patient health. The surgery is brief, less than two hours. After closing the incisions, the leg will be wrapped tightly and the patient is taken to recovery. For most same-day surgeries, individuals are allowed to leave once the anesthetic effects have worn off. Patients are not allowed to drive. Arrangements for pick up after surgery are mandated.

Unlike open surgery, arthroscopic surgery generally does not require a hospital stay. Patients usually go home the same day. Any crutches or canes required prior to surgery will be needed after surgery. Follow-up visits will be scheduled within about a week, at which point dressings will be removed.

Aftercare

Ligament- and patella-tracking surgeries

Arthroscopic surgery for severe ligament damage or knee displacement often involves ligament grafting. In some cases, this includes taking tissue from a tendon to use for the graft and drilling holes in the femur or tibia or both. Aftercare involves the use of crutches for six to eight weeks. A rehabilitation program for strengthening

---

QUESTIONS TO ASK THE DOCTOR

- Are there rehabilitation alternatives to this surgery?
- Will this surgery allow me to return to sports?
- How much success have you had with this surgery in eliminating pain?
- Is this injury one that I can live with if I pursue a change in lifestyle?
- How long will post-operative rehabilitation take and how can I help in moving it along faster?

---

is usually suggested. Recovery times for resumed athletic activity are highly dependent on age and health. The surgeon often makes very careful assessments about recovery and the need for rehabilitation.

Patella-tracking surgeries offer about a 90% chance that the patella will no longer dislocate. However, many people have continued swelling and pain after surgery. These seem to be dependent upon how carefully the rehabilitation plan is developed and/or adhered to by the patient.

Lavage and debridement surgeries

Elevation of the leg after surgery is usually required for a short period. A crutch or knee immobilizer adds additional stability and assurance when walking. Physical therapy is usually recommended to strengthen the muscles around the knee and to provide extra support. Special attention should be paid to any changes to the leg a few days after surgery. Swelling and pain to the leg can mean a blood clot has been dislodged. If this occurs, the physician should be notified immediately. Getting out of bed shortly after surgery decreases the risk of blood clots.

Risks

The risks of arthroscopic surgery are much less than open surgery, but they are not nonexistent. The risk of any surgery carries with it danger in the use of anesthesia, including heart attacks, strokes, pneumonia, and blood clots. The risks are rare, but they increase with the age of the patient. Blood clots are the most common dangers, but they occur infrequently in arthroscopic surgery. Other risks include infections at the surgery site or at the skin level, bleeding, and skin scars.

Risks related specifically to arthroscopic surgery are largely ones related to injury at the time of surgery. Arteries, veins, and nerves can be injured, resulting in discomfort in minor cases and leg weakness or decreased sensation in more serious complications. These injuries are rare. One major risk of arthropscopic surgery to the knee for conditions related to tissue tears is that the pain may not be relieved by the operation; it may even become worse.

Normal results

Normal results of ligament surgery are pain, initial immobility and inflexibility, bracing of the leg, crutch dependence, with increasing mobility and flexibility with rehabilitation. Full recovery to the level of prior physical activity can take up to three months. With ACL surgery, pain in the front of the knee occurs in 10–20% of individuals. Limited range of motion occurs in less than 5% due to inadequate placement of the graft. A second surgery may be necessary.

Research indicates that the pain-relieving effects for arthroscopic partial menisectomy (removal of torn parts of cartilage) and debridement (the abrasion of cartilage to make it smooth) are not very reliable. Pain relief varies between 50% and 75%, depending upon the age, activity level, degree of damage, and extent of follow-up. One study indicates that the two surgical procedures, lavage and debridement, fared no better than no surgical procedure in relieving pain. The participants were divided into three groups for arthroscopic surgery: one third underwent debridement, a second third underwent lavage, and the remaining third likewise were anesthetized and had three incisions made in the knee area, though no procedure was performed. All three groups reported essentially the same results. Each had slightly less pain and better knee movement. The non-procedure had the best results. Debates about normal expectations from minor arthroscopic surgery continue with many surgeons believing that arthroscopic surgery of the knee should be restricted to acute injuries.

Morbidity and mortality rates

Complications occur in less than 1% of arthroscopic surgeries. Different procedures have different complications. In general, morbidity results mostly from medically induced nerve and vascular damage; death or amputations almost never occur. Graft infection may occur, along with other types of infection largely due to microbes introduced with instruments. The latter cases are becoming increasingly rare as the science of arthroscopic surgery develops.

Alternatives

Whether or not surgical treatment is the best choice depends on a number of factors and alternatives. Age and

the degree of injury or damage are key to deciding whether to have surgery or rehabilitation. The physician calibrates the severity of acute injuries and either proceeds to a determined treatment plan immediately or recommends surgery. Alternatives for acute ligament injuries depend on the severity of injury and whether the patient can make lifestyle changes and is willing to move away from athletic activities. This decision becomes paramount for many people with collateral and cruciate injuries.

According to the American Association of Orthopedic Surgeons, conservative treatment for acute injuries involves RICE: Rest, Ice, Compression, Elevation, as well as a follow-up rehabilitation plan. The RICE protocol involves resting the knee to allow the ligament to heal, applying ice two or three times a day for 15–20 minutes, compression with a bandage or brace, and elevation of the knee whenever possible. Rehabilitation requires range-of-motion exercises to increase flexibility, braces to control joint immobility, **exercise** for quadriceps to support the front of the thigh, and upper thigh exercise with a bicycle.

For arthritis-related damage and pain management, anti-inflammatory medication, weight loss, and exercise can all be crucial to strengthening the knee to relieve pain. Evidence suggests that these alternatives work as well as surgery.

Resources

BOOKS

Canale, S. Terry. "Arthroscopic Surgery of Meniscus." In *Campbell's Operative Orthopaedics*. 9th ed. St. Louis: Mosby, Inc., 1998.

PERIODICALS

Alleyne, K. R., and M. T. Galloway. "Osteochondral Injuries of the Knee." *Clinics in Sports Medicine* 20, no. 2 (April 2001).

Brown, C. H., and E. W. Carson. "Revision Anterior Cruciate Ligament Surgery." *Clinics in Sports Medicine* 18, no. 1 (January 1999).

Heges, M. S., M. W. Richardson, and M. D. Miller. "The Dislocated Knee." *Clinics in Sports Medicine* 19, no. 3 (July 2000).

Moseley, J. B, et al. "A Controlled Trial of Arthroscopic Surgery for Osteoarthritis of the Knee." *New England Journal of Medicine* 347, no. 2 (July 11, 2002): 81–88.

Vangsness, C. T., Jr. "Overview of Treatment Options for Arthritis in the Active Patient." *Clinical Sports Medicine* 18, no. 1 (January 1999): 1–11.

ORGANIZATIONS

American Academy of Orthopaedic Surgeons (AAOS). 6300 North River Rd. Suite 200, Rosemont, IL 60018. (847) 823-7186 or (800) 346-2267; Fax: (847) 823-8125. <http://www.aaos.org>.

Arthritis Foundation. P.O. Box 7669, Atlanta, GA 30357-0669. (800) 283-7800. <http://www.arthritis.org>.

National Institute of Arthritis and Musculoskeletal and Skin Diseases Information Clearinghouse. 1 AMS Circle, Bethesda, MD 20892-3675. (301) 495-4484 or (877) 226-4267; Fax: (301) 718-6366; TTY: (301) 565-2966. <http://www.nih.gov/niams>.

OTHER

"Arthroscopic Knee Surgery No Better Than Placebo Surgery." *Medscape Medical News.* July 11, 2002. <http://www.medscape.com>.

"Arthroscopic Surgery." *Harvard Medical School Consumer Health. InteliHealth.* <http://www.intelihealth.com>.

"Knee Arthroscopy Summary." Patient Education Institute, *National Library of Medicine/NIH/MedlinePlus.* <http://www.nlm.nih.gov/medlineplus/tutorials/kneearthroscopy>.

Nancy McKenzie, PhD

Knee osteotomy

Definition

Knee osteotomy is surgery that removes a part of the bone of the joint of either the bottom of the femur (upper leg bone) or the top of the tibia (lower leg bone) to increase the stability of the knee. Osteotomy redistributes the weight-bearing force on the knee by cutting a wedge of bone away to reposition the knee. The angle of deformity in the knee dictates whether the surgery is to correct a knee that angles inward, known as a varus procedure, or one that angles outward, called a valgus procedure. Varus osteotomy involves the medial (inner) section of

> ## WHO PERFORMS THE PROCEDURE AND WHERE IS IT PERFORMED?
>
> An orthropedic surgeon speciliazing in knee reconstruction surgery performs the operation. Surgery takes place in a general hospital.

the knee at the top of the tibia. Valgus osteotomy involves the lateral (outer) compartment of the knee by shaping the bottom of the femur.

Purpose

Osteotomy surgery changes the alignment of the knee so that the weight-bearing part of the knee is shifted off diseased or deformed cartilage to healthier tissue in order to relieve pain and increase knee stability. Osteotomy is effective for patients with arthritis in one compartment of the knee. The medial compartment is on the inner side of the knee. The lateral compartment is on the outer side of the knee. The primary uses of osteotomy occur as treatment for:

- Knee deformities such as bowleg in which the knee is varus-leaning (high tibia osteotomy, or HTO) and knock-knee (tibial valgus osteotomy), in which the knee is valgus leaning.

- A torn anterior cruciate ligament (ACL), which is a set of ligaments that connects the femur to the tibia behind the patella and offers stability to the knee on the left-right or medial-lateral axis. If this ligament is injured, it must be repaired by surgery. Many ACL injuries cause inflammation of the cartilage of the knee and result in bones extrusions, as well as instability of the knee due to malalignment. Osteotomy is performed to cut cartilage and increase the fit and alignment of the ends of the femur and tibia for smooth articulation. As one very common knee injury that often occurs in athletic activity, HTO is often performed when ACL surgery is used to repair the ligament. The combination of the two surgeries occurs primarily in young people who wish to return to a highly athletic life.

- Osteoarthritis that includes loss of range of motion, stiffness, and roughness of the articular cartilage in the knee joint secondary to the wear and tear of motion, especially in athletes, as well as cartilage breakdown resulting from traumatic injuries to the knee. Surgery for progressive osteoarthritis or injury-induced arthritis is often used to stave off total joint replacement.

Demographics

According to Healthy People 2000, Final Review, published by the Centers for Disease Control and Prevention, the various forms of arthritis "the leading cause of disability in the United States" affect more than 15% of the total U.S. population (43 million persons) and more than 20% of the adult population. Osteoarthritis (OA) is the most common form of knee arthritis and involves a slowly progressive degenerative disease in which the joint cartilage gradually wears away. It most often affects middle-aged and older people. The most common source of ACL injury is skiing. Approximately 250,000 people sustain a torn or ruptured ACL in the United States each year. Research indicates that ACL injuries are on the rise in the United States due to the increase in sport activity.

Description

Osteotomy is performed as open surgery to the knee assisted by pre-operative arthropscopic diagnostic techniques. Surgery takes place on the tibia end or the femoral end at the knee according to whether the malalignment to be corrected is varus, or inward leaning, or valgus, outward leaning. The surgery involves the gaping or wedging of a piece of bone and its removal to change the pressure points of weight-bearing activity. The cut surfaces of the bone are held together with two staples, or a plate and screws. Other devices may be used, especially in tibial osteotomy where a fracture is involved. After surgery, a small plastic suction drain is left in the wound during recovery and early postoperative hospitalization.

Diagnosis/Preparation

Severe or chronic pain and/or knee instability brings the patient to an orthopedic physician. From there, the decision is made for surgery or for rehabilitation. Patients will undergo an examination and history with their physician. Once rehabilitation or other treatments are ruled out and surgery is indicated, the physician must assess for three factors: pain, instability, and knee alignment. Osteotomy is indicated if malalignment is a factor. **Debridement**, or the shaving of cartilage on the articulate femur or tibia, can usually resolve pain with instability problems. It must be determined whether the instability is related to malalignment and not to other sources such as ACL injury. Since the goal of osteotomy is to shift weight from a symptomatic cartilage to an unsymptomatic area to relieve both an instability and pain due to excessive contact, alignment of the knee is assessed for pressure distribution along the mechanical axis and the loading axis. This requires an analysis of gait pattern, range of motion, localized areas of pain, and neurological factors, as well as other technical tests for anterior instability. A diagnostic arthroscopy—examination of the knee joint with a long tube attached to a video camera—is usually indicated before all knee osteotomies. Cartilage surfaces are examined for degenerative or late-stage arthritis. **Magnetic resonance imaging** (MRI) is useful in evaluating any intra-articular pathology such as bone chips, padding tears, or injuries to ligaments.

Aftercare

After surgery, patients are placed in a hinged brace. Toe-touching is the only weight-bearing activity allowed for four weeks in order to allow the osteotomy to hold its place. Continuous passive motion is begun immediately after surgery and physical therapy is used to establish full range of motion, muscle strengthening, and gait training. After four weeks, patients can begin weight-bearing movement. The brace is worn for eight weeks or until the surgery site is healed and stable. X rays are performed at intervals of two weeks and eight weeks after surgery.

Risks

The usual general surgical risks of thrombosis and heart attack are possible in this open surgery. Osteotomy surgery itself involves some risk of infection or injury during the procedure. Combined surgery for ACL and osteotomy has higher morbidity rates.

Normal results

Varus malalignment correction with osteotomy through the high tibia (HTO) is a proven and satisfactory operation. Success rates are high when the patient has a small angle deformity (<10°). Knees with more severe deformity have less satisfactory results. Tibial osteotomy for the less common valgus deformity is less satisfactory. Research indicates that only a few individuals are able to return to their previous level of high sports activity after a knee osteotomy, whether done with an ACL repair or not. However, more than half of patients in one study were able to return to leisure sports activities. Reports also indicate that those individuals who had osteotomy without ACL reconstruction had no differences in results with respect to measures of stability. It may take up to a year for the knee to be fully aligned and adapted to its new position after surgery. Most patients, more than 50%, gain stability and are able to walk further than they could walk before osteotomy. However, according to one report, 13% of patients had severe pain or needed a total **knee replacement** after five years. In one European review, the results were better. Osteoarthritis was arrested in 105 cases (69%), with 47 cases showing deterioration. The main factors associated with further deterioration were insufficient correction and persistence of malalignment.

Morbidity and mortality rates

Morbidity rates include bleeding, inflammation of joint tissues, nerve damage, and infection.

Alternatives

For those individuals suffering from osteoarthritis, muscle-strengthening **exercise**, weight loss, and rehabilitation can be helpful in relieving pain and gaining stability. Anti-inflammatory medications can also be effective in helping pain and stability. For severe varus or valgus deformities, osteotomy or knee replacement may be indicated. For those with severe ACL injury with secondary

trauma to knee cartilage, complete knee replacement may be suggested.

Resources

BOOKS

Ruddy, Shaun, et al., eds. *Ruddy: Kelly's Textbook of Rheumatology, 6th Edition.* Philadelphia: WB Saunders Publishing, 2001.

PERIODICALS

Alleyne, K. R., and M. T. Galloway. "Management of Osteochrondral Injuries of the Knee." *Clinics in Sports Medicine* 20, No. 2 (April 2001).

Shubin Stein, B. E., R. J. William, and T. L. Wickiewicz. "Arthritis and Osteotomies in Anterior Cruciate Ligament Reconstruction." *Orthopedic Clinics of North America* 34, no. 1 (January 2003).

ORGANIZATIONS

American Academy of Orthopaedic Surgeons (AAOS). 6300 North River Rd., Suite 200, Rosemont, IL 60018. (847) 823-7186. (800) 346-2267, Fax (847) 823-8125. <http://www.aaos.org/>.

Arthritis Foundation. P.O. Box 7669, Atlanta, GA 30357-0669. (800) 283-7800. <http://www.arthritis.org>.

National Institute of Arthritis and Musculoskeletal and Skin Diseases Information Clearinghouse. 1 AMS Circle, Bethesda, MD 20892-3675. (301) 495-4484, Toll-Free (877) 226-4267. Fax: (301) 718-6366. TTY: (301) 565-2966. <www.nih.gov/niams>.

OTHER

"Osteotomy for Osteoarthritis." *WebMD Health.* <http://www.webmd.com.>.

Nancy McKenzie, PhD

Knee prosthesis surgery *see* **Knee revision surgery**

Knee replacement

Definition

Knee replacement is a procedure in which the surgeon removes damaged or diseased parts of the patient's knee joint and replaces them with new artificial parts. The operation itself is called knee **arthroplasty**. Arthroplasty comes from two Greek words, *arthros* or joint and *plassein*, "to form or shape." The artificial joint itself is called a prosthesis. Most knee prostheses have four components or parts, and are made of a combination of metal and plastic, or metal and ceramic in some newer models.

Purpose

Knee arthroplasty has two primary purposes: pain relief and improved functioning of the knee joint. Because of the importance of the knee to a person's ability to stand upright, improved joint functioning includes greater stability in the knee.

Pain relief

Total knee replacement, or TKR, is considered major surgery. Therefore, it is usually not considered a treatment option until the patient's pain cannot be managed any longer by more conservative treatment. Alternatives to surgery are described below.

Pain in the knee may be either a sudden or gradual development, depending on the cause of the pain. Knee pain resulting from osteoarthritis and other degenerative disorders may develop gradually over a period of years. On the other hand, pain resulting from an athletic injury or other traumatic damage to the knee, or from such conditions as infectious arthritis or gout, may come on suddenly. Because the structure of the knee is complex and many different disorders or conditions can cause knee pain, the cause of the pain must be diagnosed before joint replacement surgery can be discussed as an option.

Joint function

Restoration of joint function and stability is the other major purpose of knee replacement surgery. It is helpful to have a brief outline of the major structures in the knee joint in order to understand the types of disorders and injuries that can make joint replacement necessary as well as to understand the operation itself.

The knee is the largest joint in the human body, as well as one of the most vulnerable. Unlike the hip joint, which is partly protected by the bony structures of the pelvis, the knee joint is not shielded by any other parts of the skeleton. In addition, the knee joint must bear the weight of the upper body as well as the stresses and shocks carried upward through the feet when a person walks or runs. Moreover, the knee is essentially a hinge joint, designed to move primarily backwards and forwards; it is not a ball-and-socket joint like the hip, which can swivel and rotate in a variety of directions. Many knee injuries result from stresses caused by twisting or turning movements, particularly when the foot remains in one position while the upper body changes direction rapidly, as in basketball, tennis, or skiing.

The normal knee joint consists of a bone, the patella or kneecap, and a set of tendons, ligaments, and cartilage disks that connect the femur, or thighbone, to the lower leg. There are two bones in the lower leg, the tibia, which is sometimes called the shinbone; and the fibula, a smaller bone on the outside of the lower leg. There are two collateral ligaments on the outside of the knee joint that connect the femur to the tibia and fibula respectively. These ligaments help to control the stresses of side-to-side movements on the knee. The patella—a triangular bone at the front of the knee—is attached by tendons to the quadriceps muscles of the thigh. This tendon allows a person to straighten the knee. Two additional tendons inside the knee stretch between the femur and the tibia to prevent the tibia from moving out of alignment with the femur. Cartilage, which is a whitish elastic tissue that allows bones to glide smoothly against each other, covers the ends of the femur, tibia, and fibula as well as the surfaces of the patella. In addition to the cartilage that covers the bones, the knee joint also contains two crescent-shaped disks of cartilage known as menisci (singular, meniscus), which lie between the lower end of the femur and the upper end of the tibia and act as shock absorbers or cushions. The entire joint is surrounded by a thick layer of protective tissue known as the joint capsule.

Disorders and conditions that may lead to knee replacement surgery include:

- Osteoarthritis (OA). Osteoarthritis is a disorder in which the cartilage in the knee joint gradually breaks down, allowing the surfaces of the bones to rub directly against each other. The patient experiences swelling, pain, inflammation, and increasing loss of mobility. OA most often affects adults over age 45, and is thought to result from a combination of wear and tear on the joint, lifestyle, and genetic factors. As of 2003, OA is the most common cause of joint damage requiring knee replacement.

- Rheumatoid arthritis (RA). Rheumatoid arthritis is a disease that begins earlier in life than OA and affects the whole body. Women are three times as likely as men to develop RA. Its symptoms are caused by the immune system's attacks on the body's own cells and tissues. Patients with RA often suffer intense pain even when they are not putting weight on the affected joints.

- Trauma. Damage to the knee from a fall, automobile accident, or workplace or athletic injury may trigger the process of cartilage breakdown inside the joint. Trauma is a common cause of damage to the knee joint. Some traumatic injuries are caused by repetitive motion or overuse of the knee joint; these types of injury include bursitis, or housemaid's knee, and so-called runner's knee. Other traumatic injuries are caused by sudden twisting of the knee, a direct blow to a bent knee, or being tackled from the side in football.

There are several factors that increase a person's risk of eventually requiring knee replacement surgery.

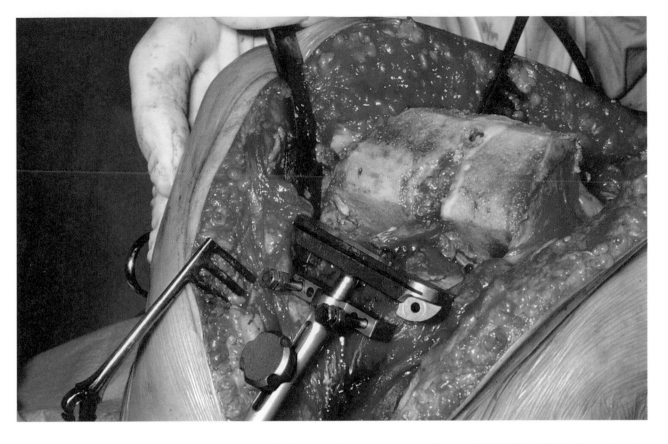

Surgeons exposing the bones in the knee area during knee replacement surgery. *(Custom Medical Stock Photo. Reproduced by permission.)*

While some of these factors cannot be avoided, others can be corrected through lifestyle changes:

- Genetic. Both OA and RA tend to run in families. One study done in France reported that the genetic factors affecting osteoarthritis in the knee can be traced back almost 8,000 years. Both OA and RA, however, are polygenic disorders, which means that more than one gene is involved in transmitting susceptibility to these forms of arthritis.

- Age. Knee cartilage becomes thinner and weaker with age, even in people who have no family history of arthritis.

- Sex. Women athletes have three times as many knee injuries as men. At present, orthopedic specialists are conducting studies to determine the cause(s) of this difference. Some doctors think it is related to the fact that most women have wider hips than most men, which results in a different pattern of stresses on the knee joint. Others think that the ligaments in women's knees tend to loosen more easily.

- Biomechanical. Biomechanics refers to the study of body structures in terms of the laws of mechanics, such

as measuring the forces that affect the operation of a joint. Biomechanical studies have shown that people with certain types of leg or foot deformities, such as bowlegs or difference in leg length, are at increased risk of knee disorders because the stresses on the knee joint are not distributed normally.

- Gait-related factors. Gait refers to a person's pattern of motion when walking or running. Some people walk with their feet turned noticeably outward or inward; others tend to favor either the heel or the toe when they walk, which makes their gait irregular. Any of these factors can increase strain on the knee joint.

- Shoes. Poorly fitted or worn-out shoes contribute to knee strain by increasing the force transmitted upward to the knee when the foot strikes the sidewalk or other hard surface. They also introduce or increase irregularities in gait. Women's high-heeled shoes are particularly harmful to the knee joint because they do not cushion the foot; and they cause prolonged tightening and fatigue of the leg muscles.

- Work or other activities that involve jumping, jogging, or squatting. Jogging tends to loosen the ligaments that hold the parts of the knee joint in alignment, while jumping increases the shock on the knee joint and the risk of twisting or tearing the knee joint when the person lands. Squatting can increase the forces on the knee joint as much as eight times body weight.

Demographics

According to the American Academy of Orthopaedic Surgeons (AAOS), there are about 270,000 knee replacement operations performed each year in the United States. Although about 70% of these operations are performed in people over the age of 65, a growing number of knee replacements are being done in younger patients. A Canadian survey released in January 2003 stated that the number of knee replacements performed in patients younger than 55 rose 90% between 1994 and 2001. Most surgeons expect to see the proportion of knee arthroplasties performed in younger patients continue to rise. One reason for this trend is improvements in surgical technique, as well as the design and construction of knee prostheses since the first knee replacement was performed in 1968. Although most knee prostheses are still cemented in place as of 2003, cementless prostheses were introduced in the 1980s. A second reason is people's changing attitudes toward aging and their expectations of an active life after retirement. Fewer are willing to endure years of discomfort or resign themselves to a restricted level of activity.

In terms of gender and racial differences, women are slightly more likely to seek knee replacement surgery than men, and Caucasians in the United States are more likely to have the operation than African Americans. Researchers have suggested that one reason for the racial difference is a difference in social networks. People in general are influenced in their health care decisions by the experiences and opinions of friends or family members, and Caucasians are more likely than African Americans to know someone who has had knee replacement surgery.

Description

The length and complexity of a total knee replacement operation depend in part on whether both knee joints are replaced during the operation or only one. Such disorders as osteoarthritis usually affect both knees, and some patients would rather not undergo surgery twice. Replacement of both knees is known as bilateral TKR, or bilateral knee arthroplasty. Bilateral knee replacement seems to work best for patients whose knees are equally weak or damaged. Otherwise most surgeons recommend operating on the more painful knee first so that the patient will have one strong leg to help him or her through the recovery period following surgery

on the second knee. The disadvantages of bilateral knee replacement include a longer period of time under anesthesia; a longer hospital stay and recovery period at home; and a greater risk of severe blood loss and other complications during surgery.

If the operation is on only one knee, it will take two to four hours. The patient may be given a choice of general, spinal, or epidural anesthesia. An epidural anesthetic, which is injected into the space around the spinal cord to block sensation in the lower body, causes less blood loss and also lowers the risk of blood clots or breathing problems after surgery. After the patient is anesthetized, the surgeon will make an incision in the skin over the knee and cut through the joint capsule. He or she must be careful in working around the tendons and ligaments inside the joint. Knee replacement is a more complicated operation than **hip replacement** because the hip joint does not depend as much on ligaments for stability. The next step is cutting away the damaged cartilage and bone at the ends of the femur and tibia. The surgeon reshapes the end of the femur to receive the femoral component, or shell, which is usually made of metal and attached with bone cement.

After the femoral part of the prosthesis has been attached, the surgeon inserts a metal component into the upper end of the tibia. This part is sometimes pressed rather than cemented in place. If it is a cementless prosthesis, the metal will be coated or textured so that new bone will grow around the prosthesis and hold it in place. A plastic plate called a spacer is then attached to the metal component in the tibia. The plastic allows the femur and tibia to move smoothly against each other.

Lastly, another plastic component is glued to the rear of the patella, or kneecap. This second piece of plastic prevents friction between the kneecap and the other parts of the prosthesis. After all the parts of the prosthesis have been implanted, the surgeon will check them for proper positioning, make certain that the tendons and ligaments have not been damaged, wash out the incision with sterile saline solution, and close the incision.

Diagnosis/Preparation

Patient history

The first part of a diagnostic interview for knee pain is the careful taking of the patient's history. The doctor will ask not only for a general medical history, but also about the patient's occupation, **exercise** habits, past injuries to the knee, and any gait-related problems. The doctor will also ask detailed questions about the patient's ability to move or flex the knee; whether specific movements or activities make the pain worse; whether the

Knee replacement

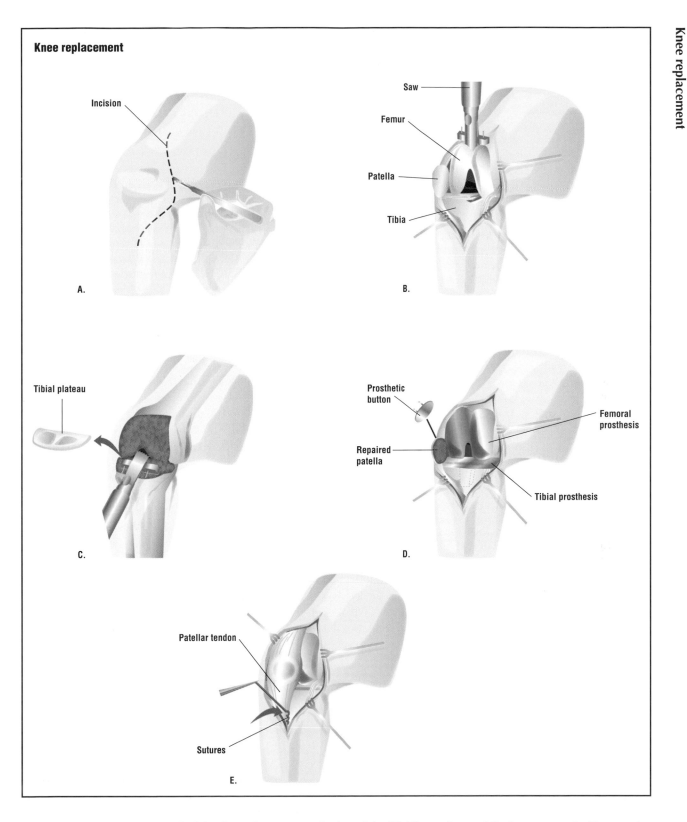

In a total knee replacement, an incision is made to expose the knee joint (A). The surfaces of the femur are cut with a saw to receive the prosthesis (B). The tibia is cut to create a plateau (C). The prostheses for the femur, tibia, and patella are put in place (D). The incision is closed (E). *(Illustration by GGS Inc.)*

pain is sharp or dull; its location in the knee; whether the knee ever buckles or catches; and whether there are clicking or popping sounds inside the joint.

Diagnostic tests

PHYSICAL EXAMINATION OF THE KNEE. Following the history, the doctor will examine the knee itself. The knee will be checked for swelling, reddening, bruises, breaks in the skin, lumps, or other unusual features while the patient is standing. The doctor will also make note of the patient's posture, including whether the patient is bowlegged or knock-kneed. The patient may be asked to walk back and forth so that the doctor can check for gait abnormalities.

In the second part of the **physical examination**, the patient lies on an examining table while the doctor palpates (feels) the structures of the knee and evaluates the strength or tightness of the tendons and ligaments. The patient may be asked to flex one knee and straighten the leg or turn the knee inward and outward so that the doctor can measure the range of motion in the joint. The doctor will also ask the patient to lie still while he or she moves the knee in different directions.

IMAGING STUDIES. The doctor will order one or more imaging studies in order to narrow the diagnosis. A radiograph or x ray is the most common, but is chiefly useful in showing fractures or other damage to bony structures. X-ray studies are usually supplemented by other imaging techniques in diagnosing knee disorders. A computed tomography, or CAT scan, which is a specialized type of x ray that uses computers to generate three-dimensional images of the knee joint, is often helpful in evaluating malformations of the joint. **Magnetic resonance imaging** (MRI) uses a large magnet, radio waves, and a computer to generate images of the knee joint. The advantage of an MRI is that it reveals injuries to ligaments, tendons, and menisci as well as damage to bony structures.

ASPIRATION. Aspiration is a procedure in which fluid is withdrawn from the knee joint by a needle and sent to a laboratory for analysis. It is done to check for infection in the joint and to draw off fluid that is causing pain. Aspiration is most commonly done when the knee has swelled up suddenly, but may be performed at any time. Blood in the fluid usually indicates a fracture or torn ligament; the presence of bacteria indicates infection; the presence of uric acid crystals indicates gout. Clear, straw-colored fluid suggests osteoarthritis.

ARTHROSCOPY. Arthroscopy can be used to treat knee problems as well as diagnose them. An arthroscope consists of a miniature camera and light source mounted on a flexible fiberoptic tube. It allows the surgeon to look into the knee joint. To perform an arthroscopy, the surgeon will make two to four small incisions known as ports. One port is used to insert the arthroscope; the second port allows insertion of miniaturized **surgical instruments**; the other ports drain fluid from the knee. Sterile saline fluid is pumped into the knee to enlarge the joint space and make it easier for the surgeon to view the knee structures and to cut, smooth, or repair damaged tissue.

Preoperative preparation

Knee replacement surgery requires extensive and detailed preparation on the patient's part because it affects so many aspects of life.

LEGAL AND FINANCIAL CONSIDERATIONS. In the United States, physicians and hospitals are required to verify the patient's insurance benefits before surgery and to obtain precertification from the patient's insurer or from **Medicare**. Without health insurance, the total cost of a knee replacement as of early 2003 can run as high as $38,000. In addition to insurance documentation, patients are legally required to sign an **informed consent** form prior to surgery. Informed consent signifies that the patient is a knowledgeable participant in making health-care decisions. The doctor will discuss all of the following with the patient before he or she signs the form: the nature of the surgery; reasonable alternatives to the surgery; and the risks, benefits, and uncertainties of each option. Informed consent also requires the doctor to make sure that the patient understands the information that has been given.

MEDICAL CONSIDERATIONS. Patients are asked to do the following in preparation for knee replacement surgery:

- Get in shape physically by doing exercises to strengthen or increase flexibility in the knee joint. Specific exercises are described in the books listed below. Many clinics and hospitals also distribute illustrated pamphlets of preoperation exercises.

- Lose weight if the surgeon recommends it.

- Quit smoking. Smoking weakens the cardiovascular system and increases the risks that the patient will have breathing difficulties under anesthesia.

- Make donations of one's own blood for storage in case a **transfusion** is necessary during surgery. This procedure is known as **autologous blood donation**; it has the advantage of avoiding the risk of transfusion reactions or transmission of diseases from infected blood donors.

- Check the skin of the knee and lower leg for external infection or irritation, and check the lower leg for signs of swelling. If either is noted, the surgeon should be contacted for instructions about preparing the skin for the operation.

- Have necessary dental work completed before the operation. This precaution is necessary because small numbers of bacteria enter the bloodstream whenever a dentist performs any procedure that causes the gums to bleed. Bacteria from the mouth can be carried to the knee area and cause an infection.

- Discontinue taking birth control pills and any anti-inflammatory medications (**aspirin** or NSAIDs) two weeks before surgery. Most doctors also recommend discontinuing any alternative herbal preparations at this time, as some of them interact with anesthetics and pain medications.

LIFESTYLE CHANGES. Knee replacement surgery requires a long period of **recovery at home** after leaving the hospital. Since the patient's physical mobility will be limited, he or she should do the following before the operation:

- Arrange for leave from work, help at home, help with driving, and similar tasks and commitments.

- Obtain a handicapped parking permit.

- Check the house or apartment thoroughly for needed adjustments to furniture, appliances, lighting, and personal conveniences. People recovering from knee replacement surgery must avoid kneeling, and minimize bending, squatting, and any risk of falling. There are several good guides available that describe household safety and comfort considerations in detail.

- Stock up on nonperishable groceries, cleaning supplies, and similar items in order to minimize shopping.

- Have a supply of easy-care clothing with elastic waistbands and simple fasteners in front rather than complicated ties or buttons in the back. Women may find knit dresses that pull on over the head or wraparound skirts easier to put on than slacks or skirts that must be pulled up over the knees. Shoes should be slip-ons or fastened with Velcro.

Many hospitals and clinics now have "preop" classes for patients scheduled for knee replacement surgery. These classes answer questions about the operation and what to expect during recovery, but in addition they provide an opportunity for patients to share concerns and experiences. Studies indicate that patients who have attended preop classes are less anxious before surgery and generally recover more rapidly.

Aftercare

Aftercare following knee replacement surgery begins while the patient is still in the hospital. Most patients will remain there for five to 10 days after the operation. During this period the patient will be given fluids

and antibiotic medications intravenously to prevent infection. Medications for pain will be given every three to four hours, or through a device known as a PCA (patient-controlled anesthesia). The PCA is a small pump that delivers a dose of medication into the IV when the patient pushes a button. To get the lungs back to normal functioning, a respiratory therapist will ask the patient to cough several times a day or breathe into blow bottles.

Aftercare during the hospital stay is also intended to lower the risk of a venous thromboembolism (VTE), or blood clot in the deep veins of the leg. Prevention of VTE involves medications to thin the blood; exercises for the feet and ankles while lying in bed; and wearing thromboembolic deterrent (TED) or deep vein thrombosis (DVT) stockings. TED stockings are made of nylon (usually white) and may be knee-length or thigh-length; they help to reduce the risk of a blood clot forming in the leg vein by putting mild pressure on the veins.

Physical therapy is also begun during the patient's hospital stay, often on the second day after the operation. The physical therapist will introduce the patient to using a cane or crutches and explain how to manage such activities as getting out of bed or showering without dislocating the new prosthesis. In most cases the patient will spend some time each day on a continuous passive motion (CPM) machine, which is a device that repeatedly bends and straightens the leg while the patient is lying in bed. In addition to increasing the patient's level of physical activity each day, the physical therapist will help the patient select special equipment for recovery at home. Commonly recommended devices include tongs or reachers for picking up objects without bending too far; a sock cone and special shoehorn; and bathing equipment.

Following **discharge from the hospital**, the patient may go to a skilled nursing facility, rehabilitation center, or home. Patients who have had bilateral knee replacement are unlikely to be sent directly home. Ongoing physical therapy is the most important part of recovery for the first four to five months following surgery. Most HMOs in the United States allow home visits by a home health aide, visiting nurse, and physical therapist for three to four weeks after surgery. Some hospitals allow patients to borrow a CPM machine for use at home for a few weeks. The physical therapist will monitor the patient's progress as well as suggest specific exercises to improve strength and range of motion. After the home visits, the patient is encouraged to take up other forms of low-impact physical activity in addition to the exercises; swimming, walking, and pedaling a stationary bicycle are all good ways to speed recovery. The patient may take a mild medication for pain (usually aspirin or ibuprofen) 30–45 minutes before an exercise session if needed.

The patient will be instructed to notify his or her dentist about the knee replacement so that extra precautions can be taken against infection resulting from bacteria getting into the bloodstream during dental work. Some surgeons ask patients to notify them whenever the dentist schedules a **tooth extraction**, root canal, or periodontal work.

Risks

Serious risks associated with TKR include the following:

- Loosening or dislocation of the prosthesis. The risk of dislocation varies, depending on the type of prosthesis used, the patient's level of activity, and the previous condition of the knee joint.

- Deep vein thrombosis (DVT). There is some risk (about 1.5% in the United States) of a clot developing in the deep vein of the leg after knee replacement surgery because the blood supply to the leg is cut off by a tourniquet during the operation. The blood-thinning medications and TED stockings used after surgery are intended to minimize the risk of DVT.

- Infection. The risk of infection is minimized by storing autologous blood for transfusion and administering intravenous **antibiotics** after surgery. The rate of infection following knee replacement is about 1.89%. Factors that increase the risk of infection after TKR include poor nutritional status, diabetes, obesity, a weakened immune system, and a history of smoking.

- Heterotopic bone. Heterotopic bone is bone that develops at the lower end of the femur after knee replacement surgery. It is most likely to develop in patients whose knee joints developed an infection. Heterotopic bone can cause stiffness and pain, and usually requires revision surgery.

Normal results

Normal results include relief of chronic pain in the knee and greater range of motion in the knee joint. Realistically, however, the patient should not expect complete restoration of function in the knee, and will usually be advised to avoid contact sports, skiing, jogging, or other athletic activities that strain the knee joint.

Mild swelling of the leg may occur for as long as three to six months after surgery. It can be treated by elevating the leg, applying an ice pack, and wearing compression stockings.

One commonplace side effect of TKR is that knee prostheses sometimes set off metal detectors in airports and high-security buildings because of their large metal content. Patients who fly frequently or whose occupations require security clearance should ask their doctor for a wallet card certifying that they have a knee prosthesis.

The patient can expect a cemented knee prosthesis to last about 10–15 years, although many still function well as long as 20 years later. Cementless prostheses have not been in use long enough for reliable evaluations of their long-term durability. When the prosthesis wears out or becomes loose, it is replaced in a procedure known as **knee revision surgery**.

Morbidity and mortality rates

A study published in 2002 reported that the 30-day mortality rate following total knee arthroplasty was 0.5%. The overall frequency of serious complications in this time period was 2.2%. This figure included 0.4%

heart attack; 0.7% pulmonary embolism; and 1.5% deep venous thrombosis. The rate of complications was highest in patients over 70, and male patients were more likely to have heart attacks than women.

A 2001 study published by the Mayo Clinic reviewed the records of 22,540 patients who had had knee replacements between 1969 and 1997. The mortality rate within 30 days of surgery was 0.21%, or 47 patients. Forty-three of the 47 patients had had preexisting cardiovascular or lung disease. Patients who had had bilateral knee operations had a higher mortality rate than those who had not.

Alternatives

Nonsurgical alternatives

MEDICATION. The most common conservative alternatives to knee replacement surgery are **analgesics**, or painkilling medications. Most patients who try medication for knee pain begin with an over-the-counter NSAID such as ibuprofen (Advil). If the pain cannot be controlled by nonprescription analgesics, the doctor may give the patient cortisone injections, which relieve the pain of arthritis by reducing inflammation. Unfortunately, the relief provided by cortisone tends to diminish with each injection; moreover, the drug can produce serious side effects.

If the knee pain is caused by rheumatoid arthritis, a group of medications known as disease-modifying antirheumatic drugs, or DMARDs, may help to slow or stop the progress of the disease. They work by suppressing or interfering with the immune system. DMARDs include such drugs as penicillamine, methotrexate, oral or injectable gold, hydroxychloroquine, leflunomide, and sulfasalazine. DMARDs are not suitable for all patients with RA, however, as they sometimes have serious side effects. In addition, some of them are slow-acting and may take several months to work before the patient feels some relief.

LIFESTYLE CHANGES. A second alternative to knee surgery is lifestyle changes. Losing weight helps to reduce stress on the knee joint. Giving up specific sports or other activities that damage the knee, such as jogging, tennis, high-impact aerobics, or stair-climbing exercise machines, may control the pain enough to make surgery unnecessary. Wearing properly fitted shoes and avoiding high heels and other extreme styles can also help to control pain and minimize further damage to the knee.

BRACES AND ORTHOTICS. Some patients with unstable knees are helped by functional braces or knee supports that are designed to keep the kneecap from slipping out of place. Orthotics, which are inserts placed inside shoes, are often helpful to patients whose knee problems are related to their gait. Orthotics are designed either to correct the position of the foot in order to keep it from turning too far outward or inward, or to correct problems in the arch of the foot. Some orthotics are made of soft material that cushions the foot and are particularly helpful for patients with osteoarthritis or diabetes.

Complementary and alternative (CAM) approaches

Complementary and alternative therapies are not substitutes for arthroscopy or joint replacement surgery, but some have been shown to relieve physical pain before or after surgery, or to help patients cope more effectively with the emotional and psychological stress of a major operation. Acupuncture, chiropractic, hypnosis, and mindfulness meditation have been used successfully to relieve the pain of osteoarthritis as well as postoperative discomfort. According to Dr. Marc Darrow, author of *The Knee Sourcebook*, a plant extract called RA-1, which is used in Ayurvedic medicine to treat arthritis, relieved pain and leg swelling in patients participating in a randomized trial. Alternative approaches that have helped patients maintain a positive mental attitude include meditation, biofeedback, and various relaxation techniques.

Alternative surgical procedures

Arthroscopy is the most common surgical alternative to knee replacement. It should be understood, however, as a way to postpone TKR rather than avoid it completely. The arthroscopic procedure most often used to treat knee pain from osteoarthritis is debridement, in which the surgeon cuts or scrapes away damaged structures or tissues until healthy tissue is reached. Most patients who have had arthroscopic débridement have been able to postpone TKR for three to five years.

Cartilage transplantation is a procedure in which small bone plugs with cartilage are removed from a part of the patient's knee where the cartilage is still healthy and transplanted to the area in which cartilage has been damaged. Another form of cartilage transplantation involves two operations, one to remove cartilage cells from the patient's knee for culture in a laboratory, and a second operation to place the new cells within the damaged part of the knee. The cultured cells are covered with a thin layer of tissue to hold them in place. After surgery, the cartilage cells multiply to form new cartilage inside the knee. Unfortunately, as of 2003 neither form of cartilage transplantation is usually beneficial to patients with osteoarthritis; transplantation has been most successful in treating patients whose knee cartilage was damaged by sudden trauma rather than by gradual degeneration.

See also Arthroscopic surgery; Knee revision surgery.

KEY TERMS

Analgesic—A medication given to relieve pain.

Arthroplasty—The medical term for surgical replacement of a joint. Arthroplasty can refer to hip as well as knee replacement.

Arthroscope—An instrument that contains a miniature camera and light source mounted on a flexible tube. It allows a surgeon to see the inside of a joint or bone during surgery.

Autologous blood—The patient's own blood, drawn and set aside before surgery for use during surgery in case a transfusion is needed.

Biomechanics—The application of mechanical laws to the structures in the human body, such as measuring the force and direction of stresses on a joint.

Bursitis—Inflammation of a bursa, which is a sac-like cavity filled with fluid that protects the tissues around certain joints in the body from friction. Bursitis of the knee frequently develops as a result of activities requiring frequent bending and kneeling, such as housecleaning.

Cartilage—A whitish elastic connective tissue that allows the bones forming the knee joint to move smoothly against each other.

Cortisone—A steroid compound used to treat autoimmune diseases and inflammatory conditions. It is sometimes injected into a joint to relieve the pain of arthritis.

Debridement—The surgical removal of foreign material and dead or contaminated tissue from a wound or the area of an incision.

Disease-modifying antirheumatic drugs (DMA RDs)—A group of medications that can be given to slow or stop the progression of rheumatoid arthritis. DMARDs include such drugs as oral or injectable gold, methotrexate, leflunomide, and penicillamine.

Fibula—The smaller of the two bones in the lower leg.

Ligament—A band of fibrous tissue that connects bones to other bones or holds internal organs in place.

Meniscus (plural, menisci)—One of two crescent-shaped pieces of cartilage attached to the upper surface of the tibia. The menisci act as shock absorbers within the knee joint.

Nonsteroidal anti-inflammatory drugs (NSAIDs)—A term used for a group of analgesics that also reduce inflammation when used over a period of time. NSAIDs are often given to patients with osteoarthritis.

Orthopedics (sometimes spelled orthopaedics)—The branch of surgery that treats deformities or disorders affecting the musculoskeletal system.

Orthotics—Shoe inserts that are intended to correct an abnormal or irregular gait or walking pattern. They are sometimes prescribed to relieve gait-related knee pain.

Patella—The medical term for the knee cap. The patella is a triangular bone located at the front of the knee.

Prosthesis (plural, prostheses)—An artificial device that substitutes for or supplements a missing or damaged body part. Prostheses may be either external or implanted inside the body.

Quadriceps muscles—A set of four muscles on each leg located at the front of the thigh. The quadriceps straighten the knee and are used every time a person takes a step.

Tibia—The larger of two leg bones that lie beneath the knee. The tibia is sometimes called the shin bone.

Resources

BOOKS

Darrow, Marc, MD, JD. *The Knee Sourcebook*. Chicago and New York: Contemporary Books, 2002.

Nohava, Ann. *My Bilateral Knee Replacement: A Personal Story*. San Jose, CA and New York: Writers Club Press, 2001.

Silber, Irwin. *A Patient's Guide to Knee and Hip Replacement: Everything You Need to Know*. New York: Simon & Schuster, 1999.

PERIODICALS

Alemparte, J., G. V. Johnson, R. L. Worland, et al. "Results of Simultaneous Bilateral Total Knee Replacement: A Study of 1208 Knees in 604 Patients." *Journal of the Southern Orthopaedic Association* 11 (Fall 2002): 153–156.

Blake, V. A., J. P. Allegrante, L. Robbins, et al. "Racial Differences in Social Network Experience and Perceptions of Benefit of Arthritis Treatments Among New York City Medicare Beneficiaries with Self-Reported Hip and Knee

Pain." *Arthritis and Rheumatism* 47 (August 15, 2002): 366–371.

Chernajovsky, Y., P. G. Winyard, and P. S. Kabouridis. "Advances in Understanding the Genetic Basis of Rheumatoid Arthritis and Osteoarthritis: Implications for Therapy." *American Journal of Pharmacogenomics* 2 (2002): 223–234.

Crubezy, E., J. Goulet, J. Bruzek, et al. "Epidemiology of Osteoarthritis and Enthesopathies in a European Population Dating Back 7700 Years." *Joint, Bone, Spine: Revue du Rhumatisme* 69 (December 2002): 580–588.

Gunther, K. P. "Surgical Approaches to Osteoarthritis." *Best Practice and Research: Clinical Rheumatology* 15 (October 2001): 627–643.

Hasegawa, M., T. Ohashi, and A. Uchida. "Heterotopic Ossification Around Distal Femur After Total Knee Arthroplasty." *Archives of Orthopaedic and Trauma Surgery* 122 (June 2002): 274–278.

Johnson, L. L. "Arthroscopic Abrasion Arthroplasty: A Review" *Clinical Orthopaedics and Related Research* 391 Supplement (October 2001): S306–S317.

Lombardi, A. V., T. H. Mallory, R. A. Fada, et al. "Simultaneous Bilateral Total Knee Arthroplasty: Who Decides?" *Clinical Orthopaedics and Related Research* 392 (November 2001): 319–329.

Mantilla, C. B., T. T. Horlocker, D. R. Schroeder, et al. "Frequency of Myocardial Infarction, Pulmonary Embolism, Deep Venous Thrombosis, and Death Following Primary Hip or Knee Arthroplasty." *Anesthesiology* 96 (May 2002): 1140–1146.

Parvisi, J., T. A. Sullivan, R. T. Trousdale, and D. G. Lewallen. "Thirty-Day Mortality After Total Knee Arthroplasty." *Journal of Bone and Joint Surgery, American Volume* 83-A (August 2001): 1157–1161.

Peersman, G., R. Laskin, J. Davis, and M. Peterson. "Infection in Total Knee Replacement: A Retrospective Review of 6489 Total Knee Replacements." *Clinical Orthopaedics and Related Research* 392 (November 2002): 15–23.

Shah, S. N., D. J. Schurman, and S. B. Goodman. "Screw Migration from Total Knee Prostheses Requiring Subsequent Surgery." *Journal of Arthroplasty* 17 (October 2002): 951–954.

Silva, M., R. Tharani, and T. P. Schmalzried. "Results of Direct Exchange or Debridement of the Infected Total Knee Arthroplasty." *Clinical Orthopaedics and Related Research* 404 (November 2002): 125–131.

Wai, E. K., H. J. Kreder, and J. I. Williams. "Arthroscopic Debridement of the Knee for Osteoarthritis in Patients Fifty Years of Age or Older: Utilization and Outcomes in the Province of Ontario." *Journal of Bone and Joint Surgery, American Volume* 84-A (January 2002): 17–22.

ORGANIZATIONS

American Academy of Orthopaedic Surgeons (AAOS). 6300 North River Road, Rosemont, IL 60018. (847) 823-7186 or (800) 346-AAOS. <http://www.aaos.org>.

American Physical Therapy Association (APTA). 1111 North Fairfax Street, Alexandria, VA 22314. (703) 684-APTA or (800) 999-2782. <http://www.apta.org>.

Canadian Institute for Health Information/Institut canadien d'information sur la santé (CIHI). 377 Dalhousie Street, Suite 200, Ottawa, ON K1N 9N8. (613) 241-7860. <http://secure.cihi.ca/cihiweb>.

National Center for Complementary and Alternative Medicine (NCCAM) Clearinghouse. P.O. Box 7923, Gaithersburg, MD 20898. (888) 644-6226. TTY: (866) 464-3615. Fax: (866) 464-3616. <http://www.nccam.nih.gov.>.

National Institute of Arthritis and Musculoskeletal and Skin Diseases (NIAMS) Information Clearinghouse. National Institutes of Health, 1 AMS Circle, Bethesda, MD 20892. (301) 495-4484. TTY: (301) 565-2966. <http://www.niams.nih.gov>.

Rush Arthritis and Orthopedics Institute. 1725 West Harrison Street, Suite 1055, Chicago, IL 60612. (312) 563-2420. <http://www.rush.edu>.

OTHER

American Academy of Orthopaedic Surgeons (AAOS) Patient Education Booklet #03057. *Total Knee Replacement.* Rosemont, IL: AAOS, 2001.

Canadian Institute for Health Information/Institut canadien d'information sur la santé (CIHI). *Total Hip and Total Knee Replacements in Canada, 2000/01.* Toronto, ON: Canadian Joint Replacement Registry, 2003.

Questions and Answers About Knee Problems. Bethesda, MD: National Institutes of Health, 2001. NIH Publication No. 01-4912.

University of Iowa Department of Orthopaedics. *Total Knee Replacement: A Patient Guide.* Iowa City, IA: University of Iowa Hospitals and Clinics, 1999.

Rebecca Frey, Ph.D.

Knee revision surgery

Definition

Knee revision surgery, which is also known as revision total knee **arthroplasty**, is a procedure in which the surgeon removes a previously implanted artificial knee joint, or prosthesis, and replaces it with a new prosthesis. Knee revision surgery may also involve the use of bone grafts. The bone graft may be an autograft, which means that the bone is taken from another site in the patient's own body; or an allograft, which means that the bone tissue comes from another donor.

Purpose

Knee revision surgery has three major purposes: relieving pain in the affected hip; restoring the patient's mobility; and removing a loose or damaged prosthesis before irreversible harm is done to the joint. Knee pros-

A knee prosthesis that has become infected or completely dislocated must be removed and replaced to prevent permanent damage to the patient's knee.

Demographics

The demographics of knee revision surgery are somewhat difficult to evaluate because the procedure is performed much less frequently than total **knee replacement** (TKR). TKR itself is a relatively new operation; the first total knee replacement was performed in the United Kingdom in 1968 and the first TKR in the United States in 1970. As of 2003, it is estimated that 98% of knee prostheses are still functioning well 10 years after surgery, with 94% still working after 20 years. Because of this high success rate, the number of patients who have had knee revision surgery yields a much smaller database than those who have had TKR. It is estimated that about 22,000 knee revision operations are performed in the United States each year; over half of them are done within two years of the patient's TKR.

Another difficulty in evaluating the demographics of knee revision surgery is the growing trend toward TKR in younger patients. A Canadian survey released in January 2003 stated that the number of knee replacements performed in patients below the age of 55 rose 90% between 1994 and 2001. As the number of knee replacement procedures done in younger patients continues to rise, the number of revision surgeries will increase as well. A study done in the United States in 1996 reported that women were almost twice as likely as men to have knee revision surgery, and that Caucasians were 1.5 times as likely as African Americans to have the procedure. This study, however, was limited to patients over the age of 65, so that its findings are not likely to be an accurate picture of younger patient populations.

theses can come loose for one of two reasons. One is mechanical and is related to the fact that the knee joint bears a great deal of weight when a person is walking or running. It is unusual for the metal part of a knee prosthesis to simply break. This part, however, is inserted into the upper part of the tibia, the larger of the two bones in the lower leg, after the surgeon has removed the upper surface of the tibia. The bone tissue that receives the metal implant is softer than the bone that was removed, which means that the metal implant may sink into the softer bone and gradually loosen.

The second reason for loosening of a knee prosthesis is related to the development of inflammation in the knee joint. The plastic part of a knee prosthesis is made of a material called polyethylene, which can form small particles of debris as a result of wear on the prosthesis over time. If the patient has an uneven gait, or pattern of walking, the debris particles tend to form at a faster rate because one side of the prosthesis will tend to pull away from the bone and the other side will be pushed further into the bone. These tiny fragments of plastic are absorbed by tissue cells around the knee joint, which become inflamed. The inflammatory response begins to dissolve the bone around the prosthesis in a process known as osteolysis. As the osteolysis continues, bone loss accelerates and the prosthesis eventually comes loose.

Description

Most knee revision operations take about three hours to perform and are similar to knee replacement procedures. After the patient has been anesthetized, the surgeon opens the knee joint by cutting through the joint capsule. The first step in revision surgery is the removal of the old femoral component of the knee prosthesis. After the metal shell has been removed, the damaged bone at the end of the femur is scraped off and the femur is reshaped. If the bone is weak, the surgeon may decide to fill the cavity inside the femur with bone grafts. In some cases, metal wedges may be used to strengthen the attachment of the new femoral component.

After the new femoral component has been glued in place with bone cement, the old implant in the tibia is removed and the bone is reshaped to receive a new implant.

If the old implant had loosened because it had moved downward into the softer tissue inside the tibia, the surgeon will pack the space with morselized bone from a donor before putting in the new implant. This technique is known as impaction grafting. The impaction grafting may be reinforced with wire mesh. If the tibia has been shortened by the removal of damaged bone, the surgeon will insert a wedge along with the new tibial implant and secure them to the end of the tibia with bone cement. A new plastic plate will be fastened to the tray at the top of the tibial implant so that the patient's femur can move smoothly over the tibia. If the patient's patella (kneecap) has been damaged, the surgeon will resurface its back surface and attach a plastic component to protect the patella from further bone loss. The tibial and femoral components of the prosthesis are then fitted together, the kneecap is replaced, and the knee tendons reattached with surgical wire. The knee joint is washed out with sterile saline fluid and the various layers of the incision closed.

Revision surgery on an infected knee requires two separate operations. In the first operation, the old prosthesis is taken out and a block of polyethylene cement known as a spacer block is inserted in the joint. The spacer block has been treated with **antibiotics** to fight the infection. The incision is closed and the spacer block remains inside the patient's knee for about six weeks. The patient is also given intravenous antibiotics during this period. After the infection has cleared, the knee is reopened and the new revision prosthesis is implanted.

Diagnosis/Preparation

In most cases, increasing pain, stiffness, and loss of mobility in the knee joint are early indications that the patient may benefit from revision surgery. The location of the pain may point to the part of the prosthesis that has been affected by osteolysis. Pain around or in the kneecap is not always significant by itself because many TKR patients have occasional discomfort in that area after their knee replacement. If the pain is diffuse (felt throughout the knee rather than in only one part of the knee), it may indicate either an infection or loosening of the prosthesis. Pain felt throughout the knee accompanied by tissue fluid accumulating in the joint points to a problem with the polyethylene part of the prosthesis. Pain in the lower thigh or in the part of the leg just below the knee suggests that the metal plate attached to the femur or the metal implant in the tibia may have come loose.

The doctor may take risk factors into account in assessing the likelihood of a failed knee prosthesis. Six factors have been identified as increasing a patient's risk of needing revision surgery within two years of knee replacement surgery:

QUESTIONS TO ASK THE DOCTOR

- How many knee revision operations do you perform each year?
- Would I be likely to benefit from arthroscopy?
- What lifestyle changes can I make to extend the life of the new prosthesis?
- What are my chances of needing another revision operation in the future?

- age (Younger patients tend to be more active and to wear out knee prostheses more rapidly than older ones.)
- a long hospital stay for the original knee surgery
- concurrent diseases or disorders
- any type of arthritis
- surgical complications during the first knee operation
- having the first knee operation performed at an urban hospital

The doctor will then usually order a series of imaging tests to determine the location of the problem and the extent of bone loss. X-ray studies can be used to check for complete dislocation of the prosthesis as well as loosening. Computed tomography appears to be more effective in detecting the early stages of osteolysis than x-ray studies. If the doctor suspects that the knee prosthesis has become infected, he or she will aspirate the joint. Aspiration is a procedure in which fluid is withdrawn from a joint through a needle and sent to a laboratory for analysis. The fluid will be cultured in order to identify the specific organism causing the infection.

Aftercare

Aftercare following knee revision surgery is essentially the same as for knee replacement, consisting of a combination of physical therapy, rehabilitation exercises, pain medication when necessary, and a period of home health care or assistance.

The length of recovery after revision knee surgery varies in comparison to the patient's first knee replacement. Some patients take longer to recover from revision surgery, but others recover more rapidly than they did from TKR, and they experience less discomfort. The reasons for this variation are not yet known. As of 2003, the Hip and Knee Center at Columbia University is conducting a study of 100 knee revision patients at five different sites in the United States in order to evaluate the outcomes of revision surgery. The patients will be examined at three-month, six-month, 12-month, and 24-month intervals in order to measure their progress after surgery.

Risks

The complications that may follow knee revision surgery are similar to those for knee replacement. They include:

• Deep vein thrombosis.

• Infection in the new prosthesis.

• Loosening of the new prosthesis. The risk of this complication is increased considerably if the patient is overweight.

• Formation of heterotopic bone. Heterotopic bone is bone that develops at the lower end of the femur following knee replacement or knee revision surgery. Patients who have had an infection in the joint have an increased risk of heterotopic bone formation.

• Bone fractures during the operation. These are caused by the force or pressure that the surgeon must sometimes apply to remove the old prosthesis and the cement that may be attached to it.

• Dislocation of the new prosthesis. The risk of dislocation is twice as great for revision surgery as for TKR.

• Difference in leg length resulting from shortening of the leg with the prosthesis.

• Additional or more rapid loss of bone tissue.

Normal results

Normal results of knee revision surgery are quite similar to those for TKR. Patients have less pain and greater mobility in the affected knee, but not complete restoration of the function of a normal knee. Between 5% and 20% of patients report some pain following either TKR or revision surgery for several years after their operation. Most patients, however, have considerably less discomfort in the knee after surgery than they did before the procedure. A recent British study found that revision knee surgery patients had the same positive results at six-month follow-up as patients who had had primary knee replacement surgery.

As with knee replacement surgery, patients who have had revision surgery may experience mild swelling of the leg for as long as three to six months after surgery. Swelling can be treated by elevating the leg, applying an ice pack, and wearing compression stockings.

Morbidity and mortality rates

The 30-day mortality rate following knee revision surgery is low, between 0.1% and 0.2%. The estimated rates of complications are as follows:

• deep infection: 0.97%

• loosening of the new prosthesis: 10–15%.

• dislocation of the new prosthesis: 2–5%.

• deep venous thrombosis: 1.5%

Alternatives

Nonsurgical alternatives

LIFESTYLE CHANGES. The American Association of Orthopaedic Surgeons (AAOS) has published a fact sheet about the effects of aging on the knee joint aimed at the baby boomer generation. Many adults in their 40s and 50s have been influenced by the contemporary emphasis on youthfulness to keep up athletic activities and forms of exercise that are hard on the knee joint. Some of them try to return to a high level of activity even after TKR. As a result, some surgeons are suggesting that adults in this age bracket scale back their athletic workouts or substitute low-impact forms of exercise. Good choices include water aerobics, tai chi, yoga, swimming, cycling, and walking.

COMPLEMENTARY AND ALTERNATIVE (CAM) APPROACHES. Complementary and alternative therapies are not substitutes for knee revision surgery, but some have been shown to relieve physical pain before or after surgery, or to help patients cope more effectively with the emotional and psychological stress of a major operation. Acupuncture, chiropractic, hypnosis, and mindfulness meditation have been used successfully to relieve postoperative discomfort following revision surgery. Alternative approaches that have helped patients maintain a positive mental attitude include meditation, biofeedback, and various relaxation techniques.

Alternative surgical procedures

Arthroscopy is the most common surgical alternative to knee revision surgery. It is a procedure in which a surgeon makes three or four small incisions in the knee in order to insert a device that allows him or her to see the inside of the joint, insert miniaturized instruments to remove or repair damaged tissue, and drain fluid from the joint. Arthroscopy has been used successfully to treat stiffness in the knee following TKR and improve range of motion in the joint. It is not successful in treating infected prostheses unless it is used very early.

Other surgical alternatives to knee revision surgery include manipulation of the joint while the patient is under general anesthesia, and arthrodesis of the knee. Arthrodesis is a procedure in which the joint is fixed in place with a long surgical nail until the growth of new bone tissue fuses the knee. It is generally considered a less preferable alternative to knee revision surgery, but is sometimes used in the treatment of elderly patients with infected prostheses or weakened bone structure.

See also Arthroscopic surgery.

Resources

BOOKS

Darrow, Marc, MD, JD. *The Knee Sourcebook*. Chicago and New York: Contemporary Books, 2002.

Silber, Irwin. *A Patient's Guide to Knee and Hip Replacement: Everything You Need to Know.* New York: Simon & Schuster, 1999.

PERIODICALS

Barrack, R. I., C. S. Brumfield, C. H. Rorabeck, et al. "Heterotopic Ossification After Revision Total Knee Arthroplasty." *Clinical Orthopaedics and Related Research* 404 (November 2002): 208–213.

Djian, P., P. Christel, and J. Witvoet. "Arthroscopic Release for Knee Joint Stiffness After Total Knee Arthroplasty." [in French] *Revue de chirurgie orthopedique et reparatrice de l'appareil moteur* 88 (April 2002): 163–167.

Hartley, R. C., N. G. Barton-Hanson, R. Finley, and R. W. Parkinson. "Early Patient Outcomes After Primary and Revision Total Knee Arthroplasty. A Prospective Study." *Journal of Bone and Joint Surgery, British Volume* 84 (September 2002): 994–999.

Hasegawa, M., T. Ohashi, and A. Uchida. "Heterotopic Ossification Around Distal Femur After Total Knee Arthroplasty." *Archives of Orthopaedic and Trauma Surgery* 122 (June 2002): 274–278.

Heck, D. A., C. A. Melfi, L. A. Mamlin, et al. "Revision Rates After Knee Replacement in the United States." *Medical Care* 36 (May 1998): 661–669.

Incavo, S. J., J. W. Lilly, C. S. Bartlett, and D. L. Churchill. "Arthrodesis of the Knee: Experience with Intramedullary Nailing." *Journal of Arthroplasty* 15 (October 2000): 871–876.

Katz, B. P., D. A. Freund, D. A. Heck, et al. "Demographic Variation in the Rate of Knee Replacement: A Multi-Year Analysis." *Health Services Research* 31 (June 1996): 125–140.

Lonner, J. H., P. A. Lotke, J. Kim, and C. Nelson. "Impaction Grafting and Wire Mesh for Uncontained Defects in Revision Knee Arthroplasty." *Clinical Orthopaedics and Related Research* 404 (November 2002): 145–151.

Peersman, G., R. Laskin, J. Davis, and M. Peterson. "Infection in Total Knee Replacement: A Retrospective Review of 6489 Total Knee Replacements." *Clinical Orthopaedics and Related Research* 392 (November 2002): 15–23.

Shah, S. N., D. J. Schurman, and S. B. Goodman. "Screw Migration from Total Knee Prostheses Requiring Subsequent Surgery." *Journal of Arthroplasty* 17 (October 2002): 951–954.

Sharkey, P. F., W. J. Hozack, R. H. Rothman, et al. "Insall Award Paper: Why Are Total Knee Arthroplasties Failing Today?" *Clinical Orthopaedics and Related Research* 404 (November 2002): 7–13.

Teng, H. P., Y. C. Lu, C. J. Hsu, and C. Y. Wong. "Arthroscopy Following Total Knee Arthroplasty." *Orthopedics* 25 (April 2002): 422–424.

Vidil, A., and P. Beaufils. "Arthroscopic Treatment of Hematogenous Infected Total Knee Arthroplasty: 5 Cases." [in French] *Revue de chirurgie orthopedique et reparatrice de l'appareil moteur* 88 (September 2002): 493–500.

ORGANIZATIONS

American Academy of Orthopaedic Surgeons (AAOS). 6300 North River Road, Rosemont, IL 60018. (847) 823-7186 or (800) 346-AAOS. <http://www.aaos.org>.

American Physical Therapy Association (APTA). 1111 North Fairfax Street, Alexandria, VA 22314. (703)684-APTA or (800) 999-2782. <http://www.apta.org>.

KEY TERMS

Arthrodesis—A procedure that is sometimes used as an alternative to knee revision surgery, in which the joint is first fixed in place with a surgical nail and then fused as new bone tissue grows in.

Arthroscope—An instrument that contains a miniature camera and light source mounted on a flexible tube. It allows a surgeon to see the inside of a joint or bone during surgery.

Femur—The medical name for the thighbone.

Gait—A person's habitual pattern of walking. An irregular gait is a risk factor for knee revision surgery.

Heterotopic bone—Bone that develops as an excess growth around a joint following joint replacement surgery.

Impaction grafting—The use of crushed bone from a donor to fill in the central canal of the tibia during knee revision surgery.

Osteolysis—Dissolution and loss of bone resulting from inflammation caused by particles of polyethylene debris from a prosthesis.

Patella—The medical term for the knee cap. The patella is a triangular bone located at the front of the knee.

Prosthesis (plural, prostheses)—An artificial device that substitutes for or supplements a missing or damaged body part. Prostheses may be either external or implanted inside the body.

Tibia—The larger of two leg bones that lie beneath the knee. The tibia is sometimes called the shin bone.

Canadian Institute for Health Information/Institut canadien d'information sur la santé (CIHI). 377 Dalhousie Street, Suite 200, Ottawa, ON K1N 9N8. (613) 241-7860. <http://secure.cihi.ca/cihiweb>.

Center for Hip and Knee Replacement, Columbia University. Department of Orthopaedic Surgery, Columbia Presbyterian Medical Center, 622 West 168th Street, PH11-Center, New York, NY 10032. (212) 305-5974. <www.hipnknee. org>.

National Center for Complementary and Alternative Medicine (NCCAM) Clearinghouse. P.O. Box 7923, Gaithersburg, MD 20898. (888) 644-6226. TTY: (866) 464-3615. Fax: (866) 464-3616. <http://www.nccam.nih.gov.>.

National Institute of Arthritis and Musculoskeletal and Skin Diseases (NIAMS) Information Clearinghouse. National Institutes of Health, 1 AMS Circle, Bethesda, MD 20892. (301) 495-4484. TTY: (301) 565-2966. <http://www. niams.nih.gov>.

Rothman Institute of Orthopaedics. 925 Chestnut Street, Philadelphia, PA 19107-4216. (215) 955-3458. <http:// www.rothmaninstitute.com>.

OTHER

Questions and Answers About Knee Problems. Bethesda, MD: National Institutes of Health, 2001. NIH Publication No. 01-4912.

University of Iowa Department of Orthopaedics. *Total Knee Replacement: A Patient Guide.* Iowa City, IA: University of Iowa Hospitals and Clinics, 1999.

Rebecca Frey, Ph.D.

Kneecap removal

Definition

Kneecap removal, or patellectomy, is the partial or total surgical removal of the patella, commonly called the kneecap.

Purpose

Kneecap removal is performed under three circumstances:

• The kneecap is fractured or shattered.

• The kneecap dislocates easily and repeatedly.

• Degenerative arthritis of the kneecap causes extreme pain.

Demographics

A person of any age can break a kneecap in an accident. When the bone is shattered beyond repair, the kneecap has to be removed. No prosthesis or artificial replacement part is put in its place.

WHO PERFORMS THE PROCEDURE AND WHERE IS IT PERFORMED?

Kneecap removal surgery is usually performed in an outpatient setting and hospital stays, if any, are short, not exceeding more than a day. An orthopedic surgeon performs the surgery. Orthopedics is the medical specialty that focuses on the diagnosis, care, and treatment of patients with disorders of the bones, joints, muscles, ligaments, tendons, nerves, and skin.

Dislocation of the kneecap is most common in young girls between the ages of 10–14. Initially, the kneecap will pop back into place of its own accord, but pain may continue. If dislocation occurs too often, or the kneecap does not go back into place correctly, the patella may rub the other bones in the knee, causing an arthritis-like condition. Some people are also born with birth defects that cause the kneecap to dislocate frequently.

Degenerative arthritis of the kneecap, also called patellar arthritis or chondromalacia patellae, can cause so much pain that it becomes necessary to remove the kneecap. As techniques of joint replacement have improved, arthritis in the knee is more frequently treated with total **knee replacement**.

People who have had their kneecap removed for degenerative arthritis and then later require a total knee replacement are more likely to have problems with the stability of their artificial knee than those who only have total knee replacement. This occurs because the realigned muscles and tendons provide less support once the kneecap is removed.

Description

General anesthesia is typically used for kneecap removal surgery, though in some cases a spinal or epidural anesthetic is used. The surgeon makes a linear incision over the front of the kneecap. The damaged kneecap is examined. If a part or the entire kneecap is so severely damaged that it cannot be repaired, it may be partially removed (partial patellectomy) or totally removed (full patellectomy). If kneecap removal is total, the muscles and tendons attached to the kneecap are cut and the kneecap is removed. However, the quadriceps tendon above the kneecap, the patellar tendon below, and the other soft tissues around the kneecap are preserved so that the patient may still be able to extend the knee after surgery. Next, the muscles are sewn together, and the

814

QUESTIONS TO ASK THE DOCTOR

- How is the kneecap removed?
- What type of anesthesia will be used?
- How long will it take for the knee to recover from the surgery?
- When will I be able to walk without crutches?
- What are the risks associated with kneecap removal surgery?
- How many kneecap removal procedures do you perform in a year?

KEY TERMS

Degenerative arthritis, or osteoarthritis—A non-inflammatory type of arthritis, usually occurring in older people, characterized by degeneration of cartilage, enlargement of the margins of the bones, and changes in the membranes in the joints.

Patella—The knee cap; the quadriceps tendon attaches to it above and the patellar tendon below.

Patellectomy—Surgical removal of the patella, or kneecap removal.

skin is closed with sutures or clips that stay in place for about two weeks.

Diagnosis/Preparation

Prior to surgery, x rays and other diagnostic tests are done on the knee to determine if removing the kneecap is the appropriate treatment. Preoperative blood and urine tests are also done.

Patients are asked not to eat or drink anything after midnight on the night before surgery. On the day of surgery, patients are directed to the hospital or clinic holding area where the final preparations are made. The knee area is usually shaved and the patient is asked to change into a hospital gown and to remove all jewelry, watches, dentures, and glasses.

Aftercare

Pain medication may be prescribed for a few days. The patient will initially need to use a cane or crutches to walk. Physical therapy exercises to strengthen the knee should start as soon as tolerated after surgery. Driving should be avoided for several weeks. Full recovery can take months.

Risks

Risks involved with kneecap removal are similar to those associated with any surgical procedure, mainly allergic reaction to anesthesia, excessive bleeding, and infection.

Kneecap removal is very delicate surgery because the kneecap is part of the extensor mechanism of the leg, meaning the muscles and ligaments, the patella, the quadriceps tendon, and the patellar tendon; which all allow the knee to extend and remain stable when extended. When the kneecap is removed, the extensor assembly becomes more lax, and it may be impossible to ever regain full extension.

Normal results

People who undergo kneecap removal because of a broken bone or repeated dislocations have the best chance for complete recovery. Those who have this operation because of arthritis may have less successful results, and later need a total knee replacement.

Resources

BOOKS

Harner, C. D., K. G. Vince, and F. H. Fu, eds. *Techniques in Knee Surgery.* Philadelphia: Lippincott, Williams & Wilkins, 2001.

Winter Griffith, H., et al., eds. "Kneecap Removal." In *The Complete Guide to Symptoms, Illness and Surgery,* 3rd edition. New York: Berkeley Publishing, 1995.

PERIODICALS

Juni, P., et al. "Population Requirement for Primary Knee Replacement Surgery: A Cross-sectional Study." *Rheumatology* 42 (April 2003): 516–521.

Meijer, O. G., and Van Den Dikkenberg. "Levels of Analysis in Knee Surgery." *Knee Surgery Sports Traumatology Arthroscopy* 11 (January 2003): 53–54.

Petersen, W., C. Beske, V. Stein, and H. Laprell. "Arthroscopical Removal of a Projectile from the Intra-articular Cavity of the Knee Joint." *Archives of Orthopaedic Trauma Surgery* 122 (May 2002): 235–236.

ORGANIZATIONS

The American Academy of Orthopaedic Surgeons. 6300 North River Road, Rosemont, IL 60018-4262. (847) 823-7186, (800) 346-AAOS. <http://www.aaos.org>.

The American Association of Hip and Knee Surgeons (AAHKS). 704 Florence Drive, Park Ridge, IL 60068-2104. (847) 698-1200. <hhttp://www.aahks.org>.

OTHER

"Patellectomy." *The Knee Guru Page.* <http://www.kneeguru.
co.uk/html/step_05_patella/step_05_patellectomy.html>.
"Patellectomy or Partial Patellectomy." *Pro Team Physicians.*
<http://www.proteamphysicians.com/Patient/Treat/knee/
kneefracture/patellectomy_procedure.asp>.

Tish Davidson, AM
Monique Laberge, PhD

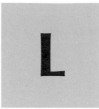

Laceration repair

Definition

Laceration repair includes all the steps required to treat a wound in order to promote healing and minimize the risks of infection, premature splitting of sutures (dehiscence), and poor cosmetic result.

Purpose

A laceration is a wound caused by a sharp object producing edges that may be jagged, dirty, or bleeding. Lacerations most often affect the skin, but any tissue may be lacerated, including subcutaneous fat, tendon, muscle, or bone.

A laceration should be repaired if it:

• Continues to bleed after application of pressure for 10–15 minutes.

• Is more than one-eighth to one-fourth inch deep.

• Exposes fat, muscle, tendon, or bone.

• Causes a change in function surrounding the area of the laceration.

• Is dirty or has visible debris in it.

• Is located in an area where an unsightly scar is undesirable.

Lacerations are less likely to become infected if they are repaired soon after they occur. Many physicians will not repair a laceration that is more than eight hours old because the risk of infection is too great.

Description

Laceration repair mends a tear in the skin or other tissue. The four goals of laceration repair are to stop bleeding, prevent infection, preserve function, and restore appearance.

The laceration is cleaned by removing any foreign material or debris. Removing foreign objects from penetrating wounds can sometimes cause bleeding, so this type of wound must be cleaned very carefully. The wound is then irrigated with saline solution and a disinfectant. The disinfecting agent may be mild soap or a commercial preparation. An antibacterial agent may be applied.

Once the wound has been cleansed, the physician anesthetizes the area of the repair. Most lacerations are anesthetized by local injection of lidocaine, with or without epinephrine, into the wound edges. Lidocaine without epinephrine is used in areas with limited blood supply such as fingers, toes, ears, penis, and nose, because epinephrine could cause constriction of blood vessels (vasoconstriction) and interfere with the supply of blood to the laceration site. Alternatively, a topical anesthetic combination such as lidocaine, epinephrine, and tetracaine may also be used.

The physician may trim edges that are jagged or extremely uneven. Tissue that is too damaged to heal must be removed (**debridement**) to prevent infection. If the laceration is deep, several absorbable stitches (sutures) are placed in the tissue under the skin to help bring the tissue layers together. Suturing also helps eliminate any pockets where tissue fluid or blood can accumulate. The skin wound is closed with sutures. Suture material used on the surface of a wound is usually non-absorbable and will have to be removed later. A light dressing or an adhesive bandage is applied for 24–48 hours. In areas where a dressing is not feasible, an antibiotic ointment can be applied. If the laceration is the result of a human or animal bite, if it is very dirty, or if the patient has a medical condition that alters wound healing, a broad-spectrum antibiotic may be prescribed.

Diagnosis/Preparation

Preparation for laceration repair involves inspecting the wound and the underlying tendons or nerves to evaluate the risk of infection, the degree of tissue damage, the need for debridement, and its complexity. If hair is located in or around the wound, it is usually removed to minimize contamination and allow for good visibility of the wound. If nerves or tendons have been injured, a surgeon may be needed to complete the repair.

Aftercare

The laceration is kept clean and dry for at least 24 hours after the repair. Light bathing is generally permitted after 24 hours if the wound is not soaked. The physician will provide directions for any special **wound care**. Sutures are removed three to 14 days after the repair is completed. Timing of suture removal depends on the location of the laceration and physician preference.

The repair should be examined frequently for signs of infection, which include redness, swelling, tenderness, drainage from the wound, red streaks in the skin surrounding the repair, chills, or fever. If any of these occur, the physician should be contacted immediately.

Risks

The most serious risk associated with laceration repair is infection. Risk of infection depends on the nature of the wound and the type of injury sustained. Infection risks are increased in wounds that are contaminated with soil or fecal matter, are the result of bites, have been open longer than one hour, or are located on the extremities or on the region between the thighs, genitalia, or other areas where opposing skin surfaces touch and may rub.

Normal results

All lacerations will heal with a scar. Wounds that are repaired with sutures are less likely to develop scars that are unsightly, but it cannot be predicted how wounds will heal and who will develop unsightly scars. Plastic surgery can improve the appearance of many scars.

Alternatives

The only alternative to laceration repair is to leave the wound without medical treatment. This increases the risk of infection, poor healing, and an undesirable cosmetic result.

See also Debridement.

Resources

BOOKS

Snell, George. "Laceration Repair." In *Procedures for Primary Care Physicians,* edited by John L. Pfenninger and Grant C. Fowler. St. Louis: Mosby, 1994.

PERIODICALS

Beredjiklian, P. K. "Biologic Aspects of Flexor Tendon Laceration and Repair." *The Journal of Bone and Joint Surgery* 85-A (March 2003): 539–550.

Gordon, C. A. "Reducing Needle-stick Injuries with the Use of 2-octyl Cyanoacrylates for Laceration Repair." *Journal of the American Academy of Nurse Practitioners* 13 (January 2001): 10–12.

Klein, E. J., D. S. Diekema, C. A. Paris, L. Quan, M. Cohen, and K. D. Seidel. "A Randomized, Clinical Trial of Oral Midazolam Plus Placebo Versus Oral Midazolam Plus Oral Transmucosal Fentanyl for Sedation during Laceration Repair." *Pediatrics* 109 (May 2002): 894–897.

Pratt, A. L., N. Burr, and A. O. Grobbelaar. "A Prospective Review of Open Central Slip Laceration Repair and Rehabilitation." *The Journal of Hand Surgery: Journal of the British Society for Surgery of the Hand* 27 (December 2002): 530–534.

KEY TERMS

Debridement—The act of removing any foreign material and damaged or contaminated tissue from a wound to expose surrounding healthy tissue.

Dehiscence—A premature bursting open or splitting along natural or surgical suture lines. A complication of surgery that occurs secondary to poor wound healing.

Laceration—A torn, ragged, mangled wound.

Sutures—Materials used in closing a surgical or traumatic wound.

Vasoconstriction—The diminution of the diameter of blood vessels, leading to decreased blood flow to a part of the body.

Singer, A. J., J. V. Quinn, H. C. Thode Jr., and J. E. Hollander. "Determinants of Poor Outcome after Laceration and Surgical Incision Repair." *Plastic and Reconstructive Surgery* 110 (August 2002): 429–437.

ORGANIZATIONS

The Association of Perioperative Registered Nurses, Inc. (AORN). 2170 South Parker Rd, Suite 300, Denver, CO 80231-5711. (800) 755-2676. <http://www.aorn.org/>.

OTHER

"Cuts and Scrapes." *Mayo Clinic Online.* <http://www.mayoclinic.com/invoke.cfm?objectid=FDEFD23A-F29F-47FB-9A7CD4CF4427D590>.

"A Systematic Approach to Laceration Repair." *Postgraduate Medicine Page.* <http://www.postgradmed.com/issues/2000/04_00/wilson.htm>.

"Wound Repair." *Family Practice Notebook.* <http://www.fp-notebook.com/SUR18.htm>.

Mary Jeanne Krob, MD, FACS
Monique Laberge, PhD

Lactate dehydrogenase isoenzymes test *see* **Liver function tests**

Laminectomy

Definition

A laminectomy is a surgical procedure in which the surgeon removes a portion of the bony arch, or lamina, on the dorsal surface of a vertebra, which is one of the bones that make up the human spinal column. It is done to relieve back pain that has not been helped by more conservative treatments. In most cases a laminectomy is an elective procedure rather than **emergency surgery**. A laminectomy for relief of pain in the lower back is called a lumbar laminectomy or an open decompression.

Purpose

Structure of the spine

In order to understand why removal of a piece of bone from the arch of a vertebra relieves pain, it is helpful to have a brief description of the structure of the spinal column and the vertebrae themselves. In humans, the spine comprises 33 vertebrae, some of which are fused together. There are seven vertebrae in the cervical (neck) part of the spine; 12 vertebrae in the thoracic (chest) region; five in the lumbar (lower back) region; five vertebrae that are fused to form the sacrum; and four vertebrae that are fused to form the coccyx, or tailbone. It is the vertebrae in the lumbar portion of the spine that are most likely to be affected by the disorders that cause back pain.

The 24 vertebrae that are not fused are stacked vertically in an S-shaped column that extends from the tailbone below the waist up to the back of the head. This column is held in alignment by ligaments, cartilage, and muscles. About half the weight of a person's body is carried by the spinal column itself and the other half by the muscles and ligaments that hold the spine in alignment. The bony arches of the laminae on each vertebra form a canal that contains and protects the spinal cord. The spinal cord extends from the base of the brain to the upper part of the lumbar spine, where it ends in a collection of nerve fibers known as the cauda equina, which is a Latin phrase meaning "horse's tail." Other nerves branching out from the spinal cord pass through openings formed by adjoining vertebrae. These openings are known as foramina (singular, foramen).

Between each vertebra is a disk that serves to cushion the vertebrae when a person bends, stretches, or twists the spinal column. The disks also keep the foramina between the vertebrae open so that the spinal nerves can pass through without being pinched or damaged. As people age, the intervertebral disks begin to lose moisture and break down, which reduces the size of the foramina between the vertebrae. In addition, bone spurs may form inside the vertebrae and cause the spinal canal itself to become narrower. Either of these processes can compress the spinal nerves, leading to pain, tingling sensations, or weakness in the lower back and legs. A lumbar laminectomy relieves pressure on the spinal nerves by removing the disk, piece of bone, tumor, or other structure that is causing the compression.

Causes of lower back pain

The disks and vertebrae in the lower back are particularly vulnerable to the effects of aging and daily wear and tear because they bear the full weight of the upper body, even when one is sitting quietly in a chair. When a person bends forward, 50% of the motion occurs at the hips, but the remaining 50% involves the lumbar spine. The force exerted in bending is not evenly divided among the five lumbar vertebrae; the segments between the third and fourth lumbar vertebrae (L3-L4) and the fourth and fifth (L4-L5) are most likely to break down over time. More than 95% of spinal disk operations are performed on the fourth and fifth lumbar vertebrae.

Specific symptoms and disorders that affect the lower back include:

- Sciatica. Sciatica refers to sudden pain felt as radiating from the lower back through the buttocks and down the back of one leg. The pain, which may be experienced as weakness in the leg, a tingling feeling, or a "pins and needles" sensation, runs along the course of the sciatic nerve. Sciatica is a common symptom of a herniated disk.

- Spinal stenosis. Spinal stenosis is a disorder that results from the narrowing of the spinal canal surrounding the spinal cord and eventually compressing the cord. It may result from hereditary factors, from the effects of aging, or from changes in the pattern of blood flow to the lower back. Spinal stenosis is sometimes difficult to diagnose because its early symptoms can be caused by a number of other conditions and because the patient usually has no history of back problems or recent injuries. Imaging studies may be necessary for accurate diagnosis.

- Cauda equina syndrome (CES). Cauda equina syndrome is a rare disorder caused when a ruptured disk, bone fracture, or spinal stenosis put intense pressure on the cauda equina, the collection of spinal nerve roots at the lower end of the spinal cord. CES may be triggered by a fall, automobile accident, or penetrating gunshot injury. It is characterized by loss of sensation or altered sensation in the legs, buttocks, or feet; pain, numbness, or weakness in one or both legs; difficulty walking; or loss of control over bladder and bowel functions. *Cauda equina syndrome is a medical emergency requiring immediate treatment.* If the pressure on the nerves in the cauda equina is not relieved quickly, permanent paralysis and loss of bladder or bowel control may result.

- Herniated disk. The disks between the vertebrae in the spine consist of a fibrous outer part called the annulus and a softer inner nucleus. A disk is said to herniate when the nucleus ruptures and is forced through the outer annulus into the spaces between the vertebrae. The material that is forced out may put pressure on the nerve roots or compress the spinal cord itself. In other cases, the chemicals leaking from the ruptured nucleus may irritate or inflame the spinal nerves. More than 80% of herniated disks affect the spinal nerves associated with the L5 vertebra or the first sacral vertebra.

- Osteoarthritis (OA). OA is a disorder in which the cartilage in the hips, knees, and other joints gradually breaks down, allowing the surfaces of the bones to rub directly against each other. In the spine, OA may result in thickening of the ligaments surrounding the spinal column. As the ligaments increase in size, they may begin to compress the spinal cord.

Factors that increase a person's risk of developing pain in the lower back include:

- Hereditary factors. Some people are born with relatively narrow spinal canals and may develop spinal stenosis fairly early in life.

- Sex. Men are at greater risk of lower back problems than women, in part because they carry a greater proportion of their total body weight in the upper body.

- Age. The intervertebral disks tend to lose their moisture content and become thinner as people get older.

- Occupation. Jobs that require long periods of driving (long-distance trucking; bus, taxi, or limousine operation) are hard on the lower back because of vibrations from the road surface transmitted upward to the spine. Occupations that require heavy lifting (nursing, child care, construction work, airplane maintenance) put extra stress on the lumbar vertebrae. Other high-risk occupations include professional sports, professional dance, assembly line work, foundry work, mining, and mail or package delivery.

- Lifestyle. Wearing high-heeled shoes, carrying heavy briefcases or shoulder bags on one side of the body, or sitting for long periods of time in one position can all throw the spine out of alignment.

- Obesity. Being overweight, particularly if the extra pounds are concentrated in the abdomen, adds to the strain on the muscles and ligaments that support the spinal column.

- Trauma. Injuries to the back from contact sports, falls, criminal assaults, or automobile accidents may lead to misalignment of the vertebrae or a ruptured disk. Traumatic injuries may also trigger the onset of cauda equina syndrome.

Laminectomy

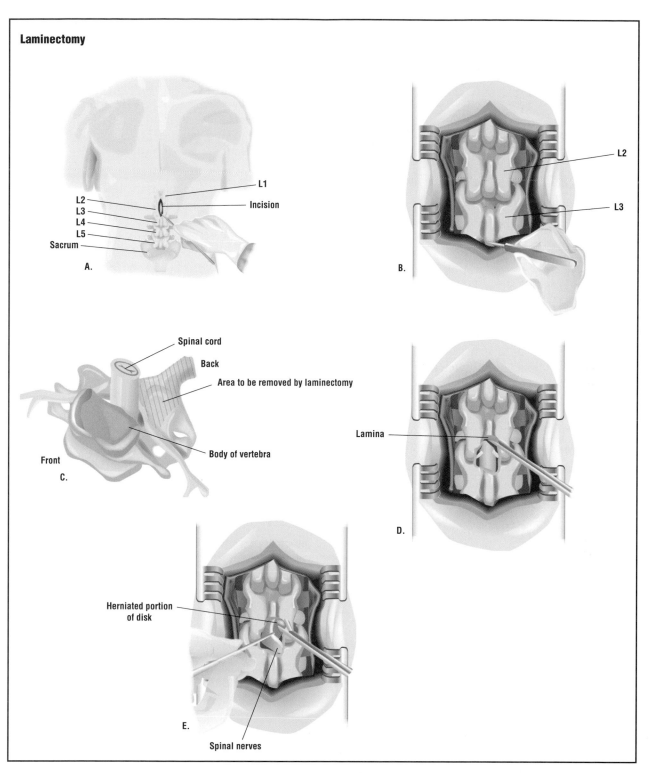

A.

L1
L2
L3
L4
L5
Sacrum
Incision

B.
L2
L3

Spinal cord
Back
Area to be removed by laminectomy
Front
C.
Body of vertebra

Lamina
D.

Herniated portion
of disk
E.
Spinal nerves

In this posterior (from the back) lumbar laminectomy, an incision is made in the patient's back over the lumbar vertebrae (A). The wound is opened with retractors to expose the L2 and L3 vertebrae (B). A piece of bone at the back of the vertebrae is removed (C and D), allowing a damaged disk to be repaired (E). *(Illustration by GGS Inc.)*

WHO PERFORMS THE PROCEDURE AND WHERE IS IT PERFORMED?

A lumbar laminectomy is performed by an orthopedic surgeon or a neurosurgeon. It is performed as an inpatient procedure in a hospital with a department of **orthopedic surgery**. Minimally invasive laminotomies and microdiscectomies are usually performed in **outpatient surgery** facilities.

Demographics

Pain in the lower back is a chronic condition that has been treated in various ways from the beginnings of human medical practice. The earliest description of disorders affecting the lumbar vertebrae was written in 3000 B.C. by an ancient Egyptian surgeon. In the modern world, back pain is responsible for more time lost from work than any other cause except the common cold. Between 10% and 15% of workers' compensation claims are related to chronic pain in the lower back. It is estimated that the direct and indirect costs of back pain to the American economy range between $75 and $80 billion per year.

In the United States, about 13 million people seek medical help each year for the condition. According to the Centers for Disease Control, 14% of all new visits to primary care doctors are related to problems in the lower back. The CDC estimates that 2.4 million adults in the United States are chronically disabled by back pain, with another 2.4 million temporarily disabled. About 70% of people will experience pain in the lower back at some point in their lifetime; on a yearly basis, one person in every five will have some kind of back pain.

Back pain primarily affects the adult population, most commonly people between the ages of 45 and 64. It is more common among men than women, and more common among Caucasians and Hispanics than among African Americans or Asian Americans.

Description

A laminectomy is performed with the patient under general anesthesia, usually positioned lying on the side or stomach. The surgeon begins by making a small straight incision over the damaged vertebra.

The surgeon next uses a retractor to spread apart the muscles and fatty tissue overlying the spine. When the laminae have been reached, the surgeon cuts away part of the bony arch in order to expose the ligamentum flavum, which is a band of yellow tissue attached to the vertebra that helps to support the spinal column and closes in the spaces between the vertebral arches. The surgeon then cuts an opening in the ligamentum flavum in order to reach the spinal canal and expose the compressed nerve. At this point the cause of the compression (herniated disk, tumor, bone spur, or a fragment of the disk that has separated from the remainder) will be visible.

Bone spurs, if any, are removed in order to enlarge the foramina and the spinal canal. If the disk is herniated, the surgeon uses the retractor to move the compressed nerve aside and removes as much of the disk as necessary to relieve pressure on the nerve. The space that was occupied by the disk will be filled eventually by new connective tissue.

If necessary, a **spinal fusion** is performed to stabilize the patient's lower back. A small piece of bone taken from the hip is grafted onto the spine and attached with metal screws or plates to support the lumbar vertebrae.

Following completion of the spinal fusion, the surgeon closes the incision in layers, using different types of sutures for the muscles, connective tissues, and skin. The entire procedure takes one to three hours.

Diagnosis/Preparation

Diagnosis

The differential diagnosis of lower back pain is complicated by the number of possible causes and the patient's reaction to the discomfort. In many cases the patient's perception of back pain is influenced by poor-quality sleep or emotional issues related to occupation or family matters. A primary care doctor will begin by taking a careful medical and occupational history, asking about the onset of the pain as well as its location and other characteristics. Back pain associated with the lumbar spine very often affects the patient's ability to move, and the muscles overlying the affected vertebrae may feel sore or tight. Pain resulting from heavy lifting usually begins within 24 hours of the overexertion. Most patients who do not have a history of chronic pain in the lower back feel better after 48 hours of bed rest with pain medication and either a heating pad or ice pack to relax muscle spasms.

If the patient's pain is not helped by rest and other conservative treatments, he or she will be referred to an orthopedic surgeon for a more detailed evaluation. An orthopedic evaluation includes a **physical examination**, neurological workup, and imaging studies. In the physical examination, the doctor will ask the patient to sit, stand, or walk in order to see how these functions are affected by the pain. The patient may be asked to cough or to lie on a table and lift each leg in turn without bending the knee, as these maneuvers can help to diagnose nerve root disorders. The doctor will also palpate (feel) the patient's spinal column and the overlying muscles and ligaments to determine the external location of any tender spots, bruises, thickening of the ligaments, or other structural abnormalities. The neurological workup will focus on the patient's reflexes and the spinal nerves that affect the functioning of the legs. Imaging studies for lower back pain typically include an x ray study and CT scan of the lower spine, which will reveal bone deformities, narrowing of the intervertebral disks, and loss of cartilage. An MRI may be ordered if spinal stenosis is suspected. In some cases the doctor may order a myelogram, which is an x ray or CT scan of the lumbar spine performed after a special dye has been injected into the spinal fluid.

Lower back pain is one of several common general medical conditions that require the doctor to assess the possibility that the patient has a concurrent psychiatric disorder. Such diagnoses as somatization disorder or pain disorder do not mean that the patient's physical symptoms are imaginary or that they should not receive surgical or medical treatment. Rather, a psychiatric diagnosis indicates that the patient is allowing the back pain to become the central focus of life or responding to it in other problematic ways. Some researchers in Europe as well as North America think that the frequency of lower back problems in workers' disability claims reflect emotional dissatisfaction with work as well as physical stresses related to specific jobs.

Preparation

Most hospitals require patients to have the following tests before a laminectomy: a complete physical examination; **complete blood count (CBC)**; an electrocardiogram (EKG); a urine test; and tests that measure the speed of blood clotting.

Aspirin and arthritis medications should be discontinued seven to 10 days before a laminectomy because they thin the blood and affect clotting time. Patients should provide the surgeon and anesthesiologist with a complete list of all medications, including over-the-counter and herbal preparations, that they take on a regular basis.

The patient is asked to stop smoking at least a week before surgery and to take nothing by mouth after midnight before the procedure.

Aftercare

Aftercare following a laminectomy begins in the hospital. Most patients will remain in the hospital for one

---

QUESTIONS TO ASK THE DOCTOR

- What conservative treatments would you recommend for my lower back pain?
- How much time should I allow for conservative therapies to demonstrate effectiveness before considering surgery?
- Am I a candidate for a laminotomy and microdiscectomy?
- How many laminectomies have you performed?

---

to three days after the procedure. During this period the patient will be given fluids and antibiotic medications intravenously to prevent infection. Medications for pain will be given every three to four hours, or through a device known as a PCA (patient-controlled anesthesia). The PCA is a small pump that delivers a dose of medication into the IV when the patient pushes a button. To get the lungs back to normal functioning, a respiratory therapist will ask the patient to do some simple breathing exercises and begin walking within several hours of surgery.

Aftercare during the hospital stay is also intended to lower the risk of a venous thromboembolism (VTE), or blood clot in the deep veins of the leg. Prevention of VTE involves medications to thin the blood and wearing compression stockings or boots.

Most surgeons prefer to see patients one week after surgery to remove stitches and check for any postoperative complications. Patients should not drive or return to work before their checkup. A second follow-up examination is usually done four to eight weeks after the laminectomy.

Patients can help speed their recovery by taking short walks on a daily basis; avoiding sitting or standing in the same position for long periods of time; taking brief naps during the day; and sleeping on the stomach or the side. They may take a daily bath or shower without needing to cover the incision. The incision should be carefully patted dry, however, rather than rubbed.

Risks

Risks associated with a laminectomy include:
- bleeding
- infection
- damage to the spinal cord or other nerves
- weakening or loss of function in the legs

KEY TERMS

Cauda equina—The collection of spinal nerve roots that lie inside the spinal column below the end of the spinal cord. The name comes from the Latin for "horse's tail."

Cauda equina syndrome (CES)—A group of symptoms characterized by numbness or pain in the legs and/or loss of bladder and bowel control, caused by compression and paralysis of the nerve roots in the cauda equina. CES is a medical emergency.

Chiropractic—A system of therapy based on the notion that health and disease are related to the interactions between the brain and the nervous system. Treatment involves manipulation and adjustment of the segments of the spinal column. Chiropractic is considered a form of alternative medicine.

Decompression—Any surgical procedure done to relieve pressure on a nerve or other part of the body. A laminectomy is sometimes called an open decompression.

Dorsal—Referring to a position closer to the back than to the stomach. The laminae in the spinal column are located on the dorsal side of each vertebra.

Dura—A tough fibrous membrane that covers and protects the spinal cord.

Foramen (plural, foramina)—The medical term for a natural opening or passage. The foramina of the spinal column are openings between the vertebrae for the spinal nerves to branch off from the spinal cord.

Laminae (singular, lamina)—The broad plates of bone on the upper surface of the vertebrae that fuse together at the midline to form a bony covering over the spinal canal.

Laminotomy—A less invasive alternative to a laminectomy in which a hole is drilled through the lamina.

- blood clots
- leakage of spinal fluid resulting from tears in the dura, the protective membrane that covers the spinal cord
- worsening of back pain

Normal results

Normal results depend on the cause of the patient's lower back pain; most patients can expect considerable relief from pain and some improvement in functioning. There is some disagreement among surgeons about the success rate of laminectomies, however, which appears to be due to the fact that the operation is generally done to improve quality of life—cauda equina syndrome is the only indication for an emergency laminectomy. Different sources report success rates between 26% and 99%, with 64% as the average figure. According to one study, 31% of patients were dissatisfied with the results of the operation, possibly because they may have had unrealistic expectations of the results.

Morbidity and mortality rates

The mortality rate for a lumbar laminectomy is between 0.8% and 1%. Rates of complications depend partly on whether a spinal fusion is performed as part of the procedure; while the general rate of complications following a lumbar laminectomy is given as 6–7%, the rate rises to 12% of a spinal fusion has been done.

Alternatives

Conservative treatments

Surgery for lower back pain is considered a treatment of last resort, with the exception of cauda equina syndrome. Patients should always try one or more conservative approaches before consulting a surgeon about a laminectomy. In addition, most health insurers will require proof that the surgery is necessary, since the average total cost of a lumbar laminectomy is $85,000.

Some conservative approaches that have been found to relieve lower back pain include:

- Analgesic or muscle relaxant medications. **Analgesics** are drugs given to relieve pain. The most commonly prescribed pain medications are aspirin or NSAIDs. **Muscle relaxants** include methocarbamol, cyclobenzaprine, or diazepam.

- Epidural injections. Epidural injections are given directly into the space surrounding the spinal cord. **Corticosteroids** are the medications most commonly given by this route, but preliminary reports indicate that epidural injections of indomethacin are also effective in relieving recurrent pain in the lower back.

- Rest. Bed rest for 48 hours usually relieves acute lower back pain resulting from muscle strain.

KEY TERMS (contd.)

Ligamenta flava (singular, ligamentum flavum)—A series of bands of tissue that are attached to the vertebrae in the spinal column. They help to hold the spine straight and to close the spaces between the laminar arches. The Latin name means "yellow band(s)."

Lumbar—Pertaining to the part of the back between the chest and the pelvis.

Myelogram—A special type of x ray study of the spinal cord, made after a contrast medium has been injected into the space surrounding the cord.

Osteopathy—A system of therapy that uses standard medical and surgical methods of diagnosis and treatment while emphasizing the importance of proper body alignment and manipulative treatment of musculoskeletal disorders. Osteopathy is considered mainstream primary care medicine rather than an alternative system.

Pain disorder—A psychiatric disorder in which pain in one or more parts of the body is caused or made worse by psychological factors. The lower back is one of the most common sites for pain related to this disorder.

Retractor—An instrument used during surgery to hold an incision open and pull back underlying layers of tissue.

Sciatica—Pain in the lower back, buttock, or leg along the course of the sciatic nerve.

Somatization disorder—A chronic condition in which psychological stresses are converted into physical symptoms that interfere with work and relationships. Lower back pain is a frequent complaint of patients with somatization disorder.

Spinal stenosis—Narrowing of the canals in the vertebrae or around the nerve roots, causing pressure on the spinal cord and nerves.

Vertebra (plural, vertebrae)—One of the bones of the spinal column. There are 33 vertebrae in the human spine.

- Appropriate **exercise**. Brief walks are recommended as a good form of exercise to improve blood circulation, particularly after surgery. In addition, there are several simple exercises that can be done at home to strengthen the muscles of the lower back. A short pamphlet entitled *Back Pain Exercises* may be downloaded free of charge from the American Academy of Orthopedic Surgeons (AAOS) web site.

- Losing weight. People who are severely obese may wish to consider weight reduction surgery to reduce the stress on their spine as well as their heart and respiratory system.

- Occupational modifications or change. Lower back pain related to the patient's occupation can sometimes be eased by taking periodic breaks from sitting in one position; by using a desk and chair proportioned to one's height; by learning to use the muscles of the thighs when lifting heavy objects rather than the lower back muscles; and by maintaining proper posture when standing or sitting. In some cases the patient may be helped by changing occupations.

- Physical therapy. A licensed physical therapist can be helpful in identifying the patient's functional back problems and planning a course of treatment to improve flexibility, strength, and range of motion.

- Osteopathic manipulative treatment (OMT). Osteopathic physicians (DOs) receive the same training in medicine and surgery as MDs; however, they are also trained to evaluate postural and spinal abnormalities and to perform several different manual techniques for relief of back pain. An article published in the *New England Journal of Medicine* in 1999 reported that OMT was as effective as physical therapy and standard medication in relieving lower back pain, with fewer side effects and lower health care costs. OMT is recommended in the United Kingdom as a very low-risk treatment that is more effective than bed rest or mild analgesics.

- Transcutaneous electrical nerve stimulation (TENS). TENS is a treatment technique developed in the late 1960s that delivers a mild electrical current to stimulate nerves through electrodes attached to the skin overlying a painful part of the body. It is thought that TENS works by stimulating the production of endorphins, which are the body's natural painkilling compounds.

Surgical alternatives

The most common surgical alternative to laminectomy is a minimally invasive laminotomy and/or microdiscectomy. In this procedure, which takes about an hour, the surgeon makes a 0.5-in (1.3-cm) incision in the lower back and uses a series of small dilators to separate the layers of muscle and fatty tissue over the spine rather than cutting through them with a scalpel. A tube-shaped retractor is inserted to expose the part of the lamina over the nerve root. The surgeon then uses a power drill to make a small hole in the lamina to expose the nerve itself. After the nerve has been moved aside with the retractor, a small grasping device is used to remove the herniated portion or fragments of the damaged spinal disk.

The advantages of these minimally invasive procedures are fewer complications and a shortened recovery time for the patient. The average postoperative stay is three hours. In addition, 90% of patients are pleased with the results.

Complementary and alternative (CAM) approaches

Two alternative methods of treating back disorders that have been shown to help many patients are acupuncture and chiropractic. Chiropractic is based on the belief that the body has abilities to heal itself provided that nerve impulses can move freely between the brain and the rest of the body. Chiropractors manipulate the segments of the spine in order to bring them into proper alignment and restore the nervous system to proper functioning. Many are qualified to perform acupuncture as well as chiropractic adjustments of the vertebrae and other joints. Several British and Swedish studies have reported that acupuncture and chiropractic are at least as effective as other conservative measures in relieving pain in the lower back.

Movement therapies, including yoga, tai chi, and gentle stretching exercises, may be useful in maintaining or improving flexibility and range of motion in the spine. A qualified yoga instructor can work with the patient's doctor before or after surgery to put together an individualized set of beneficial stretching and breathing exercises. The Alexander technique is a type of movement therapy that is often helpful to patients who need to improve their posture.

See also Disk removal.

Resources

BOOKS

American Psychiatric Association. "Somatoform Disorders." In *Diagnostic and Statistical Manual of Mental Disorders.* 4th ed. Revised text. Washington, DC: American Psychiatric Association, 2000.

"Low Back Pain." In *The Merck Manual of Diagnosis and Therapy*, edited by Mark H. Beers, MD, and Robert Berkow, MD. Whitehouse Station, NJ: Merck Research Laboratories, 1999.

"Nerve Root Disorders." In *The Merck Manual of Diagnosis and Therapy*, edited by Mark H. Beers, MD, and Robert Berkow, MD. Whitehouse Station, NJ: Merck Research Laboratories, 1999.

"Osteoarthritis." In *The Merck Manual of Diagnosis and Therapy*, edited by Mark H. Beers, MD, and Robert Berkow, MD. Whitehouse Station, NJ: Merck Research Laboratories, 1999.

Pelletier, Kenneth R., MD. "Acupuncture." In *The Best Alternative Medicine.* New York: Simon & Schuster, 2002.

Pelletier, Kenneth R., MD. "Chiropractic." In *The Best Alternative Medicine.* New York: Simon & Schuster, 2002.

PERIODICALS

Aldrete, J. A. "Epidural Injections of Indomethacin for Postlaminectomy Syndrome: A Preliminary Report." *Anesthesia and Analgesia* 96 (February 2003): 463–468.

Braverman, D. L., J. J. Ericken, R. V. Shah, and D. J. Franklin. "Interventions in Chronic Pain Management. 3. New Frontiers in Pain Management: Complementary Techniques." *Archives of Physical Medicine and Rehabilitation* 84 (March 2003) (3 Suppl 1): S45–S49.

Carlsson, C. P., and B. H. Sjolund. "Acupuncture for Chronic Low Back Pain: A Randomized Placebo-Controlled Study with Long-Term Follow-Up." *Clinical Journal of Pain* 17 (December 2001): 296–305.

Harvey, E., A. K. Burton, J. K. Moffett, and A. Breen. "Spinal Manipulation for Low-Back Pain: A Treatment Package Agreed to by the UK Chiropractic, Osteopathy and Physiotherapy Professional Associations." *Manual Therapy* 8 (February 2003): 46–51.

Hurwitz, E. L., H. Morgenstern, P. Harber, et al. "A Randomized Trial of Medical Care With and Without Physical Therapy and Chiropractic Care With and Without Physical Modalities for Patients with Low Back Pain: 6-Month Follow-Up Outcomes from the UCLA Low Back Pain Study." *Spine* 27 (October 15, 2002): 2193–2204.

Nasca, R. J. "Lumbar Spinal Stenosis: Surgical Considerations." *Journal of the Southern Orthopedic Association* 11 (Fall 2002): 127–134.

Pengel, H. M., C. G. Maher, and K. M. Refshauge. "Systematic Review of Conservative Interventions for Subacute Low Back Pain." *Clinical Rehabilitation* 16 (December 2002): 811–820.

Sleigh, Bryan C., MD, and Ibrahim El Nihum, MD. "Lumbar Laminectomy." *eMedicine.* August 8, 2002 [cited May 3, 2003]. <http://www.emedicine.com/aaem/topic500.htm>.

Wang, Michael Y., Barth A. Green, Sachin Shah, et al. "Complications Associated with Lumbar Stenosis Surgery in Patients Older Than 75 Years of Age." *Neurosurgical Focus* 14 (February 2003): 1–4.

ORGANIZATIONS

American Academy of Neurological and Orthopedic Surgeons (AANOS). 2300 South Rancho Drive, Suite 202, Las Vegas, NV 89102. (702) 388-7390. <http://www.aanos.org>.

American Academy of Neurology. 1080 Montreal Avenue, Saint Paul, MN 55116. (800) 879-1960 or (651) 695-2717. <http://www.aan.com>.

American Academy of Orthopedic Surgeons (AAOS). 6300 North River Road, Rosemont, IL 60018. (847) 823-7186 or (800) 346-AAOS. <http://www.aaos.org>.

American Chiropractic Association. 1701 Clarendon Blvd., Arlington, VA 22209. (800) 986-4636. <http://www.amerchiro.org>.

American Osteopathic Association (AOA). 142 East Ontario Street, Chicago, IL 60611. (800) 621-1773 or (312) 202-8000. <http://www.aoa-net.org>.

American Physical Therapy Association (APTA). 1111 North Fairfax Street, Alexandria, VA 22314. (703)684-APTA or (800) 999-2782. <http://www.apta.org>.

National Institute of Arthritis and Musculoskeletal and Skin Diseases (NIAMS) Information Clearinghouse. National Institutes of Health, 1 AMS Circle, Bethesda, MD 20892. (301) 495-4484. TTY: (301) 565-2966. <http://www.niams.nih.gov>.

OTHER

American Academy of Orthopedic Surgeons (AAOS). *Back Pain Exercises.* March 2000 [cited May 5, 2003]. <http://www.orthoinfo.aaos.org>.

American Physical Therapy Association. *Taking Care of Your Back.* 2003 [cited May 4, 2003]. <http://www.apta.org/Consumer/ptandyourbody/back>.

Waddell, G., A. McIntosh, A. Hutchinson, et al. *Clinical Guidelines for the Management of Acute Low Back Pain.* London, UK: Royal College of General Practitioners, 2000.

Rebecca Frey, Ph.D.

Laparoscopic cholecystectomy *see*
Cholecystectomy

Laparoscopy

Definition

Laparoscopy is a minimally invasive procedure used as a diagnostic tool and surgical procedure that is performed to examine the abdominal and pelvic organs, or the thorax, head, or neck. Tissue samples can also be collected for biopsy using laparoscopy and malignancies treated when it is combined with other therapies. Laparoscopy can also be used for some cardiac and vascular procedures.

Purpose

Laparoscopy is performed to examine the abdominal and pelvic organs to diagnose certain conditions and—depending on the condition—can be used to perform surgery. Laparoscopy is commonly used in gynecology to examine the outside of the uterus, the fallopian tubes, and the ovaries—particularly in pelvic pain cases

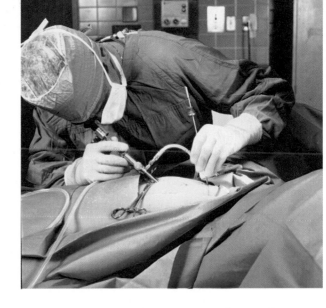

This surgeon is performing a laparoscopic procedure on a patient. *(Photo Researchers, Inc. Reproduced by permission.)*

where the underlying cause cannot be determined using diagnostic imaging (ultrasound and computed tomography). Examples of gynecologic conditions diagnosed using laparoscopy include endometriosis, ectopic pregnancy, ovarian cysts, pelvic inflammatory disease [PID], infertility, and cancer. Laparoscopy is used in **general surgery** to examine the abdominal organs, including the gallbladder, bile ducts, the liver, the appendix, and the intestines.

During the laparoscopic surgical procedure, certain conditions can be treated using instruments and devices specifically designed for laparoscopy. Medical devices that can be used in conjunction with laparoscopy include surgical lasers and electrosurgical units. Laparoscopic surgery is now preferred over open surgery for several types of procedures because of its minimally invasive nature and its association with fewer complications.

Microlaparoscopy can be performed in the physician's office using smaller laparoscopes. Common clinical applications in gynecology include pain mapping (for endometriosis), sterilization, and fertility procedures. Common applications in general surgery include evaluation of chronic and acute abdominal pain (as in appendicitis), basic trauma evaluation, biopsies, and evaluation of abdominal masses.

Laparoscopy is commonly used by gynecologists, urologists, and general surgeons for abdominal and pelvic applications. Laparoscopy is also being used by orthopedic surgeons for spinal applications and by cardiac surgeons for **minimally invasive heart surgery**. As of 2003, procedures under investigation for possible laparoscopy included **thyroidectomy** and **parathyroidectomy**.

Demographics

At first, laparoscopy was only been performed on young, healthy adults, but the use of this technique has greatly expanded. Populations on whom laparoscopies are now performed include infants, children, the elderly, the obese, and those with chronic disease states, such as cancer. The applications of this type of surgery have grown considerably over the years to include a variety of patient populations, and will continue to do so with the refinement of laparascopic techniques.

Description

Laparoscopy is typically performed in the hospital under general anesthesia, although some laparoscopic procedures can be performed using local anesthetic agents. Once under anesthesia, a urinary catheter is inserted into the patient's bladder for urine collection. To begin the procedure, a small incision is made just below the navel and a cannula or trocar is inserted into the incision to accommodate the insertion of the laparoscope. Other incisions may be made in the abdomen to allow the insertion of additional laparoscopic instrumentation. A laparoscopic insufflation device is used to inflate the abdomen with carbon dioxide gas to create a space in which the laparoscopic surgeon can maneuver the instruments. After the laparoscopic diagnosis and treatment are completed, the laparoscope, cannula, and other instrumentation are removed, and the incision is sutured and bandaged.

Laparoscopes have integral cameras for transmitting images during the procedure, and are available in various sizes depending upon the type of procedure performed. The images from the laparoscope are transmitted to a viewing monitor that the surgeon uses to visualize the internal anatomy and guide any surgical procedure. Video and photographic equipment are also used to document the surgery, and may be used postoperatively to explain the results of the procedure to the patient.

Robotic systems are available to assist with laparoscopy. A robotic arm, attached to the operating table may be used to hold and position the laparoscope. This serves to reduce unintentional camera movement that is common when a surgical assistant holds the laparoscope. The surgeon controls the robotic arm movement by foot pedal with voice-activated command, or with a handheld control panel.

Microlaparoscopy has become more common over the past few years. The procedure involves the use of smaller laparoscopes (that is, 2 mm compared to 5–10

mm for hospital laparoscopy), with the patient undergoing local anesthesia with conscious sedation (during which the patient remains awake but very relaxed) in a physician's office. Video and photographic equipment, previously explained, may be used.

Laparoscopy has been explored in combination with other therapies for the treatment of certain types of malignancies, including pelvic and aortic lymph node dissection, ovarian cancer, and early cervical cancer. Laparoscopic radiofrequency ablation is a technique whereby laproscopy assists in the delivery of radiofrequency probes that distribute pulses to a tumor site. The pulses generate heat in malignant tumor cells and destroys them.

The introduction of items such as temperature-controlled instruments, **surgical instruments** with greater rotation and articulation, improved imaging systems, and multiple robotic devices will expand the utility of laparoscopic techniques in the future. The skills of surgeons will be enhanced as well with further development of training simulators and computer technology.

Diagnosis/Preparation

Before undergoing laparoscopic surgery, the patient should be prepared by the doctor for the procedure both psychologically and physically. It is very important that the patient receive realistic counseling before surgery and prior to giving **informed consent**. This includes discussion about further open abdominal surgery (laparotomy) that may be required during laparoscopic surgery, information about potential complications during surgery, and the possible need for blood transfusions. In the case of diagnostic laparoscopy for chronic pelvic pain, the procedure may simply indicate that all organs are normal and the patient should be prepared for this possibility. The surgery may be explained using pictures, models, videotapes, and movies. It is especially important for the patient to be able to ask questions and express concerns. It may be helpful, for the patient to have a family member or friend present during discussions with the doctor. Such conversations could understandably cause anxiety, and information relayed may not be adequately recalled under such circumstances.

There is usually a presurgical exam two weeks before the surgery to gather a medical history and obtain blood and urine samples for laboratory testing. It is important that the patient inform the doctor completely about any prior surgeries, medical conditions, or medications taken on a regular basis, including such **nonsteroidal anti-inflammatory drugs** (NSAIDs) as **aspirin**. Patients taking blood thinners like Coumadin or Heparin (generic name: warfarin) should not adjust their medication themselves, but should speak with their prescribing doctors regarding

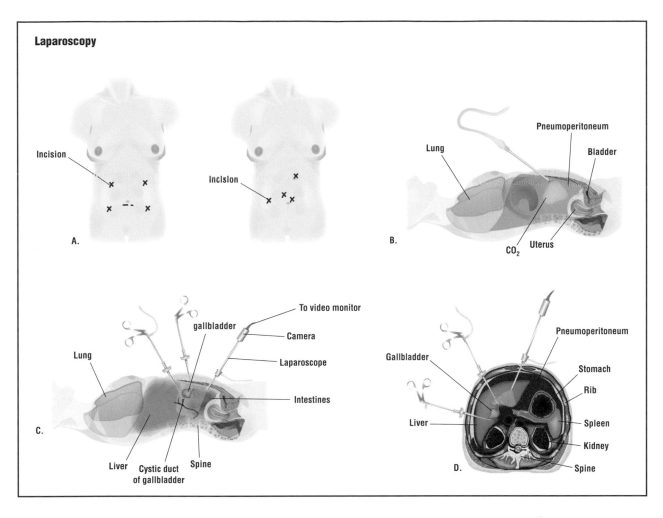

Laparoscopy

The surgeon has a choice of incision options for laparoscopy, depending on the needs of the procedure (A). In this abdominal procedure, carbon dioxide is pumped into the cavity to create a condition called pneumoperitoneum, which allows the surgeon easier access to internal structures. The laparoscope is connected to a video monitor, and special forceps are used to carry out any necessary procedure (C and D) *(Illustration by GGS Inc.)*

their upcoming surgery. (Patients should never adjust dosage without their doctors' approval. This is especially important for elderly patients, asthmatics, those with hypertension, or those who are on ACE inhibitors.) If a tubal dye study is planned during the procedure, the patient may also be required to provide information on menstrual history. For some procedures, an autologous (self) blood donation may be suggested prior to the surgery to replace blood that may be lost during the procedure. Chest x rays may also be required. For some obese patients, weight loss may be necessary prior to surgery.

Immediately before to surgery, there are several preoperative steps that the patient may be advised to take. The patient should shower at least 24 hours prior to the surgery, and gently but thoroughly cleanse the umbilicus (belly button) with antibacterial soap and water using a cotton-tipped swab. Because laparoscopy requires general anesthesia in most cases, the patient may be asked to eat lightly 24 hours prior to surgery and fast at least 12 hours prior to surgery. Bowel cleansing with a laxative may also required, allowing the it to be more easily visualized and to prevent complications in the unlikely event of bowel injury. Those who are have diabetes or have hypoglycemia may wish to schedule their procedures early in the morning to avoid low blood sugar reactions. The patient should follow the directions of the hospital staff, arriving early on the day of surgery to sign paperwork and to be screened by the anesthesiology staff. Questions will be asked regarding current medications and dosages, allergies to medication, previous experiences with anesthesia (that is, allergic reactions, and previous experiences regarding time-to-consciousness), and a variety of other questions. It is often helpful for the patient to make a list of this information beforehand so that the information can be easily retrieved when requested by the hospital staff.

Aftercare

Following laparoscopy, patients are required to remain in a recovery area until the immediate effects of anesthesia subside and until normal voiding is accomplished (especially if a urinary catheter was used during the surgery). **Vital signs** are monitored to ensure that there are no reactions to anesthesia or internal injuries present. There may be some nausea and/or vomiting, which may be reduced by the use of the propofol anesthetic for healthy patients undergoing elective procedures such as **tubal ligation**, diagnostic laparoscopy, or hernia repair. Laparoscopy is usually an outpatient procedure and patients are discharged from the recovery area within a few hours after the procedure. For elderly patients and those with other medical conditions, recovery may be slower. Patients with more serious medical conditions, or patients undergoing emergency laparoscopy, an overnight hospital stay or a stay of several days may be required.

Discharged patients will receive instructions regarding activity level, medications, postoperative dietary modifications, and possible side effects of the procedure. It may be helpful to have a friend or family member present when these instructions are given, as the after-effects of anesthesia may cause some temporary confusion. Postoperative instructions may include information on when one might resume normal activities such as bathing, housework, and driving. Depending on the nature of the laparoscopic procedure and the patient's medical condition, daily activity may be restricted for a few days and strenuous during administration of anesthesia may cause some soreness. Additionally, shoulder pain may persist as long as 36 hours after surgery. Pain-relieving medications and **antibiotics** may be prescribed for several days postoperatively.

Patients will be instructed to watch for signs of a urinary tract infection (UTI) or unusual pain; either may indicate organ injury. It is important to understand the difference between normal discomfort and pain, because pain may indicate a problem. Patients may also experience an elevated temperature, and occasionally "postlaparoscopy syndrome"; this condition is similar in appearance to peritonitis (marked by abdominal pain, constipation, vomiting, and fever) that disappears shortly after surgery without antibiotics. However, any postoperative symptoms that cause concern for the patient should be discussed with the doctor, so that any fears can be alleviated and recovery can be accomplished. Due to the after-effects of anesthesia, patients should not drive themselves home.

It is advisable for someone to stay with the patient for a few hours following the procedure, in case complications arise. Injury to an organ might not be readily apparent for several days after the procedure. The physical signs that should be watched for and reported immediately include:

- fever and chills
- abdominal distension
- vomiting
- difficulty urinating
- sharp and unusual pain in the abdomen or bowel
- redness at the incision site, which indicate infection
- discharge from any places where tubes were inserted or incisions were made

Additional complications may include a urinary tract infection (resulting from catheterization) and minor infection of the incision site. An injury to the ureter may be indicated by abdominal distention or a pain in the flank. Additional testing may be required if a complication is suspected.

Risks

Complications may be associated with the laparoscopy procedure in general, or may be specific to the type of operation that is performed. Patients should consult with their doctors regarding the types of risks that are specific for their procedures. The most serious complication that can occur during laparoscopy is laceration of a major abdominal blood vessel resulting from improper positioning, inadequate insufflation (inflation) of the abdomen, abnormal pelvic anatomy, and too much force exerted during scope insertion. Thin patients with well-developed abdominal muscles are at higher risk, since the aorta may only be an inch or so below the skin. Obese patients are also at higher risk because more forceful and deeper needle and scope penetration is required. During laparoscopy, there is also a risk of bleeding from blood vessels, and adhesions may require repair by open surgery if bleeding cannot be stopped using laparoscopic instrumentation. In laparoscopic procedures that use electrosurgical devices, burns to the incision site are possible due to passage of electrical current through the laparoscope caused by a fault or malfunction in the equipment.

Complications related to insufflation of the abdominal cavity include gas inadvertently entering a blood vessel and causing an embolism, pneumothorax, or subcutaneous emphysema. One common but not serious side effect of insufflation is pain in the shoulder and upper chest area for a day or two following the procedure.

Any abdominal surgery, including laparoscopy, carries the risk of unintentional organ injury (punctures and perforations). For example, the bowel, bladder, ureters, or fallopian tubes may be injured during the laparoscopic procedure. Many times these injuries are unavoidable due to the patient's anatomy or medical condition. Patients at higher risk for bowel injury include those with chronic bowel disease, PID, a history of pervious abdominal surgery, or severe endometriosis. Some types of laparoscopic procedures have a higher risk of organ injury. For instance, during laparoscopic removal of endometriosis adhesions or ovaries, the ureters may be injured due to their proximity to each other.

Several clinical studies have shown that the complication rate during laparoscopy is associated with inadequate surgeon experience. Surgeons who are more experienced in laparoscopic procedures have fewer complications than those performing their first 100 cases.

Normal results

In diagnostic laparoscopy, the surgeon will be able to see signs of a disease or condition (for example, endometriosis adhesions; ovarian cysts; diseased gallbladder)immediately, and can either treat the condition surgically or proceed with appropriate medical management. In diagnostic laparoscopy, biopsies may be taken of tissue in questionable areas, and laboratory results will govern medical treatment. In therapeutic laparoscopy, the surgeon performs a procedure that rectifies a known medical problem, such as hernia repair or appendix removal. Because laparoscopy is minimally invasive compared to open surgery, patients may experience less trauma and postoperative discomfort, have fewer procedural complications, have a shorter hospital stay, and return more quickly to daily activities. The results will vary, however, depending on the patients's condition and type of treatment.

Morbidity and mortality rates

Laparoscopic surgery, like most surgeries, is not without risk. Risks should be thoroughly explained to the patient. Complications from laparoscopic surgeries arise in 1–5% of the cases, with a mortality of about 0.05%. Complications may arise from the laparoscopic entry during procedure, and the risks vary depending on the elements specific to a particular procedure. For example, the risk of injury to the common bile duct in laparoscopic biliary surgery is 0.3–0.6% of cases. The factors that contribute to morbidity are currently under study and debate. Injury may occur to blood vessels and internal organs. Some studies examining malpractice data indicate that trocar injury to the bowel or blood vessels may account up to one-fourth of laparoscopic medical claims. It has been suggested that these injuries can be reduced by alterations in the placement and use of the Verses needle, or by using an open technique of trocar insertion in which a blunt cannula (non-bladed) is inserted into the abdominal cavity through an incision. The insertion of

---

QUESTIONS TO ASK THE DOCTOR

- Will this surgery be covered by my insurance? Will any postsurgical care that I require also be covered?

- What do I need to do to prepare for the surgery? Are there any restrictions on diet, fluid intake, or other measures?

- Are there any medications that should be stopped prior to the surgery?

- Does my medical history pose any potential problems that need to be considered before undergoing this procedure?

- What is your (the doctor's) training in performing this surgery? Will you perform the actual surgery or will a trainee?

- What aftereffects can I expect?

- Are there any post-surgical symptoms that might indicate a complication that I should report, and to whom should these questions be directed? What post-surgical symptoms should be considered "normal" and how might discomfort be relieved?

- What is the expected recovery period from this procedure?

- What special care or self-care is required following this surgery?

---

secondary trocars may be of particular interest as a risk factor. There is still some debate, however, as to which method of trocar insertion is most appropriate in a particular situation, as no technique is without risk. The most commonly cited injury in laparoscopic malpractice claims has been injury to the bile duct (66%). Proper identification of this structure by an experienced surgeon, or by a cholangiogram, may reduce this type of injury. Other areas of the body may be injured during access including the stomach, bladder, and liver. Hemorrhages may also occur during the operation.

Laparoscopic entry injuries have been the subject of recent study. Data collected from insurance companies and medical device regulation indicate that bowel and vascular injuries may account for 76% of the injuries that occur when a primary port is created. Delayed recognition of bowel injuries was noted to be an important factor in mortality. The risk of possible injury or death in laparoscopy depends on such factors as the

WHO PERFORMS THE PROCEDURE AND WHERE IS IT PERFORMED?

Laparoscopy may be performed by a gynecologist, general surgeon, gastroenterologist, or other physician—depending upon the patient's condition. An anesthesiologist is required during the procedure to administer general and/or local anesthesia and to perform patient monitoring. Nurses and surgical technicians/assistants are needed during the procedure to assist with scope positioning, video system adjustments and image recording, and laparoscopic instrumentation.

anatomy of the patient, the force of entry, and the type operative procedure being performed.

Alternatives

The alternatives to laparoscopy vary, depending on the medical condition being treated. Laparotomy (open abdominal surgery with larger incision) may be pursued when further visualization is needed to treat the condition, such as in the case of pain of severe endometriosis with deeper lesions. For those female patients with pelvic masses, transvaginal sonography may be a helpful technique in obtaining information about whether such masses are malignant, assisting in the choice between laparoscopy or laparotomy.

Resources

BOOKS

Merrell, Ronald C., ed. *Laparoscopic Surgery.* New York: Springer-Verlag New York, Inc., 1999.

Pasic, Resad P., Ronald L. Levine. *A Practical Manual of Laparoscopy: A Clinical Cookbook.* New York: The Parthenon Publishing Group, 2002.

Schier, Felix. *Laparoscopy in Children.* Berlin: Springer, 2003.

Soderstrom, Richard M., ed. *Operative Laparoscopy,* 2nd ed. Philadelphia: Lippincott-Raven, 1998.

Webb, Maurice, ed. J. *Mayo Clinic Manual of Pelvic Surgery,* 2nd ed. Philadelphia, 2000.

Zucker, Karl A., ed. *Surgical Laparoscopy,* 2nd ed. Philadelphia, 2001.

PERIODICALS

Abu-Rustum, Nadeem R. "Laparoscopy 2003: Oncologic Perspective." *Clinical Obstetrics and Gynecology* 46, no.1 (March 2003): 61-69.

Bieber, Eric. "Laparoscopy: Past, Present, and Future." *Clinical Obstetrics and Gynecology* 46, no.1 (March 2003): 3–14.

Boike, Guy M., and Brian Dobbins. "New Equipment for Operative Laparoscopy." *Contemporary OB/GYN,* no. 2 (April 1998). <http://consumer.pdr.net/consumer/psrecord.htm>.

KEY TERMS

Ascites—Accumulation of fluid in the abdominal cavity; laparoscopy may be used to determine its cause.

Cholecystitis—Inflammation of the gallbladder, often diagnosed using laparoscopy.

Electrosurgical device—A medical device that uses electrical current to cauterize or coagulate tissue during surgical procedures; often used in conjunction with laparoscopy.

Embolism—Blockage of an artery by a clot, air or gas, or foreign material. Gas embolism may occur as a result of insufflation of the abdominal cavity during laparoscopy.

Endometriosis—A disease involving occurrence of endometrial tissue (lining of the uterus) outside the uterus in the abdominal cavity; often diagnosed and treated using laparoscopy.

Hysterectomy—Surgical removal of the uterus; often performed laparoscopically.

Insufflation—Inflation of the abdominal cavity using carbon dioxide; performed prior to laparoscopy to give the surgeon space to maneuver surgical equipment.

Oophorectomy—Surgical removal of the ovaries; often performed laparoscopically.

Pneumothorax—Air or gas in the pleural space (lung area) that may occur as a complication of laparoscopy and insufflation.

Subcutaneous emphysema—A pathologic accumulation of air underneath the skin resulting from improper insufflation technique.

Trocar—A small sharp instrument used to puncture the abdomen at the beginning of the laparoscopic procedure.

Chandler, J.G., S.L. Corson, L.W. Way. "Three Spectra of Laparoscopic Entry Access Injuries." *Journal of American College of Surgeons* 192, no.4 (April 2001):478–490.

ORGANIZATIONS

American College of Obstetricians and Gynecologists. 409 12th Street SW, P.O. Box 96920, Washington, DC 20090-6920. <http://www.acog.org>.

Society of American Gastrointestinal Endoscopic Surgeons (SAGES). 2716 Ocean Park Boulevard, Suite 3000, Santa Monica, CA 90405. (310) 314-2404. <http://www.endoscopy-sages.com>.

Society of Laparoendoscopic Surgeons. 7330 SW 62nd Place, Suite 410, Miami, FL 33143-4825. (305) 665-9959. <http://www.sls.org>.

OTHER

Agency for Healthcare Research and Quality. <http://www.
    webmm.ahrq.gov/cases.aspx?ic=3>.
"Diagnostic Laparoscopy." Society of Gastrointestinal Endo-
    scopic Surgeons. <http://www.sages.org/pi_diaglap.html>.
"Laparoscopy." WebMD.com. October 24, 2002). <http://my.
    webmd.com/content/healthwise/21/5199.htm?lastselected
    guid={5FE84E90-BC77-4056-A91C-9531713CA348}>.

Jennifer E. Sisk, M.A.
Jill Granger, M.S.

Laparoscopy for endometriosis

Definition

Laparoscopy is a surgical procedure in which a laparoscope, a telescope-like instrument, is inserted into the abdomen through a small incision and used to diagnose or treat various diseases. Specifically, laparoscopy may be used to diagnose and treat endometriosis, a condition in which the tissue that lines the uterus grows elsewhere in the body, usually in the abdominal cavity.

Purpose

The endometrium is the inner lining of the uterus; it is where a fertilized egg will implant during the early days of pregnancy. The endometrium normally sheds during each menstrual cycle if the egg released during ovulation has not been fertilized. Endometriosis is a condition that occurs when cells from the endometrium begin growing outside the uterus. The outlying endometrial cells respond to the hormones that control the menstrual cycle, bleeding each month the way the lining of the uterus does. This causes irritation of the surrounding tissue, leading to pain and scarring.

Endometrial growths are most commonly found on the pelvic organs, including the ovaries (the most common site), fallopian tubes, bladder, rectum, cervix, vagina, and the outer surface of the uterus. Growths are also sometimes found in other areas of the body, including the skin, lungs, brain, or surgical scars. There are numerous theories as to the cause of endometriosis; these include retrograde menstruation (movement of menstrual blood up through the fallopian tubes), movement of endometrial tissue through the blood or lymph system, or surgical transplantation (when endometriosis is found in surgical scars).

There are a number of reasons why laparoscopy is used to treat endometriosis. It is useful as both a diagnostic tool (to visualize structures in the abdominal cavity

---

WHO PERFORMS THE PROCEDURE AND WHERE IS IT PERFORMED?

Laparoscopy for endometriosis is performed by a surgeon or gynecologist who has been trained in laparoscopic techniques. A gynecologist is a medical doctor who has completed specialized training in the areas of women's general and reproductive health, pregnancy, labor and delivery, and prenatal testing. Laparoscopy is usually performed in a hospital on an outpatient basis.

---

and examine them for endometrial growths) and as an operative tool (to excise or destroy endometrial growths). A patient's recovery time following laparoscopic surgery is shorter and less painful than following a traditional laparotomy (a larger surgical incision into the abdominal cavity). A disadvantage to laparoscopy is that some growths may be too large or extensive to remove with laparoscopic instruments, necessitating a laparotomy.

Demographics

Endometriosis has been estimated to affect up to 10% of women. Approximately four out of every 1,000 women are hospitalized as a result of endometriosis each year. Women ages 25–35 are most affected, with 27 being the average age at diagnosis. The incidence of endometriosis is higher among white women and among women who have a family history of the disease.

Description

The patient is given anesthesia before the procedure commences. The method of anesthesia depends on the type and duration of surgery, the patient's preference, and the recommendation of the physician. General anesthesia is most common for operative laparoscopy, while diagnostic laparoscopy is often performed under regional or local anesthesia. A catheter is inserted into the bladder to empty it of urine; this is done to minimize the risk of injury to the bladder.

A small incision is first made into the patient's abdomen in or near the belly button. A gas such as carbon dioxide is used to inflate the abdomen to allow the surgeon a better view of the surgical field. The laparoscope is a thin, lighted tube that is inserted into the abdominal cavity through the incision. Images taken by the laparoscope may be seen on a video monitor connected to the scope.

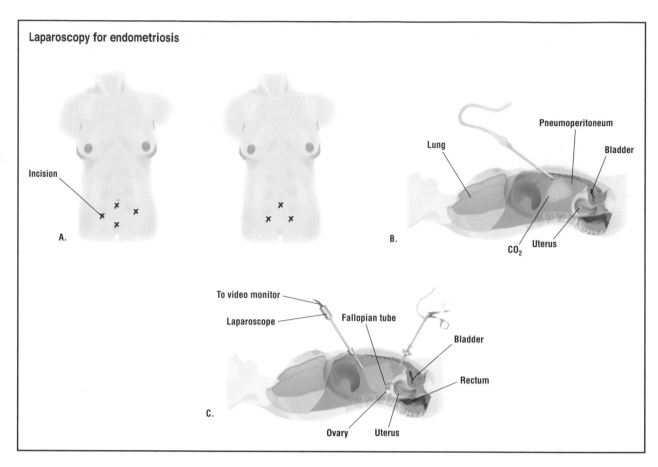

Laparoscopy for endometriosis

For this procedure, three or four incisions may be made in the woman's lower abdomen (A). Carbon dioxide is pumped into the abdomen to create a condition called pneumoperitoneum, which gives the surgeon more room to work (B). A laparoscope with video monitor is used to view the internal structures, while endometrial growths are removed with other tools (C). *(Illustration by GGS Inc.)*

The surgeon will examine the pelvic organs for endometrial growths or adhesions (bands of scar tissue that may form after surgery or trauma). Other incisions may be made to insert additional instruments; this would allow the surgeon to better position the internal organs for viewing. To remove or destroy endometrial growths, a laser or electric current (electrocautery) may be used. Alternatively, implants may be cut away with a scalpel (surgical knife). After the procedure is completed, any incisions are closed with stitches.

Diagnosis/Preparation

Some of the symptoms of endometriosis include pelvic pain (constant or during menstruation), infertility, painful intercourse, and painful urination and/or bowel movements during menstruation. Such symptoms, however, are also exhibited by a number of other diseases. A definitive diagnosis of endometriosis may only be made by laparoscopy or laparotomy.

Prior to surgery, the patient may be asked to refrain from eating or drinking after midnight on the day of surgery. An intravenous (IV) line will be placed for administration of fluids and/or medications.

Aftercare

After the procedure is completed, the patient will usually spend several hours in the **recovery room** to ensure that she recovers from the anesthesia without complication. After leaving the hospital, she may experience soreness around the incision, shoulder pain from the gas used to inflate the abdomen, cramping, or constipation. Most symptoms resolve within one to three days.

Risks

Risks that are associated with laparoscopy include complications due to anesthesia, infection, injury to organs or other structures, and bleeding. There is a risk that endometriosis will reoccur or that not all of the endometrial implants will be removed with surgery.

QUESTIONS TO ASK THE DOCTOR

- Why is laparoscopic surgery recommended for my particular case?
- Will operative laparoscopy be performed if endometriosis is diagnosed?
- What options do I have in terms of anesthesia and pain relief?
- What are the risks if I decide against surgical treatment?
- What alternatives to laparoscopy are available to me?

KEY TERMS

Acupuncture—The insertion of tiny needles into the skin at specific spots on the body for curative purposes.

Fallopian tubes—The structures that carry a mature egg from the ovaries to the uterus.

Ovulation—A process in which a mature female egg is released from one of the ovaries (egg-shaped structures located to each side of the uterus) every 28 days.

Sub-fertility—A decreased ability to become pregnant.

Normal results

After laparoscopy for endometriosis, a woman should recover quickly from the surgery and experience a significant improvement in symptoms. Some studies suggest that surgical treatment of endometriosis may improve a sub-fertile woman's chance of getting pregnant.

Morbidity and mortality rates

The overall rate of risks associated with laparoscopy is approximately 1–2%, with serious complications occurring in only 0.2% of patients. The rate of reoccurrence of endometrial growths after laparoscopic surgery is approximately 19%. The mortality rate associated with laparoscopy is less than five per 100,000 cases.

Alternatives

While laparoscopy remains the definitive approach to diagnosing endometriosis, some larger endometrial growths may be located by ultrasound, a procedure that uses high-frequency sound waves to visualize structures in the human body. Ultrasound is a noninvasive technique that may detect endometriomas (cysts filled with old blood) larger than 0.4 in (1 cm).

A physician may recommend noninvasive measures to treat endometriosis before resorting to surgical treatment. Over-the-counter or prescription pain medications may be recommended to relieve pain-related symptoms. Oral contraceptives or other hormone drugs may be prescribed to suppress ovulation and menstruation. Some women seek alternative medical therapies such as acupuncture, management of diet, or herbal treatments to reduce pain.

Severe endometriosis may need to be treated by more extensive surgery. Conservative surgery consists of excision of all endometrial implants in the abdominal cavity, with or without removal of bowel that is involved by the disease. Semi-conservative surgery involves removing some of the pelvic organs; examples are **hysterectomy** (removal of the uterus) and **oophorectomy** (removal of the ovaries). Radical surgery involves removing the uterus, cervix, ovaries, and fallopian tubes (called a total hysterectomy with bilateral **salpingo-oophorectomy**).

See also Laparoscopy.

Resources

PERIODICALS

Prentice, Andrew. "Endometriosis." *British Medical Journal* 323 (July 14, 2001): 93–95.

Wellbery, Caroline. "Diagnosis and Treatment of Endometriosis." *American Family Physician* 60 (October 1, 1999): 1753–68.

ORGANIZATIONS

American Association of Gynecologic Laparoscopists. 13021 East Florence Ave., Sante Fe Springs, CA 90670-4505. (800) 554-AAGL. <http://www.aagl.com>.

Endometriosis Association. 8585 North 76th Place, Milwaukee, WI 53223. (414) 355-2200. <http://www.endometriosis assn.org>.

OTHER

"Endometriosis." *UC Davis Health System.* 2002 [cited March 22, 2003]. <http://www.ucdmc.ucdavis.edu/ucdhs/health/a-z/74Endometriosis__/>.

Hurd, William W., and Janice M. Duke. "Gynecologic Laparoscopy." *eMedicine.* November 27, 2002 [cited March 22, 2003]. <http://www.emedicine.com/med/topic3299.htm>.

Kapoor, Dharmesh. "Endometriosis." *eMedicine.* September 17, 2002 [cited March 22, 2003]. <http://www.emedicine.com/med/topic3419.htm>.

"What is Endometriosis?" *Endometriosis Association.* 2002 [cited March 22, 2003]. <http://www.endometriosisassn.org/endo.html>.

Stephanie Dionne Sherk

Laparotomy, exploratory

Definition

A laparotomy is a large incision made into the abdomen. Exploratory laparotomy is used to visualize and examine the structures inside of the abdominal cavity.

Purpose

Exploratory laparotomy is a method of abdominal exploration, a diagnostic tool that allows physicians to examine the abdominal organs. The procedure may be recommended for a patient who has abdominal pain of unknown origin or who has sustained an injury to the abdomen. Injuries may occur as a result of blunt trauma (e.g., road traffic accident) or penetrating trauma (e.g., stab or gunshot wound). Because of the nature of the abdominal organs, there is a high risk of infection if organs rupture or are perforated. In addition, bleeding into the abdominal cavity is considered a medical emergency. Exploratory laparotomy is used to determine the source of pain or the extent of injury and perform repairs if needed.

Laparotomy may be performed to determine the cause of a patient's symptoms or to establish the extent of a disease. For example, endometriosis is a disorder in which cells from the inner lining of the uterus grow elsewhere in the body, most commonly on the pelvic and abdominal organs. Endometrial growths, however, are difficult to visualize using standard imaging techniques such as x ray, ultrasound technology, or computed tomography (CT) scanning. Exploratory laparotomy may be used to examine the abdominal and pelvic organs (such as the ovaries, fallopian tubes, bladder, and rectum) for evidence of endometriosis. Any growths found may then be removed.

Exploratory laparotomy plays an important role in the staging of certain cancers. Cancer staging is used to describe how far a cancer has spread. A laparotomy enables a surgeon to directly examine the abdominal organs for evidence of cancer and remove samples of tissue for further examination. When laparotomy is used for this use, it is called staging laparotomy or pathological staging.

Some other conditions that may be discovered or investigated during exploratory laparotomy include:

- cancer of the abdominal organs
- peritonitis (inflammation of the peritoneum, the lining of the abdominal cavity)
- appendicitis (inflammation of the appendix)
- pancreatitis (inflammation of the pancreas)
- abscesses (a localized area of infection)

WHO PERFORMS THE PROCEDURE AND WHERE IS IT PERFORMED?

Depending on the reason for performing an exploratory laparotomy, the procedure may be performed by a general or specialized surgeon in a hospital **operating room**. In the case of trauma to the abdomen, laparotomy may be performed by an emergency room physician.

- adhesions (bands of scar tissue that form after trauma or surgery)
- diverticulitis (inflammation of sac-like structures in the walls of the intestines)
- intestinal perforation
- ectopic pregnancy (pregnancy occurring outside of the uterus)
- foreign bodies (e.g., a bullet in a gunshot victim)
- internal bleeding

Demographics

Because laparotomy may be performed under a number of circumstances to diagnose or treat numerous conditions, no data exists as to the overall incidence of the procedure.

Description

The patient is usually placed under general anesthesia for the duration of surgery. The advantages to general anesthesia are that the patient remains unconscious during the procedure, no pain will be experienced nor will the patient have any memory of the procedure, and the patient's muscles remain completely relaxed, allowing safer surgery.

Incision

Once an adequate level of anesthesia has been reached, the initial incision into the skin may be made. A scalpel is first used to cut into the superficial layers of the skin. The incision may be median (vertical down the patient's midline), paramedian (vertical elsewhere on the abdomen), transverse (horizontal), T-shaped, or curved, according to the needs of the surgery. The incision is then continued through the subcutaneous fat, the abdominal muscles, and finally, the peritoneum. Electrocautery is often used to cut through the subcutaneous tissue as it

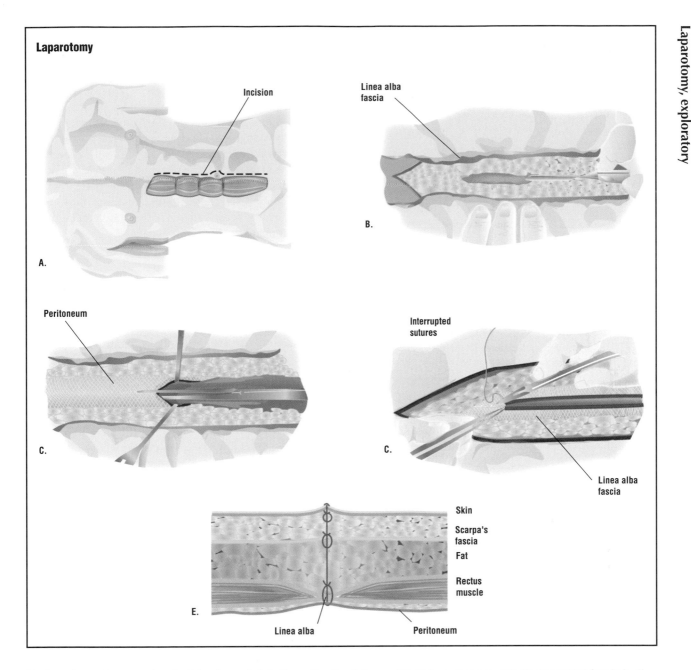

Laparotomy

A.

Incision

B.

Linea alba
fascia

C.

Peritoneum

C.

Interrupted
sutures

Linea alba
fascia

E.

Skin

Scarpa's
fascia

Fat

Rectus
muscle

Linea alba

Peritoneum

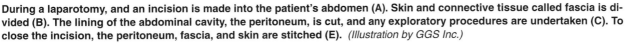

During a laparotomy, and an incision is made into the patient's abdomen (A). Skin and connective tissue called fascia is divided (B). The lining of the abdominal cavity, the peritoneum, is cut, and any exploratory procedures are undertaken (C). To close the incision, the peritoneum, fascia, and skin are stitched (E). *(Illustration by GGS Inc.)*

has the ability to stop bleeding as it cuts. Instruments called retractors may be used to hold the incision open once the abdominal cavity has been exposed.

Abdominal exploration

The surgeon may then explore the abdominal cavity for disease or trauma. The abdominal organs in question will be examined for evidence of infection, inflammation, perforation, abnormal growths, or other conditions.

Any fluid surrounding the abdominal organs will be inspected; the presence of blood, bile, or other fluids may indicate specific diseases or injuries. In some cases, an abnormal smell encountered upon entering the abdominal cavity may be evidence of infection or a perforated gastrointestinal organ.

If an abnormality is found, the surgeon has the option of treating the patient before closing the wound or initiating treatment after exploratory surgery. Alternatively, samples of various tissues and/or fluids may be removed for further analysis. For example, if cancer is suspected, biopsies may be obtained so that the tissues can be examined microscopically for evidence of abnormal cells. If no abnormality is found, or if immediate treatment is not needed, the incision may be closed without performing any further surgical procedures.

During exploratory laparotomy for cancer, a pelvic washing may be performed; sterile fluid is instilled into the abdominal cavity and washed around the abdominal organs, then withdrawn and analyzed for the presence of abnormal cells. This may indicate that a cancer has begun to spread (metastasize).

Closure

Upon completion of any exploration or procedures, the organs and related structures are returned to their normal anatomical position. The incision may then be sutured (stitched closed). The layers of the abdominal wall are sutured in reverse order, and the skin incision closed with sutures or staples.

Diagnosis/Preparation

Various diagnostic tests may be performed to determine if exploratory laparotomy is necessary. Blood tests or imaging techniques such as x ray, computed tomography (CT) scan, and **magnetic resonance imaging** (MRI) are examples. The presence of intraperitoneal fluid (IF) may be an indication that exploratory laparotomy is necessary; one study indicated that IF was present in nearly three-quarters of patients with intra-abdominal injuries.

Directly preceding the surgical procedure, an intravenous (IV) line will be placed so that fluids and/or medications may be administered to the patient during and after surgery. A Foley catheter will be inserted into the bladder to drain urine. The patient will also meet with

the anesthesiologist to go over details of the method of anesthesia to be used.

Aftercare

The patient will remain in the postoperative **recovery room** for several hours where his or her recovery can be closely monitored. **Discharge from the hospital** may occur in as little as one to two days after the procedure, but may be later if additional procedures were performed or complications were encountered. The patient will be instructed to watch for symptoms that may indicate infection, such as fever, redness or swelling around the incision, drainage, and worsening pain.

Risks

Risks inherent to the use of general anesthesia include nausea, vomiting, sore throat, fatigue, headache, and muscle soreness; more rarely, blood pressure problems, allergic reaction, heart attack, or stroke may occur. Additional risks include bleeding, infection, injury to the abdominal organs or structures, or formation of adhesions (bands of scar tissue between organs).

Normal results

The results following exploratory laparotomy depend on the reasons why it was performed. The procedure may indicate that further treatment is necessary; for example, if cancer was detected, chemotherapy, radiation therapy, or more surgery may be recommended. In some cases, the abnormality is able to be treated during laparotomy, and no further treatment is necessary.

Morbidity and mortality rates

The operative and postoperative complication rates associated with exploratory laparotomy vary according to the patient's condition and any additional procedures performed.

Alternatives

Laparoscopy is a relatively recent alternative to laparotomy that has many advantages. Also called minimally invasive surgery, laparoscopy is a surgical procedure in which a laparoscope (a thin, lighted tube) and other instruments are inserted into the abdomen through small incisions. The internal operating field may then be visualized on a video monitor that is connected to the scope. In some patients, the technique may be used for abdominal exploration in place of a laparotomy. Laparoscopy is associated with faster recovery times, shorter hospital stays, and smaller surgical scars.

Resources

BOOKS

Marx, John A., et al. *Rosen's Emergency Medicine.* St. Louis, MO: Mosby, Inc., 2002.

PERIODICALS

Hahn, David D., Steven R. Offerman, and James F. Holmes. "Clinical Importance of Intraperitoneal Fluid in Patients with Blunt Intra-abdominal Injury." *American Journal of Emergency Medicine* 20, no. 7 (November 2002).

OTHER

Awori, Nelson, et al. "Laparotomy." *Primary Surgery.* [cited April 6, 2003]. <http://www.meb.uni-bonn.de/dtc/prim-surg/index.html>.

"Surgery by Laparotomy." *Stream OR.* 2001 [cited April 6, 2003]. <http://www.streamor.com/opengyn/openindex.html>.

Stephanie Dionne Sherk

Large bowel resection *see* **Bowel resection**

Laryngectomy

Definition

A laryngectomy is the partial or complete surgical removal of the voice box (larynx).

Purpose

Because of its location, the voice box, or larynx, plays a critical role in breathing, swallowing, and speaking. The larynx is located above the windpipe (trachea) and in front of the food pipe (esophagus). It contains two small bands of muscle called the vocal cords that close to prevent food from entering the lungs and vibrate to produce the voice. If cancer of the larynx develops, a laryngectomy is performed to remove tumors or cancerous tissue. In rare cases, the procedure may also be performed when the larynx is badly damaged by gunshot, automobile injuries, or other traumatic accidents.

Demographics

The American Cancer Society estimates that, in 2003, about 9,500 people in the United States will be found to have laryngeal cancer. Laryngeal cancer occurs 4.4 times more frequently in men than in women, although, like lung cancer, it is becoming increasingly common in women. Tobacco smoking is by far the greatest risk factor for laryngeal cancer. Others include alcohol abuse, radiation exposure, asbestos exposure, and genetic factors. In the United Kingdom, cancer of the larynx is quite rare, affecting under 3,000 people each year.

Description

Laryngectomies may be total or partial. In a total laryngectomy, the entire larynx is removed. If the cancer has spread to other surrounding structures in the neck, such as the lymph nodes, they are removed at the same time. If the tumor is small, a partial laryngectomy is performed, by which only a part of the larynx, usually one vocal chord, is removed. Partial laryngectomies are also often performed in conjunction with other cancer treatments, such as radiation therapy or chemotherapy.

During a laryngectomy, the surgeon removes the larynx through an incision in the neck. The procedure also requires the surgeon to perform a tracheotomy, because air can no longer flow into the lungs. He makes an artificial opening called a stoma in the front of the neck. The upper portion of the trachea is brought to the stoma and secured, making a permanent alternate way for air to get to the lungs. The connection between the throat and the esophagus is not normally affected, so after healing, the person whose larynx has been removed (called a laryngectomee) can eat normally.

Diagnosis/Preparation

A laryngectomy is performed after cancer of the larynx has been diagnosed by a series of tests that allow the otolaryngologist (a physician often called an ear, nose & throat or ENT specialist) to examine the throat and take tissue samples (biopsies) to confirm and stage the cancer. People need to be in good general health to undergo a laryngectomy, and will have standard pre-operative blood work and tests to make sure they are able to safely withstand the operation.

As with any surgical procedure, the patient is required to sign a consent form after the procedure is thoroughly explained. Blood and urine studies, along with chest x ray and EKG may be ordered as required. If a total laryngectomy is planned, the patient meets with a speech pathologist for discussion of post-operative expectations and support.

Aftercare

A person undergoing a laryngectomy spends several days in intensive care (ICU) and receives intravenous (IV) fluids and medication. As with any major surgery, blood pressure, pulse, and respiration are monitored regularly. The patient is encouraged to turn, cough, and deep-breathe to help mobilize secretions in the lungs. One or more drains are usually inserted in the neck to remove any fluids that collect. These drains are removed after several days.

It takes two to three weeks for the tissues of the throat to heal. During this time, the laryngectomee cannot swallow food and must receive nutrition through a tube inserted through the nose and down the throat into the stomach. Normal speech is also no longer possible and patients are instructed in alternate means of vocal communication by a speech pathologist.

When air is drawn in normally through the nose, it is warmed and moistened before it reaches the lungs. When air is drawn in through the stoma, it does not have the opportunity to be warmed and humidified. In order to keep the stoma from drying out and becoming crusty, laryngectomees are encouraged to breathe artificially humidified air. The stoma is usually covered with a light cloth to keep it clean and to keep unwanted particles from accidentally entering the lungs. Care of the stoma is extremely important, since it is the person's only way to get air to the lungs. After a laryngectomy, a health-care professional will teach the laryngectomee and his or her caregivers how to care for the stoma.

There are three main methods of vocalizing after a total laryngectomy. In esophageal speech, patients learn how to "swallow" air down into the esophagus and create sounds by releasing the air. Tracheoesophageal speech diverts air through a hole in the trachea made by the surgeon. The air then passes through an implanted artificial voice. The third method involves using a hand-held electronic device that translates vibrations into sounds. The choice of vocalization

method depends on several factors including the age and health of the laryngectomee, and whether other parts of the mouth, such as the tongue, have also been removed (**glossectomy**).

Risks

Laryngectomy is often successful in curing early-stage cancers. However, it requires major lifestyle changes and there is a risk of severe psychological stress from unsuccessful adaptations. Laryngectomees must learn new ways of speaking, they must be constantly concerned about the care of their stoma. Serious problems can occur if water or other foreign material enters the lungs through an unprotected stoma. Also, women who undergo partial laryngectomy or who learn some types of artificial speech will have a deep voice similar to that of a man. For some women this presents psychological challenges. As with any major operation, there is a risk of infection. Infection is of particular concern to laryngectomees who have chosen to have a voice prosthesis implanted, and is one of the major reasons for having to remove the device.

Normal results

Ideally, removal of the larynx will remove all cancerous material. The person will recover from the operation, make lifestyle adjustments, and return to an active life.

Morbidity and mortality rates

For 2003, the American Cancer Society estimates a 40% mortality rate for laryngeal cancer, meaning that about 3,800 people will die of this disease.

Alternatives

There are two alternatives forms of treatment:

- Radiation therapy, a treatment that uses high-energy rays (such as x rays) to kill or shrink cancer cells.

- Chemotherapy, a treatment that uses drugs to kill cancer cells. Usually the drugs are given into a vein or by mouth. Once the drugs enter the bloodstream, they spread throughout the body to the cancer site.

See also Glossectomy; Tracheotomy.

Resources

BOOKS

Algaba, J., ed. *Surgery and Prosthetic Voice Restoration after Total and Subtotal Laryngectomy.* New York: Excerpta Medica, 1996.

Casper, J. K. and R. H. Colton. *Clinical Manual For Laryngectomy And Head/Neck Cancer Rehabilitation.* Independence, KY: Singular Publishing, 1998.

Singer, M. I. and R. C. Hamaker. *Tracheoesophageal Voice Restoration Following Total Laryngectomy.* Independence, KY: Singular Publishing, 1998.

Weinstein, G. S., O. Laccourreye, D. Brasnu, and H. Laccourreye. *Organ Preservation Surgery For Laryngeal Cancer.* Independence, KY: Singular Publishing, 1999.

PERIODICALS

King, A. I., B. E. Stout, and J. K. Ashby. "The Stout prosthesis: an alternate means of restoring speech in selected laryngectomy patients." *Ear Nose and Throat Journal* 82 (February 2003): 113–116.

Landis, B. N., R. Giger, J. S. Lacroix, and P. Dulguerov. "Swimming, snorkeling, breathing, smelling, and motorcycling after total laryngectomy." *American Journal of Medicine* 114 (March 2003): 341–342.

Nakahira, M., K. Higashiyama, H. Nakatani, and T. Takeda. "Staple-assisted laryngectomy for intractable aspiration." *American Journal of Otolaryngology* 24 (January-February 2003): 70–74.

ORGANIZATIONS

American Academy of Otolaryngology - Head and Neck Surgery. One Prince Street, Alexandria, VA 22314. (703) 806-4444. <http://www.entnet.org>.

American Cancer Society. National Headquarters. 1599 Clifton Road NE, Atlanta, GA 30329. (800) ACS -2345. <http://www.cancer.org>.

Cancer Information Service. National Cancer Institute. Building 31, Room 10A19, 9000 Rockville Pike, Bethesda, MD 20892. (800)4-CANCER. <http://www.nci.nih.gov/cancerinfo/index.html> .

International Association of Laryngectomees (IAL). <http://www.larynxlink.com/>.

National Institute on Deafness and Other Communication Disorders. National Institutes of Health. 31 Center Drive, MSC 2320, Bethesda, MD 20892-2320. <http://www.nidcd.nih.gov> .

> ## KEY TERMS
>
> **Larynx**—Also known as the voice box, the larynx is composed of cartilage that contains the apparatus for voice production. This includes the vocal cords and the muscles and ligaments that move the cords.
>
> **Lymph nodes**—Accumulations of tissue along a lymph channel, which produce cells called lymphocytes that fight infection.
>
> **Tracheotomy**—A surgical procedure in which an artificial opening is made in the trachea (windpipe) to allow air into the lungs.

The Voice Center at Eastern Virginia Medical School. Norfolk, VA 23507. <http://www.voice-center.com>.

OTHER

"Laryngectomy: The Operation." The Voice Center. <http://www.voice-center.com/laryngectomy.html>.

Kathleen Dredge Wright
Tish Davidson, A.M.
Monique Laberge, Ph.D.

Larynx removal *see* **Laryngectomy**

Laser coagulation therapy *see* **Photocoagulation therapy**

Laser in-situ keratomileusis (LASIK)

Definition

Laser in-situ keratomileusis (LASIK) is a non-reversible refractive procedure performed by ophthalmologists to correct myopia, hyperopia, or astigmatism. The surgeon uses an excimer laser to cut or reshape the cornea so that light will focus properly on the retina.

Purpose

LASIK is an **elective surgery** for patients who want to permanently correct myopia (nearsightedness), hyperopia (farsightedness), or astigmatism without eyeglasses,

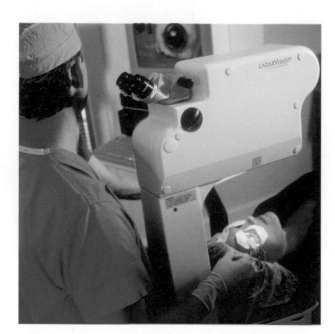

Ophthalmologist performing LASIK eye surgery on a patient. *(Custom Medical Stock Photo. Reproduced by permission.)*

contact lenses, or refractive surgical procedures. The goal for most patients is to be free of any type of corrective lenses. Some patients may find wearing eyeglasses or contact lenses interferes with their careers or hobbies. Many professional athletes have chosen LASIK to improve their performance. However, patients with higher degrees of refractive error will still need some type of corrective lens.

LASIK is most commonly performed on myopes. For myopia, the surgeon flattens the cornea; for hyperopia, the surgeon steepens the cornea. Surgeons correct astigmatism by creating a normally shaped cornea with the excimer laser.

A new type of LASIK also can treat contrast sensitivity as well as refractive error. Custom LASIK incorporates new eye mapping technology into standard LASIK. The surgeon measures the eye from front to back creating a three dimensional corneal map. This much-more detailed map gives surgeons more specific information for the excimer laser and enables them to correct other abnormalities besides refractive error.

Demographics

LASIK candidates have myopia, hyperopia, or astigmatism; are 18 or older; and have had stable vision for at least two years. The American Academy of Ophthalmology (AAO) estimated that 1.8 million refractive surgery procedures were performed in 2002. LASIK was estimated to account for 95% of those procedures.

The first LASIK patients in the late 1990s were in the upper class, or upper middle class, and in their early 30s to mid-40s. The market was limited for the elective procedure that at first could range as expensive as $5,000 per eye. The number of younger patients receiving LASIK (in their early to mid-20s) was expected to rise in 2003 and beyond. The number of procedures also was expected to increase as prices continued to stabilize, and surgery centers and physicians offered payment plans.

Description

LASIK is a relatively new procedure. In April 1985, German physician Theo Seiler was the first to use an excimer laser to attempt to correct astigmatism in blind eyes. Experiments with excimer lasers on blind eyes were also completed in the United States in the mid-1980s. The term LASIK was invented by Greek ophthalmologist Ioannis Pallikari, the first surgeon to use the hinged flap technique. Dr. Stephen Brint, as part of a clinical trial in 1991, performed the first LASIK procedure in the United States.

As of 2003, there are two types of LASIK. The standard LASIK procedure and custom LASIK, which relatively few surgeons have the technology to perform.

Standard LASIK

Standard LASIK takes from 10 to 20 minutes to perform and the results are immediate. It's standard practice in LASIK operating rooms to have a clock on the wall so patients immediately can note they are able to read a clock face or other items that previously were blurry.

Immediately before the procedure, the ophthalmologist may request corneal topography (a corneal map) to compare with previous maps to ensure the treatment plan is still correct. The surgeon may also measure the cornea's thickness if he didn't previously. After these tests, a technician or co-managing optometrist will perform a refraction to make sure the refractive correction the surgeon will program into the laser is correct.

Three sets of eye drops will be administered twice before surgery. The first drop anesthetizes the cornea, the second drop prevents infection and the third drop controls inflammation after LASIK. Patients may be given a sedative, such as Valium. This is administered to calm nervous patients or to help patients sleep after the procedure.

After the prep work is completed, the patient reclines on a laser bed and the surgeon is seated directly behind the patient. If the procedure is being done on both eyes on the same day, the surgeon will patch the second eye. An eyelid speculum is inserted in the eye to be treated first to hold the eyelids apart. The patient stares at the

Laser in situ keratomileusis

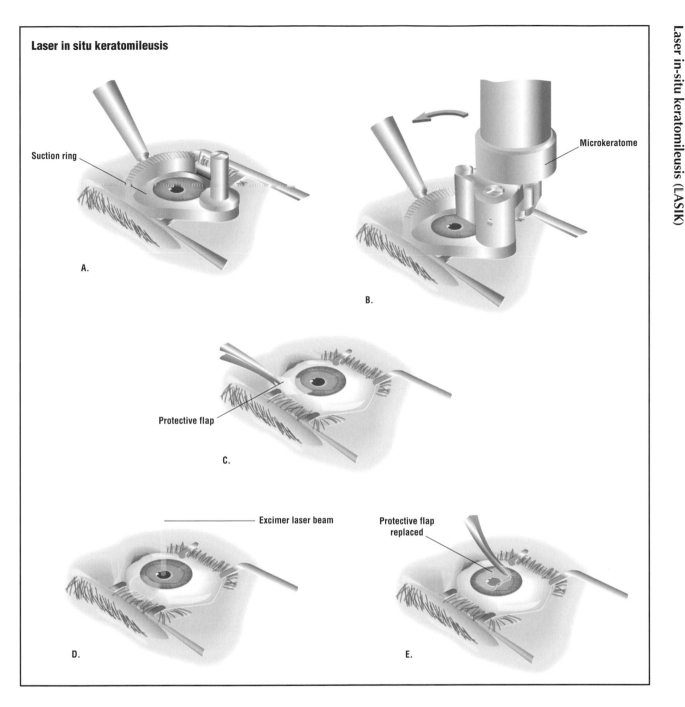

Suction ring

A.

Microkeratome

B.

Protective flap

C.

Excimer laser beam

D.

Protective flap replaced

E.

In LASIK surgery, the eye is held open with a speculum, and a suction ring is attached to the eyeball (A). A microkeratome is used to shave the protective flap off the top of the eye (B), which is then pulled back (C). A computer-controlled laser is used to reshape the cornea (D), and the protective flap is replaced (E). *(Illustration by GGS Inc.)*

blinking light of a laser microscope and must fixate his or her gaze on that light. The patient must remain still throughout the procedure.

The surgeon checks the refractive numbers on the laser. Because each patient's cornea is shaped differently, the surgeon may have to adjust the level of correction. Laser companies provide an algorithm to determine the correction level, and the surgeon may alter the level because of a patient's special needs. The adjustments are called nomograms. After the adjustments, the surgeon checks the microkeratome blade for defects.

The surgeon then indents the cornea to mark the flap location. The surgeon places a suction ring in the center of the sclera. A technician will activate the microkeratome's suction. The patient's vision dims at this point. The surgeon tests pressure by touching the cornea with a tonometer. Before using the microkeratome, sterile saline solution is squirted into the suction ring to lubricate the cornea. The microkeratome head is placed in the gear tracks of the suction ring, and the surgeon guides the microkeratome across the suction ring to create a flap. The microkeratome stops just short of traveling completely across the cornea. It leaves a hinge of tissue, commonly called a flap. After the flap is created, the surgeon removes the suction ring and slips a spatula under it and moves it to the side, exposing the stroma (inner cornea).

Once the stroma is exposed, the laser ablation begins, ranging from 30 to 60 seconds. The ablation flattens the cornea of myopic patients; steepens the cornea of hyperopic patients; and reshapes the cornea of astigmatic patients. After the ablation, the surgeon replaces the flap. More saline solution is squirted to remove any debris and enable the flap to move back into place without interruption. The surgeon ensures the flap is in place and removes any wrinkles. The surgeon places a shield over the eye to keep the flap in place. No stitches are used.

If bilateral LASIK is being performed, the patient must remain still while he is prepared for treatment on the remaining eye.

Custom LASIK

As of early 2003, a handful of ophthalmologists in the United States had the technology to perform custom LASIK. The difference between standard LASIK and custom LASIK lies in the diagnosis and who can be treated. With custom LASIK, surgeons use a wavefront analyzer (aberrometer) that beams light through the eye and finds irregularities based on how the light travels through the eye. It creates a three-dimensional corneal map to create a customized pattern for each patient. For standard LASIK, each patient with the same refractive error is treated with the same setting on the excimer laser, barring a few adjustments. The new technology individualizes treatment not only for refractive errors, but also for visual disorders that previous corneal mapping technology could not detect. As of early 2003, there was only one FDA-approved laser capable of the customized ablations, but others were awaiting approval.

Besides the customized excimer laser, the surgical procedure is the same. Surgeons now can treat patients who have higher-order aberrations, such as contrast sensitivity. Therefore, custom LASIK can successfully treat glare, night vision and other contrast problems.

Diagnosis/Preparation

Before LASIK, patients need to have a complete eye evaluation and comprehensive medical history taken. Soft contact lens wearers should stop wearing their lenses at least one week before the initial exam. Gas permeable lens wearers should not wear their lenses from three weeks to a month before the exam. Contact lens wear can alter the cornea's shape, which should be allowed to return to its natural shape before the initial exam.

The initial exam

During the first exam, the surgeon's staff will take a comprehensive medical history to determine if there are underlying medical problems that will prevent a successful surgery. This screening process will determine patients who should not have the procedure including:

• pregnant women or women who are breastfeeding

• patients with very small or very large refractive errors

• patients with low contrast sensitivity

• patients with scarred corneas or macular disease

• people with autoimmune diseases

• diabetics

• glaucoma patients

• patients with persistent blepharitis

The physician will also ask about medication. Some prescription medicines have been known to cause post-surgical scarring or cause flecks under the corneal flap. It's important for the patient to disclose any prescriptions or over-the-counter medicines taken regularly. Allergies to prescription medicine must also be discussed.

A complete eye exam will be performed to determine refractive error, uncorrected visual acuity and best corrected visual acuity. A cycloplegic refraction using eye drops to dilate the pupils also will be performed. Other examination procedures include corneal mapping, a keratometer reading to determine the curvature of the central part of the cornea, a slit lamp exam to determine any damage to the cornea and evidence of glaucoma and cataracts. A fundus exam also will be performed to check for retinal holes and macular degeneration and macular disease. Other tests are done to rule out glaucoma.

While those tests check general eye health, others more closely relate to the outcome of LASIK surgery. A corneal pachymeter measures the cornea's thickness. This is important because surgeons remove tissue during surgery. A pupilometer measures the pupil when it is naturally dilated in a dark room without drops. Patients with large pupils have been known to have complications after LASIK, such as glare and halos.

Treatment options/Informed consent

After the exam, the patient and physician discuss treatment options and expectations. Patients who expect to see perfectly after LASIK are usually not considered good candidates because they usually are dissatisfied with the results. Surgeons also discuss how patients will handle presbyopia, which occurs during the patient's 40s. LASIK does not correct for presbyopia, and patients will need reading glasses to accommodate for reading when presbyopia occurs. Sometimes patients 40 and older opt for monovision to treat presbyopia, where one eye is left untreated or one eye is only partially corrected. Monovision means one eye is for short-term vision and the other is for distance vision.

The doctor will advise the patient of any possible LASIK complications, explain the procedure and answer questions. After deciding on a treatment option, the patient is required to sign an **informed consent** form.

At this time, payment will also be discussed. Insurance usually does not cover LASIK, although some offer a limited benefit for the procedure. Some laser centers offer payment plans and some physicians have begun using credit companies to handle payments. LASIK can cost anywhere from $999 to $3,000 per eye. The cost varies greatly from surgeon to surgeon. Most of the fees are global, and cover all the pre-operative and post-operative exams as well as the procedure. Patients should be advised of what the fee covers, and if retreatments to the original surgery are included in that price.

Pre-surgery preparations

The patient is advised to discontinue contact lens wear immediately and refrain from using creams, lotions, make-up or perfume for at least two days before surgery. Patients may also be asked to scrub their eyelashes for a period of time to remove any debris. Patients also must find transportation to and from the surgery, and also to and from the first post-operative visit. Medication and distorted vision make it unsafe for the patients to drive after LASIK.

Aftercare

After LASIK, patients may experience burning, itching or a foreign body sensation. They should be advised not to touch the eye as that could damage the flap. Many physicians recommend sleeping after the surgery. Patients may also experience glare, starbursts, or halos that should improve after the first few days. Patients are advised to seek help immediately if they feel severe eye pain, or if symptoms worsen.

WHO PERFORMS THE PROCEDURE AND WHERE IS IT PERFORMED?

An ophthalmologist performs LASIK, but because it is a relatively new technology, the surgeon may not have received training as part of his residency. It is more likely the surgeon has completed continuing medical education courses or may have had training provided by the laser companies. He may also have received training as part of membership in an organization such as the American Society of Refractive Surgeons.

Before and aftercare probably will be provided by a co-managing optometrist. The optometrist usually performs the pre- and post-operative exams, and also discusses the patient's suitability for LASIK and any potential problems.

Ophthalmic technicians may perform preliminary testing, including corneal topography and corneal measuring. Laser technicians are required to have special training provided by the laser manufacturer.

Surgeons may perform LASIK in a hospital where they rely on the hospital staff for support. Because lasers are expensive, some surgeons pool their resources and purchase a laser that they share at a freestanding surgery center. LASIK is also provided by surgeons at surgery centers owned by refractive surgery companies. These businesses hire support staff, optometrists and surgeons to perform LASIK.

The first follow-up visit is from 24 to 48 hours after surgery. The physician will remove the eye shield, check the patient's vision, and may prescribe more antibiotic drops or artificial tears. Patients must refrain from strenuous activity, such as contact sports, for at least a month. The use of creams, lotions, and make-up must also be avoided for at least two weeks. Hot tubs and swimming pools should be avoided for at least two months. Patients are advised that refraining from these activities and products will help stem infection and aid healing of the cornea.

Patients will have regularly scheduled visits post-LASIK for at least six months. Vision gradually improves the first few months after surgery. In some cases, if the vision does not meet expectations and the surgeon believes it can be further corrected, he will perform an enhancement. Enhancements are usually done for undercorrection. Overcorrected patients usually need eyeglasses or contact lenses.

Risks

Surgeons separate LASIK complications into two categories.

Intraoperative risks

- Cornea perforation. This complication has almost disappeared because of advances in microkeratome design.
- Flap complications. Newer microkeratomes also have reduced the likelihood of "free caps," where the cap becomes unhinged. An experienced surgeon replaces the cap after ablation. In some cases, the procedure must be aborted while the eye heals.
- Laser hot spots. Higher energy surrounding the laser beam can cause irregular astigmatism. Proper laser testing before the procedure eliminates this risk.
- Central islands. This refers to a raised area in the central part of the treated zone that receives insufficient laser treatment. Any raised area can decrease the laser's effectiveness. The island either shrinks by itself or can be remedied with retreatment.
- Decentered ablation. This occurs when the laser beam is aimed incorrectly. This can result in permanent halos and ghost images.

Post-operative complications

- Undercorrection or overcorrection. Undercorrection can usually be treated with an enhancement, but overcorrection will require the use of eyeglasses or contact lenses.
- Debilitating symptoms. These can be permanent or transient, and include glare, halos, double vision and poor nighttime vision. Some patients may also lose contrast sensitivity.
- Dry eye. This also can be permanent or transient. Most patients experience some dry eye immediately after surgery. Some patients continue to experience dry eye and are treated with artificial tears or punctal plugs.
- Displaced flap. Occurs after the eye is hit or rubbed. If immediate attention is given by the surgeon, who must lift the flap and clean under it, no long-term effects occur.
- Nonspecific diffuse intralamellar keratitis. Commonly known as Sands of the Sahara, this complication can range from corneal haze to eye clouding that resembles swirling sand. It is treated with topical steroids, although severe cases may require eye irrigation.
- Epithelial ingrowth. The cells of the lower cornea migrate under the corneal cap. The surgeon must lift the cap and remove the cells. If untreated, vision is impaired.
- Striae. These are wrinkles in the flap that can reduce visual acuity. The surgeon must lift the corneal flap and smooth the wrinkles.
- Photophobia. Extreme sensitivity to light can last a few days or a week after surgery.
- Infection. This rarely occurs after LASIK. It is treated with **antibiotics**.

Normal results

After LASIK, most patients are able to see well enough to pass a driver's license exam without glasses or contact lenses. Some patients will still need corrective lenses, but the lenses won't need to be as powerful.

Because LASIK is a relatively new procedure, there is limited information on long-term regression. If patients are being treated for myopia, they should be aware they will have to rely on spectacles with the onset of presbyopia.

Morbidity and mortality rates

Information about mortality rates following LASIK is limited because the procedure is elective. Complications that can lead to more serious conditions, such as in-

KEY TERMS

Ablation—During LASIK, the vaporization of eye tissue.

Astigmatism—Asymmetric vision defects due to irregularities in the cornea.

Cornea—The clear, curved tissue layer in front of the eye. It lies in front of the colored part of the eye (iris) and the black hole in the center of the iris (pupil).

Corneal topography—Mapping the cornea's surface with a specialized computer that illustrates corneal elevations.

Dry eye—Corneal dryness due to insufficient tear production.

Enhancement—A secondary refractive procedure performed in an attempt to achieve better visual acuity.

Excimer laser—An instrument that is used to vaporize tissue with a cold, coherent beam of light with a single wavelength in the ultraviolet range.

Hyperopia—The inability to see near objects as clearly as distant objects, and the need for accommodation to see objects clearly.

Intraocular lens (IOL) implant—A small, plastic device (IOL) that is usually implanted in the lens capsule of the eye to correct vision after the lens of the eye is removed. This is the implant used in cataract surgery.

Macular degeneration—A condition usually associated with age in which the area of the retina called the macula is impaired due to hardening of the arteries (arteriosclerosis). This condition interferes with vision.

Microkeratome—A precision surgical instrument that can slice an extremely thin layer of tissue from the surface of the cornea.

Myopia—A vision problem in which distant objects appear blurry. Myopia results when the cornea is too steep or the eye is too long, and the light doesn't focus properly on the retina. People who are myopic, or nearsighted, can usually see near objects clearly, but not far objects.

Nomogram—A surgeon's adjustment of the excimer laser to fine-tune results.

Presbyopia—A condition affecting people over the age of 40 where the system of accommodation that allows focusing of near objects fails to work because of age-related hardening of the lens of the eye.

Retina—The sensory tissue in the back of the eye that is responsible for collecting visual images and sending them to the brain.

Stroma—The thickest part of the cornea between Bowman's membrane and Decemet's membrane.

---

fection, are treated with topical antibiotics after LASIK. The most serious possible complication from LASIK is blindness from an untreated complication. As of 2000, there had been no reports of blindness-induced LASIK. One incidence of legal blindness was reported after a severely myopic patient had retinal hemorrhages. However, it was inconclusive whether or not LASIK was the causative agent.

Alternatives

Nonsurgical alternatives

Nonsurgical alternatives to LASIK are contact lenses and eyeglasses, which can also correct refractive errors. Continuous-wear contact lenses, which a patient can sleep in for as long as 30 days, can provide the same effect as LASIK if the patient wants good vision upon waking. Orthokeratology involves a rigid gas permeable contact lens the patient wears for a predetermined amount of time to reshape the cornea. After removing the lens, it takes weeks for the cornea to return to its normal shape. At that time, the patient repeats the process.

Corneal rings and implants are another alternative for myopes. These require surgery without lasers and involve a corrective lens surgically implanted in the eye. One of the biggest benefits to these procedures is that they are reversible. However, they may not provide the crisp vision of a successful LASIK. There also are several different types of intraocular lenses being tested to treat myopia and hyperopia.

Surgical alternatives

There also are surgical alternatives to LASIK. They include:

- Conductive keratoplasty. This uses radio frequency waves to shrink corneal collagen. It is used to treat mild to moderate hyperopia.

- Photorefractive keratectomy (**PRK**). PRK also uses an excimer laser and is similar to LASIK. However, in PRK, the surface of the cornea is removed by the laser. PRK patients have a longer recovery time and may need steroidal eye drops for months after surgery. Its success rate is similar to that of LASIK.

- Radial keratotomy (RK). RK was the first widely used surgical correction for mild to moderate myopia. The surgeon alters the shape of the cornea without a laser. This is one of the oldest refractive procedures, and has proved successful on lower and moderate corrections.

- Astigmatic keratotomy (AK). AK is a variation of RK used to treat mild to moderate astigmatism. AK has proved successful if the errors are mild to moderate.

- Laser thermal keratoplasty (LTK). LTK was approved as to treat hyperopia in 2000. An LTK patient's vision is overcorrected for one to three months, and the effect of improved near vision may diminish over time as distance vision improves. Some regression has been noted.

Resources

BOOKS

Brint, Stephen F., M.D., Dennis Kennedy, O.D., and Corinne Kuypers-Denlinger. *The Laser Vision Breakthrough* Roseville, CA: Prima Health, 2000.

Caster, Andrew I., M.D., F.A.C.S. *The Eye Laser Miracle: The Complete Guide to Better Vision* New York, NY: Ballantine Books, 1997.

Slade, Stephen G., M.D., Richard Baker, O.D., and Dorothy Kay Brockman. *The Complete Book of Laser Eye Surgery* Naperville, ILL: Sourcebooks, Inc., 2000.

ORGANIZATIONS

American Academy of Ophthalmology. PO Box 7424, San Francisco, CA 94120-7424 (415) 561-8500. <http://www.aao.org>

American Society of Cataract and Refractive Surgery. 4000 Legato Road, Suite 850, Fairfax, VA 22033-4055. (703) 591-2220. <ascrs@ascrs.org>. <http://www.ascrs.org>.

OTHER

"Basik Lasik: Tips on LASIK Eye Surgery." Federal Trade Commission. August 2000 [cited February 22, 2003] <http://www.ftc.gov/bcp/conline/pubs/health/lasik.htm>.

Croes, Keith. "Custom LASIK: The Next Generation in Laser Eye Surgery." *All About Vision* [cited February 22, 2003]. <http://www.allaboutvision.com/visionsurgery/custom_lasik.htm>.

Gonzalez, Jeanne Michelle. "To Increase LASIK Volume, Know Your Market." *Ocular Surgery News.* September 1, 2002 [cited February 23, 2003]. <http://www.osnsupersite.com/view.asp?ID=3473>.

Gottlieb, Howard O.D. "The Changing LASIK Patient." *Ophthalmology Management.* February 2001 [cited February 22, 2003]. <http://www.ophmanagement.com/archive_results.asp?loc=archive/2001/february/0201038.htm>.

"LASIK Eye Surgery." U.S. Food and Drug Administration Center for Devices and Radiological Health. October 1, 2002 [cited February 20, 2003]. <http://www.fda.gov/cdrh/lasik>.

"Refractive Errors and Refractive Surgery." American Academy of Ophthalmology [cited February 23, 2003]. <http://www.aao.org/aao/newsroom/facts/errors.cfm>.

Mary Bekker

Laser iridotomy

Definition

Laser iridotomy is a surgical procedure that is performed on the eye to treat angle closure glaucoma, a condition of increased pressure in the front chamber (anterior chamber) that is caused by sudden (acute) or slowly progressive (chronic) blockage of the normal circulation of fluid within the eye. The block occurs at the angle of the anterior chamber that is formed by the junction of the cornea with the iris. All one needs to do to see this angle is to look at a person's eye from the side. Angle closure of the eye occurs when the trabecular meshwork, the drainage site for ocular fluid, is blocked by the iris. Laser iridotomy was first used to treat angle closures in 1956. During this procedure, a hole is made in the iris of the eye, changing its configuration. When this occurs, the iris moves away from the trabecular meshwork, and proper drainage of the intraocular fluid is enabled.

The angle of the eye refers to a channel in which the trabecular meshwork is located. To maintain the integrity of the eye, fluid must always be present in the anterior (front) and posterior (back) chambers of the eye. The fluid, known as aqueous fluid, is made in the ciliary processes, which are located behind the iris. Released continuously into the posterior chamber of the eye, aqueous fluid circulates throughout the eye. Eventually the fluid returns to the general circulation of the body, first passing through a space between the iris and the lens, then flowing into the anterior chamber of the eye and down the angle, where the trabecular meshwork is located. Finally, the fluid leaves the eye. An angle closure occurs when drainage of the aqueous fluid through the trabecular meshwork is blocked and the intraocular pressure builds up as a result.

For most types of angle closure, or narrow angle glaucoma, laser iridotomy is the procedure of choice. Changes in intraocular pressure (IOP) can alter the name of the condition when the IOP in the eye becomes elevated above 22 mm/Hg as a result of an angle closure. Then,

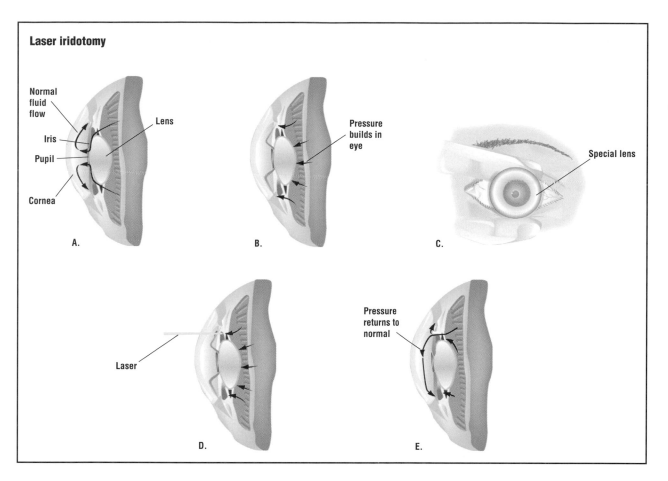

Laser iridotomy

Normal fluid flow

Iris

Pupil

Lens

Cornea

A.

Pressure builds in eye

B.

Special lens

C.

Laser

D.

Pressure returns to normal

E.

Normally intraocular fluid flows freely between the anterior and posterior sections of the eye (A). As pressure builds in the eye, this circulation is cut off (B). In laser iridotomy, a special lens is placed on the eye (C). A laser is used to create a hole in part of the iris (D), allowing fluid to flow more normally and intraocular pressure to return to normal (E). *(Illustration by GGS Inc.)*

angle closure becomes angle closure glaucoma. Lowering of the IOP is important because extreme elevations in IOP can damage the retina and the optic nerve permanently. The lasers used to perform this surgery are either the Nd:Yag laser or, if a patient has a bleeding disorder, the argon laser. The majority of patients with glaucoma do not have angle closure glaucoma, but rather have an open angle glaucoma, a type of glaucoma in which the angle of the eye is open.

An angle closure occurs when ocular anomalies (abnormalities) temporarily or permanently block the trabecular meshwork, restricting drainage of the ocular fluid. The anatomical anomalies that make an individual susceptible to an angle closure are, for example, an iris that is bent forward in the anterior chamber (front) of the eye, a small anterior chamber of the eye, and a narrow entrance to the angle of the eye. Some conditions that cause an angle closure are a pupillary block, a plateau iris, phacolytic glaucoma, and malignant glaucoma. The end re-

sult of all of these situations is an elevation of the IOP due to a build-up of aqueous fluid in the back part of the eye. The IOP rises quickly when an acute angle attack occurs and within an hour the pressure can be dangerously elevated. The sclera or white of the affected eye becomes red or injected. The patient will usually experience decreased vision and ocular pain with an acute angle closure. In severe cases of acute angle glaucoma, the patient may experience nausea and vomiting. Individuals with neurovascular glaucoma caused by uncontrolled diabetes or hypertension may have similar symptoms, but treatment for this type of glaucoma is very different.

Within a normal eye, the iris is in partial contact with the lens of the eye behind it. Individuals with narrow angles are at greater risk of angle closure by pupillary block because their anterior chamber is shallow; thus, the iris is closer to the lens and more likely to adhere completely to the lens, creating a pupillary block. Patients who experience a pupillary block may have had occasionally temporary blocks prior to a complete angle closure. Pupillary block can be started by prolonged exposure to dim light. Therefore, it not uncommon for an acute angle closure to occur as an individual with a narrow angle emerges from a dark environment such as a theater into bright light. It can also be brought on by neurotransmitter release during emotional stress or by medications taken for other medical conditions. Pupil dilation may be a side effect of one or more of those medications. However, pupillary block is the most common cause of angle closure, and laser iridotomy effectively treats this condition.

The irises of individuals with plateau iris is bunched up in the anterior chamber, and it is malpositioned along the trabecular meshwork. Plateau iris develops into glaucoma when the iris bunches up further; this occurs on dilation of the iris, which temporarily closes off the angle of the eye. Laser iridotomy is often performed as a preventive measure in these patients, but is not a guarantee against future angle closure. This is because changes within the eye, such as narrowing of the angle and increase in lens size can lead to iris plateau syndrome, where the iris closes the angle of the eye even if a laser iridotomy has already been performed. Peripheral laser iridoplasty and other surgical techniques can be performed if the angle still closes after iridotomy.

Other causes of narrow angle glaucoma are not as common. Phacolytic glaucoma results when a cataract becomes hypermature and the proteins of the lens with the cataract leak out to block the angle and the trabecular meshwork. Laser iridotomy is not effective for this type of angle closure. Malignant glaucoma exists secondary to prior ocular surgery, and is the result of the movement of anatomical structures within the eye such that the meshwork is blocked. Patients who have no intraocular lens (aphakic) are at increased risk for angle closure, as well.

Laser iridotomy is also performed prophylactically (preventively) on asymptomatic individuals with narrow angles and those with pigment dispersion. Individuals with a narrow angle are at higher risk of an acute angle closure, especially upon dilation of the eye. Pigment dispersion is a condition in which the iris pigment is shed and is dispersed throughout the anterior part of the eye. If the dispersion occurs because of bowing of the iris (the case in 60% of patients with pigment dispersion) a laser iridotomy will decrease the bowing or concavity of the iris and subsequent pigment dispersion. This decreases the risk of these individuals to develop pigmentary glaucoma, a condition in which the dispersed pigment may clog the trabecular meshwork. Laser iridotomy is also done on the fellow eye of a patient who has had an angle closure of one eye, as the probability of an angle closure in the second eye is 50%.

There are other indications for laser iridotomy. It is performed on patients with nanophthalmos, or small eyes. Laser iridotomy may be also be indicated for patients with malignant glaucoma to help identify the etiology of elevated IOP. Because laser iridotomy changes the configuration of the iris, it is sometimes used to open the angle of the eye prior to performing a laser argon laser trabeculoplasty, if the angle is narrow. Laser trabeculoplasty is another laser procedure used to treat pigmentary and pseudoexfoliation glaucoma.

Laser iridotomy cannot be performed if the cornea is edematous or opacified, nor if the angle is completely closed. If an inflammation (such as uveitis or neovascular glaucoma) has caused the angle to close, laser iridotomy cannot be performed.

Purpose

The purpose of a laser iridotomy is to allow an equalization of pressure between the anterior (front) and posterior (back) chambers of the eye by making a hole in the superior peripheral iris. Once the laser iridotomy is completed, the intraocular fluid flows freely from the posterior to the anterior part of the eye, where it is drained via the trabecular meshwork. The result of this surgery is a decrease in IOP.

When laser iridotomy is performed on patients with chronic angle closure, or on patients with narrow angles with no history of angle closure, the chances of future pupillary blocks are decreased.

Demographics

Acute angle glaucoma occurs in one in 1,000 individuals. Angle-closure glaucoma generally expresses itself in populations born with a narrow angle. Individuals of Asian and Eskimo ancestry appear to be at greater risk of developing it. Family history, as well as age, are risk factors. Older women are more often affected than are others. Laser iridotomy is performed on the same groups of individuals as those likely to experience angle closures due to pupillary block or plateau iris. They are performed more often on females (whose eyes are smaller than those of males), and more often performed on the smaller eyes of farsighted people than on those of the nearsighted because angle closures occur more frequently in those who are farsighted. Most laser iridotomies are performed on those over age 40 with a family history of plateau iris or narrow angles. However, preventative plateau iris laser iridotomies are performed on patients in their 30s. Individuals who are aphakic (have no intraocular lens) are at greater risk of angle closure and undergo laser iridotomy more frequently than phakic patients. Phakic patients are those who either have an intact lens or who are psuedophakic (have had a lens implant after the removal of a cataract removal).

Description

After the cornea swelling has subsided and the IOP has been lowered, which is usually 48 hours after an acute angle closure, laser iridotomy can be performed. Pilocarpine is applied topically to the eye to constrict the pupil prior to surgery. When the pupil is constricted, the iris is thinner and it is easier for the surgeon to form a penetrating hole. If the eye is still edematous (swollen)—often the situation when the IOP is extremely high—glycerin is applied to the eye to enable the surgeon to visualize the iris. Apraclonidine, an IOP-lowering drop, is applied one hour before surgery. Immediately prior to surgery, an anesthetic is applied to the eye.

Next, an iridotomy contact lens, to which methylcellulose is added for patient comfort, is placed on the upper part of the front of the eye. This lens increases magnification and helps the surgeon to project the laser beam accurately. The patient is asked to look downwards as the surgeon applies laser pulses to the iris, until a hole is formed. Once the hole has penetrated the iris, iris material bursts through the opening, followed by aqueous fluid. At this point, the surgeon can also see the anterior part of the lens capsule through the opening. The hole, or iridotomy, is formed on the upper section of the iris at an 11:00 or 1:00 position, so that the hole is covered by the eyelid. In an aphakic eye, the hole may be made on the inferior iris. After performing the laser iridotomy, the surgeon may place a gonioscopy lens on the eye if the angle has been opened. There is no pain associated with this surgery, although heat may be felt at the site of the lasering.

If a patient has a tendency to bleed, the argon laser will be used to pre-treat the patient prior to completing the procedure with an Nd:Yag laser, or the argon laser alone may be used. The argon laser is capable of photocoagulation, and, thus, minimizes any bleeding that occurs as the iris is penetrated. Formation of a hole is more difficult with the argon laser because it operates with a decreased power density and the tissue response to the argon laser has greater variability. The argon laser can be used with more patients who have medium-brown irises, however, since the energy of this laser is readily absorbed by irises of this color.

Diagnosis/Preparation

To determine if laser iridotomy is indicated, the surgeon must first determine if and how the angle is occluded. The eye is anesthetized and the aonioscopic lens, which enables the surgeon to see the interior of the eye,

is placed on the front of the eye. This is done at the slit lamp biomicroscope in a dark room. In cases of prophylactic surgery, an image of the eye is taken with a ultrasound biomicroscope in both dim and bright light; this shows the doctor how the patient's iris moves with dilation and constriction, and how this movement can close an angle if the patient has ocular features that predispose the eye to an angle closure.

When an angle is completely occluded (blocked), the elevated IOP usually causes corneal edema (swelling). Because this swelling can obscure the surgeon's view of the iris, prior to performing a laser iridotomy, the IOP must be lowered. One technique to lower the IOP is corneal indentation, in which the gentle pressure is applied several times to the cornea with a lens or hook to open the angle. This pressure on the cornea causes a shift in the internal structures of the eye, enhances aqueous drainage, and lowers the IOP.

The doctor can attempt to lower the IOP medically, as well. One drug that lowers the pressure is acetazolamide, which is given either orally or by intravenous(IV) to decrease aqueous production in the eye. This may be administered up to four times a day, until the adhesion is broken. Another method of lowering the IOP, if acetazolamide is not effective, is with the use of hyperosmotic agents, which through osmosis causes drainage of the aqueous fluid from the eye into the rest of the body. Hyperosmotic agents are given orally; an example of such an agent is glycerine. Given by IV (intravenous administration), mannitol can be used. As the fluid drains from the eye, the vitreous—the jelly-like substance behind the lens in the posterior chamber—shrinks. As it shrinks, the lens in the eye pulls away from the vitreous, creating an opening to the anterior chamber such that aqueous fluid can flow to the anterior chamber. The success of this procedure is increased, due to gravity, if the patient is laying supine.

Once the IOP has begun to decrease, the pressure is further decreased using topical glaucoma medications, such as pilocarpine, or beta blockers. Any inflammation that occurs because of the iridotomy must be controlled with steroid eye drops.

If glaucomatous-like visual field is present prior to surgical intervention, the prognosis for the patient is not as good as if the visual field were completely intact. Thus, a visual field test may be done prior to surgery.

Aftercare

Immediately after the procedure, another drop of apro-clonidine is applied to the eye. The IOP is checked every hour for a several hours postsurgery. If the IOP increases dramatically, then the increased IOP is treated until lowered. Because of inflammation is inherent in this procedure, **corticosteroids** are applied to the eye every five minutes for 30 minutes, then hourly for six hours. This therapy is then continued four times a day for a week. Thereafter, the patient is seen by the surgeon at one week post-surgery and again at two to six weeks post-surgery. If there are complications, the patient is seen more frequently.

After the pressure has been stabilized, a visual field test to determine the extent of damage to the optic nerve may be performed again.

Risks

The greatest risk of laser iridotomy is an increase in intraocular pressure. Usually, the IOP spike is transient and of concern to the surgeon only during the first 24 hours after surgery. However, if there is damage to the trabecular meshwork during **laser surgery**, the intraocular pressure may not be lowered enough and extended medical intervention or filtration surgery is required. Patients who undergo preventative laser iridotomy do not experience as great an elevation in IOP.

The second greatest risk of this procedure is anterior uvetis, or inflammation within the eye. Usually the in-flammation subsides within several days, but can persist for up to 30 days. Thus, the follow-up care for laser iridotomy includes the application of topical corticosteroids. A posterior synechia, in which the iris may again adhere to the lens, may occur if intraocular inflammation is not properly managed.

Other risks of this procedure include the following: swelling of, abrasions to, or opacification of the cornea; and damage to the corneal endothelium (the part of the cornea that pumps oxygen and nutrients into the iris); bleeding of the iris during surgery, which is controlled during surgery by using the iridotomy lens to increase pressure on the eye; and macular edema, which can be avoided by careful aim of the laser during surgery to avoid the macula. The macula is the part of the eye where the highest concentration of photoreceptors is found. Perforations of the retina are rare. Distortion of the pupil and rupture of the lens capsule are other possible complications. Opacification of the anterior part of the lens is common, but this does not increase the risk of cataract formation when compared with the general population.

When the iridotomy hole is large, or if the eyelid does not completely cover the opening, some patients report such side effects as glare and double vision. The argon laser produces larger holes. Patients may also complain of an intermittent horizontal line in their vision. This may occur when the eyelid is raised just enough such that a small section of the inferior part of the hole is exposed, and disappears when the eyelid is lowered. Blurred vision may occur as well, but usually disappears 30 minutes after surgery.

Normal results

In successful laser iridotomy, the IOP differential between the anterior and posterior chambers is relieved and IOP is decreased, and the pupil is able to constrict normally. These are the results of the flatter configuration of the iris after laser iridotomy. If an angle closure is treated promptly, the patient will have minimal or no loss of vision. This procedure is successful in up to 44% of patients treated.

Morbidity and mortality rates

For up to 64% of patients, one to three years after laser iridotomy, the IOP will rise above 21 mmHg, and long-term medical treatment is required. One-third of argon laser iridotomies will close within six to 12 weeks after surgery and will require a repeat laser iridotomy. Approximately 9% of Nd:Yag laser iridotomies must be redone for this reason. Closure of the iridotomy site is more likely if a uveitis presented after surgery. Up to

KEY TERMS

Angle—A channel in the anterior part of the eye in which the trabecular meshwork is located.

Angle closure—A blockage of the angle of the eye, causing an increase in pressure in the eye and possible glaucoma.

Aphakic—Having no lens in the eye.

Cataract—Condition that causes the lens to become opaque.

Glaucoma—A group of diseases of the eye, often caused by increased pressure (IOP), which can cause blindness if not treated.

Gonioscopy—Examination of the anterior chamber of the eye using a special instrument called a gonioscope.

Hyperosmotic agents—Causing abnormally rapid osmosis.

Iridectomy—Removal of a portion of the iris.

Iridoplasty—Surgery to alter the iris.

Iris—The colored part of the eye that is located in the anterior chamber.

Malignant glaucoma—Glaucoma the gets worse even after iridectomy.

Mannitol—A type of diuretic.

Laser iridotomy—A procedure, using either the Nd:Yag laser or the argon laser, to penetrate the iris, such that a hole, through which the fluid in the eye can drain, is formed.

Osmosis—Passage of a solvent through a membrane from an area of greater concentration to an area of lesser concentration.

Phacolytic glaucoma—Type of glaucoma causing dissolution of the lens.

Photocoagulation—Condensation of material by laser.

Pilocarpine—Drug used to treat glaucoma.

Trabecular meshwork—Area of fibrous tissue that forms a canal between the iris and cornea, through which aqueous humor flows.

Uveitis—Inflammation of the iris and ciliary bodies.

45% of patients will have anterior lens opacities after laser iridotomy, but these opacifications do not put the patient at an increased risk of cataracts.

Alternatives

An alternative to laser iridotomy is surgical **iridectomy**, a procedure in which part of the iris is removed surgically. This was the procedure of choice prior to the development of laser iridotomy. The risks for iridectomy are greater than for the laser iridotomy, because it involves an incision through the sclera, the white tunic covering of the eye that surrounds the cornea. The most common complication of an iridectomy is cataract formation, occurring in more than 50% of patients who have had a surgical iridectomy. Since an incision in the eye is required for surgical iridectomy, other procedures, such as filtration surgery—if needed in the future—will be more difficult to perform. Studies comparing the visual outcomes and IOP control of laser iridotomy with surgical iridectomy show equivalent results.

In the case of acute angle closures that occur because of reasons other than, or in addition to pupillary block, argon laser peripheral iridoplasty is performed. During this procedure, several long burns of low power are placed in the periphery of the iris. The iris contracts and pulls away from the angle, opening it up and relieving the IOP.

Resources

BOOKS

Albert, Daniel M., M.D. *Ophthalmic Surgery Principles and Techniques.* Oxford, England: Blackwell Science, 1999.

Albert, Daniel M., M.D. *Principles and Practice of Ophthalmology,* 2nd ed. Philadelphia, PA: W. B. Saunders Company, 2000.

Azuara-Blanco, Augusto, M.D, Ph.D., et. al. *Handbook of Glaucoma.* London, England: Martin Dunitz Ltd, 2002.

Kanski, Jack J. M. D., et. al. *Glaucoma A Colour Manual of Diagnosis and Treatment.* Oxford, England: Butterworth-Heinemann, 1996.

Ritch, Robert, M. D., et. al. *The Glaucomas.* St. Louis, MO: 1996.

PERIODICALS

Breingan, Peter J. M. D., et. al. "Iridolenticular Contact Decreases Following Laser Iridotomy For Pigment Dispersion Syndrome." *Archives of Ophthalmology* 117 (March 1999): 325-28.

Brown, Reay H.,M. D., et. al. "Glaucoma Laser Treatment Parameters and Practices of ASCRS Members–1999 Survey." *Journal of Cataract and Refractive Surgery* 26 (May 2000): 755-65.

Nolan, Winifred P., et. el. "YAG Laser Iridotomy Treatment for Primary Angle Closure in East Asian Eyes." *British Journal of Ophthalmology* 84 (2000): 1255-59.

Wu, Shiu-Chen, M. D., et. al. "Corneal Endothelial Damage After Neodymium: YAG Laser Iridotomy." *Ophthalmic Surgery and Lasers* 31 (October 2000): 411-16.

OTHER

"Narrow Angle Glaucoma and Acute Angle Closure Glaucoma." <http://www.M.D.eyedocs.com/edacuteglaucoma.htm>.
"Laser Iridotomy and Iridoplasty." <http://cuth.cataegu.ac.kr/~jwkim/glaucoma/doctor/LI.htm>.
"Lasers in the Treatment of Anterior Segment Disorders." <http:www.tnoa.net/articles/1.HTM>.
"Plateau Iris Glaucoma." <http://emedicine.com/OPH/topics574.htm>.

Martha Reilly, OD

Laser posterior capsulotomy

Definition

Laser posterior capsulotomy, or YAG laser capsulotomy, is a noninvasive procedure performed on the eye to remove the opacification (cloudiness) that develops on the posterior capsule of the lens of the eye after extraction of a cataract. This differs from the anterior capsulotomy that the surgeon makes during cataract extraction to remove a cataract and implant an intraocular lens (IOL). Laser posterior capsulotomy is performed with Nd:YAG laser, which uses a wavelength to disrupt the opacification on the posterior lens capsule. The energy emitted from the laser forms a hole in the lens capsule, removing a central area of the opacification. This posterior capsule opacification (PCO) is also referred to as a secondary cataract.

PCO formation is an attempt by the eye to make a new lens from remaining lens material. One form of PCO is a fibrosis that forms inside the capsule by lens epithelial (covering) cells that migrate from the anterior capsule to the posterior capsule when the anterior lens capsule is opened to remove the primary cataract and insert the IOL. Opacification is also be formed by residual lens cortex cells. The epithelial cells can transform into myofibroblasts and proliferate; myofibroblasts are precursors to muscle cells and capable of contraction. The deposit of collagen on these cells leaves the posterior lens capsule with a white, fibrous appearance. This type of opacification can appear within days of cataract surgery. The greatest capsule opacification is found around the edges of the IOL, where the anterior and posterior lens capsules adhere and form a seam, called Soemmering's ring.

Elschnig's pearls are a proliferation of cells on the outside of the capsule. This type of PCO can be several layers thick and develops months to years after cataract surgery. Elschnig's pearls can also appear along the margins of a previously performed laser capsulotomy.

A secondary cataract will also form from wrinkling of the lens capsule, either secondary to contraction of the myofibroblasts on the capsule or because of stretching of the capsule by haptics, or hooks, used to hold the IOL in place.

Posterior capsule opacification is the most common complication of cataract removal or extraction. It does not occur when an anterior chamber lens is implanted, because in this procedure the capsule is usually extracted along with the cataract, and a lens is attached to the iris in the front part of the eye, called the anterior chamber. This technique for cataract removal is not often performed.

Purpose

The purpose of a laser capsulotomy is to remove a PCO. This procedure dramatically improves visual acuity and contrast sensitivity and decreases glare. The visual acuity before capsulotomy can be as poor as 20/400, but barring any other visual or ophthalmologic conditions, the patient will see as well after a laser posterior capsulotomy as after removal of the original cataract. Laser capsulotomies are usually performed once a patient's vision is 20/30.

Demographics

Approximately 20% of patients who undergo cataract extraction with placement of an intraocular lens into the posterior lens capsule will eventually undergo a laser capsulotomy, although a PCO may appear in up to 50% of patients who have undergone cataract surgery. The average time after cataract extraction for this procedure to be performed is two years, but it may be performed as early as three months after cataract removal, or as late as five years afterward.

Patients who fall into groups with an increased incidence of a secondary cataract formation have an increased rate of YAG capsulotomy. Patients who are younger when undergoing cataract removal are more likely to develop a PCO than are geriatric patients. This is particularly true of pediatric patients who are experiencing ocular growth. The incidence of PCO is higher in women than in men. Fifty percent of patients who experience papillary, or iris capture, of the IOL, which occurs if the IOL moves through the pupil (a hole in the iris) from its position in the posterior chamber of the eye to the anterior chamber, will form a PCO and benefit from laser capsulotomy.

The degree and incidence of capsule opacification also varies with the type of implant used in the initial cataract operation. Larger implants are associated with decreased opacification, and round-edged silicone implants are associated with a greater incidence of opacification than are acrylic implants, which have a square-edged design. These two types of IOLs are called foldable implants because they unfold after being placed in the eye, allowing for a smaller incision on the front of the eye during cataract surgery. Also, the incidence of PCO is less with a silicone IOL than with a rigid IOL. The greater the amount of remaining lens material after extraction, especially in the area of Soemmering's ring, the greater the probability of PCO formation and laser capsulotomy. Also, diabetic patients are more likely to require a YAG capsulotomy than are non-diabetic patients. This is especially true for YAG capsulotomies performed on diabetics 18 months or later after cataract removal. The extent of diabetic retinopathy does not correlate with incidence of PCO or laser capsulotomy. Finally, insufficient dilation of the pupil during cataract surgery and inexperience of the surgeon doing cataract removal contribute to an increased risk of secondary cataract formation.

Description

Laser capsulotomy is usually performed in an ophthalmologist's office as an outpatient procedure. Before beginning the capsulotomy, the patient is given an **informed consent** for the procedure. An hour before the laser capsulotomy, a drop of a pressure-lowering drug such as timoptic or apraclonidine is administered. A weak dilating drop to enlarge the pupil is applied to the eye. The eye may be anesthetized locally if the doctor uses a special contact lens for the procedure.

The patient then puts the head in the chinrest of a slit lamp microscope, to which a laser is attached. The doctor then may place a special lens on the front of the eye. It is important that the patient remain still as the doctor focuses on the posterior capsule. A head strap to help keep the patient's head in place may be used. While focusing on the posterior capsule, the doctor, with repeated bursts from the Nd:Yag laser in a circular manner, disrupts the PCO. An opening forms on the posterior part of the lens capsule as part of the PCO falls off of the posterior capsule and into the vitreous. Another drop of apraclonidine, or other pressure-lowering eyedrop, is applied to the eye as a preventative measure for increased pressure in the eye, which is experienced by most patients after the procedure. This is a brief procedure lasting only a few minutes and is not associated with pain.

Diagnosis/Preparation

Prior to performing a posterior capsulotomy, the doctor will perform a thorough ophthalmic examination

and review any systemic medical problems. The ophthalmologic includes evaluation of visual acuity, slit-lamp biomicroscope examination of the eye to assess the extent and type of opacification and rule out inflammation or swelling in the front of the eye, measurement of intraocular pressure, and a thorough evaluation of the fundus or back of the eye to check for retinal detachments and macular problems, which would limit the extent to which the YAG capsulotomy could improve vision. A potential acuity meter (PAM) may be used to ascertain best expected visual acuity after YAG capsulotomy, and brightness acuity testing will determine the extent of glare experienced by the patient. Contrast sensitivity testing is employed by some doctors.

This procedure cannot be performed in the presence of certain preexisting ophthalmologic conditions. For example, irregularities of the cornea would interfere with the ability of the doctor to see the posterior capsule. Also, a laser capsulotomy could not be performed if there is ongoing inflammation in the eye, or if swelling of the macula (a part of the retina) is present. A laser capsulotomy would be contraindicated with glass IOLs. If macular edema is suspected, which can occur in up to 30% of patients who have undergone cataract surgery, a test called a fluoroscein **angiography** may also be performed.

Aftercare

After a laser capsulotomy, the patient will remain in the office for one to four hours so that the pressure in the eye can be evaluated. The patient can then resume normal everyday activities. After surgery, pressure-lowering eyedrops may be used for a week, if the intraocular pressure is raised significantly after the

QUESTIONS
TO ASK THE DOCTOR

- What are the alternatives to laser capsulotomy?
- Am I a good candidate for this procedure?
- What will my vision be like afterwards?
- How many of these procedures have you done?

procedure. Cycloplegic agents to keep the pupil dilated and to prevent spasm of the muscles in the iris, and steroids to reduce inflammation may also be prescribed for up to a week. Follow-up visits are scheduled at one day, one week, one month, three months, and six months after capsulotomy.

Risks

One risk of laser capsulotomy is damage to the intraocular implant. Factors that determine the extent of damage to the IOL include the inherent resistance of a particular IOL to damage by the laser, the amount of energy used in the procedure, the position of the IOL within the lens capsule, and the focusing accuracy of the surgeon. The thicker the opacification of the lens capsule, the greater the amount of energy needed to remove it. The accuracy of the surgeon is improved when there is less opacification on the lens capsule.

In addition, during laser capsulotomy the IOL can be displaced into the eye's vitreous. This happens more often in eyes with a rigid implant, rather than with acrylic or silicone IOLs, and also if a larger implant is used. If the posterior capsule ruptures during extraction of the primary cataract, risk of lens displacement is also increased. Displacement risk is also increased if the area over which the laser capsulotomy is done is large. The most serious complication of a capsulotomy would be IOL damage so extensive that extraction would be required. This is a rare complication.

Another risk of this surgery is the re-formation of Elschnig's pearls over the opening created by the capsulotomy. This occurs in up to 80% of patients within two years of laser capsulotomy. Most of time, these PCOs will resolve over time without treatment, but 20% of patients will require a second laser capsulotomy. This secondary opacification by Elschnig pearls represents a spatial progression of the opacification that caused the initial secondary cataract.

Other risks to take into account when considering a posterior capsulotomy are macular edema, macular holes, corneal edema, inflammation of the iris, retinal detachment, and increased pressure in the eye, as well as glaucoma. These risks escalate with increased laser energy and with increased size of the capsulotomy area. Retinal detachments are usually treated with removal of the vitreous behind the lens capsule. Macular edema is treated by application of topical anti-inflammatory drops or intraocular steroid injections. Steroids control iritis (inflammation of the iris), either topically or intraocularly. Macular holes are also treated by removal of the vitreous (the substance that fills the main area of the eyeball), followed by one to three weeks of facedown positioning. Elevated intraocular pressure and glaucoma are treated with anti-glaucoma drops or glaucoma surgery, if necessary.

Finally, increased glare at night may result when the size of the capsulotomy is smaller than the diameter of the pupil during dark conditions.

Normal results

Within one to two days after surgery, maximum visual acuity will be attained by almost 99% of patients. Once the opacification is removed, most patients will not need a change in spectacle prescription. However, patients who have undergone implantation of a rigid IOL may experience an increase in hyperopia, or far-sightedness, after a capsulotomy. For a few weeks after surgery, the presence of visual floaters, which are pieces of the excised capsule, is normal. But, the presence of floaters months after this timeframe, especially if accompanied by flashes of light, may signal a retinal tear or detachment and require immediate attention. Also, if vision suddenly or gradually worsens after an initial improvement, further follow-up to determine the cause of a decrease in visual function is imperative.

Morbidity and mortality rates

The probability of a retinal detachment after capsulotomy is 1.6–1.9%. This represents a two-fold increase of retinal detachment over the rate for all patients undergoing cataract surgery, regardless if a posterior capsulotomy was done or not. Macular edema occurs in up to 2.5% of patients who undergo a laser capsulotomy and is more likely to occur when the capsulotomy is performed soon after cataract extraction, or in younger individuals. Rarely does glaucoma develop after laser capsulotomy, although as many as two-thirds of patients will experience transient increased intraocular pressure.

Alternatives

The alternative to laser capsulotomy is surgical capsulotomy of the PCO and the adjacent anterior vitreous.

KEY TERMS

Anterior chamber—The part of the eye located behind the cornea and in front of the iris and lens; it is filled with aqueous fluid.

Cataract—An opacification of the lens in the eye. There are three types of cataracts: subcapsular, which forms inside the capsule in which the lens is located; nuclear, which is a natural yellowing of the lens nucleus; cortical, which refers to spoke-type opacities within the cortex layer of the lens.

Lens capsule—The "bag" is a membrane that holds the lens in place and holds a posterior lens implant when a cataract is removed.

Macula—This is the part of the retina in which the highest concentration of photoreceptors are found.

Posterior chamber—This is the part of the eye located behind the lens of the eye and includes the retina, where the photoreceptors are located.

Posterior capsule opacification (PCO)—This refers to the opacities that form on the back of the lens capsule after cataract removal or extraction. It is synonymous with a secondary cataract.

Vitreous—This is the jelly-like substance that fills the space between the lens capsule and the retina.

There is an increased risk of retinal detachment when this invasive intraocular surgery is employed. The other alternative is to leave the PCO in place. This leaves the patient with permanent decreased visual acuity.

Resources

BOOKS

Albert, Daniel M., et al. *Principles and Practice of Ophthalmology, 2nd Edition.* Philadelphia, PA: W. B. Saunders Co., 2000.

Gills, James P. *Cataract Surgery: The State of the Art.* Thorofare, NJ: Slack Inc., 1998.

Jaffe, Norman. *Atlas of Ophthalmic Surgery.* London: Mosby-Wolfe, 1996.

Jaffe, Norman, et al. *Cataract Surgery and Its Complications.* St Louis, MO: Mosby, 1997.

Steinert, Roger F. *Cataract Surgery: Technique, Complications, & Management.* Philadelphia, PA: W. B. Saunders, 1995.

PERIODICALS

Baratz, K. H., et al. "Probability of Nd:YAG Laser Capsulotomy After Cataract Surgery in Olmsted County, Minnesota." *American Journal of Ophthalmology* 131 (February 2001): 161–166.

Charles, Steve. "Vitreoretinal Complications of YAG Laser Capsulotomy." *Ophthalmology Clinics of North America* 14 (December 2001): 705–9.

Chua, C. N, et al. "Refractive Changes following Nd:YAG Capsulotomy." *Eye* 15 (June 2001): 303–5.

Hayashi, Ken. "Posterior Capsule Opacification After Surgery In Patients With Diabetes Mellitus." *American Journal of Ophthalmology* 134 (July 2002): 10–16.

Hu, Chao-Yu., et al. "Change in the Area of Laser Posterior Capsulotomy: 3 Month Follow-Up." *Journal of Cataract and Refractive Surgery* 27 (April 2001): 537–42.

Kurosaka, Daijiro, et al. "Elschnig Pearl Formation Along the Neodymium:YAG Laser Posterior Capsulotomy Margin." *Journal of Cataract and Refractive Surgery* 28 (October 2002): 1809–1813.

O'Keefe, Michael, et al. "Visual Outcomes and Complications of Posterior Chamber Intraocular Lens Implantation in the First Year of Life." *Journal of Cataract and Refractive Surgery* 27 (December 2001): 2006–11.

Sundelin, Karin, and Johan Sjostrand. "Posterior Capsule Opacification 5 Years After Extracapsular Cataract Extraction." *Journal of Cataract and Refractive Surgery* 25 (February 1999): 246–50.

Trinavarant, A., et al. "Neodymium: YAG laser Damage Threshold of Foldable Intraocular Lenses." *Journal of Cataract and Refractive Surgery* 27 (May 2001): 775–880.

Martha Reilly, OD

Laser skin resurfacing

Definition

Laser skin resurfacing involves the application of laser light to the skin in order to remove fine wrinkles and tighten the skin surface. It is most often used on the skin of the face.

Purpose

The purpose of laser skin resurfacing is to use the heat generated by extremely focused light to remove the upper to middle layers of the skin. This procedure eliminates superficial signs of aging and softens the appearance of other lesions such as scars. Upon healing, the surface of the skin has a younger appearance. Microscopic analysis of skin after laser resurfacing shows that the healed surface more closely resembles younger, healthier skin in many aspects.

Demographics

According to the American Society for Aesthetic Plastic Surgery, there were more than 72,000 laser skin resurfacing procedures performed in the United States in 2002. Almost all persons of sufficient age have one or more symptoms of aging or damaged skin that can be treated by this procedure, including fine lines in the skin, known as rhytides; discoloration of the skin; acne scarring; and surgical or other types of scars.

Description

A central component of the laser skin resurfacing technique is the laser device. Laser is an acronym for light amplification by stimulated emission of radiation. This device produces an intense beam of light of a specific, known wavelength. Laser light is produced by high-energy stimulation of different substances such as crystals, liquid dyes, and gases. For skin resurfacing, two types of lasers produce light that is well absorbed by the upper to middle layers of the skin: light produced from carbon dioxide gas (CO_2) and light produced from a crystal made of eribium, yttrium, aluminum, and garnet (Er:YAG). Combination lasers are also commercially available.

There are as yet no standard parameters for laser use in all skin resurfacing procedures. Settings are determined on a case-by-case basis by the laser surgeon who relies on his or her own experience.

Before the procedure begins, medication is often given to relax the patient and reduce pain. For small areas, local topical (surface-applied) anesthetics are often used to numb the area to be treated. Alternatively, for large areas, nerve block-type anesthesia is used. Some laser surgeons use conscious sedation (twilight anesthesia) alone or in combination with other techniques.

During the procedure, the patient lies on his or her back on the surgical table, eyes covered to protect them from the laser light. Laser passes are performed over the area being treated, utilizing computer control of the laser for precise results. In general, more passes are needed with Er:YAG lasers than carbon dioxide laser treatment.

Because areas of the body other than the face have relatively low numbers of the cells central to the healing process, laser skin resurfacing is not generally used anywhere but on the face, as elsewhere the healing process may be so slow as to result in scarring.

Diagnosis/Preparation

An initial consideration is to determine which laser would be best for any particular skin resurfacing procedure. Carbon dioxide lasers have been in use longer and have been shown to produce very good results. However, the healing times tend to be long and redness can persist for several months. In contrast, because the light produced by the Er:YAG laser is more efficiently absorbed by the skin, less light energy and shorter pass times can be used, which significantly shortens the healing time. Unfortunately, the results obtained with this laser have not been as consistently good as with a carbon dioxide laser. Patients should therefore discuss the two laser types and the condition of their skin with their doctor to determine which would be better for their particular situation.

Although controversial, some studies have reported abnormal scarring in patients previously treated with 13 cis-retinoic acid (Accutane), so many surgeons will require a six-month break from the medication before performing laser skin resurfacing.

Laser skin resurfacing does increase the chance of recurrent or initial herpes simplex virus infection (cold sores) during the healing process. Even with no patient history of the problem, it is important that anti-viral medicine is administered before, the morning of, and following laser skin resurfacing.

Aftercare

After the procedure, any treated areas are dressed for healing. Surgeons are divided on whether the wound should remain open or closed (covered) during the healing process. For example, surgeons that adopt a closed procedure can use a dressing that is primarily hydrogel held on a mesh support to cover the wound. This kind of dressing is changed daily while the epithelium (outer layer) is restored. Open **wound care** involves frequent soaks in salt water or dilute acetic acid, followed by application of ointment. Whatever wound treatment is used, it is important to keep the healing skin hydrated.

Full restoration of the epithelial layer occurs in seven to 10 days after treatment with a carbon dioxide laser and three to five days after treatment with a Er:YAG laser, although redness can persist for many weeks afterward.

Risks

Risks of this procedure include skin redness that persists beyond the initial healing period, swelling, burning sensations, or itching. These risks tend to be short term and lessen over time. More long-term problems can include scarring, increased or decreased pigmentation of the skin, and infection during healing. Finally, the formation of milia, bumps that form due to obstruction of the sweat glands, can occur, although this can be treated after healing with retinoic acid.

Normal results

Normal results of this procedure include reduction in the fine lines found in aging skin, improving skin texture, making skin coloration more consistent, and softening the appearance of scars. In a recent study, more than 93% of patients subjectively rated their results from the procedure either very good or excellent.

Morbidity and mortality rates

The morbidity and mortality rates for this cosmetic procedure are close to zero.

Alternatives

Surgical techniques such as facelifts or **blepharoplasty** (eyelid surgery) are often recommended when facial aging is beyond the restorative powers of a laser treatment and the most common alternative technique. Patients should also consider other skin resurfacing techniques such as **dermabrasion** or chemical peels, as these are more effective than laser resurfacing for certain skin conditions and certain skin types.

Resources

BOOKS

Roberts, Thomas L. III, and Jason N. Pozner. "Aesthetic Laser Surgery." In *Plastic Surgery: Indications, Operations, and*

KEY TERMS

Acetic acid—Vinegar; very dilute washes of the treated areas with a vinegar solution are suggested by some surgeons after laser skin resurfacing.

Carbon dioxide—Abbreviated CO_2; a gas that produces light that is well absorbed by the skin, so is commonly used for skin resurfacing treatments.

Erbium:YAG—A crystal made of erbium, yttrium, aluminum, and garnet that produces light that is well absorbed by the skin, so it is used for skin resurfacing treatments.

Hydrogel—A gel that contains water, used as a dressing after laser skin resurfacing.

Milia—Small bumps on the skin that are occur when sweat glands are clogged.

Rhytides—Very fine wrinkles, often of the face.

Topical—Applied to the skin surface.

Outcomes, Volume 5, edited by Craig A. Vander Kolk, et al. St. Louis, MO: Mosby, 2000.

PERIODICALS

Bisson, M. A., R. Grover, and A.O. Grobbelaar. "Long-term Results of Facial Rejuvenation by Carbon Dioxide Laser Resurfacing Using a Quantitative Method of Assessment." *British Journal of Plastic Surgery* 55 (2002): 652–656.

ORGANIZATIONS

American Society for Aesthetic Plastic Surgery. 11081 Winners Circle, Los Alamitos, CA 90720. (800) 364-2147 or (562) 799-2356. <www.surgery.org>.

American Society of Plastic Surgeons. 444 E. Algonquin Rd., Arlington Heights, IL 60005. (800) 475-2784. <www.plasticsurgery.org>.

OTHER

Tanzi, Elizabeth L. "Cutaneous Laser Resurfacing: Erbuim: YAG." *eMedicine,* January 10, 2002.

Michelle Johnson, MS, JD

Laser surgery

Definition

The term laser means light amplification by stimulated emission of radiation, and it uses a laser light source (laser beam) to remove tissues that are diseased or to treat blood vessels that are bleeding. Laser beams are strong beams of light produced by electrically stimulating a particular material. A solid, a liquid, or a gas is used. Alternatively, the laser is used cosmetically; it can remove wrinkles, birthmarks, or tattoos.

The special light beam is focused to treat tissues by heating the cells until they burst. There are a number of different laser types. Each has a different use and color. The color, or the light beam, relates to the type of surgery that is being performed and the color of the tissue that is being treated. There are three types of laser: the carbon dioxide (CO_2) laser; the YAG laser (yttrium aluminum garnet); and the pulsed dye laser.

Purpose

Laser surgery is used to:

• cut or destroy tissue that is abnormal or diseased without harming healthy, normal tissue

• shrink or destroy tumors and lesions

• close off nerve endings to reduce postoperative pain

• cauterize (seal) blood vessels to reduce blood loss

• seal lymph vessels to minimize swelling and decrease spread of tumor cells

• remove moles, warts, and tattoos

• decrease the appearance of skin wrinkles

Precautions

Anyone who is thinking about having laser surgery should ask the surgeon to:

• explain why laser surgery is likely to be of greater benefit than traditional surgery

• describe the surgeon's experience in performing the laser procedure the patient is considering

Because some lasers can temporarily or permanently discolor the skin of blacks, Asians, and Hispanics, a dark-skinned patient should make sure that the surgeon has successfully performed laser procedures on people of color. Potential problems include infection, pain, scarring, and changes in skin color.

Some types of laser surgery should not be performed on pregnant women or on patients with severe cardiopulmonary disease or other serious health problems.

Additionally, because some laser surgical procedures are performed under general anesthesia, its risks should be fully discussed with the anesthesiologist. The patient should fully disclose all over-the-counter and prescription medications that are being taken, as well as the foods and beverages that are generally consumed; some can interact with agents used in anesthesia.

Description

Lasers can be used to perform almost any surgical procedure. In fact, general surgeons employ the various laser wavelengths and laser delivery systems to cut, coagulate, vaporize, and remove tissue. In most "laser surgeries," they actually use genuine laser devices in place of conventional surgical tools—scalpels, cryosugery probes, electrosurgical units, or microwave devices—to carry out standard procedures, like mastectomy (breast surgery). With the use of lasers, the skilled and trained surgeon can accomplish tasks that are more complex, all the while reducing blood loss, decreasing postoperative patient discomfort, decreasing the chances of infection to the wound, reducing the spread of some cancers, minimizing the extent of surgery (in some cases), and achieving better outcomes in wound healing. Also, because lasers are more precise, the laser can penetrate tissue by adjusting the intensity of the light.

Lasers are also extremely useful in both open and laparoscopic procedures. Common surgical uses include breast surgery, removal of the gallbladder, hernia repair, **bowel resection**, **hemorrhoidectomy**, solid organ surgery, and treatment of pilonidal cyst.

The first working laser was introduced in 1960. Initially used to treat diseases and disorders of the eye, the device was first used to treat diseases and disorders of the eye, whose transparent tissues gave ophthalmic surgeons a clear view of how the narrow, concentrated beam was being directed. Dermatologic surgeons also helped to pioneer laser surgery, and developed and improved upon many early techniques and more refined surgical procedures.

Types of lasers

The three types of lasers most often used in medical treatment are the:

• Carbon dioxide (CO_2) laser. Primarily a surgical tool, this device converts light energy to heat strong enough to minimize bleeding, while cutting through or vaporizes tissue.

• Neodymium:yttrium-aluminum-garnet (Nd:YAG) laser. Capable of penetrating tissue more deeply than other lasers, the Nd:YAG laser enables blood to clot quickly, allowing surgeons to see and can enable surgeons to see and touch body parts that could otherwise be reached only through open (invasive) surgery.

• Argon laser. This laser provides the limited penetration needed for eye surgery and superficial skin disorders. In a special procedure known as photodynamic therapy (PDT), this laser uses light-sensitive dyes to shrink or dissolve tumors.

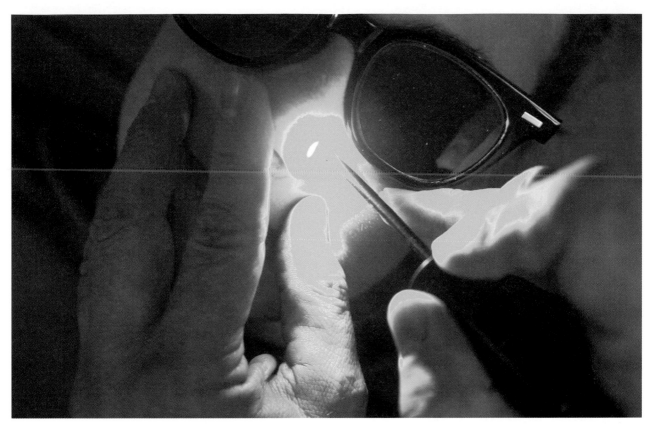

Cosmetic laser surgery in progress. The wavelengths of the laser's light can be matched to a specific target, enabling the physician to destroy the capillaries near the skin's surface without damaging the surrounding tissue. *(Photograph by Will & Deni McIntyre, Photo Researchers, Inc. Reproduced by permission.)*

Laser applications

Sometimes described as "scalpels of light," lasers are used alone or with conventional **surgical instruments** in a array of procedures that:

- improve appearance
- relieve pain
- restore function
- save lives

Laser surgery is often standard operating procedure for specialists in:

- cardiology (branch of medicine which deals with the heart and its diseases)
- dentistry (branch of medicine which deals with the anatomy and development and diseases of the teeth)
- dermatology (science which treats the skin, its structure, functions, and its diseases)
- gastroenterology (science which treats disorders of the stomach and intestines)
- gynecology (science which treats of the structure and diseases of women)

- neurosurgery (surgery of the nervous system)
- oncology (cancer treatment)
- ophthalmology (treatment of disorders of the eye)
- orthopedics (treatment of disorders of bones, joints, muscles, ligaments, and tendons)
- otolaryngology (treatment of disorders of the ears, nose, and throat)
- pulmonology (treatment of disorders of the respiratory system)
- urology (treatment of disorders of the urinary tract and of the male reproductive system)

Routine uses of lasers, include eliminating birthmarks, skin discoloration, and skin changes due to aging, and removing benign, precancerous, or cancerous tissues or tumors. Lasers are used to stop a patient's snoring, remove tonsils, remove or transplant hair, and relieve pain and restore function in patients who are too weak to undergo major surgery. Lasers are also used to treat:

- angina (chest pain)
- cancerous or noncancerous tumors that cannot be removed or destroyed

- cold and canker sores, gum disease, and tooth sensitivity or decay
- ectopic pregnancy (development of a fertilized egg outside the uterus)
- endometriosis
- fibroid tumors
- gallstones
- glaucoma, mild-to-moderate nearsightedness and astigmatism, and other conditions that impair sight
- migraine headaches
- noncancerous enlargement of the prostate gland
- nosebleeds
- ovarian cysts
- ulcers
- varicose veins
- warts
- numerous other conditions, diseases, and disorders

Advantages of laser surgery

Often referred to as "bloodless surgery," laser procedures usually involve less bleeding than conventional surgery. The heat generated by the laser keeps the surgical site free of germs and reduces the risk of infection. Because a smaller incision is required, laser procedures often take less time (and cost less money) than traditional surgery. Sealing off blood vessels and nerves reduces bleeding, swelling, scarring, pain, and the length of the recovery period.

Disadvantages of laser surgery

Although many laser surgeries can be performed in a doctor's office, rather than in a hospital, the person guiding the laser must be at least as thoroughly trained and highly skilled as someone performing the same procedure in a hospital setting. The American Society for Laser Medicine and Surgery urges that:

- All operative areas be equipped with oxygen and other drugs and equipment required for **cardiopulmonary resuscitation** (CPR).
- Non-physicians performing laser procedures be properly trained, licensed, and insured.
- A qualified and experienced supervising physician be able to respond to and manage unanticipated events or other emergencies within five minutes of the time they occur.
- Emergency transportation to a hospital or other acute care facility (ACF) be available whenever laser surgery is performed in a non-hospital setting.

Diagnosis/Preparation

Because laser surgery is used to treat so many diverse conditions, the patient should ask the physician for detailed instructions about how to prepare for a specific procedure. Diet, activities, and medications may not have to be limited prior to surgery, but some procedures require a **physical examination**, a medical history, and conversation with the patient that:

- enables the doctor to evaluate the patient's general health and current medical status
- provides the doctor with information about how the patient has responded to other illnesses, hospital stays, and diagnostic or therapeutic procedures
- clarifies what the patient expects the outcome of the procedure to be

Aftercare

Most laser surgeries can be performed on an outpatient basis, and patients are usually permitted to leave the hospital or medical office when their **vital signs** have stabilized. A patient who has been sedated should not be discharged until recovery from the anesthesia is complete, unless a responsible adult is available to accompany the patient home.

The doctor may prescribe analgesic (pain-relieving) medication, and should provide easy-to-understand, written instructions on how to take the medication. The doctor should also be able to give the patient a good estimate of how the patient's recovery should progress, the recovery time, and what to do in case complications or emergency arise. The amount of time it takes for the patient to recover from surgery depends on the surgery and on the individual. Recovery time for laser surgery is, for the most part, faster than for traditional surgery.

Risks

Like traditional surgery, laser surgery can be complicated by:

- hemorrhage
- infection
- perforation (piercing) of an organ or tissue

Laser surgery can also involve risks that are not associated with traditional surgical procedures. Being careless or not practicing safe surgical techniques can severely burn the patient's lungs or even cause them to explode. Patients must wear protective eye shields while undergoing laser surgery on any part of the face near the eyes or eyelids, and the United States Food and Drug Administration has said that both doctors and patients

KEY TERMS

Argon—A colorless, odorless gas.

Astigmatism—A condition in which one or both eyes cannot filter light properly and images appear blurred and indistinct.

Canker sore—A blister-like sore on the inside of the mouth that can be painful but is not serious.

Carbon dioxide—A heavy, colorless gas that dissolves in water.

Cardiopulmonary disease—Illness of the heart and lungs.

Cardiopulmonary resuscitation (CPR)—An emergency procedure used to restore circulation and prevent brain death to a person who has collapsed, is unconscious, is not breathing, and has no pulse.

Cauterize—To use heat or chemicals to stop bleeding, prevent the spread of infection, or destroy tissue.

Cornea—The outer, transparent lens that covers the pupil of the eye and admits light.

Endometriosis—An often painful gynecologic condition in which endometrial tissue migrates from the inside of the uterus to other organs inside and beyond the abdominal cavity.

Glaucoma—A disease of the eye in which increased pressure within the eyeball can cause gradual loss of vision.

Invasive surgery—A form of surgery that involves making an incision in the patient's body and inserting instruments or other medical devices into it.

Laparoscopic procedures—Surgical procedures during which surgeons rely on a laparoscope—a pencil-thin instrument that has its own lighting system and miniature video camera. To perform surgeries, only small incisions are needed to insert the instruments and the miniature camera.

Nearsightedness—A condition in which one or both eyes cannot focus normally, causing objects at a distance to appear blurred and indistinct. Also called myopia.

Ovarian cyst—A benign or malignant growth on an ovary. An ovarian cyst can disappear without treatment or become extremely painful and have to be surgically removed.

Pilonidal cyst—A special kind of abscess that occurs in the cleft between the buttocks. Forms frequently in adolescence after long trips that involve sitting.

Vaporize—To dissolve solid material or convert it into smoke or gas.

Varicose veins—Swollen, twisted veins, usually occurring in the legs, that occur more often in women than in men.

must use special wavelength-specific, protective eyewear whenever a CO_2 laser is used.

There are other kinds of dangers that laser surgery can impose of which the patient should be aware. Laser beams have the capacity to do a great deal of damage when coupled with high enough energy and absorption. They can ignite clothing, paper, and hair. Further, the risk of fire from lasers increases in the presence of oxygen. Hair should be protected and clothing should be tied back, or removed, within the treatment areas. It is important to guard against electric shock, as lasers require the use of high voltage. Critically, installation must ensure proper wiring.

Laser beams can burn or destroy healthy tissue, cause injuries that are painful and sometimes permanent, and actually compound problems they are supposed to solve. Errors or inaccuracies in laser surgery can worsen a patient's vision, for example, and lasers can scar and even change the skin color of some patients.

All of the above risks, precautions, and potential complications should be discussed by the doctor with the patient.

Normal results

The nature and severity of the problem, the skill of the surgeon performing the procedure, and the patient's general health and realistic expectations are among the factors that influence the outcome of laser surgery. Successful procedures can enable patients to feel better, look younger, and enjoy longer, fuller, more active lives.

A patient who is considering any kind of laser surgery should ask the doctor to provide detailed information about what the outcome of the surgery is expected to be, what the recovery process will involve, and how long it will probably be before a normal appearance is regained and the patient can resume normal activities.

A person who is considering any type of laser surgery should ask the doctor to provide specific and detailed information about what could go wrong during the procedure and what the negative impact on the patient's health or appearance might be.

Lighter or darker skin may appear, for example, when a laser is used to remove sun damage or age spots from an olive- or dark-skinned individual. This abnormal pigmentation may or may not disappear over time.

Scarring or rupturing of the cornea is uncommon, but laser surgery on one or both eyes can:

• increase sensitivity to light or glare

• reduce night vision

• permanently cloud vision, or cause sharpness of vision to decline throughout the day

Signs of infection following laser surgery include:

• burning

• crusting of the skin

• itching

• pain

• scarring

• severe redness

• swelling

Resources

BOOKS

Carlson, Karen J., et. al. *The Harvard Guide to Women's Health.* Cambridge, MA: Harvard University Press, 1996.

PERIODICALS

"Laser Procedures for Nearsightedness." *FDA Consumer* (Jan./Feb. 1996): 2.

"Laser Resurfacing Slows the Hands of Time." *Harvard Health Letter* (Aug. 1996): 4-5.

"Lasers." *Mayo Clinic Health Letter* (July 1994): 1-3.

"Lasers: Bright Lights of the Medical World." *Cosmopolitan* (May 1995): 262-265.

"Lasers for Skin Surgery." *Harvard Women's Health Watch* (Mar. 1997): 2-3.

"Lasers–Hope or Hype?" *American Health* (June 1994): 68-72, 103.

"New Cancer Therapies That Ease Pain, Extend Life." *Cancer Smart* (June 1997): 8-10.

"New Laser Surgery for Angina." *HealthNews* (6 May 1997): 3-4.

"Saving Face." *Essence* (Aug. 1997), 24, 26, 28.

ORGANIZATIONS

American Society for Dermatologic Surgery. 930 N. Meacham Road, P.O. Box 4014, Schaumburg, IL 60168-4014. (847) 330-9830. <http://www.asds-net.org>.

American Society for Laser Medicine and Surgery. 2404 Stewart Square, Wausau, WI 54401.(715) 845-9283. <http://www.aslms.org>.

Cancer Information Service. 9000 Rockville Pike, Building 31, Suite 10A18, Bethesda, MD 20892. 1-800-4-CANCER. <http://wwwicic.nci.nih.gov>.

Mayo Clinic. Division of Colon and Rectal Surgery. 200 First Street. SW, Rochester, MN 55905. (507) 284-2511. <http://www.mayoclinic.org/colorectalsurgery-rst/laparo scopicsurgery.html>.

Mayo Clinic. Mayo Foundation for Medical Education and Research, 200 First Street. SW, Rochester, MN 55905. (507) 284-2511. <http://http://www.mayoclinic.com>.

National Cancer Institute. Building 31, Room 10A31, 31 Center Drive, MSC 2580, Bethesda, MD 20892-2580. (800) 422-6237. <http://www.nci.nih.gov>.

OTHER

"Complications of Dermatologic Laser Surgery." 2 Nov. 2001 <http://www.emedicine.com/derm/topic525.htm>.

"Facts About Laser Surgery." *Glaucoma Research Foundation Page.* 12 Mar. 1998 <http://www.glaucoma.org/fs-laser-sur.html>.

Haggerty, Maureen. "ASLMS Guidelines for Office-Based Laser Procedures." *A Healthy Me Page.* 19 Mar. 1998 <http://www.ahealthyme.com/topic/topic100587070>.

"Refractive Eye Surgery." *Mayo Clinic Online.* 15 Mar. 1998 <http://www.mayohealth.org/mayo/9707/htm/refract. htm>.

"What is Laser?" *The American Society for Dermatologic Surgery Page.* 19 Mar. 1998 <http://www.asds-net.org>.

Laith Farid Gulli,M.D., M.S.
Randi B. Jenkins, B.A.
Bilal Nasser,M.D., M.S.
Robert Ramirez, B.S.

LASIK *see* **Laser in-situ keratomileusis (LASIK)**

Lateral release *see* **Knee arthroscopic surgery**

Laxatives

Definition

Laxatives are products that promote bowel movements.

Purpose

Laxatives are used to treat constipation—the passage of small amounts of hard, dry stools, usually fewer than three times a week. Before recommending use of laxatives, differential diagnosis should be performed. Pro-

KEY TERMS

Carbohydrates—Compounds such as cellulose, sugar, and starch that contain only carbon, hydrogen, and oxygen, and are a major part of the diets of people and other animals.

Cathartic colon—A poorly functioning colon, resulting from the chronic abuse of stimulant cathartics.

Colon—The large intestine.

Diverticulitis—Inflammation of the part of the intestine known as the diverticulum.

Fiber—Carbohydrate material in food that cannot be digested.

Hyperosmetic—Hypertonic, containing a higher concentration of salts or other dissolved materials than normal tissues.

Osteomalacia—A disease of adults, characterized by softening of the bone; similar to rickets, which is seen in children.

Pregnancy category—A system of classifying drugs according to their established risks for use during pregnancy: category A: controlled human studies have demonstrated no fetal risk; category B: animal studies indicate no fetal risk, and there are no adequate and well-controlled studies in pregnant women; category C: no adequate human or animal studies, or adverse fetal effects in animal studies, but no available human data; category D: evidence of fetal risk, but benefits outweigh risks; category X: evidence of fetal risk, which outweigh any benefits.

Steatorrhea—An excess of fat in the stool.

Stool—The solid waste that is left after food is digested. Stool forms in the intestines and passes out of the body through the anus.

longed constipation may be evidence of a significant problem such as localized peritonitis or diverticulitis. Complaints of constipation may be associated with obsessive-compulsive disorder. Use of laxatives should be avoided in these cases. Patients should be aware that patterns of defecation are highly variable, and may vary from two to three times daily to two to three times weekly.

Laxatives may also be used prophylacticly for patients such as those recovering from a myocardial infarction (heart attack) or those who have had recent surgery and should not strain during defecation.

Description

Laxatives may be grouped by mechanism of action.

Saline cathartics include dibasic sodium phosphate (Phospo-Soda), magnesium citrate, magnesium hydroxide (milk of magnesia), magnesium sulfate (Epsom salts), sodium biphosphate, and others. They act by drawing to and holding water in the intestinal tissues, and may produce a watery stool. Magnesium sulfate is the most potent of the laxatives in this group.

Stimulant and irritant laxatives increase the peristaltic movement of the intestine. Product examples include cascara and bisadocyl (Dulcolax). Castor oil works in a similar fashion.

Bulk-producing laxatives increase the volume of the stool, and will both soften the stool and stimulate intestinal motility. Psyllium (Metamucil, Konsil) and methyl-cellulose (Citrucel) are examples of this type. The overall effect is similar to that of eating high-fiber foods, and this class of laxative is most suitable for regular use.

Docusate (Colace) is the only representative example of the stool softener class. It holds water within the fecal mass, providing a larger, softer stool. Docusate has no effect on acute constipation, since it must be present before the fecal mass forms to have any effect, but may be useful for prevention of constipation in patients with recurrent problems, or those who are about to take a constipating drug such as narcotic **analgesics**.

Mineral oil is an emollient laxative. It acts by retarding intestinal absorption of fecal water, thereby softening the stool.

The hyperosmotic laxatives are glycerin and lactulose (Chronulac, Duphalac), both of which act by holding water within the intestine. Lactulose may also increase peristaltic action of the intestine.

Precautions

Short-term use of laxatives is generally safe except in cases of appendicitis, fecal impaction, or intestinal obstruction. Lactulose is composed of two sugar molecules, galactose and fructose, and should not be administered to patients who require a low-galactose diet.

Chronic use of laxatives may result in fluid and electrolyte imbalances, steatorrhea, osteomalacia, diarrhea, cathartic colon, and liver disease. Excessive intake of mineral oil may cause impaired absorption of oil soluble vitamins, particularly A and D. Excessive use of magnesium salts may cause hypermanesemia.

Lactulose and magnesium sulfate are pregnancy category B. Casanthranol, cascara sagrada, danthron, docusate sodium, docusate calcium, docusate potassium, mineral oil, and senna are category C. Casanthranol, cascara sagrada, and danthron are excreted in breast milk, resulting in a potential increased incidence of diarrhea in the nursing infant.

Interactions

Mineral oil and docusate should not be used in combination. Docusate is an emulsifying agent that will increase the absorption of mineral oil.

Bisacodyl tablets are enteric coated, and so should not be used in combination with antacids. The antacids will cause premature rupture of the enteric coating.

Recommended dosage

The consumer is advised to see specific resources for each product.

Resources

PERIODICALS

"Constipation, Laxatives and Dietary Fiber." *HealthTips* (April 1993): 9.
"Overuse Hazardous: Laxatives Rarely Needed." *FDA Consumer* (April 1991): 33.

ORGANIZATIONS

National Digestive Diseases Information Clearinghouse. 2 Information Way, Bethesda, MD 20892-3570. <nddic@ aerie. com>. <http://www.niddk.nih.gov/Brochures/NDDIC.htm>.

OTHER

"Effectiveness of Laxatives in Adults." Centre for Reviews and Dissemination, University of York. [cited June 2003] <http://www.york.ac.uk/inst/crd/ehc71.htm>.
"Laxatives (Oral)." Medline Plus Drug Information. [cited June 2003] <http://www.nlm.nih.gov/medlineplus/druginfo/uspdi/202319.html>.

Samuel D. Uretsky, PharmD

Leg lengthening/shortening

Definition

Leg lengthening or shortening involves a variety of surgical procedures used to correct legs of unequal lengths, a condition referred to as limb length discrepancy (LLD). LLD occurs because a leg bone grows more slowly in one leg than on the other leg. Surgical treatment is indicated for discrepancies exceeding 1 in (2.5 cm).

Purpose

Leg lengthening or shortening surgery, also known as bone lengthening, bone shortening, correction of unequal bone length, femoral lengthening, or femoral shortening, has the goal of correcting LLD and associated deformities while preserving function of muscles and joints. It is performed to:

- Lengthen an abnormally short leg (bone lengthening or femoral lengthening). Leg lengthening is usually recommended for children whose bones are skeletally immature, meaning that they are still growing. The surgery can add up to 6 in (15.2 cm) in length. The leg lengthening and deformity correction process is based on the principle of distraction osteogenesis, meaning that a bone that has been cut during surgery can be gradually distracted (pulled apart), leading to new bone formation (osteogenesis) at the site of the lengthening. The procedure basically involves breaking a bone of the leg and attaching pins through the leg into the bone. The pins pull the bones apart by about 0.4 in (1 mm) each day and the bone grows new bone to try to mend the gap. It takes about a month to grow an inch (2.5 cm).

- Shorten an abnormally long leg (bone shortening or femoral shortening). Shortening a longer leg is usually indicated for patients who have achieved skeletal maturity, meaning that their bones are no longer growing. This surgery can produce a very precise degree of correction.

- Limit the growth of a normal leg to allow a short leg to grow to a matching length (epiphysiodesis). During childhood and adolescence, the long bones—femur (thighbone) or tibia and fibula (lower leg bones)—each consist of a shaft (diaphysis) and end parts (epiphyses). The epiphyses are separated from the shaft by a layer of cartilage called the epiphyseal or growth plate. As the limbs grow during childhood and adolescence, the epiphyseal plates absorb calcium and develop into bone. By adulthood, the plates have been replaced by bone. Epiphysiodesis is an operation performed on the epiphyseal plate in one of the patient's legs that slows down the growth of a specific bone.

Leg lengthening or shortening surgery is usually recommended for severe unequal leg lengths resulting from:

- poliomyelitis, cerebral palsy, or septic arthritis

- small, weak (atrophied) muscles

- short, tight (spastic) muscles

- hip diseases, such as Legg-Perthes disease

- previous injuries or bone fractures that may have stimulated excessive bone growth

- scoliosis (abnormal spine curvature)

- birth defects of bones, joints, muscles, tendons, or ligaments

Guidelines for treatment are tailored to patient needs and are usually as follows:

- LLD < 0.79 in (2 cm): Orthotics (lift in shoe)

- LLD – 0.79-3.2 in (2-6 cm): Epiphysiodesis or shortening procedure

- LLD > 3.2 in (6 cm): Lengthening procedure

- LLD > 5.9-7.9 in (15-20 cm): Lengthening procedure, staged or combined with epiphysiodesis (**Amputation** is done if the procedure fails.)

Demographics

According to the Maryland Center for Limb Lengthening and Reconstruction, the rate of increase of the leg length difference is progressive in the United States with one-fourth of the LLD present at birth, one-third by age one year, and one-half by age three years in girls and four years in boys.

LLD is common in the general population, with 23% of the population having a discrepancy of 0.4 in (1 cm) or more. One person out of 1000 requires a corrective device such as a shoe lift.

Description

Leg lengthening

Leg lengthening is performed under general anesthesia, so that the patient is deep asleep and can't feel pain. Of the several surgical techniques developed, the Ilizarov method, or variation thereof, is the one most often used. An osteotomy is performed, meaning that the bone to be lengthened is cut, usually the lower leg bone (tibia) or upper leg bone (femur). Metal pins or screws are inserted through the skin and into the bone. Pins are placed above and below the cut in the bone and the skin incision is stitched closed. An external fixator is attached to the pins in the bone, which is used after surgery to gradually pull the cut bone apart, creating a gap between the ends of the cut bone in which new bone growth can occur. The fixator functions much like a bone scaffold and will be used very gradually, so that the bone lengthens in extremely small steps. The original Ilizarov external fixator consists of stainless steel rings connected by threaded rods. Each ring is attached to the underlying bone segment by two or more wires, placed under tension to increase stability, yet maintain axial motion. Titanium pins are also used for

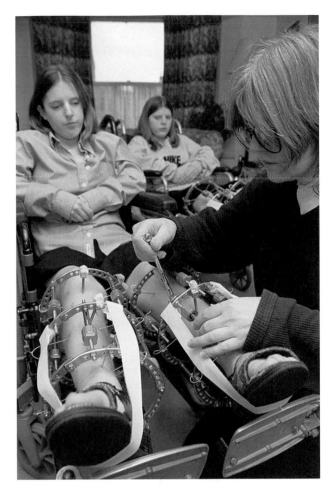

These twin sisters are undergoing leg lengthening treatment. Their mother turns bolts on the external fixators of the leg to increase the distance between the two parts of the the surgically broken bone 1 millimeter a day. *(Custom Medical Stock Photo. Reproduced by permission.)*

supporting the bone segments. Several fixators are available and the choice depends on the desired goal and on specific patient requirements.

Other surgical techniques, such as the Wagner method, or acute lengthening, are used much less commonly. The Wagner technique features more rapid lengthening followed by **bone grafting** and plating. The advantage of the Ilizarov technique is that it does not require an additional procedure for grafting and plating. However, there are reports indicative of higher pain scores associated with the Ilizarov method and conflicting reports concerning the level of complications associated with each technique.

Leg shortening

Leg shortening surgery is also performed under general anesthesia. Generally, femoral shortening is preferred to

Leg lengthening

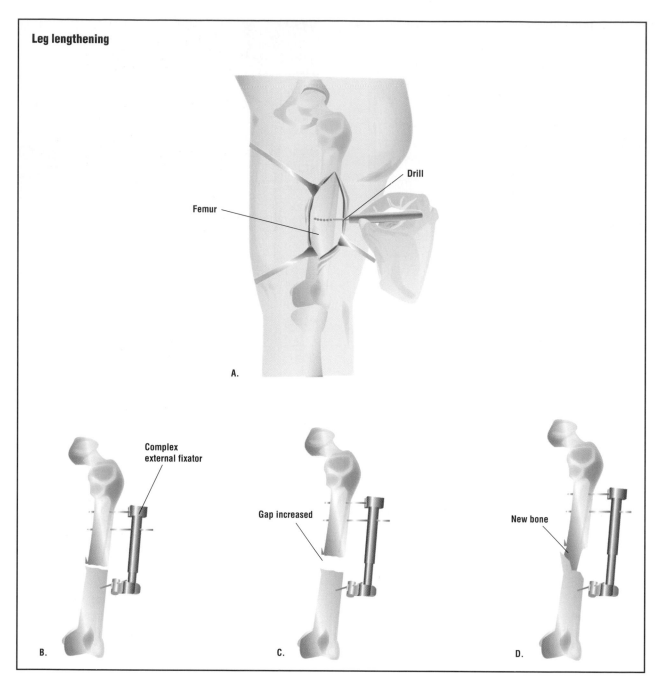

To lengthen a leg surgically, an incision is made in the leg to access the femur (A). A surgical drill is used to weaken the femur so the surgeon can break it. During the operation, screws are drilled into the bone on both sides of the break, and an external fixator is applied (B). The gap between the two pieces of bone is increased gradually (C), so new bone growth results in a longer leg (D). *(Illustration by GGS Inc.)*

tibial shortening, as larger resections are possible. Femoral shortening can be performed by open or closed methods at various femur locations. The bone to be shortened is cut, and a section is removed. The ends of the cut bone are joined together, and a metal plate with screws or an intermedullary rod down the center of the bone is placed across the bone incision to hold it in place during healing.

Epiphysiodesis

Epiphysiodesis is also performed under general anesthesia. The surgeon makes an incision over the epiphyseal plate at the end of the bone in the longer leg. He then proceeds to destroy the epiphyseal plate by scraping or drilling it to restrict further growth.

Diagnosis/Preparation

LLD is a common problem that is frequently discovered during the growing years. A medical history specific to the problem of limb length discrepancy, is taken by the treating physician to provide information as to the cause of discrepancy, previous treatment, and neuromuscular status of the limb. The patient is first evaluated standing on both legs to assess pelvic obliquity, relative height of the knees, presence of angular deformity, foot size, and heel pad thickness. Overall discrepancy is assessed by having the patient stand with the shorter leg on graduated blocks until the pelvis is leveled. Examination is then performed with the patient prone, hips extended and knees flexed to 90 degrees. In this position, the respective lengths of the femur and tibia segments of the two legs can be compared, and the relative contribution of the difference within each segment to the overall LLD can be roughly assessed.

Imaging studies, such as x rays, are the diagnostic tool of choice to fully evaluate the patient. A leg series of x rays shows the overall picture of the affected leg. The extent of LLD and required alignment can be measured with precision, and bone abnormalities involving specific parts of the leg can also be seen. The x rays are usually repeated at six to 12 month intervals to establish the growth pattern of the limbs. When several determinations of limb length have been compiled, the remaining growth and the ultimate discrepancy between the legs can be calculated, and a treatment plan selected based on predicting future growth and discrepancy, which is in turn dependent on an accurate record of past and present growth. Treatment is rarely started solely on the basis of a single determination of the existing discrepancy in a skeletally immature child. **CT scans** are not performed routinely but may be helpful in confirming the diagnosis or more accurately measure the amount of discrepancy.

For LLD patients with a nonfunctional foot, most physicians recommend amputation. In patients with a functional foot, the surgical procedure recommendations generally fall into one of the following three groups:

- The first group involves patients with a leg discrepancy less than 10%. There is little disagreement that these patients can benefit from lengthening procedures.

- The second group involves patients with a leg discrepancy exceeding 30%. Amputation is usually recommended for these patients.

- The third group involves patients a discrepancy ranging between 10 and 30%. Lengthening more than 4 in (10 cm) in a leg with associated knee, ankle, and foot abnormalities is very complex. At skeletal maturity, an average lower-extremity length is often 31.5–39.4 in (80–110 cm) and a 10% discrepancy represents 3.1–4.3 in (8–11 cm).

In the case of leg lengthening, the patient is also seen and evaluated for the design of the external fixator before surgery.

One week before surgery, patients are usually scheduled for a blood and urine test. They are asked to have nothing at all to eat or drink after midnight on the night before surgery.

Aftercare

After the operation, nursing staff teach patients how to clean and care for the skin around the pins that attach the external fixator to the limb (pinsite care). Patients are also shown how to recognize and treat early signs of infection and not to neglect pinsite care, which takes about 30 minutes every day until the apparatus is removed. It is very important in preventing infection from developing.

After an epiphysiodesis procedure, hospitalization is required for about a week. Occasionally, a cast is placed on the operated leg for some three to four weeks. Healing usually requires from eight to 12 weeks, at which time full activities can be resumed.

In the case of leg shortening surgery, two to three weeks of hospitalization is common. Occasionally, a cast is placed on the leg for three to four weeks. Muscle weakness is common, and muscle-strengthening therapy is started as soon as tolerated after surgery. Crutches are required for six to eight weeks. Some patients may require from six to 12 months to regain normal knee control and function. The intramedullary rod is usually removed after a year.

In the case of leg lengthening surgery, hospitalization may require a week or longer. Intensive physical

**QUESTIONS
TO ASK THE DOCTOR**

- Is surgery the best solution?
- How long does bone lengthening take?
- What is an external fixator?
- What are the major risks of the procedure?
- What kind of pain is to be expected after surgery and for how long?
- What are the risks associated with the surgery?
- How long will it take to resume normal walking?
- When will I be fitted with the external fixator?

therapy is required to maintain a normal range of leg motion. Frequent visits to the treating physician are also required to adjust the external fixator and attentive care of the pins holding the device is essential to prevent infection. Healing time depends on the extent of lengthening. A rule of thumb is that each 0.4 in (1 cm) of lengthening requires some 36 days of healing. A large variety of external fixators are now available for use. Today's fixators are very durable, and are generally capable of holding full weight. Most patients can continue many normal activities during the three to six months the device is worn.

Metal pins, screws, staples, rods, or plates are used in leg lengthening/shortening surgery to stabilize bone during healing. Most orthopedic surgeons prefer to plan to remove any large metal implants after several months to a year. Removal of implanted metal devices requires another surgical procedure under general anesthesia.

During the recovery period, physical therapy plays a very important role in keeping the patient's joints flexible and in maintaining muscle strength. Patients are advised to eat a nutritious diet and to take calcium supplements. To speed up the bone healing process, gradual weight-bearing is encouraged. Patients are usually provided with an external system that stimulates bone growth at the site, either an ultrasound device or one that creates a painless electromagnetic field.

Risks

All the risks associated with surgery and the administration of anesthesia exist, including adverse reactions to medications, bleeding and breathing problems.

Specific risks associated with LLD surgery include:

- osteomyelitis (bone infection)

- nerve injury that can cause loss of feeling in the operated leg
- injury to blood vessels
- poor bone healing (non-union)
- avascular necrosis (AVN) of the femoral head as a result of vascular damage during surgery
- chondrolysis (destruction of cartilage) following insertion of rods and pins
- hardware failure, failure of epiphysiodesis, failure of slip progression
- unequal limb lengths if one leg fails to heal properly (The physician may need to reverse the direction of the external fixator device to strengthen it, causing a slight discrepancy between the two legs.)
- joint stiffness (contractures) may occur during lengthening, especially significant lengthenings
- pin loosening in the anchor sites

Another serious specific risk associated with leg lengthening/shortening surgery is infection of the pins or wires going through the bone and/or resting on the skin that may result in further bone or skin infections (osteomyelitis, cellulitis, staph infections).

Normal results

Epiphysiodesis usually has good outcomes when performed at the correct time in the growth period, though it may result in an undesirable short stature. Bone shortening may achieve better correction than epiphysiodesis, but requires a much longer convalescence. Bone lengthening is completely successful only 40% of the time and has a much higher rate of complications. Recovery time from leg lengthening surgery varies among patients, with the consolidation phase sometimes lasting a long period, especially in adults. Generally speaking, children heal in half the time as it takes an adult patient. For example, when the desired goal is 1.5 in (3.8 cm) of new bone growth, a child will wear the fixation device for some three months while an adult will need to wear it for six months.

Alternatives

A LLD of 0.8 in (2 cm) or less is usually not a functional problem and non-surgical treatment options are preferred. The simplest forms do not involve surgery:

- Orthotics. Often leg length can be equalized with a sole or heel lift attached to or inserted inside the shoe. This measure can effectively level a difference of 0.4–2.0 in (1.0–5.0 cm) and correct about two thirds of the LLD. Up to 0.4 in (1 cm) can be inserted in a shoe. Beyond

Arthrodesis—The surgical immobilization of a joint, also called joint fusion.

Cerebral palsy—Group of disorders characterized by loss of movement or loss of other nerve functions. These disorders are caused by injuries to the brain that occur during fetal development or near the time of birth.

Diaphysis—The shaft of a long bone.

Epiphysiodesis—An surgical procedure that partially or totally destroys an epiphysis and may incorporate a bone graft to produce fusion of the epiphysis or premature cessation of its growth; usually performed to equalize leg length.

Epiphysis—A part of a long bone where bone growth occurs from.

Fibula—The long bone in the lower leg that is next to the tibia. It supports approximately one-sixth of the body weight and produces the outer prominence of the ankle.

Femur—The thighbone. The large bone in the thigh that connects with the pelvis above and the knee below.

Fixator—A device providing rigid immobilization

through external skeletal fixation by means of rods (attached to pins which are placed in or through the bone.

Ilizarov method—A bone fixation technique using an external fixator for lengthening limbs, correcting deformities, and assisting the healing of fractures and infections. The method was designed by the Russian orthopedic surgeon Gavriil Abramovich Ilizarov (1921-1992).

Medullary cavity—The marrow cavity in the shaft of a long bone.

Non-union—Bone fracture or defect induced by disease, trauma, or surgery that fails to heal within a reasonable time span.

Osteotomy—The surgical cutting of a bone.

Poliomyelitis—Disorder caused by a viral infection (poliovirus) that can affect the whole body, including muscles and nerves.

Septic arthritis—A pus-forming bacterial infection of a joint.

Tibia—The large bone between the knee and foot that supports five-sixths of the body weight.

this, the lift gets heavy, awkward, and can cause problems such as ankle sprains and falls. The shoes look unsightly and patients complain of gait instability with such a large lift. A foot-in-foot prosthesis can be used for larger LLDs but they tend to be bulky and used as a temporary measure.

• Physical therapy. LLD results in the pelvis tilting sideways since one side of the body is higher than the other side. In turn, this causes a "kink" in the spine known as a scoliosis. Thus, leg length discrepancies can alter the mechanics of the pelvis so that the normal stabilizing and controlling action of specific muscles is altered. A common approach is to use exercises designed to modify the mechanics through specific strengthening of muscles that are weak and stretching of muscles that are restricting movement.

See also Amputation.

Resources

BOOKS

Golyakhovsky, V. and V. H. Frankel. *Operative Manual of Ilizarov Techniques.* Chicago: Year Book Medical Publishers, 1993.

Maiocchi, A. B. *Operative Principles of Ilizarov: Fracture, Treatment, Nonunion, Osteomyelitis, Lengthening Deformity Correction.* Phildalephia: Lippincott, Williams & Wilkins, 1991.

Menelaus, M. B., ed. *The Management of Limb Inequality.* Edinburgh: Churchill Livingstone, Pub., 1997.

Watts, H., Williams, M. *Who Is Amelia?: Caring for Children With Limb Difference.* Rosemont, IL: American Academy of Orthopedic Surgeons, 1998.

PERIODICALS

Aarnes, G. T., H. Steen, P. Ludvigsen, L. P. Kristiansen, and O. Reikeras. "High frequency distraction improves tissue adaptation during leg lengthening in humans." *Journal of Orthopedic Research* 20 (July 2002): 789–792.

Barker, K. L., A. H. Simpson, and S. E. Lamb. "Loss of knee range of motion in leg lengthening." *Journal of Orthopedics Sports and Physical Therapy* 31 (May 2001): 238–144.

Bidwell, J. P., G. C. Bennet, M. J. Bell, and P. J. Witherow. "Leg lengthcning for short stature in Turner's syndrome." *Journal of Bone and Joint Surgery (British)* 82 (November 2000): 1174–1176.

Choi, I. H., J. K. Kim, C. Y. Chung, et al. "Deformity correction of knee and leg lengthening by Ilizarov method in hypophosphatemic rickets: outcomes and significance of serum phosphate level." *Journal of Pediatric Orthopedics* 22 (September-October 2002): 626–631.

Kocaoglu, M., L. Eralp, A. C. Atalar, and F. E. Bilen. "Correction of complex foot deformities using the Ilizarov external fixator." *Journal of Foot and Ankle Surgery* 41 (January-February 2002): 30–39.

Lee, S. H., G. Szoke, and H. Simpson. "Response of the physis to leg lengthening." *Journal of Pediatric Orthopedics* 10 (October 2001): 339–343.

Lindsey, C. A., M. R. Makarov, S. Shoemaker, et al. "The effect of the amount of limb lengthening on skeletal muscle." *Clinical Orthopedics and Related Research* 402 (September 2002): 278–287.

Nanchahal, J. and M. F. Pearse. "Management of soft-tissue problems in leg trauma in conjunction with application of the Ilizarov fixator assembly." *Plastic and Reconstructive Surgery* 111 (March 2003): 1359–1360.

ORGANIZATIONS

American Academy of Orthopedic Surgeons. 6300 North River Road, Rosemont, Illinois 60018-4262. (847) 823-7186. <http://www.aaos.org>

American College of Foot and Ankle Surgeons. 515 Busse Highway, Park Ridge, Illinois, 60068. (847) 292-2237. (800) 421-2237. <http://www.acfas.org/>.

OTHER

"Epiphysiodesis." Institute of Child Health. [cited April 2003]. <http://www.ich.ucl.ac.uk/factsheets/test_procedure_operations/epiphysiodesis/index.html>.

"Ilizarov Method." Northwestern orthopedics. [cited April 2003]. <http://www.orthopedics.northwestern.edu/orthopedics/nmff/ilizarov.htm>.

"Leg lengthening/shortening." MedlinePlus. [cited April 2003]. <http://www.nlm.nih.gov/medlineplus/ency/article/002965.htm>.

Monique Laberge, Ph.D.

Leg veins x ray *see* **Phlebography**

Ligation for varicose veins *see* **Vein ligation and stripping**

Limb salvage

Definition

Limb salvage surgery is a type of surgery primarily performed to remove bone and soft-tissue cancers occurring in limbs in order to avoid **amputation**.

Purpose

Limb salvage surgery is performed to remove cancer and avoid amputation, while preserving the patient's appearance and the greatest possible degree of function in the affected limb. The procedure is most commonly performed for bone tumors and bone sarcomas, but is also performed for soft tissue sarcomas affecting the extremities. This complex alternative to amputation is used to cure cancers that are slow to spread from the limb where they originate to other parts of the body, or that have not yet invaded soft tissue.

Twenty years ago, the standard of care for a patient with a cancer in a limb was to amputate the affected extremity. Limb salvage surgery was an exception to the rule. Today, it is the exception that a patient loses a limb as part of cancer treatment. This is due to improvements in surgical technique, both resection and reconstruction, imaging methods (computed tomography [CT scan] and **magnetic resonance imaging** [MRI]), and survival rates of patients treated with chemotherapy.

In recent years, limb salvage has been extended more and more to patients severely affected by chronic degenerative bone and joint diseases, such as rheumatoid arthritis, or those facing diabetic limb amputation or acute and chronic limb wounds.

Demographics

According to the National Cancer Institute, primary bone cancer is rare, with only 2,500 new cases diagnosed each year in the United States. More commonly, bones are the site of tumors that result from the spread of other primary cancers—that is, from cancers that spread other organs, such as the breasts, lungs, and prostate. Bone cancers occur more frequently in children and young adults.

Description

Also called limb-sparing surgery, limb salvage involves removing the cancer and about an inch of healthy tissue surrounding it. In addition, if had been removed, the removed bone is replaced. The replacement can be made with synthetic metal rods or plates (prostheses), pieces of bone (grafts) taken from the patient's own body (autologous transplant), or pieces of bone removed from a donor body (cadaver) and frozen until needed for transplant (allograft). In time, transplanted bone grows into the patient's remaining bone. Chemotherapy, radiation, or a combination of both treatments may be used to shrink the tumor before surgery is performed.

Limb salvage is performed in three stages. Surgeons remove the cancer and a margin of healthy tissue, implant a prosthesis or bone graft (when necessary), and close the wound by transferring soft tissue and muscle from other parts of the patient's body to the surgical site. This treatment cures some cancers as successfully as amputation.

Surgical techniques

BONE TUMORS. Surgeons remove the malignant lesion and a cuff of normal tissue (wide excision) to cure low-grade tumors of bone or its components. To cure high-grade tumors, they also remove muscle, bone, and other tissues affected by the tumor (radical resection).

SOFT TISSUE SARCOMAS. Surgeons use limb-sparing surgery to treat about 80% of soft tissue sarcomas affecting extremities. The surgery removes the tumor, lymph nodes, or tissues to which the cancer has spread, and at least 1 in (2.54 cm) of healthy tissue on all sides of the tumor.

Radiation and/or chemotherapy may be administered before or after the operation. Radiation may also be administered during the operation by placing a special applicator against the surface from which the tumor has just been removed, and inserting tubes containing radioactive pellets at the site of the tumor. These tubes remain in place during the operation and are removed several days later.

To treat a soft tissue sarcoma that has spread to the patient's lung, the doctor may remove the original tumor, administer radiation or chemotherapy treatments to shrink the lung tumor, and surgically remove the lung tumor.

Diagnosis/Preparation

Before deciding that limb salvage is appropriate for a particular patient, the treating doctor considers what type of cancer the patient has, the size and location of the tumor, how the illness has progressed, and the patient's age and general health.

After determining that limb salvage is appropriate for a particular patient, the doctor makes sure that the patient understands what the outcome of surgery is likely to be, that the implant may fail, and that additional surgery—even amputation—may be necessary.

Physical and occupational therapists help prepare the patient for surgery by introducing the muscle-strengthening, ambulation (walking), and range of motion (ROM) exercises the patient will begin performing right after the operation.

Aftercare

During the five to 10 days the patient remains in the hospital following surgery, nurses monitor sensation and blood flow in the affected extremity and watch for signs that the patient may be developing pneumonia, pulmonary embolism, or deep-vein thrombosis.

The doctor prescribes broad-spectrum **antibiotics** for at least the first 48 hours after the operation and often prescribes medication (prophylactic anticoagulants) and

> ## WHO PERFORMS THE PROCEDURE AND WHERE IS IT PERFORMED?
>
> Limb salvage surgery is performed in a hospital setting by experienced orthopedic surgeons with demonstrated expertise in limb salvage.

antiembolism stockings to prevent blood clots. A drainage tube placed in the wound for the first 24–48 hours prevents blood (hematoma) and fluid (seroma) from accumulating at the surgical site. As postoperative pain becomes less intense, mild narcotics or anti-inflammatory medications replace the epidural catheter or patient-controlled analgesic pump used to relieve pain immediately after the operation.

Exercise intervention

Limb salvage requires extensive surgical incisions, and patients who have these operations need extensive rehabilitation. The amount of bone removed and the type of reconstruction performed dictate how soon and how much the patient can **exercise**, but most patients begin muscle-strengthening, continuous passive motion (CPM), and ROM exercises the day after the operation and continue them for the next 12 months.

A patient who has had upper-limb surgery can use the opposite side of the body to perform hand and shoulder exercises. Patients should not do active elbow or shoulder exercises for two to eight weeks after having surgery involving the bone between the shoulder and elbow (humerus). Rehabilitation following lower-extremity limb salvage focuses on strengthening the muscles that straighten the legs (quadriceps), maintaining muscle tone, and gradually increasing weight-bearing so that the patient is able to stand on the affected limb within three months of the operation. A patient who has had lower-extremity surgery may have to learn a new way of walking (gait retraining) or wear a lift in one shoe.

Goals of rehabilitation

Physical and occupational therapy regimens are designed to help the patient move freely, function independently, and accept changes in body image. Even patients who look the same after surgery as they did previously may feel that the operation has altered their appearance.

Before a patient goes home from the hospital or rehabilitation center, the doctor decides whether the patient needs a walker, brace, cane, or other device, and

QUESTIONS TO ASK THE DOCTOR

- What are the possible complications involved in limb salvage surgery?
- How do I prepare for surgery?
- What type of anesthesia will be used?
- How is the surgery performed?
- How long will I be in the hospital?
- How much limb salvage surgery do you perform in a year?
- Why do you think limb salvage will be successful in my case?
- How will I look and feel after the operation?
- Will I be able to enjoy my favorite sports and other activities after the operation?

should make sure that the patient can climb stairs. Also, the doctor should emphasize the life-long importance of preventing infection and give the patient written instructions about how to prevent and recognize infection, as well as what steps to take if infection does develop.

Risks

The major risks associated with limb salvage are: superficial or deep infection at the site of the surgery; loosening, shifting, or breakage of implants; rapid loss of blood flow or sensation in the affected limb; and severe blood loss and anemia from the surgery.

Postoperative infection is a serious problem. Chemotherapy or radiation can weaken the immune system, and extensive bone damage can occur before the infection is identified. Tissue may die (necrosis) if the surgeon used a large piece of tissue (flap) to close the wound. This is most likely to occur if the surgical site was treated with radiation before the operation. Treatment for postoperative infection involves removing the graft or implant, inserting drains at the infected site, and giving the patient oral or intravenous (IV) antibiotic therapy for as long as 12 months. Doctors may have to amputate the affected limb.

Normal results

A patient who has had limb salvage surgery will remain disease-free as long as a patient whose affected extremity has been amputated.

Salvaged limbs always function better than artificial ones. However, it takes a year for patients to learn to walk again following lower-extremity limb salvage, and patients who have undergone upper-extremity salvage must master new ways of using the affected arm or hand.

Successful surgery reduces the frequency and severity of patient falls and fractures that often result from disease-related changes in bone. Although successful surgery results in limbs that look and function very much like normal, healthy limbs, it is not unusual for patients to feel that their appearance has changed.

Some patients may also need additional surgery within five years of the first operation.

Morbidity and mortality rates

Orthopedic oncologists recognize that an operation to remove a tumor that spares the limb is associated with an incidence of tumor recurrence higher than that following an amputation. However, because there is no significant difference in overall survival rates, the increased rate of recurrence in patients who undergo limb salvage surgery is considered acceptable.

Alternatives

If the cancer's location makes it impossible to remove the malignancy without damaging or removing vital organs, essential nerves, or key blood vessels, or if it is impossible to reconstruct a limb that will function satisfactorily, salvage surgery may not be an appropriate treatment and amputation of the limb becomes the only alternative treatment.

See also Amputation.

Resources

BOOKS

Brown, K., ed. *Complications of Limb Salvage: Prevention Management and Outcome.* UK: International Society of Limb Salvage, 1991.

Greenhalgh, R. M. and C.W. Jamieson. *Limb Salvage and Amputation for Vascular Disease.* Philadelphia: W. B. Saunders Co., 1988.

Groenwald, Susan L., et al., eds. *Cancer Nursing,* 4th ed. Sudbury, MA: Jones and Bartlett, 1997.

PERIODICALS

Nehler, M. R., Hiatt, W. R., and L. M. Taylor Jr. "Is revascularization and limb salvage always the best treatment for critical limb ischemia?" *Journal of Vascular Surgery* 37 (March 2003): 704–708.

Neville, R. F. "Diabetic revascularization: Improving limb salvage in the absence of autogenous vein." *Seminars in Vascular Surgery* 16 (March 2003): 19-26.

KEY TERMS

Resection—Remove of a part of an organ.

Sarcoma—A form of cancer that arises in the supportive tissues such as bone, cartilage, fat, or muscle.

Plotz, W., Rechl, H., Burgkart, R., Messmer, C., Schelter, R., Hipp, E., and R. Gradinger. "Limb salvage with tumor endoprostheses for malignant tumors of the knee." *Clinical Orthopedics* 405 (December 2002): 207-215.

Tefera, G., Turnipseed, W., and T. Tanke. "Limb salvage angioplasty in poor surgical candidates." *Vascular and Endovascular Surgery* 37 (March-April 2003): 99–104.

Teodorescu, V. J., Chun, J. K., Morrisey, N. J., Faries, P. L., Hollier, L. H., and M. L. Marin. "Radial artery flow-through graft: A new conduit for limb salvage." *Journal of Vascular Surgery* 37 (April 2003): 816-820.

van Etten, B., van Geel, A. N., de Wilt, J. H., and A. M. Eggermont. "Fifty tumor necrosis factor-based isolated limb perfusions for limb salvage in patients older than 75 years with limb-threatening soft tissue sarcomas and other extremity tumors." *Annals of Surgical Oncology* 10 (January-February 2003): 32-37.

ORGANIZATIONS

American Academy of Orthopedic Surgeons (AAOS). 6300 North River Road, Rosemont, Illinois 60018-4262. (847) 823-7186. <www.aaos.org>

American Diabetes Association (ADA). 1701 North Beauregard Street, Alexandria, VA 22311. (800) DIABETES <www.diabetes.org>.

International Society of Limb Salvage (ISOLS). E-mail: rjesusgarcia.dot@epm.br (UK) <www.isols.org>.

OTHER

"Adult Soft Tissue Sarcoma." "Bone Cancer." *CancerNet* 2000. [cited July 11, 2001] <www.cancernet.nci.nih.gov>.

"Bone Cancer." *ACS Cancer Resource Center* American Cancer Society. 2000. [cited July 11, 2001] <www3.cancer.org>.

"Limb salvage after osteosarcoma resection." *AAOS.* <www.aaos.org/wordhtml/bulletin/apr97/temple.htm>.

Limb Salvage Center. <www.limbsalvagecentre.com/>.

Maureen Haggerty
Monique Laberge, Ph.D.

Lipid tests

Definition

Lipid tests are routinely performed on plasma, which is the liquid part of blood without the blood cells. Lipids themselves are a group of organic compounds that are greasy and cannot be dissolved in water, although they can be dissolved in alcohol. Lipid tests include measurements of total cholesterol, triglycerides, high-density lipoprotein (HDL) cholesterol, and low-density lipoprotein (LDL) cholesterol. Lipid tests may also be performed on amniotic fluid, which is the fluid that surrounds the fetus during pregnancy. Prenatal lipid tests include tests for lecithin and other pulmonary (lung) surfactants that cover the air spaces in the lungs with a thin film.

Purpose

Blood tests

The purpose of blood lipid testing is to determine whether abnormally high or low concentrations of a specific lipid are present. Low levels of cholesterol are associated with liver failure and inherited disorders of cholesterol production. Cholesterol is a primary component of the plaques that form in atherosclerosis and is therefore the major risk factor for the rapid progression of coronary artery disease (CAD). High blood cholesterol may be inherited or result from such other conditions as biliary obstruction, diabetes mellitus, hypothyroidism, and nephrotic syndrome. In addition, cholesterol levels may be increased in persons who eat foods that are rich in saturated fats and cholesterol, and who lead a sedentary lifestyle.

Low levels of triglyceride are seen in persons with malnutrition or malabsorption. Increased levels are associated with diabetes mellitus, hypothyroidism, pancreatitis, glycogen storage diseases, and estrogens. Diets rich in either carbohydrates or fats may cause elevated triglyceride levels in some persons. Although triglycerides are not a component of the plaque associated with atherosclerosis, they increase the viscosity (thickness) of the blood and promote obesity, which can contribute to coronary disease. The majority of cholesterol and triglyceride testing is performed to screen persons at increased risk of coronary artery disease.

Amniotic fluid tests

Lipid tests are performed on amniotic fluid to determine the maturity of the fetal lungs. These tests are performed prior to delivery to ensure that there is sufficient pulmonary surfactant to prevent collapse of the lungs when the baby exhales (breathes out).

Description

Cholesterol screening can be performed with or without fasting, but it should include tests of total and HDL cholesterol levels. The frequency of cholesterol testing depends on the patient's risk of developing CAD. Adults over 20 with total cholesterol levels below 200 mg/dL should be tested once every five years. People with higher levels should be tested for LDL cholesterol levels, and tested at least once per year thereafter if their LDL cholesterol is 130 mg/dL or higher. The National Cholesterol Education Program (NCEP) suggests further evaluation when the patient has any of the symptoms of CAD, or if she or he has two or more of the following risk factors for CAD:

• high blood pressure

• history of cigarette smoking

• diabetes

• low HDL levels

• family history of CAD

• age over 45 years (men) or 55 years (women)

Measurements of cholesterol and triglyceride levels are routinely performed in all patients.

Measurement of pulmonary surfactants

Lecithin is the principal pulmonary surfactant secreted by the alveolar cells of the lung. Lecithin and the other surfactants prevent collapse of the air sacs when the baby exhales. During the first half of gestation, the levels of lecithin and another lipid known as sphingomyelin in the amniotic fluid are approximately equal. During the second half of pregnancy, however, lecithin production increases while the sphingomyelin level remains constant. Infants born prematurely may suffer from respiratory distress syndrome (RDS) because the levels of pulmonary surfactant in their lungs are insufficient to prevent collapse of the air sacs. Tests for RDS are called fetal lung maturity (FLM) tests. The reference method for determining fetal lung maturity is the ratio between lecithin and sphingomyelin in the amniotic fluid, or the L/S ratio.

Precautions

Tests for triglycerides and LDL cholesterol must be performed following a 12-hour fast. Acute illness, high fever, starvation, or recent surgery lowers the blood cholesterol and triglyceride levels. If possible, patients should also stop taking any medications that may affect the accuracy of the test.

Amniotic fluid is collected by a process called **amniocentesis**. This procedure is usually performed after the 30th week of gestation to evaluate the maturity of the baby's lungs. A miscarriage (spontaneous abortion) may occur as a consequence of this procedure, although its overall incidence following amniocentesis is less than

1%. Possible complications of amniocentesis include premature labor and placental bleeding. The fluid that is withdrawn may be contaminated with blood or meconium (a dark-green material in the intestines of a fetus), which may interfere with some fetal lung maturity tests.

Preparation

Patients who are scheduled for a lipid profile test should fast (except for water) for 12 to 14 hours before the blood sample is drawn. If the patient's LDL cholesterol is to be measured, he or she should also avoid alcohol for 24 hours before the test. When possible, patients should also stop taking any medications that may affect the accuracy of the test results. These drugs include **corticosteroids**; estrogen or androgens; oral contraceptives; some **diuretics**; antipsychotic medications, including haloperidol; some **antibiotics**; and niacin. Antilipemics are drugs that lower the concentration of fatty substances in the blood. When these medications are taken by the patient, blood testing may be done frequently to evaluate liver function as well as lipid levels.

Aftercare

Aftercare following blood lipid tests includes routine care of the skin around the needle puncture. Most patients have no aftereffects, but some may have a small bruise or swelling. A washcloth soaked in warm water usually relieves any discomfort. In addition, the patient can resume taking any prescription medications that were discontinued before the test.

Care after amniocentesis requires that the clinician monitor the patient for any signs of infection or possible injury to the fetus. Some things to look for are fever, vaginal bleeding, or vaginal discharge. The patient may feel sick and there may be some cramping. She should be advised to rest and avoid strenuous activity. If the mother appears to be going into labor, she should be given supportive care. She may be given medications known as tocolytic agents to prevent the premature birth of the baby.

Risks

The primary risk to the patient from blood tests of lipid levels is a mild stinging or burning sensation during the venipuncture, with minor swelling or bruising afterward.

Although amniocentesis is much safer in the third trimester, and is less risky when it is performed with the guidance of ultrasound technology, does present a risk of miscarriage and fetal injury. The mother should be monitored for any signs of bleeding, infection, or impending labor.

KEY TERMS

Amniocentesis—A procedure for removing amniotic fluid from the womb using a fine needle.

Atherosclerosis—A disease of the coronary arteries in which cholesterol is deposited in plaques on the arterial walls. The plaque narrows or blocks blood flow to the heart. Atherosclerosis is sometimes called coronary artery disease, or CAD.

High-density lipoprotein (HDL)—A type of lipoprotein that protects against CAD by removing cholesterol deposits from arteries or preventing their formation.

Hypercholesterolemia—The presence of excessively high levels of cholesterol in the blood.

Hypertriglyceridemia—The presence of excessively high levels of TAG in the blood.

Lecithin—A phospholipid found in high concentrations in surfactant.

Lipid—Any organic compound that is greasy, insoluble in water, but soluble in alcohol. Fats, waxes, and oils are examples of lipids.

Lipoprotein—A complex molecule that consists of a protein membrane surrounding a core of lipids. Lipoproteins carry cholesterol and other lipids from the digestive tract to the liver and other body tissues. There are five major types of lipoproteins.

Low-density lipoprotein (LDL)—A type of lipoprotein that consists of about 50% cholesterol and is associated with an increased risk of CAD.

Plaque—An abnormal deposit on the wall of an artery. Plaque is made of cholesterol, triglyceride, dead cells, lipoproteins and calcium.

Sedentary—Characterized by inactivity and lack of exercise. A sedentary lifestyle is a risk factor for high blood cholesterol levels.

Surfactant—A compound made of fats and proteins that is found in a thin film along the walls of the air sacs of the lungs. Surfactant keeps the surface pressure low so that the sacs can inflate easily and not collapse.

Tocolytic drug—A compound given to women to stop the progression of labor.

Triglyceride (TAG)—A chemical compound that forms about 95% of the fats and oils stored in animal and vegetable cells. TAG levels are sometimes measured as well as cholesterol levels when a patient is screened for heart disease.

Results

The normal values for serum lipids depend on the patient's age, sex, and race. Normal values for people in Western countries are usually given as 140–220 mg/dL for total cholesterol in adults, although as many as 5% of the population have a total cholesterol higher than 300 mg/dL. Among Asians, the figures are about 20% lower. As a rule, both total and LDL cholesterol levels rise as people get older. Normal values for HDL cholesterol are also age- and sex-dependent. The range for males between 20 and 29 years is approximately 30–63 mg/dL; for females of the same age group it is 33–83 mg/dL. Normal values for fasting triglycerides are also age- and sex-dependent. The reference range for adult males 20 to 29 years is 45–200 mg/dL; for females of the same age group it is 37–144 mg/dL. As with cholesterol, the normal range rises with age.

Since a person's diet and lifestyle affect normal values, which are determined by the interval between the 5th and 95th percentile of the group, it is more helpful to evaluate cholesterol and triglycerides from the perspective of desirable plasma levels. The desirable values defined by the Nation Cholesterol Education Program (NCEP) in 2001 are as follows:

- Total cholesterol: Less than 200 mg/dL; 200–239 mg/dL is considered borderline high and greater than 240 mg/dL is high.

- HDL cholesterol: Less than 40mg/dL is low.

- LDL cholesterol: Less than 100 mg/dL is optimal; near-optimal is 100–129 mg/dL; borderline high is 130-159 mg/dL; high is 160–189 mg/dL; and very high is any value over 190 mg/dL.

- Total cholesterol: HDL ratio: Under 4.0 in males; 3.8 in females.

Fetal lung maturity tests

Low levels of surfactant in amniotic fluid are denoted by an L/S ratio lower than 2.0 or a lecithin level lower than or equal to 0.10 mg/dL. Lung development can be delayed in premature births and in babies whose mothers have diabetes.

Patient education

Nurses should explain the results of abnormal blood lipid tests to patients and advise them on lifestyle changes. Patient education is important in fetal lung maturity testing. The situation faced by the expectant parents may be very critical; the more information they are given, the better choices they can make.

Resources

BOOKS

Henry, J. B. *Clinical Diagnosis and Management by Laboratory Methods*, 20th ed. Philadelphia, PA: W. B. Saunders Company, 2001.

"Hyperlipidemia." Section 2, Chapter 15 in *The Merck Manual of Diagnosis and Therapy*, edited by Mark H. Beers, MD, and Robert Berkow, MD. Whitehouse Station, NJ: Merck Research Laboratories, 1999.

"Prenatal Diagnostic Techniques: Amniocentesis." Section 18, Chapter 247 in *The Merck Manual of Diagnosis and Therapy*, edited by Mark H. Beers, MD, and Robert Berkow, MD. Whitehouse Station, NJ: Merck Research Laboratories, 1999.

Wallach, Jacques. *Interpretation of Diagnostic Tests*, 7th ed. Philadelphia, PA: Lippincott Williams & Wilkens, 2000.

ORGANIZATIONS

American Dietetic Association. (800) 877-1600. <www.eatright.org.>.

National Cholesterol Education Program. National Heart, Lung, and Blood Institute (NHLBI), National Institutes of Health. PO Box 30105, Bethesda, MD, 20824-0105. (301) 251-1222. May 2001 [cited April 4, 2003]. <www.nhlbi.nih.gov/guidelines/cholesterol/atglance.pdf>.

OTHER

National Institutes of Health. [cited April 5, 2003]. <www.nlm.nih.gov/medlineplus/encyclopedia.html>.

Jane E. Phillips
Mark A. Best

Liposuction

Definition

Liposuction, also known as lipoplasty or suction-assisted lipectomy, is cosmetic surgery performed to remove unwanted deposits of fat from under the skin. The surgeon sculpts and re-contours a person's body by removing excess fat deposits that have been resistant to reduction by diet or **exercise**. The fat is permanently removed from under the skin with a suction device.

Purpose

Liposuction is intended to reduce and smooth the contours of the body and improve a person's appearance.

WHO PERFORMS THE PROCEDURE AND WHERE IS IT PERFORMED?

Many liposuction surgeries are performed by plastic surgeons or by dermatologists. Any licensed physician may legally perform liposuction. Liposuction may be performed in a private professional office, an outpatient center, or in a hospital.

Its goal is cosmetic improvement. It is the most commonly performed cosmetic procedure in the United States.

Liposuction does not remove large quantities of fat and is not intended as a weight reduction technique. The average amount of fat removed is about a quart (liter). Although liposuction is not intended to remove cellulite (lumpy fat), some doctors believe that it improves the appearance of areas that contain cellulite, including thighs, hips, buttocks, abdomen, and chin. A new technique called liposhaving shows more promise at reducing cellulite.

Demographics

Liposuction is the most commonly performed cosmetic procedure in the United States. In 2002, there were 372,831 liposuction procedures performed in the United States, approximately 13% of all plastic surgical procedures.

Description

Most liposuction procedures are performed under local anesthesia (loss of sensation without loss of consciousness) by the tumescent, or wet, technique. In this technique, large volumes of very dilute local anesthetic (a substance that produces anesthesia) are injected under the person's skin, making the tissue swollen and firm. Epinephrine is added to the solution to reduce bleeding, which allows the removal of larger amounts of fat.

The physician first numbs the skin with an injection of local anesthetic. After the skin is desensitized, the doctor makes a series of tiny incisions, usually 0.12–0.25 in (3–6 mm) in length. Flooding the area with a larger amount of local anesthetic, fat is then extracted with suction through a long, blunt hollow tube called a cannula. The doctor repeatedly pushes the cannula through the fat layers in a radiating pattern creating tunnels, thus removing fat and re-contouring the area. Large quantities of intravenous fluid (IV) are given during the procedure to replace lost body fluid. Blood transfusions might be necessary.

Some newer modifications to the procedure include the use of a cutting cannula called a liposhaver and the use of ultrasound to help break up the fat deposits. The person is awake and comfortable during these procedures.

The length of time required to perform the procedure varies with the amount of fat that is to be removed and the number of areas to be treated. Most operations take from 30 minutes up to two hours, but extensive procedures can take longer. The length of time required also varies with the manner in which the anesthetic is injected.

The cost of liposuction can vary depending upon the standardized fees in the region of the country where it is performed, the extent of the area being treated, and the person performing the procedure. Generally, small areas such as the chin or knees can be done for as little as $500, while more extensive treatment such as when hips, thighs, and abdomen are done simultaneously can cost as much as $10,000. These procedures are cosmetic and are not covered by most insurance policies.

Diagnosis/Preparation

Liposuction is most successful when performed on persons who have firm, elastic skin and concentrated pockets of fat in areas that are characterized by cellulite. To get good results after fat removal, the skin must contract to conform to the new contours without sagging. Older persons have less elastic skin and, consequently, may not be good candidates for this procedure. People with generalized fat distribution, rather than localized pockets, are not good candidates. People with poor circulation or who have had recent surgery at the intended site of fat reduction are not good candidates.

Candidates should be in good general health and free of heart or lung disease.

The doctor will conduct a **physical examination** and may order blood work to determine clotting time and hemoglobin level for transfusions, in case the need should arise. The person may be placed on **antibiotics** immediately prior to surgery to ward off potential infection.

Aftercare

After the surgery, the person will need to wear a support garment continuously for two to three weeks. If ankles or calves were treated, support hose will need to be worn for up to six weeks. The support garments can be removed during bathing 24 hours after surgery. A drainage tube under the skin in the area of the procedure may be inserted to prevent fluid build-up.

Mild side effects can include a burning sensation at the site of the surgery for up to one month. The candi-

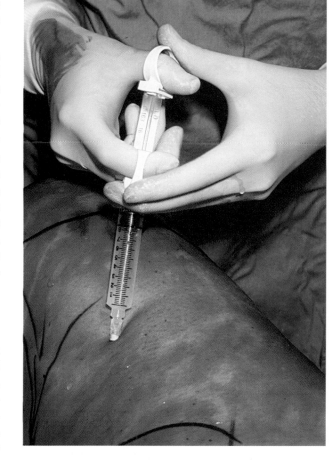

Surgeon injecting anesthetic into an area to be treated with liposuction. *(Custom Medical Stock Photo. Reproduced by permission.)*

date should be prepared for swelling of the tissues below the site of the operation for up to six to eight weeks after surgery. Wearing the special elastic garments will help reduce this swelling and help to achieve the desired final results.

The incisions involved in this procedure are tiny, but the surgeon may close them with metal stitches or staples. These will be removed the day after surgery. However, three out of eight doctors use no sutures, relying on dressings to cover the incisions. Minor bleeding or seepage through the incision site(s) is common after this procedure. Wearing the elastic bandage or support garment helps reduce fluid loss.

Liposuction is virtually painless. However, for the first postoperative day, there may be some discomfort that will require light pain medication. Soreness or aching may persist for several days. A person can usually return to normal activity within a week. Postoperative bruising will go away within 10 to 14 days. Postopera-

Liposuction

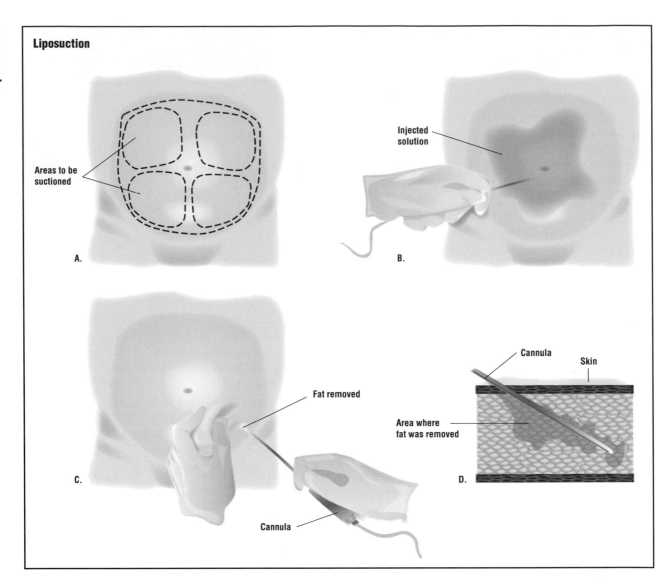

A.

B.

Areas to be suctioned

Injected solution

C.

D.

Fat removed

Cannula

Cannula

Skin

Area where fat was removed

The areas to be treated during liposuction are marked before surgery (A) and then injected with a solution to aid in fat removal (B). The surgeon inserts a cannula into the areas (C), then suctions out fat with a back and forth motion (D). *(Illustration by GGS Inc.)*

tive swelling begins to go down after a week. It may take three to six months for the final contour to be reached.

Risks

Liposuction under local anesthesia using the tumescent (wet) technique is exceptionally safe. Two recent large studies reached similar conclusions. One concluded that there were no serious complications or deaths with liposuction. The other study calculated the risk of any complication to be 1%. However, as with any surgery, there are some risks and serious complications. Death is possible, but extremely unlikely.

The main hazards associated with liposuction surgery involve migration of a blood clot or fat globule to the heart, brain, or lungs. Such an event can cause a heart attack, stroke, or serious lung damage. However, this complication is exceedingly rare. The risk of blood clot formation is reduced by wearing a special girdle-like compression garment after the surgery, and with the resumption of normal mild activity soon after surgery.

Remaining in bed increases the risk of clot formation, but not getting enough rest can also result in increased swelling of the surgical area. Such swelling is a result of excess fluid and blood accumulation, and generally comes from not wearing the compression garments. If necessary, this excess fluid can be drained off with a needle in the doctor's office.

Infection is another complication, but this rarely occurs. If the physician is skilled and works in a sterile environment, infection should not be a concern.

If too much fat is removed, the skin may peel in that area. Smokers are at increased risk for shedding skin because their circulation is impaired. Another and more serious hazard of removing too much fat is that the person may go into shock. Fat tissue has an abundant blood supply and removing too much of it at once can cause shock if the fluid is not replaced.

A rare complication is perforation, or puncture, of an organ. The procedure involves pushing a cannula vigorously through the fat layer. If the doctor pushes too hard or if the tissue gives way too easily under the force, the blunt hollow tube could possibly injure internal organs.

Liposuction can damage superficial nerves. Some persons lose sensation in the area that has been suctioned, but most feeling usually returns with time.

Normal results

The loss of fat cells is permanent. The person should have smoother, more pleasing body contours without excessive bulges. However, if a person overeats, the remaining fat cells will grow in size. Although lost weight may be regained, the body should retain the new proportions and the suctioned area should remain proportionally smaller.

Tiny scars about 0.25–0.5 in (6–12 mm) long at the site of incision are normal. The doctor usually makes the incisions in concealed places such as along skin folds, where the scars are not likely to show.

In some instances, the skin may appear rippled, wavy, or baggy after surgery. Pigmentation spots may develop. The re-contoured area may be uneven. This unevenness is common, occurring in 5–20% of the cases, and can be corrected with a second liposuction procedure that is less extensive than the first.

Morbidity and mortality rates

The morbidity rate from liposuction is under 1%. Mortality is exceedingly rare.

Alternatives

Some of the alternatives to liposuction include modifying diet to lose excess body fat, exercise, accepting one's body and appearance as it is, or using clothing or makeup to downplay or emphasize body or facial features.

See also Breast reduction; Face lift; Plastic, cosmetic, and reconstructive surgery.

QUESTIONS TO ASK THE DOCTOR

- What will be the resulting appearance?
- Is the surgeon board certified in plastic and reconstructive surgery?
- How many liposuction procedures has the surgeon performed?
- What is the surgeon's complication rate?

Resources

BOOKS

Engler, Alan M. *BodySculpture: Plastic Surgery of the Body for Men and Women,* 2nd Edition. New York: Hudson Publishing, 2000.

Irwin, Brandith, and Mark McPherson. *Your Best Face: Looking Your Best without Plastic Surgery.* Carlsbad, CA: Hay House, Inc., 2002.

Klein, Jeffrey A. *Tumescent Technique: Tumescent Anesthesia and Microcannular Liposuction.* St. Louis: Mosby-Year Book, 2000.

Man, Daniel, and L. C. Faye. *New Art of Man: Faces of Plastic Surgery: Your Guide to the Latest Cosmetic Surgery Procedures, 3rd Edition.* New York: BeautyArt Press, 2003.

Sandhu, Baldev S. *Doctor, Is Liposuction Right for Me?* New York: Universe Publishers, 2001.

PERIODICALS

Field, L. M. "Tumescent Axillary Liposuction and Curretage with Axillary Scarring: Not an Important Sequela." *Dermatologic Surgery* 29, no.3 (2003): 317–319.

Goyen, M. R. "Lifestyle Outcomes of Tumescent Liposuction Surgery." *Dermatologic Surgery* 28, no.6 (2002): 459–462.

Housman, T. S., et al. "The Safety of Liposuction: Results of a National Survey." *Dermatologic Surgery* 28, no.11 (2002): 971–978.

Lowe, N. J. "On the Safety of Liposuction." *Journal of Dermatologic Treatment* 12, no.4 (2001): 189–190.

ORGANIZATIONS

American Board of Plastic Surgery. Seven Penn Center, Suite 400, 1635 Market Street, Philadelphia, PA 19103-2204. (215) 587-9322. <http://www.abplsurg.org/>.

American College of Plastic and Reconstructive Surgery. <http://www.breast-implant.org>.

American College of Surgeons. 633 North Saint Claire Street, Chicago, IL 60611. (312) 202-5000. <http://www.facs.org/>.

American Society for Aesthetic Plastic Surgery. 11081 Winners Circle, Los Alamitos, CA 90720. (800) 364-2147 or (562) 799-2356. <http://www.surgery.org/>.

KEY TERMS

Cellulite—Dimpled skin that is caused by uneven fat deposits beneath the surface.

Epinephrine—A drug that causes blood vessels to constrict or narrow; it is used in local anesthetics to reduce bleeding.

Hemoglobin—The component of blood that carries oxygen to the tissues.

Liposhaving—Involves removing fat that lies closer to the surface of the skin by using a needle-like instrument that contains a sharp-edged shaving device.

Tumescent technique—A technique of liposuction involves swelling, or tumescence, of the tissue with large volumes of dilute anesthetic.

American Society for Dermatologic Surgery. 930 N. Meacham Road, P.O. Box 4014, Schaumburg, IL 60168-4014. (847) 330-9830. <http://www.asds-net.org>.

American Society of Plastic and Reconstructive Surgeons. 444 E. Algonquin Rd., Arlington Heights, IL 60005. (847) 228-9900. <http://www.plasticsurgery.org>.

Lipoplasty Society of North America. 444 East Algonquin Road, Arlington Heights, IL 60005. (708) 228-9273; (800) 848-1991, ext. 1126. <http://www.lipoplasty.com/business/lsna/index.htm>.

OTHER

Covenant Health. [cited March 21, 2003] <http://www.covenanthealth.com/Features/Health/Cosm/COSM4355.cfm>.

Liposuction Surgery Network. [cited March 21, 2003] <http://www.liposuction-surgery.org/>.

University of Washington. [cited March 21, 2003] <http://faculty.washington.edu/danberg/bergweb/page2.htm>.

U.S. Food and Drug Administration. [cited March 21, 2003] <http://www.fda.gov/cdrh/liposuction/>.

L. Fleming Fallon, Jr, MD, DrPH

Lithotripsy

Definition

Lithotripsy is the use of high-energy shock waves to fragment and disintegrate kidney stones. The shock wave, created by using a high-voltage spark or an electromagnetic impulse outside of the body, is focused on the stone. The shock wave shatters the stone, allowing the fragments to pass through the urinary system. Since the shock wave is generated outside the body, the procedure is termed extracorporeal shock wave lithotripsy (ESWL). The name is derived from the roots of two Greek words, *litho*, meaning stone, and *trip*, meaning to break.

Purpose

ESWL is used when a kidney stone is too large to pass on its own, or when a stone becomes stuck in a ureter (a tube that carries urine from the kidney to the bladder) and will not pass. Kidney stones are extremely painful and can cause serious medical complications if not removed.

Demographics

For an unknown reason, the number of persons in the United States developing kidney stones has been increasing over the past 20 years. White people are more prone to develop kidney stones than are persons of color. Although stones occur more frequently in men, the number of women who develop them has been increasing over the past 10 years, causing the ratio to change. Kidney stones strike most people between the ages of 20 and 40. Once persons develop more than one stone, they are more likely to develop others. Lithotripsy is not required for treatment in all cases of kidney stones.

Description

Lithotripsy uses the technique of focused shock waves to fragment a stone in the kidney or the ureter. The affected person is placed in a tub of water or in contact with a water-filled cushion. A sophisticated machine called Lithotripter produces the focused shock waves. A high-voltage electrical discharge is passed through a spark gap under water. The shock waves thus produced are focused on the stone inside the person's body. The shock waves are created and focused on the stone with the help of a machine called C-Arm Image Intensifier. The wave shatters and fragments the stone. The resulting debris, called gravel, can then pass through the remainder of the ureter, through the bladder, and through the urethra during urination. There is minimal chance of damage to skin or internal organs because biologic tissues are resilient, not brittle, and because the shock waves are not focused on them.

The shock wave is characterized by a very rapid pressure increase in the transmission medium and is quite different from ultrasound. The shock waves are transmitted through a person's skin and pass harmlessly through soft tissues. The shock wave passes through the

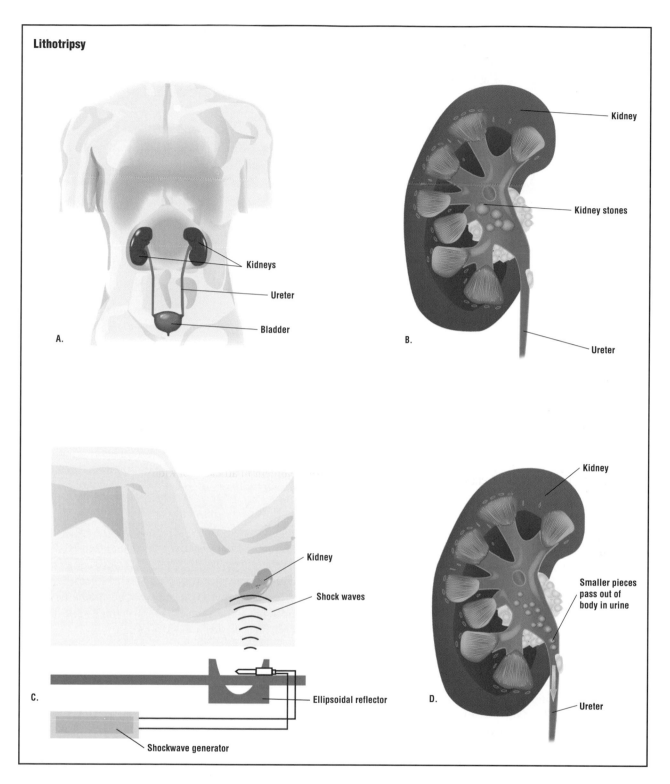

Lithotripsy

A. Kidneys / Ureter / Bladder

B. Kidney / Kidney stones / Ureter

C. Kidney / Shock waves / Ellipsoidal reflector / Shockwave generator

D. Kidney / Smaller pieces pass out of body in urine / Ureter

Kidney stones that are too big to pass through the ureter become very painful (B). During lithotripsy, the patient is put in a tub of water, or on a water-filled blanket. Shock waves are used to break up the stone (C). These smaller pieces are able to pass out of the body (D). *(Illustration by GGS Inc.)*

kidney and strikes the stone. At the edge of the stone, energy is transferred into the stone, causing small cracks to form on the edge of the stone. The same effect occurs when the shock wave exits the stone. With successive shock waves, the cracks open up. As more cracks form, the size of the stone is reduced. Eventually, the stone is reduced to small particles, which are then flushed out of the kidneys or ureter naturally during urination.

Diagnosis/Preparation

ESWL should not be considered for persons with severe skeletal deformities, people weighing more than 300 lb (136 kg), individuals with abdominal aortic aneurysms, or persons with uncontrollable bleeding disorders. Women who are pregnant should not be treated with ESWL. Individuals with cardiac **pacemakers** should be evaluated by a cardiologist familiar with ESWL. The cardiologist should be present during the ESWL procedure in the event the pacemaker needs to be overridden.

Prior to the lithotripsy procedure, a complete **physical examination** is performed, followed by tests to determine the number, location, and size of the stone or stones. A test called an intravenous pyelogram (IVP) is used to locate the stones, which involves injecting a dye into a vein in the arm. This dye, which shows up on x ray, travels through the bloodstream and is excreted by the kidneys. The dye then flows down the ureters and into the bladder. The dye surrounds the stones. In this manner, x rays are used to evaluate the stones and the anatomy of the urinary system. Blood tests are performed to determine if any potential bleeding problems exist. For women of childbearing age, a pregnancy test is done to make sure they are not pregnant. Older persons have an EKG test to make sure that no potential heart problems exist. Some individuals may have a stent placed prior to the lithotripsy procedure. A stent is a plastic tube placed in the ureter that allows the pas-

sage of gravel and urine after the ESWL procedure is completed.

The process of lithotripsy generally takes about one hour. During that time, up to 8,000 individual shock waves are administered. Depending on a person's pain tolerance, there may be some discomfort during the treatment. **Analgesics** may be administered to relieve this pain.

Aftercare

Most persons pass blood in their urine after the ESWL procedure. This is normal and should clear after several days to a week. Lots of fluids should be taken to encourage the flushing of any gravel remaining in the urinary system. Treated persons should follow up with a urologist in about two weeks to make sure that everything is progressing as planned. If a stent has been inserted, it is normally removed at this time.

Risks

Abdominal pain is fairly common after ESWL, but it is usually not a cause for worry. However, persistent or severe abdominal pain may imply an unexpected internal injury. Occasionally, stones may not be completely fragmented during the first ESWL treatment and further lithotripsy procedures may be required.

Some people are allergic to the dye material used during an IVP, so it cannot be used. For these people, focused sound waves, called ultrasound, can be used to identify where the stones are located.

Normal results

In most cases, stones are reduced to gravel and passed within a few days. Individuals may return to work whenever they feel able.

Morbidity and mortality rates

Colicky renal pain is very common when gravel is being passed. Other problems may include perirenal

KEY TERMS

Aneurysm—A dilation of the wall of an artery that causes a weak area prone to rupture.

Bladder—Organ in which urine is stored prior to urination.

Bleeding disorder—A problem related to the clotting mechanism of the blood.

Cardiologist—A physician who specializes in problems of the heart.

EKG—A graphical tracing of the electrical activity of the heart.

Extracorporeal shock wave lithotripsy (ESWL)—The use of focused shock waves, generated outside the body, to fragment kidney stones.

Gravel—The debris that is formed from a fragmented kidney stone.

Intravenous pyelogram (IVP)—A type of x ray. After obtaining an x ray of the lower abdomen, a radio-opaque dye is injected into the veins. X rays are then obtained every 15 minutes for the next

hour. The dye pinpoints the location of kidney stones. It is also used to determine the anatomy of the urinary system.

Kidney stone—A hard mass that forms in the urinary tract that can cause pain, bleeding, obstruction, and/or infection. Stones are primarily composed of calcium.

Stent—A plastic tube placed in the ureter prior to the ESWL procedure, which facilitates the passage of gravel and urine.

Ultrasound—A diagnostic imaging modality that uses sound waves to determine internal structures of the body.

Ureter—A tube that carries urine from the kidney to the bladder.

Urethra—A tube that carries urine from the bladder to the outside of the body.

Urologist—A physician who specializes in problems of the urinary system.

---

hematomas (blood clots near the kidneys) in 66% of the cases; nerve palsies; pancreatitis (inflammation of the pancreas); and obstruction by stone fragments. Death is extremely rare and usually due to an undiagnosed associated or underlying condition that is aggravated by the lithotripsy procedure.

Alternatives

Before the advent of lithotripsy, surgery was used to remove kidney stones. This approach is uncommon today, but occasionally used when other conditions prevent the use of lithotripsy. Attempts are occasionally made to change the pH of urine so as to dissolve kidney stones. This treatment has limited success.

See also Cystoscopy.

Resources

BOOKS

Field, Michael, David Harris, and Carol Pollock. *The Renal System.* London: Churchill Livingstone, 2001.

Parker, James N. *The 2002 Official Patient's Source Book on Kidney Stones.* Logan, UT: ICON Health, 2002.

Tanagho, Emil A., and Jack W. McAninch. *Smith's General Urology, 15th ed.* New York: McGraw-Hill, 2000.

Walsh, Patrick C., and Alan B. Retik. *Campbell's Urology, 8th ed.* Philadelphia: Saunders, 2002.

PERIODICALS

Ather, M. H., and M. A. Noor. "Does Size and Site Matter for Renal Stones Up to 30 mm in Size in Children Treated by Extracorporeal Lithotripsy?" *Urology* 61, no.1 (2003): 212–215.

Downey, P., and D. Tolley. "Contemporary Management of Renal Calculus Disease." *Journal of the Royal College of Surgery (Edinburgh)* 47, no.5 (2002): 668–675.

Hochreiter, W. W., H. Danuser, M. Perrig, and U. E. Studer. "Extracorporeal Shock Wave Lithotripsy for Distal Ureteral Calculi." *Journal of Urology* 169, no.3 (2003): 878–880.

Rajkumar, P., and G. F. Schmitgen. "Shock Waves Do More Than Just Crush Stones: Extracorporeal Shock Wave Therapy in Plantar Fasciitis." *International Journal of Clinical Practice* 56, no.10 (2002): 735–737.

ORGANIZATIONS

American Foundation for Urologic Disease. 1128 North Charles Street, Baltimore, MD 21201. (800) 242-2383 or (410) 468-1800. <admin@afud.org>. <http://www.afud.org>.

American Lithotripsy Society. 305 Second Avenue, Suite 200, Waltham, MA 02451.

American Medical Association. 515 N. State Street, Chicago, IL 60610. (312) 464-5000. <http://www.ama-assn.org>.

American Urological Association. 1120 North Charles Street, Baltimore, MD 21201-5559. (410) 727-1100. <http://www.auanet.org/index_hi.cfm>.

National Kidney Foundation. 30 East 33rd Street, New York, NY 10016. (800) 622-9010. (781) 895-9098. Fax: (781)

895-9088. E-mail: <als@lithotripsy.org>. <http://www.kidney.org>.

OTHER

Case Western Reserve University. [cited March 17, 2003] <http://www.cwru.edu/artsci/dittrick/artifactspages/b-2lithotripsy.htm>.

Global Lithotripsy Services. [cited March 17, 2003] <http://www.gls-lithotripsy.com/Howdoes.html>.

Lifespan. [cited March 17, 2003] <http://www.lifespan.org/mininvasive/revised/patient/gallstones/lithotripsy.htm>.

National Institute of Diabetes and Digestive and Kidney Diseases. [cited March 17, 2003] <http://www.niddk.nih.gov/health/urolog/pubs/stonadul/stonadul.htm#whogets>.

National Library of Medicine. [cited March 17, 2003] <http://www.nlm.nih.gov/medlineplus/ency/article/007113.htm>.

L. Fleming Fallon, Jr, MD, DrPH

Liver biopsy

Definition

A liver biopsy is a medical procedure performed to obtain a small piece of liver tissue for diagnostic testing. The sample is examined under a microscope by a pathologist, a doctor who specializes in the effects of disease on body tissues; in this case, to detect abnormalities of the liver. Liver biopsies are sometimes called percutaneous liver biopsies, because the tissue sample is obtained by going through the patient's skin. This is a useful diagnostic procedure with very low risk and little discomfort to the patient.

Purpose

A liver biopsy is usually done to evaluate the extent of damage that has occurred to the liver because of chronic and acute disease processes or toxic injury. Biopsies are often performed to identify abnormalities in liver tissues after other techniques have failed to yield clear results. In patients with chronic hepatitis C, liver biopsy may be used to assess the patient's prognosis and the likelihood of responding to antiviral treatment.

A liver biopsy may be ordered to diagnose or stage any of the following conditions or disorders:

- jaundice
- cirrhosis
- repeated abnormal results from liver function tests
- alcoholic liver disease
- unexplained swelling or enlargement of the liver (hepatomegaly)
- suspected drug-related liver damage such as **acetaminophen** poisoning
- hemochromatosis, a condition of excess iron in the liver
- intrahepatic cholestasis, the build up of bile in the liver
- hepatitis
- primary cancers of the liver such as hepatomas, cholangiocarcinomas, and angiosarcomas
- metastatic cancers of the liver (more than 20 times as common in the United States as primary cancers)
- post-liver transplant to measure graft rejection
- fever of unknown origin
- suspected tuberculosis, sarcoidosis, or amyloidosis
- genetic disorders such as Wilson's disease (a disorder in which copper accumulates in the liver, brain, kidneys, and corneas)

Demographics

According to the American Liver Foundation, liver disease affects approximately 25 million (one in 10) Americans annually. Cirrhosis accounts for over 27,000 deaths each year. Liver disease is the third most common cause of death among individuals between the ages of 25 and 59, and the seventh most common cause of all disease-related deaths.

Description

Percutaneous liver biopsy is sometimes called aspiration biopsy or fine-needle aspiration (FNA) because it is done with a hollow needle attached to a suction syringe. The special needles used to perform a liver biopsy are called Menghini or Jamshedi needles. The amount of specimen collected should be about 0.03–0.7 fl oz (1–2 cc). In many cases, the biopsy is done by a radiologist, doctor who specializes in x rays and imaging studies. The radiologist will use computed tomography (CT) scan or ultrasound to guide the needle to the target site for the biopsy. Some ultrasound-guided biopsies are performed using a biopsy gun that has a spring mechanism that contains a cutting sheath. This type of procedure gives a greater yield of tissue.

An hour or so before the biopsy, the patient will be given a sedative to aid in relaxation. The patient is then asked to lie on the back with the right elbow to the side and the right hand under the head. The patient is instructed to lie as still as possible during the procedure. He or she is warned to expect a sensation resembling a pinch in the right shoulder when the needle passes a certain nerve

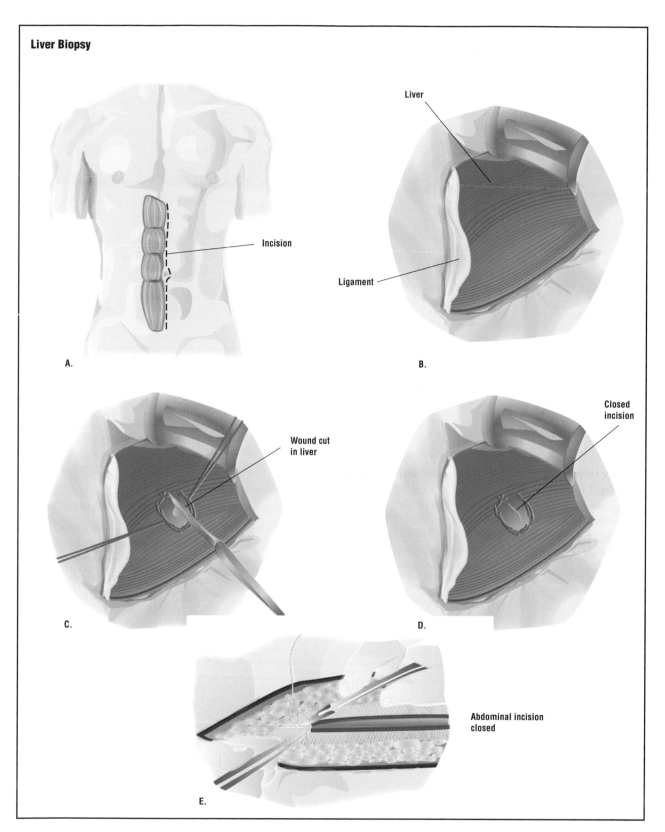

Liver Biopsy

A.
Incision

B.
Liver
Ligament

C.
Wound cut
in liver

D.
Closed
incision

E.
Abdominal incision
closed

In a traditional liver biopsy, access to the liver is gained through an incision in the abdomen (A). The liver is exposed (B). A wedge-shaped section is cut into the liver and removed (C). The liver incision is stitched (D). The abdominal incision is then repaired (E). *(Illustration by GGS Inc.)*

The liver biopsy requires the skill of many clinicians, including the radiologist, hepatologist, and pathologist, to make the diagnosis. Nurses will assist the physician during the biopsy procedure and in caring for the patient after the procedure. Tissues are prepared for microscopic evaluation by a histologic technician in the pathology lab. The procedure is generally performed on an outpatient basis in a hospital.

(the phrenic nerve), but to remain motionless in spite of the momentary pain.

The doctor will then mark a spot on the skin of the abdomen where the needle will be inserted. The right side of the upper abdomen is thoroughly cleansed with an antiseptic solution, generally iodine. The patient is then given a local anesthetic at the biopsy site.

The doctor prepares the needle by drawing sterile saline solution into a syringe. The syringe is then attached to the biopsy needle, which is inserted into the patient's chest wall. The doctor then draws the plunger of the syringe back to create a vacuum. At this point, the patient is asked to take a deep breath and hold it. The needle is inserted into the liver and withdrawn quickly, usually within two seconds or less. The negative pressure in the syringe draws or pulls a sample of liver tissue into the biopsy needle. As soon as the needle is withdrawn, the patient can breathe normally. This step takes only a few seconds. Pressure is applied at the biopsy site to stop any bleeding and a bandage is placed over it. The liver tissue sample is placed in a cup with a 10% formalin solution and sent to the laboratory immediately. The entire procedure takes 10–15 minutes. Test results are usually available within a day.

Most patients experience minor discomfort during the procedure (up to 50% of patients), but not severe pain. According to a medical study of adult patients undergoing percutaneous liver biopsy, pain was most often described as mild to moderate (i.e., a rating of three on a scale of one to 10). Mild medications of a non-aspirin type can be given after the biopsy if the pain persists for several hours.

Diagnosis/Preparation

Liver biopsies require some preparation by the patient. Since **aspirin** and ibuprofen (Advil, Motrin) are known to cause excessive bleeding by inhibiting platelets

and lessening clotting function, the patient should avoid taking any of these medications for at least a week before the biopsy. The doctor should check the patient's records to see whether he or she is taking any other medications that may affect blood clotting. Both a platelet count (or **complete blood count**) and a prothrombin time (to assess how well the patient's blood clots) are performed prior to the biopsy. These tests determine whether there is an abnormally high risk of uncontrolled bleeding from the biopsy site, which may contraindicate the procedure. The patient should limit food or drink for a period of four to eight hours before the biopsy.

Patients should be told what to expect in the way of discomfort pre- and post-procedure. In addition, they should be advised about what medications they should not take before or after the biopsy. It is important for the clinician to reassure the patient concerning the safety of the procedure.

Before the procedure, the patient or family member must sign a consent form. The patient will be questioned about any history of allergy to the local anesthetic, and then will be asked to empty the bladder so that he or she will be more comfortable during the procedure. **Vital signs**, including pulse rate, temperature, and breathing rate will be noted so that the doctor can tell during the procedure if the patient is having any physical problems.

When performing the liver biopsy and blood collection that precedes it, the physician and other health care providers will follow universal precautions to maintain sterility for the prevention of transmission of blood-borne pathogens.

Some patients should not have percutaneous liver biopsies. They include those with any of the following conditions:

• a platelet count below 50,000

• a prothrombin test time greater than three seconds over the reference interval, indicating a possible clotting abnormality

• a liver tumor with a large number of veins

• a large amount of abdominal fluid (ascites)

• infection anywhere in the lungs, the lining of the chest or abdominal wall, the biliary tract, or the liver

• benign tumors (angiomas) of the liver, which consist mostly of enlarged or newly formed blood vessels and may bleed heavily

• biliary obstruction (bile may leak from the biopsy site and cause an infection of the abdominal cavity)

Aftercare

Liver biopsies are now performed as outpatient procedures in most hospitals. Patients are asked to lie on their right sides for one hour and then to rest quietly for three more hours. At regular intervals, a nurse checks the patient's vital signs. If there are no complications, the patient is discharged, but will be asked to stay in an area that is within an hour from the hospital in case delayed bleeding occurs.

Patients should arrange to have a friend or relative take them home after discharge. Bed rest for a day is recommended, followed by a week of avoiding heavy work or strenuous **exercise**. The patient can immediately resume eating a normal diet.

Some mild soreness in the area of the biopsy is expected after the anesthetic wears off. Irritation of the muscle that lies over the liver can also cause mild discomfort in the shoulder for some patients. Acetaminophen can be taken for minor soreness, but aspirin and ibuprofen products are best avoided. The patient should, however, call the doctor if there is severe pain in the abdomen, chest, or shoulder; difficulty breathing; or persistent bleeding. These signs may indicate that there has been leakage of bile into the abdominal cavity, or that air has been introduced into the cavity around the lungs.

Risks

The complications associated with a liver biopsy are usually minor; most will occur in the first two hours following the procedure, and greater than 95% in the first 24 hours. The most significant risk is prolonged internal bleeding. Other complications from percutaneous liver biopsies include the leakage of bile or the introduction of air into the chest cavity (pneumothorax). There is also a small chance that an infection may occur. The risk that an internal organ such as the lung, gallbladder, or kidney might be punctured is decreased when using the ultrasound- or CT-guided procedure.

Normal results

After the biopsy, the liver sample is sent to the pathology laboratory and examined. A normal (negative) result would find no evidence of pathology in the tissue sample. It should be noted that many diseases of the liver are focal and not diffuse; an abnormality may not be detected if the sample was taken from an unaffected site. If symptoms persist, the patient may need to undergo another biopsy.

The pathologist will perform a visual inspection of the sample to note any abnormalities in appearance. In

cirrhosis, the sample will be fragmented and hard. Fatty liver, seen in heavy drinkers, will float in the formalin solution and will be yellow. Carcinomas are white. The pathologist will also look for deposition of bile pigments (green), indicating cholestasis (obstruction of bile flow). In preparation for microscopic examination, the tissue will be frozen and cut into thin sections, which will be mounted on glass slides and stained with various dyes to aid in identifying microscopic structures. Using the microscope, the pathologist will examine the tissue samples, and identify abnormal cells and any deposited substances such as iron or copper. In liver cancer, small dark malignant cells will be visible within the liver tissue. An infiltration of white blood cells may signal infection. The pathologist also checks for the number of bile ducts, and determines whether they are dilated. He or she also looks at the health of the small arteries and portal veins. Fibrosis will appear as scar tissue, and fatty changes are diagnosed by the presence of lipid droplets. Many different findings may be noted and a differential diagnosis (one out of many possibilities) can often be made. In difficult cases, other laboratory tests such as those assessing liver function enzymes will aid the clinician in determining the final diagnosis.

Morbidity and mortality rates

Post-biopsy complications that require hospitalization occur in approximately 1–3% of cases. Moderate pain is reported by 20% of patients, and 3% report pain severe enough to warrant intravenous pain relief. The mortality rate is approximately one in 10,000. In about 0.4% of cases, a patient with liver cancer will develop a fatal hemorrhage from a percutaneous biopsy. These fatalities result because some liver tumors are supplied with a large number of blood vessels and thus may bleed excessively.

Alternatives

Liver biopsy is an invasive and sometimes painful procedure that is also expensive (in 2002, direct costs associated with liver biopsy were $1,500–2,000). In some

KEY TERMS

Aspiration—The technique of removing a tissue sample for biopsy through a hollow needle attached to a suction syringe.

Bile—Liquid produced by the liver that is excreted into the intestine to aid in the digestion of fats.

Biliary—Relating to bile.

Biopsy—The surgical removal and microscopic examination of living tissue for diagnostic purposes.

Cholestasis—A blockage in the flow of bile.

Cirrhosis—A progressive disease of the liver characterized by the death of liver cells and their replacement with fibrous tissue.

Formalin—A clear solution of diluted formaldehyde that is used to preserve liver biopsy specimens until they can be examined in the laboratory.

Hepatitis—Inflammation of the liver, caused by infection or toxic injury.

Jaundice—Also termed icterus; an increase in blood bile pigments that are deposited in the skin, eyes, deeper tissue, and excretions. The skin and whites of the eye will appear yellow.

Menghini needle/Jamshedi needle—Special needles used to obtain a sample of liver tissue by aspiration.

Metastatic cancer—A cancer that has been transmitted through the body from a primary cancer site.

Percutaneous biopsy—A biopsy in which the needle is inserted and the sample removed through the skin.

Prothrombin test—A common test to measure the amount of time it takes for a patient's blood to clot; measurements are in seconds.

Vital signs—A person's essential body functions, usually defined as the pulse, body temperature, and breathing rate.

instances, blood tests may provide enough information to health care providers to make an accurate diagnosis and therefore avoid a biopsy. Occasionally, a biopsy may be obtained using a laparoscope (an instrument inserted through the abdominal wall that allows the doctor to visualize the liver and obtain a sample) or during surgery if the patient is undergoing an operation on the abdomen.

Resources

BOOKS

"Hepatobiliary Disorders: Introduction." In *Professional Guide to Diseases,* edited by Stanley Loeb, et al. Springhouse, PA: Springhouse Corporation, 2001.

Kanel, Gary C., and Jacob Korula. *Liver Biopsy Evaluation, Histologic Diagnosis and Clinical Correlations.* Philadelphia, PA: W.B. Saunders Company, 2000.

"Screening and Diagnostic Evaluation." In *The Merck Manual of Diagnosis and Therapy,* 17th Edition, edited by Robert Berkow, et al. Whitehouse Station, NJ: Merck Research Laboratories, 1999.

PERIODICALS

Castera, Laurent, Isabelle Negre, Kamran Samii, and Catherine Buffett. "Pain Experienced during Percutaneous Liver Biopsy." *Hepatology* 30, no. 6 (December 1999): 1529–30.

Dienstag, Jules L. "The Role of Liver Biopsy in Chronic Hepatitis C." *Hepatology* 36, no. 5 (November 2002): 152–60.

Moix, F. Martin, and Jean-Pierre Raufman. "The Role of Liver Biopsy in the Evaluation of Liver Test Abnormalities." *Clinical Cornerstone* 3, no. 6 (2001): 13–23.

ORGANIZATIONS

American Liver Foundation. 1425 Pompton Avenue, Cedar Grove, NJ 07009. (800) 465-4837. <http://www.liverfoundation.org>.

Jane E. Phillips, PhD
Stephanie Dionne Sherk

Liver function tests

Definition

Liver function tests, or LFTs, include tests that are routinely measured in all clinical laboratories. LFTs include bilirubin, a compound formed by the breakdown of hemoglobin; ammonia, a breakdown product of protein that is normally converted into urea by the liver before being excreted by the kidneys; proteins that are made by the liver including total protein, albumin, prothrombin, and fibrinogen; cholesterol and triglycerides, which are made and excreted via the liver; and the enzymes alanine aminotransferase (ALT), aspartate aminotransferase (AST), alkaline phosphatase (ALP), gamma-glutamyl transferase (GGT), and lactate dehydrogenase (LDH). Other liver function tests include serological tests (to demonstrate antibodies) and DNA tests for hepatitis and other viruses; and tests for antimitochondrial and smooth muscle antibodies, transthyretin (prealbumin), protein electrophoresis, bile acids, alpha-fetoprotein, and a constellation of other enzymes that help differentiate necrotic (characterized by death of tissues) versus obstructive liver disease.

Purpose

Liver function tests done individually do not give the physician very much information, but used in combination with a careful history, **physical examination**, and imaging studies, they contribute to making an accurate diagnosis of the specific liver disorder. Different tests will show abnormalities in response to liver inflammation; liver injury due to drugs, alcohol, toxins, or viruses; liver malfunction due to blockage of the flow of bile; and liver cancers.

Precautions

Blood for LFTs is collected by sticking a needle into a vein. The nurse or phlebotomist performing the procedure must be careful to clean the skin before sticking in the needle.

Bilirubin: Drugs that may cause increased blood levels of total bilirubin include anabolic steroids, **antibiotics**, antimalarials, ascorbic acid, Diabinese, codeine, **diuretics**, epinephrine, oral contraceptives, and vitamin A.

Ammonia: Muscular exertion can increase ammonia levels, while cigarette smoking produces significant increases within one hour of inhalation. Drugs that may cause increased levels include alcohol, **barbiturates**, narcotics, and diuretics. Drugs that may decrease levels include antibiotics, levodopa, lactobacillus, and potassium salts.

ALT: Drugs that may increase ALT levels include **acetaminophen**, ampicillin, codeine, dicumarol, indomethacin, methotrexate, oral contraceptives, **tetracyclines**, and verapamil. Previous intramuscular injections may cause elevated levels.

GGT: Drugs that may cause increased GGT levels include alcohol, phenytoin, and phenobarbital. Drugs that may cause decreased levels include oral contraceptives.

LDH: Strenuous activity may raise levels of LDH. Alcohol, anesthetics, **aspirin**, narcotics, procainamide, and fluoride may also raise levels. Ascorbic acid (vitamin C) can lower levels of LDH.

Description

The liver is the largest and one of the most important organs in the body. As the body's "chemical factory," it regulates the levels of most of the biomolecules found in the blood, and acts with the kidneys to clear the blood of drugs and toxic substances. The liver metabolizes these products, alters their chemical structure, makes them water soluble, and excretes them in bile. Laboratory tests for total protein, albumin, ammonia, transthyretin, and cholesterol are markers for the synthetic function of the liver. Tests for cholesterol, bilirubin, ALP, and bile salts are measures of the secretory (excretory) function of the liver. The enzymes ALT, AST, GGT, LDH, and tests for viruses are markers for liver injury.

Some liver function tests are used to determine if the liver has been damaged or its function impaired. Elevations of these markers for liver injury or disease tell the physician that something is wrong with the liver. ALT and bilirubin are the two primary tests used largely for this purpose. Bilirubin is measured by two tests, called total and direct bilirubin. The total bilirubin measures both conjugated and unconjugated bilirubin while direct bilirubin measures only the conjugated bilirubin fraction in the blood. Unconjugated bilirubin is formed in the reticuloendothelial (RE) cells in the spleen that remove old red blood cells from the circulation. The RE cells release the bilirubin into the blood, where it is bound by albumin and transported to the liver. The bilirubin is taken up by liver cells and conjugated to glucuronic acid, which makes the bilirubin water soluble. This form will react directly with a Ehrlich's diazo reagent, hence the name direct bilirubin. While total bilirubin is elevated in various liver diseases, it is also increased in certain (hemolytic) anemias caused by increased red blood cell turnover. Neonatal hyperbilirubinemia is a condition caused by an immature liver than cannot conjugate the bilirubin. The level of total bilirubin in the blood becomes elevated, and must be monitored closely in order to prevent damage to the brain caused by unconjugated bilirubin, which has a high affinity for brain tissue. Bilirubin levels can be decreased by exposing the baby to UV light. Direct bilirubin is formed only by the liver, and therefore, it is specific for hepatic or biliary disease. Its concentration in the blood is very low (0–0.2 mg/dL) and therefore, even slight increases are significant. Highest levels of direct bilirubin are seen in obstructive liver diseases. However, direct bilirubin is not sensitive to all forms of liver disease (e.g., focal intrahepatic obstruction) and is not always elevated in the earliest stages of disease; therefore, ALT is needed to exclude a diagnosis.

ALT is an enzyme that transfers an amino group from the amino acid alanine to a ketoacid acceptor (oxaloacetate). The enzyme was formerly called serum glutamic pyruvic transaminase (SGPT) after the products formed by this reaction. Although ALT is present in other tissues besides liver, its concentration in liver is far greater than any other tissue, and blood levels in nonhepatic conditions rarely produce levels of a magnitude seen in liver disease. The enzyme is very sensitive to necrotic or inflammatory liver injury. Consequently, if ALT or direct bilirubin is increased, then some form of liver disease is likely. If both are normal, then liver disease is unlikely.

These two tests along with others are used to help determine what is wrong. The most useful tests for this purpose are the liver function enzymes and the ratio of direct to total bilirubin. These tests are used to differentiate diseases characterized primarily by hepatocellular damage (necrosis, or cell death) from those characterized by obstructive damage (cholestasis or blockage of bile flow). In hepatocellular damage, the transaminases, ALT and AST, are increased to a greater extent than alkaline phosphatase. This includes viral hepatitis, which gives the greatest increase in transaminases (10–50-fold normal), hepatitis induced by drugs or poisons (toxic hepatitis), alcoholic hepatitis, hypoxic necrosis (a consequence of congestive heart failure), chronic hepatitis, and cirrhosis of the liver. In obstructive liver diseases, the alkaline phosphatase is increased to a greater extent than the transaminases (ALP>ALT). This includes diffuse intrahepatic obstructive disease which may be caused by some drugs or biliary cirrhosis, focal obstruction that may be caused by malignancy, granuloma from chronic inflamation, or stones in the intrahepatic bile ducts, or extrahepatic obstruction such as gall bladder or common bile duct stones, or pancreatic or bile duct cancer. In both diffuse intrahepatic obstruction and extrahepatic obstruction, the direct bilirubin is often greatly elevated because the liver can conjugate the bilirubin, but this direct bilirubin cannot be excreted via the bile. In such cases the ratio of direct to total bilirubin is greater than 0.4.

Aspartate aminotransferase, formerly called serum glutamic oxaloacetic transaminase (SGOT), is not as specific for liver disease as is ALT, which is increased in myocardial infarction, pancreatitis, muscle wasting diseases, and many other conditions. However, differentiation of acute and chronic forms of hepatocellular injury is aided by examining the ratio of ALT to AST, called the DeRitis ratio. In acute hepatitis, Reye's syndrome, and infectious mononucleosis the ALT predominates. However, in alcoholic liver disease, chronic hepatitis, and cirrhosis, the AST predominates.

Alkaline phosphatase is increased in obstructive liver diseases, but it is not specific for the liver. Increases of a similar magnitude (three- to five-fold normal) are commonly seen in bone diseases, late pregnancy, leukemia, and some other malignancies. The enzyme gamma-glutamyl transferase (GGT) is used to help differentiate the source of an elevated ALP. GGT is greatly increased in obstructive jaundice, alcoholic liver disease,

and hepatic cancer. When the increase in GGT is two or more times greater than the increase in ALP, the source of the ALP is considered to be from the liver. When the increase in GGT is five or more times the increase in ALP, this points to a diagnosis of alcoholic hepatitis. GGT, but not AST and ALT, is elevated in the first stages of liver inflammation due to alcohol consumption, and GGT is useful as a marker for excessive drinking. GGT has been shown to rise after acute persistent alcohol ingestion and then fall when alcohol is avoided.

Lactate dehydrogenase (LDH) is found in almost all cells in the body. Different forms of the enzyme (isoenzymes) exist in different tissues, especially in heart, liver, red blood cells, brain, kidney, and muscles. LDH is increased in megaloblastic and hemolytic anemias, leukemias and lymphomas, myocardial infarction, infectious mononucleosis, muscle wasting diseases, and both necrotic and obstructive jaundice. While LDH is not specific for any one disorder, the enzyme is elevated (two- to five-fold normal) along with liver function enzymes in both necrotic and obstructive liver diseases. LDH is markedly increased in most cases of liver cancer. An enzyme pattern showing a marked increase in LDH and to a lesser degree ALP with only slightly increased transaminases (AST and ALT) is seen in cancer of the liver (space occupying disease). Such findings should be followed-up with imaging studies and measurement of alpha-fetoprotein and carcinoembryonic antigen, two tumor markers prevalent in hepatic cancers.

Some liver function tests are not sensitive enough to be used for diagnostic purposes, but are elevated in severe or chronic liver diseases. These tests are used primarily to indicate the extent of damage to the liver. Tests falling into this category are ammonia, total protein, albumin, cholesterol, transthyretin, fibrinogen, and the prothrombin time.

Analysis of blood ammonia aids in the diagnosis of severe liver diseases and helps to monitor the course of these diseases. Together with the AST and the ALT, ammonia levels are used to confirm a diagnosis of Reye's syndrome, a rare disorder usually seen in children and associated with infection and aspirin intake. Reye's syndrome is characterized by brain and liver damage following an upper respiratory tract infection, chickenpox, or influenza. Ammonia levels are also helpful in the diagnosis and treatment of hepatic encephalopathy, a serious brain condition caused by the accumulated toxins that result from liver disease and liver failure. Ammonia levels in the blood are normally very low. Ammonia produced by the breakdown of amino acids is converted to urea by the liver. When liver disease becomes severe, failure of the urea cycle results in elevated blood ammonia and decreased urea (or blood urea nitrogen, BUN). Increasing ammonia signals end-stage liver disease and a high risk of hepatic coma.

Albumin is the protein found in the highest concentration in blood, making up over half of the protein mass. Albumin has a half-life in blood of about three weeks and decreased levels are not seen in the early stages of liver disease. A persistently low albumin in liver disease signals reduced synthetic capacity of the liver and is a sign of progressive liver failure. In the acute stages of liver disease, proteins such as transthyretin (prealbumin) with a shorter half-life may be measured to give an indication of the severity of the disease.

Cholesterol is synthesized by the liver, and cholesterol balance is maintained by the liver's ability to remove cholesterol from lipoproteins, and use it to produce bile acids and salts that it excretes into the bile ducts. In obstructive jaundice caused by stones, biliary tract scarring, or cancer, the bile cannot be eliminated and cholesterol and triglycerides may accumulate in the blood as low-density lipoprotein (LDL) cholesterol. In acute necrotic liver diseases triglycerides may be elevated due to hepatic lipase deficiency. In liver failure caused by necrosis, the liver's ability to synthesize cholesterol is reduced and blood levels may be low.

The liver is responsible for production of the vitamin K clotting factors. In obstructive liver diseases a deficiency of vitamin K-derived clotting factors results from failure to absorb vitamin K. In obstructive jaundice, intramuscular injection of vitamin K will correct the prolonged prothrombin time. In severe necrotic disease, the liver cannot synthesize factor I (fibrinogen) or factors II, VII, IX, and X from vitamin K. When attributable to hepatic necrosis, an increase in the prothrombin time by more than two seconds indicates severe liver disease.

Serum protein electrophoresis patterns will be abnormal in both necrotic and obstructive liver diseases. In the acute stages of hepatitis, the albumin will be low and the gamma globulin fraction will be elevated owing to a large increase in the production of antibodies. The alpha-1 globulin and alpha-2 globulin fractions will be elevated owing to production of acute phase proteins as a response to inflamation. In biliary cirrhosis the beta globulin may be elevated owing to an increase in beta lipoprotein. In hepatic cirrhosis the albumin will be greatly decreased, and the pattern will show bridging between the beta and gamma globulins owing to production of IgA. The albumin to globulin ratio (A/G) ratio will fall below one.

The most prevalent liver disease is viral hepatitis. Tests for this condition include a variety of antigen and antibody markers and nucleic acid tests. Acute viral hepatitis is associated initially with 20- to 100-fold increases in transaminases and is followed shortly afterward by jaundice. Such patients should be tested for hepatitis B surface antigen (HbsAg) and IgM antibodies to hepatitis B core antigen (anti-HBc IgM), and anti-hepatitis C virus (anti-HVC) to identify these causes. In addition to hepatitis A-E, viral hepatitis may be caused by Epstein-Barr virus (EBV) and cytomegalovirus (CMV) infections of the liver. Tests for these viruses such as the infectious mononucleosis antibody test, anti-viral capsid antigen test (anti-VCA), and anti-CMV test are useful in diagnosing these infections.

Liver disease may be caused by autoimmune mechanisms in which autoantibodies destroy liver cells. Autoimmune necrosis is associated with systemic lupus erythematosus and chronic viral hepatitis usually caused by hepatitis B and hepatitis C virus infections. These conditions give rise to anti-smooth muscle antibodies and anti-nuclear antibodies, and tests for these are useful markers for chronic hepatitis. Antibodies to mitochondrial antigens (antimitochondrial antibodies) are found in the blood of more than 90% of persons with primary biliary cirrhosis, and those with M2 specificity are considered specific for this disease.

Preparation

Patients are asked to fast and to inform clinicians of all drugs, even over-the-counter drugs, that they are taking. Many times liver function tests are done on an emergency basis and fasting and obtaining a medical history are not possible.

Aftercare

Patients will have blood drawn into a vacuum tube and may experience some pain and burning at the site of injection. A gauze bandage may be placed over the site to prevent further bleeding. If the person is suffering from severe liver disease, they may lack clotting factors. The nurse or caregiver should be careful to monitor bleeding in these patients after obtaining blood.

Normal results

Reference ranges vary from laboratory to laboratory and also depend upon the method used. However, normal values are generally framed by the ranges shown below. Values for enzymes are based upon measurement at 37°C.

- ALT: 5–35 IU/L. (Values for the elderly may be slightly higher, and values also may be higher in men and in African-Americans.)

- AST: 0–35 IU/L.

- ALP: 30–120 IU/LALP is higher in children, older adults and pregnant females.

- GGT: males 2–30 U/L; females 1–24 U/L.

- LDH: 0–4 days old: 290–775 U/L; 4–10 days: 545–2000 U/L; 10 days–24 months: 180–430 U/L; 24 months–12 years: 110–295 U/L; 12–60 years: 100–190 U/L; 60 years: >110–210 U/L.

- Bilirubin: (Adult, elderly, and child) Total bilirubin: 0.1–1.0 mg/dL; indirect bilirubin: 0.2–0.8 mg/dL; direct bilirubin: 0.0–0.3 mg/dL. (Newborn) Total bilirubin: 1–12 mg/dL. Note: critical values for adult: greater than 1.2 mg/dL. Critical values for newborn (requiring immediate treatment): greater than 15 mg/dL.

- Ammonia: 10–70 micrograms per dL (heparinized plasma). Normal values for this test vary widely, depending upon the age of the patient and the type of specimen.

- Albumin: 3.2–5.4 g/L.

Abnormal results

ALT: Values are significantly increased in cases of hepatitis, and moderately increased in cirrhosis, liver tumor, obstructive jaundice, and severe burns. Values are mildly increased in pancreatitis, heart attack, infectious mononucleosis, and shock. Most useful when compared with ALP levels.

AST: High levels may indicate liver cell damage, hepatitis, heart attack, heart failure, or gall stones.

ALP: Elevated levels occur in diseases that impair bile formation (cholestasis). ALP may also be elevated in many other liver disorders, as well as some lung cancers (bronchogenic carcinoma) and Hodgkin's lymphoma. However, elevated ALP levels may also occur in otherwise healthy people, especially among older people.

GGT: Increased levels are diagnostic of hepatitis, cirrhosis, liver tumor or metastasis, as well as injury from drugs toxic to the liver. GGT levels may increase with alcohol ingestion, heart attack, pancreatitis, infectious mononucleosis, and Reye's syndrome.

LDH: Elevated LDH is seen with heart attack, kidney disease, hemolysis, viral hepatitis, infectious mononucleosis, Hodgkin's disease, abdominal and lung cancers, germ cell tumors, progressive muscular dystrophy, and pulmonary embolism. LD is not normally elevated in cirrhosis.

Bilirubin: Increased indirect or total bilirubin levels can indicate various serious anemias, including hemolytic disease of the newborn and **transfusion** reaction. Increased direct bilirubin levels can be diagnostic of bile duct obstruction, gallstones, cirrhosis, or hepatitis. It is important to note that if total bilirubin levels in the newborn reach or exceed critical levels, exchange transfusion is necessary to avoid kernicterus, a condition that causes brain damage from bilirubin in the brain.

KEY TERMS

Bile acid—A detergent that is made in the liver and excreted into the intestine to aid in the absorption of fats.

Biliary—Relating to bile.

Cirrhosis—A liver disease where there is a loss of normal liver tissues, replaced by scar tissue. This is usually caused by chronic alcohol abuse, but also can be caused by blockage of the bile ducts.

Deamination—Removal of the NH_2 group from an amino compound, usually by hydrolysis.

Detoxification—A process of altering the chemical structure of a compound to make it less toxic.

Hepatitis—Inflammation of the liver.

Hepatocyte—Liver cell.

Isoenzyme—One of a group of enzymes that brings about the same reactions on the same chemicals, but are different in their physical properties.

Jaundice—Hyperbilirubinemia or too much bilirubin in the blood. Bilirubin will be deposited in the skin and the mucosal membranes. The whites of the eyes and the skin appear yellow.

Neonatal jaundice—A disorder in newborns where the liver is too premature to conjugate bilirubin, which builds up in the blood.

Ammonia: Increased levels are seen in primary liver cell disease, Reye's syndrome, severe heart failure, hemolytic disease of the newborn, and hepatic encephalopathy.

Albumin: Albumin levels are increased due to dehydration. They are decreased due to a decrease in synthesis of the protein which is seen in severe liver failure and in conditions such as burns or renal disease that cause loss of albumin from the blood.

Patient education

Health-care providers should inform the patient of any abnormal results and explain how these values reflect the status of their liver disease. It is important to guide the patient in ways to stop behaviors such as taking drugs or drinking alcohol, if these are the causes of the illness.

Resources

BOOKS

Burtis, Carl A. and Edward R. Ashwood. *Tietz Textbook of Clinical Chemistry.* Philadelphia: W. B. Saunders, 1999.

Cahill, Matthew. *Handbook of Diagnostic Tests.* 2nd ed. Springhouse, PA: Springhouse Corporation, 1999.

Henry, J. B. *Clinical Diagnosis and Management by Laboratory Methods.* 20th ed. Philadelphia: W. B. Saunders, 2001.

Wallach, Jacques. *Interpretation of Diagnostic Tests.* 7th ed. Philadelphia: Lippincott Williams & Wilkins, 2000.

OTHER

Jensen, J. E. *Liver Function Tests.* [cited April 4, 2003]. <http://www.gastromd.com/lft.html>.

National Institutes of Health. [cited April 4, 2003]. <http://www.nlm.nih.gov/medlineplus/encyclopedia.html>.

Worman, Howard J. *Common Laboratory Tests in Liver Disease.* [cited April 4, 2003]. <http://www.cpmcnet.columbia.edu/dept/gi/labtests.html>.

Jane E. Phillips, Ph.D.
Mark A. Best, M.D.

Liver removal *see* **Hepatectomy**

Liver transplantation

Definition

Liver transplantation is a surgery that removes a diseased liver and replaces it with a healthy donor liver.

Purpose

A liver transplant is needed when the liver's function is reduced to the point that the life of the patient is threatened.

Demographics

Compared to whites, those with African-American, Asian, Pacific Islander, or Hispanic descent are three times more likely to suffer from end-stage renal disease (ESRD). Both children and adults can suffer from liver failure and require a transplant.

Patients with advanced heart and lung disease, who are human immunodeficiency virus (HIV) positive, and who abuse drugs and alcohol are poor candidates for liver transplantation. Their ability to survive the surgery and the difficult recovery period, as well as their long-term prognosis, is hindered by their conditions.

Description

The liver is the body's principle chemical factory. It receives all nutrients, drugs, and toxins, which are ab-
sorbed from the intestines, and performs the final stages of digestion, converting food into energy and replacement parts for the body. The liver also filters the blood of all waste products, removes and detoxifies poisons, and excretes many of these into the bile. It further processes other chemicals for excretion by the kidneys. The liver is also an energy storage organ, converting food energy to a chemical called glycogen that can be rapidly converted to fuel.

When other medical treatment interferes with the functioning of a damaged liver, a transplant is necessary. Since 1963, when the first human liver transplant was performed, thousands more have been performed each year. Cirrhosis, a disease that kills healthy liver cells, replacing them with scar tissue, is the most common reason for liver transplantation in adults. The most frequent reason for transplantation in children is biliary atresia—a disease in which the ducts that carry bile out of the liver, are missing or damaged.

Included among the many causes of liver failure that bring patients to **transplant surgery** are:

• Progressive hepatitis, mostly due to virus infection, accounts for more than one-third of all liver transplants.

• Alcohol damage accounts for approximately 20% of transplants.

• Scarring, or abnormality of the biliary system, accounts for roughly another 20% of liver transplants.

• The remainder of transplants come from various cancers, uncommon diseases, and a disease known as fulminant liver failure.

Fulminant liver failure most commonly happens during acute viral hepatitis, but is also the result of mushroom poisoning by *Amanita phalloides* and toxic reactions to overdose of some medicines, such as acetaminophen—a medicine commonly used to relieve pain and reduce fever. The person who is the victim of mushroom poisoning is a special category of candidate for a liver transplant because of the speed of the disease and the immediate need for treatment.

As the liver fails, all of its functions diminish. Nutrition suffers, toxins build, and waste products accumulate. Scar tissue accumulates on the liver as the disease progresses. Blood flow is increasingly restricted in the portal vein, which carries blood from the stomach and abdominal organs to the liver. The resulting high blood pressure (hypertension) causes swelling of and bleeding from the blood vessels of the esophagus. Toxins build-up in the blood (liver encephalopathy), resulting in severe jaundice (yellowing of the skin and eyes), fluid accumulation in the abdomen (ascites), and deterioration of mental function. Eventually, death occurs.

There are three types of liver transplantation methods. They include:

• Orthotopic transplantation, the replacement of a whole diseased liver with a healthy donor liver.

• Heterotrophic transplantation, the addition of a donor liver at another site, while the diseased liver is left intact.

• Reduced-size liver transplantation, the replacement of a whole diseased liver with a portion of a healthy donor liver. Reduced-size liver transplants are most often performed on children.

When an orthotropic transplantation is performed, a segment of the inferior vena cava (the body's main vein to the heart) attached to the liver is taken from the donor, as well. The same parts are removed from the recipient and replaced by connecting the inferior vena cava, the hepatic artery, the portal vein, and the bile ducts.

When there is a possibility that the afflicted liver may recover, a heterotypic transplantation is performed. The donor liver is placed in a different site, but it still has to have the same connections. It is usually attached very close to the patient's original liver; if the original liver recovers, the donor liver will wither away. If the patient's original liver does not recover, that liver will dry up, leaving the donor in place.

Reduced-size liver transplantation puts part of a donor liver into a patient. A liver can actually be divided into eight pieces—each supplied by a different set of blood vessels. In the past, just two of these sections have been enough to save a patient suffering from liver failure, especially if it is a child. It is possible, therefore, to transplant one liver into at least two patients and to transplant part of a liver from a living donor—and for both the donor and recipients to survive. Liver tissue grows to accommodate its job provided that the organ is large enough initially. Patients have survived with only 15–20% of their original liver intact, assuming that that portion was healthy from the beginning.

As of 2003, the availability of organs for transplant was in crisis. In October 1997, a national distribution system was established that gives priority to patients who are most ill and in closest proximity to the donor livers. Livers, however, are available nationally. It is now possible to preserve a liver out of the body for 10 to 20 hours by flushing it with cooled solutions of special chemicals and nutrients, if necessary. This enables transport cross-country.

Description

Once a donor liver has been located and the patient is in the **operating room** and under general anesthesia, the patient's heart and blood pressure are monitored. A long cut is made alongside of the ribs; sometimes, an upwards cut may also be made. When the liver is removed, four blood vessels that connect the liver to the rest of the body are cut and clamped shut. After getting the donor liver ready, the transplant surgeon connects these vessels to the donor vessels. A connection is made from the bile duct (a tube that drains the bile from the liver) of the donor liver to the bile duct of the liver of the patient's bile duct. In some cases, a small piece of the intestine is connected to the new donor bile duct. This connection is called Roux-en-Y. The operation usually takes between six and eight hours; another two hours is spent preparing the patient for surgery. Therefore, a patient will likely be in the operating room for eight to 10 hours.

The United Network for Organ Sharing (UNOS) data indicates that patients in need of organ transplants outnumber available organs three to one.

Diagnosis/Preparation

The liver starts to fail only when more than half of it is damaged. Thus, once a person demonstrates symptoms of liver failure, there is not much liver function left. Signs and symptoms of liver failure include:

• jaundice

• muscle wasting (loss of muscle)

• forgetfulness, confusion, or coma

• fatigue

• itching

• poor blood clotting

• build-up of fluid in the stomach (ascites)

• infections

• bleeding in the stomach

A doctor will diagnose liver disease; a liver specialist, a transplant surgeon, and other doctors will have to be consulted, as well, before a patient can be considered for a liver transplant. Before transplantation takes place, the patient is first determined to be a good candidate for transplantation by going through a rigorous medical examination. Blood tests, consultations, and x rays will be needed to determine if the patient is a good candidate. Other tests that may be conducted are: computed tomography (CAT or CT) scan, magnetic resonance image (MRI), ultrasound, routine **chest x ray**, endoscopy, sclerotherapy and rubber-band ligation, transjugular intrahepatic portosystemic shunt (TIPS), creatinine clearance, cardiac testing (echocardiogram [ECHO]) and/or electrocardiogram [EKG or ECG]), and pulmonary function test [PFTs]), **liver biopsy**, and nutritional evaluation. A dietitian will evaluate the patient's nutritional needs and design an eating plan. Since a patient's emotional state is as important as their physical state, a psychosocial evaluation will be administered.

Once test results are reviewed and given to the liver transplant selection committee, the patient will be assessed for whether he or she is an appropriate candidate. Some patients are deemed too healthy for a transplant and will be followed and retested at a later date if their liver gets worse. Other patients are determined to be too sick to survive a transplant. The committee will not approve a transplant for these patients. Once a patient is approved, they will be placed on a waiting list for a donor liver. When placed on the waiting list, a patient will be given a score based on the results of the blood tests. The higher a patient's score, the sicker the patient is. This results in the patient earning a higher place on the waiting list.

Suitable candidates boost their nutritional intakes to ensure that they are as healthy as possible before surgery. Drugs are administered that will decrease organ rejection after surgery. The medical committee consults with the patient and family, if available, to explain the surgery and any potential complications. Many problems can arise during the waiting period. Medicines should be changed as needed, and blood tests should be done to assure a patient is in the best possible health for the transplant surgery. Psychological counseling during this period is recommended, as well.

When a donor is found, it is important that the transplant team be able to contact the patient. The patient awaiting the organ must not eat or drink anything from the moment the hospital calls. On the other hand, the liver may not be good enough for transplantation. Then, the operation will be cancelled, although this does not happen often.

Aftercare

Following surgery, the patient will wake up in the surgical **intensive care unit** (SICU). During this time, a

---

QUESTIONS TO ASK THE DOCTOR

- What should I do to prepare for this operation?
- Who will tell me about the transplant process?
- Can I tour the transplant center?
- Who are the members of the transplant team and what are their jobs?
- Is there a special nursing unit for transplant patients?
- How many attending surgeons are available to do my type of transplant?
- Does the hospital do living donor transplants?
- Is a living donor transplant a choice in my case? If so, where will the living donor evaluation be done?
- What is the organ recovery cost if I have a living donor?
- Will I also need to change my lifestyle?
- How long will I have to stay in the hospital?
- Why is recovery such a slow process?

---

tube will be inserted into the windpipe to facilitate breathing. It is removed when the patient is fully awake and strong enough to breathe on his or her own. There may be other tubes that are removed as the patient recovers. When safe to leave the SICU, the patient is moved to the transplant floor. Walking and eating will become the primary focus. Physical therapy may be started to help the patient become active, as it is an important part of recovery. When the patient begins to feel hungry and the bowels are working, regular food that is low in salt will be given.

A patient should expect to spend about 10 to 14 days in the hospital, although some stays may be shorter or longer. Before leaving the hospital, a patient will be advised of: signs of infection or rejection, how to take medications and change dressings, and how to understand general health problems. Infection can be a real danger, because the medications taken compromise the body's defense systems. The doctors will conduct blood tests, ultrasounds, and x rays to ensure that the patient is doing well.

The first three months after transplant are the most risky for getting such infections as the flu, so patients should follow these precautions:

KEY TERMS

Acetaminophen—A common pain reliever (e.g., Tylenol).

Anesthesia—A safe and effective means of alleviating pain during a medical procedure.

Antibody—An antibody is a protein complex used by the immune system to identify and neutralize foreign objects, such as like bacteria and viruses. Each antibody recognizes a specific antigen unique to its target

Antigen—Any chemical that provokes an immune response.

Ascites—A build-up of fluid in the stomach as a result of liver failure.

Bile ducts—Tubes carrying bile from the liver to the intestines.

Biliary atresia—A disease in which the ducts that carry bile out of the liver are missing or damaged is the most frequent reason for transplantation in children. Biliary atresia of the major bile ducts causes cholestasis and jaundice, which does not become apparent until several days after birth; periportal fibrosis develops and leads to cirrhosis,

with proliferation of small bile ducts unless these are also atretic; giant cell transformation of hepatic cells also occurs.

Biliary system—The tree of tubes that carries bile.

Cirrhosis—A disease in which healthy liver cells are killed and replaced with scar tissue. Cirrhosis is the most common reason for liver transplantation in adults and is often a result of alcoholism.

Computed tomography (CT or CAT) scan—A radiologic imaging modality that uses computer processing to generate an image of the tissue density in a "slice" as thin as 1–10 mm in thickness through the patient's body. These images are spaced at intervals of 0.5 cm–1 cm. Cross-sectional anatomy can be reconstructed in several planes without exposing the patient to additional radiation. Called also computerized axial tomography (CAT) and computerized transaxial tomography (CTAT).

Electrocardiogram (EKG)—A graphic record showing the electrical activity of the heart.

Endoscopy—An instrument (endoscope) used to visualize a hollow organ's interior.

- Avoid people who are ill.
- Wash hands frequently.
- Tell the doctor if you are exposed to any disease.
- Tell the doctor if a cold sore, rash, or water blister appears on the body or spots appear in the throat or on the tongue.
- Stay out of crowds and rooms with poor circulation.
- Do not swim in lakes or community pools during the three months following transplant.
- Eat meats that are well-cooked.
- Stay away from soil, including those in which houseplants are grown, and gardens, during the three months following transplant.
- Take all medications as directed.
- Learn to report the early symptoms of infection.

To ensure that the transplant is successful and that the patient has a long and healthy life, a patient must get good medical care, prevent and treat complications, keep in touch with doctors and nurses, and follow their advice. Nutrition plays a big part in the success of a liver

transplant, so what a patient eats after the transplant is very important.

Medications needed following liver transplantation

Successfully receiving a transplanted liver is only the beginning of a lifelong process. Patients with transplanted livers have to stay on **immunosuppressant drugs** for the rest of their lives to prevent organ rejection. Although many patients can reduce the dosage after the initial few months, virtually none can discontinue drugs altogether. For adolescent transplant recipients, post transplantation is a particularly difficult time, as they must learn to take responsibility for their own behavior and medication, as well as balance their developing sexuality in a body that has been transformed by the adverse effects of immunosuppression. Long-term outcome and tailoring of immunosuppression is of great importance.

Cyclosporine has long been the drug of experimentation in the immunosuppression regimen, and has been well-tolerated and effective. Hypertension, nephrotoxicity, and posttransplant lymphoproliferative disease (PTLD) are some of the long-term adverse effects. Tacrolimus has been

KEY TERMS (contd.)

Hepatic artery—The blood vessel supplying arterial blood to the liver.

Heterotrophic transplantation—The addition of a donor liver at another site, while the diseased liver is left intact.

Interleukin-2 (IL-2)—A cytokine derived from T helper lymphocytes that causes proliferation of T-lymphocytes and activated B lymphocytes.

Immunosuppression—A disorder or condition where the immune response is reduced or absent.

Inferior vena cava—The biggest vein in the body, returning blood to the heart from the lower half of the body.

Jaundice—Yellowing of the skin and eyes caused by a buildup of bile or excessive breakdown of red blood cells.

Leukemia—A cancer of the white blood cells (WBCs).

Lymphoma—A cancer of lymphatic tissue.

Lymphoproliferative—An increase in the number of lymphocytes. Lymphocytes are a white blood cell (WBC) formed in lymphatic tissue throughout the body—in the lymph nodes, spleen, thymus, tonsils, Peyer patches, and sometimes in bone marrow), and in normal adults, comprising approximately 22%–28% of the total number of leukocytes in the circulating blood.

Magnetic resonance imaging (MRI)—A test that provides pictures of organs and structures inside the body by using a magnetic field and pulses of radio wave energy to detect tumors, infection, and other types of tissue disease or damage, and helps to diagnose conditions that affect blood flow. The area of the body being studied is positioned inside a strong magnetic field.

Nephrotoxicity—The quality or state of being toxic to kidney cells.

Orthotopic transplantation—The replacement of a whole diseased liver with a healthy donor liver.

Portal vein—The blood vessel carrying venous blood from the abdominal organs to the liver.

Receptor—A structural protein molecule on the cell surface or within the cytoplasm that binds to a specific factor, such as a drug, hormone, antigen, or neurotransmitter.

developed more recently, and has improved the cosmetic adverse effects of cyclosporine, but has similar rates of hypertension and nephrotoxicity, and possibly a higher rate of PTLD. Prednisone, azathioprine, and tacrolimus are often combined with cyclosporine for better results. Newer immunosuppressive agents promise even better results.

There has been a recent, welcome development in renal sparing drugs, such as mycophenolate mofetil, which has no cosmetic adverse effects, does not require drug level monitoring, and is thus particularly attractive to teenagers. If started prior to irreversible renal dysfunction, recent research demonstrates recovery of renal function with mycophenolate mofetil. There is little published data on the use of sirolimus (rapamycin) in the pediatric population, but preliminary studies suggest that the future use of interleukin-2 receptor antibodies may be beneficial for immediate post-transplant induction of immunosuppression. When planning immunosuppression for adolescents, it is important to consider the effects of drug therapy on both males and females in order to maintain fertility and to ensure safety in pregnancy. Adequate practical measures and support should reduce noncompliance in this age group, and allow good, long-term function of the transplanted liver.

Risks

Early failure of the transplant occurs in every one in four surgeries and has to be repeated. Some transplants never work, some patients succumb to infection, and some suffer immune rejection. Primary failure is apparent within one or two days. Rejection usually starts at the end of the first week. There may be problems like bleeding of the bile duct after surgery, or blood vessels of the liver may become too narrow. The surgery itself may need revision because of narrowing, leaking, or blood clots at the connections. These issues may be solved with or without more surgery depending on the severity.

Infections are a constant risk while on immunosuppressive agents, because the immune system is supposed to prevent them. A method has not yet been devised to control rejection without hampering immune defenses against infections. Not only do ordinary infections pose a threat, but because of the impaired immunity, transplant patients are susceptible to the same opportunistic infections (OIs) that threaten acquired immune deficiency syndrome (AIDS) patients—pneumocystis pneumonia, herpes and cytomegalovirus (CMV) infections, fungi, and a host of bacteria.

Drug reactions are also a continuing threat. Every drug used to suppress the immune system has potential problems. As previously stated, hypertension, nephrotoxicity, and PTLD are some of the long-term adverse effects with immunosupressive drugs like cyclosporine. Immunosuppressants also hinder the body's ability to resist cancer. All drugs used to prevent rejection increase the risk of leukemias and lymphomas.

There is also a risk of the original disease returning. In the case of hepatitis C, reoccurrence is a risk factor for orthotropic liver transplants. Newer antiviral drugs hold out promise for dealing with hepatitis. In alcoholics, the urge to drink alcohol will still be a problem. Alcoholics Anonymous (AA) is the most effective treatment known for alcoholism.

Transplant recipients can get high blood pressure, diabetes, high cholesterol, thinning of the bones, and can become obese. Close medical care is needed to prevent these conditions.

Normal results

For a successful transplant, good medical care is important. Patients and families must stay in touch with their medical teams and drugs must be taken as advised to prevent infection and rejection of the new organ. However, sometimes because of the way it is preserved, the new liver doesn't function as it should, and a patient may have to go back on to the waiting list to receive a new liver.

Morbidity and mortality

Twenty-five million or one in 10 Americans are or have been afflicted with liver or biliary diseases. As of June 2003, there were 17,239 patients on the UNOS National Transplant Waiting List who were waiting for a liver transplantation. For the previous year (July 1, 2001 to June 30, 2002), there were a total of 5,261 liver transplants performed. Of those, 4,785 were cadaver donors (already deceased) and 476 living donors. For liver transplants performed from July 1, 1999 to June 30, 2001, the one-year survival rate was 86% for adults; 1,861 patients died while on the UNOS waiting list for the year ending June 30, 2002. More than 80% of children survive transplantation to adolescence and adulthood.

Since the introduction of cyclosporine and tacrolimus (drugs that suppress the immune response and keep it from attacking and damaging the new liver), success rates for liver transplantation have reached 80–90%.

Infections occur in about half of transplant patients and often appear during the first week. Biliary complica-

tions are apparent in about 22% of recipient patients (and 6% of donors), and vascular complications occur in 9.8% of recipient patients. Other complications in donors include re-operation (4.5%) and death (0.2%).

There are potential social, economic, and psychological problems, and a vast array of possible medical and surgical complications. Close medical surveillance must continue for the rest of the patient's life.

Alternatives

There is no treatment that can help the liver with all of its functions; thus, when a person reaches a certain stage of liver disease, a liver transplant may be the only way to save the patient's life.

Resources

BOOKS

Abhinav, Humar, M.D., I. Hertz Marshall, M.D., Laura J., Blakemore, M.D., eds. *Manual of Liver Transplant Medical Care.* Minneapolis, MN: Fairview Press, 2002.

Beauchamp, Daniel R., M.D., Mark B. Evers, M.D., Kenneth L. Mattox, M.D., Courtney M. Townsend, and David C. Sabiston, eds. *Sabiston Textbook of Surgery: The Biological Basis of Modern Surgical Practice,* 16th ed. London: W. B. Saunders Co., 2001.

Lawrence, Peter F., Richard M. Bell, and Merril T. Dayton, eds. *Essentials of General Surgery,* 3rd ed. Philadelphia, PA: Lippincott, Williams & Wilkins, 2000.

PERIODICALS

Brown, R.S., Jr., M. W. Russo, M. Lai, M. L. Shiffman, M. C. Richardson, J. E. Everhart, et al. "A survey of liver transplantation from living adult donors in the United States." *New England Journal of Medicine* 348, no. 9 (February, 2003):818–25.

Goldstein, M. J., E. Salame, S. Kapur, M. Kinkhabwala, D. La-Pointe-Rudow, N. P. P. Harren, et al. "Analysis of failure in living donor liver transplantation: differential outcomes in children and adults." *World Journal of Surgery* 27, no. 3 (2003):356–64.

Kelly, D. A. "Strategies for optimizing immunosuppression in adolescent transplant recipients: a focus on liver transplantation." *Paediatric Drugs* 5, no. 3 (2003):177–83.

Longheval, G., P. Vereerstraeten, P. Thiry, M. Delhaye, O. Le Moine, J. Deviere, et al. "Predictive models of short- and long-term survival in patients with nonbiliary cirrhosis." *Liver Transplantation: Official Publication of the American Association for the Study of Liver Diseases and the International Liver Transplantation Society* 9, no. 3 (March, 2003):260–7.

Neff, G. W., A. Bonham, A. G. Tzakis, M. Ragni, D. Jayaweera, E. R. Schiff, et al. "Orthotopic liver transplantation in patients with human immunodeficiency virus and end-stage liver disease." *Liver Transplantation: official publication of the American Association for the Study of*

Liver Diseases and the International Liver Transplantation Society 9, no. 3 (March, 2003):239–47.

Papatheodoridis, G. V., V. Sevastianos, and A. K. Burrouhs. "Prevention of and treatment for hepatitis B virus infection after liver transplantation in the nucleoside analogues era." *American Journal of Transplantation* 3, no. 3 (March, 2003):250–8.

Rudow, D. L., M. W. Russo, S. Haflige, J. C. Emond, and R. S. Brown, Jr. "Clinical and ethnic differences in candidates listed for liver transplantation with and without potential living donors." *Liver Transplantation: Official Publication of the American Association for the Study of Liver Diseases and the International Liver Transplantation Society* 9, no. 3 (March, 2003):254–9.

Wong, F. "Liver and kidney diseases." *Clinics in Liver Disease* 6, no. 4 (November, 2002):981–1011.

ORGANIZATIONS

American Liver Foundation. 75 Maiden Lane, Suite 603, New York, NY. 10038. (800) 465-4837 or (888) 443-7872. Fax: (212) 483.8179. info@liverfoundation.org. <http://www.liverfoundation.org>.

Hepatitis Foundation International (HFI). 504 Blick Drive, Silver Spring, MD. 20904-2901. (800) 891-0707 or (301) 622-4200. Fax: (301) 622-4702. hfi@comcast.net. <http://www.hepfi.org>

National Digestive Diseases, Information Clearinghouse. 2 Information Way, Bethesda, MD. 20892-3570. nddic@info.niddk.nih.gov.

National Institutes of Health, 9000 Rockville Pike, Bethesda, Maryland. 20892. (301) 496-4000. NIHInfo@OD.NIH.GOV. <http://www.nih.gov.>

United Network for Organ Sharing. 500-1100 Boulders Parkway, P.O. Box 13770. Richmond, VA. 23225. (888) 894-6361 or (804) 330-8500. <http://www.unos.org>

OTHER

U.S. National Library of Medicine and the National Institutes of Health. *Liver Transplantation.* 2003 [cited March 13, 2003]. < www.nlm.nih.gov/medlineplus/livertransplantation.html>.

J. Ricker Polsdorfer, M.D.
Crystal H. Kaczkowski, M.Sc.

Living will

Definition

A living will is a legal document in which patients instruct health-care providers about their wishes with respect to medical procedures should they become incapacitated. The living will and the durable medical **power of attorney** are two federally mandated parts of what is known as advanced medical directives.

Purpose

Advanced medical directives are legal mechanisms to assure that patients' wishes with respect to a number of medical procedures are carried out in their final days or when they are incapacitated. The documents reflect patients' rights of consent and medical choice under conditions whereby patients can no longer choose for themselves what medical interventions they wish to undergo.

In 1990, recognizing the importance of patient treatment wishes at the end of life, Congress enacted the Patient Self-Determination Act (PSDA). This federal law ensures that patients admitted to hospitals, **nursing homes**, home health agencies, HMOs, and **hospices** be informed of their rights under state law to prepare advance health care directives and have the documents entered into their medical record. Each state has different requirements for the living will and the power of attorney. It is important to research medical directives before an accident or illness make that an impossibility. Living wills have become customary in many parts of the country and are broadly respected by health care providers. However, a high percentage of Americans do not have a living will and/or a power of attorney to ensure its compliance.

Description

The living will can be a very broad or a very narrow document, according to the wishes of the patient. It is the patient's declaration, a written statement of what he or she wants to occur in the event of serious accident or illness. It is primarily directed to medical personnel about the type of care the patient wishes to have, or wishes not to have, under situations of terminal illness or incapacitation.

The document commonly includes the kinds of medical procedures that are usually administered to patients who are seriously ill. These may include:

• transfusions of blood and blood products

• cardiopulmonary resuscitation (CPR)

• diagnostic tests

• dialysis

• administration of drugs

• tissue and organ donation

• use of a respirator

• surgery

The living will declaration can also include issues of pain medication, food, and water. Most states recognize that relief from pain and discomfort are procedures that most people wish to have and these are not considered life-prolonging treatments. In some states, however, food and water may be considered life prolonging. and the consideration to forego them may fall within the rights of the patient to refuse. What may be included in the living will depends upon the state.

The living will—in some states called instructions, directive to physicians, or declaration—does not require a surrogate (an appointed person) to make decisions for the patient. Most states include these types of instructions in their medical durable power of attorney forms. Not all states, however, recognize separate living wills as legally binding; California, for instance, does not.

Preparation

The living will should be given careful thought, and be talked about with the patient's family, physician, and care providers. It is highly recommended that discussion of patient wishes occurs before medical treatment is necessary, because the living will involves both the patient's family and loved ones, who are expected to assist in its implementation. It should be researched for the state in which the patient is most likely to receive medical care, and be dated and signed before two witnesses.

The living will may be drafted on standardized forms, with or without the assistance of an attorney. The document may be revoked in writing, or orally, by either the patient (the person making the advance directive) or by a designated proxy (a surrogate) at any time. If the patient does not specify in the living will a particular element of treatment or treatment withdrawal, then it is not included. It is very important that living wills be as specific and detailed as possible.

Most hospitals offer a medical directives resource, commonly in the religious office attached to the hospital. Coupled with a durable medical power of attorney (a person chosen to make medical decisions on the patient's behalf if the patient cannot make his or her own decisions), the living will ensures in advance that patient wishes about the quality of death are respected.

Normal results

The living will, whether prepared prior to hospitalization or prepared once the patient is admitted, is placed in the patient's medical chart along with other documents such as the medical power of attorney declaration. Providers are required by federal law to honor this declaration of the patient's wishes. The document serves as a statement of intentions on the part of the patient and can be very important to family members, health care providers, and patient proxy during a very distressful and disconcerting time.

See also Do not resuscitate order.

Resources

PERIODICALS

Matousek, M. "Start the Conversation: The Modern Maturity Guide to End-of-Life Care." "The Last Taboo." *Modern Maturity* (September-October 2000).

ORGANIZATIONS

Partnership for Caring. 1620 Eye St., NW, Suite 202, Washington, DC 20006. (202) 296-8071. Fax: (202) 296-8352. Toll-free hotline: (800) 989-9455 <www.partnershipfor caring.org/>.

U.S. Living Will Registry. 523 Westfield Ave., P.O. Box 2789, Westfield, NJ 07091-2789. Toll-free: (800) LIV-WILL or (800) 548-9455). <www.uslivingwillregistry.com/>.

OTHER

Living Wills And Other Advance Directives. <wwww.inteli health.com>.

What You Can Cover in Your Healthcare Directives. Nolo Law for All. <wwww.nolo.com/lawcenter/ency>

Nancy McKenzie, PhD

Lobectomy, hepatic *see* **Hepatectomy**

Lobectomy, pulmonary

Definition

A lobectomy is the removal of a lobe, or section, of the lung.

Purpose

Lobectomies are performed to prevent the spread of cancer to other parts of the lung or other parts of the body, as well as to treat patients with such noncancerous diseases as chronic obstructive pulmonary disease (COPD). COPD includes emphysema and chronic bronchitis, which cause airway obstruction.

Demographics

Lung cancer

Lung cancer is the leading cause of cancer-related deaths in the United States. It is expected to claim nearly 157,200 lives in 2003. Lung cancer kills more people than cancers of the breast, prostate, colon, and pancreas combined. Cigarette smoking accounts for nearly 90% of cases of lung cancer in the United States.

Lung cancer is the second most common cancer among both men and women and is the leading cause of death from cancer in both sexes. In addition to the use of tobacco as a major cause of lung cancer among smokers, second-hand smoke contributes to the development of lung cancer among nonsmokers. Exposure to asbestos and other hazardous substances is also known to cause lung cancer. Air pollution is also a probable cause, but makes a relatively small contribution to incidence and mortality rates. Indoor exposure to radon may also make a small contribution to the total incidence of lung cancer in certain geographic areas of the United States.

In each of the major racial/ethnic groups in the United States, the rates of lung cancer among men are about two to three times greater than the rates among women. Among men, age-adjusted lung cancer incidence rates (per 100,000) range from a low of about 14 among Native Americans to a high of 117 among African Americans, an eight-fold difference. For women, the rates range from approximately 15 per 100,000 among Japanese Americans to nearly 51 among Native Alaskans, only a three-fold difference.

Chronic obstructive pulmonary disease

The following are risk factors for COPD:

- current smoking or a long-term history of heavy smoking
- employment that requires working around dust and irritating fumes
- long-term exposure to second-hand smoke at home or in the workplace
- a productive cough (with phlegm or sputum) most of the time
- shortness of breath during vigorous activity

- shortness of breath that grows worse even at lower levels of activity
- a family history of early COPD (before age 45)

Description

Lobectomies of the lung are also called pulmonary lobectomies. The lungs are a pair of cone-shaped breathing organs within the chest. The function of the lungs is to draw oxygen into the body and release carbon dioxide, which is a waste product of the body's cells. The right lung has three lobes: a superior lobe, a middle lobe, and an inferior lobe. The left lung has only two, a superior and an inferior lobe. Some lobes exchange more oxygen than others. The lungs are covered by a thin membrane called the pleura. The bronchi are two tubes which lead from the trachea (windpipe) to the right and left lungs. Inside the lungs are tiny air sacs called alveoli and small tubes called bronchioles. Lung cancer sometimes involves the bronchi.

To perform a lobectomy, the surgeon makes an incision (**thoracotomy**) between the ribs to expose the lung while the patient is under general anesthesia. The chest cavity is examined and the diseased lung tissue is removed. A drainage tube (chest tube) is then inserted to drain air, fluid, and blood out of the chest cavity. The ribs and chest incision are then closed.

Lung surgery may be recommended for the following reasons:

- presence of tumors
- small areas of long-term infection (such as highly localized pulmonary tuberculosis or mycobacterial infection)

- lung cancer
- abscesses
- permanently enlarged (dilated) airways (bronchiectasis)
- permanently dilated section of lung (lobar emphysema)
- injuries associated with lung collapse (atelectasis, pneumothorax, or hemothorax)
- a permanently collapsed lung (atelectasis)

Diagnosis/Preparation

Diagnosis

In some cases, the diagnosis of a lung disorder is made when the patient consults a physician about chest pains or other symptoms. The symptoms of lung cancer vary somewhat according to the location of the tumor; they may include persistent coughing, coughing up blood, wheezing, fever, and weight loss. Patients with a lung abscess often have symptoms resembling those of pneumonia, including a high fever, loss of appetite, general weakness, and putrid sputum. The doctor will first take a careful history and listen to the patient's breathing with a **stethoscope**. Imaging studies include x ray studies of the chest and **CT scans**. If lung cancer is suspected, the doctor will obtain a tissue sample for a biopsy. If a lung abscess is suspected, the doctor will send a sample of the sputum to a laboratory for culture and analysis.

For patients with lungs that have been damaged by emphysema or chronic bronchitis, pulmonary function tests are conducted prior to surgery to determine whether the patient will have enough healthy lung tissue remaining after surgery. A test may be used before surgery to help determine how much of the lung can safely be removed. This test is called a quantitative ventilation/perfusion scan, or a quantitative V/Q scan.

Preparation

Patients should not take **aspirin** or ibuprofen for seven to 10 days before surgery. Patients should also consult their physician about discontinuing any blood-thinning medications such as Coumadin (warfarin). The night before surgery, patients should not eat or drink anything after midnight.

Aftercare

If no complications arise, the patient is transferred from the surgical **intensive care unit** (ICU) to a regular hospital room within one to two days. Patients may need to be hospitalized for seven to 10 days after a lobectomy. A tube in the chest to drain fluid will probably be required, as well as a mechanical ventilator to help the patient breathe. The chest tube normally remains in place until the lung has fully re-expanded. Oxygen may also be required, either on a temporary or permanent basis. A respiratory therapist will visit the patient to teach him or her deep breathing exercises. It is important for the patient to perform these exercises in order to re-expand the lung and lower the risk of pneumonia or other infections. The patient will be given medications to control postoperative pain. The typical recovery period for a lobectomy is one to three months following surgery.

Risks

The specific risks of a lobectomy vary depending on the specific reason for the procedure and the general state of the patient's health; they should be discussed with the surgeon. In general, the risks for any surgery requiring a general anesthetic include reactions to medications and breathing problems. As previously mentioned, patients having part of a lung removed may have difficulty breathing and may require the use of oxygen. Excessive bleeding, wound infections, and pneumonia are possible complications of a lobectomy. The chest will hurt for some time after surgery, as the surgeon must cut through the patient's ribs to expose the lung. Patients with COPD may experience shortness of breath after surgery.

Normal results

The outcome of lobectomies depends on the general condition of the patient's lung. This variability is related to the fact that lung tissue does not regenerate after it is removed. Therefore, removal of a large portion of the lung may require a person to need oxygen or ventilator support for the rest of his or her life. On the other hand, removal of only a small portion of the lung may result in very little change to the patient's quality of life.

Morbidity and mortality rates

A small percentage of patients undergoing lung lobectomy die during or soon after the surgery. This percentage varies from about 3–6% depending on the amount of lung tissue removed. Of cancer patients with completely removable stage-1 non-small cell cancer of the lung (a disease in which malignant cancer cells form in the tissues of the lung), 50% survive five years after the procedure.

Alternatives

Lung cancer

The treatment options for lung cancer are surgery, radiation therapy, and chemotherapy, either alone or in combination, depending on the stage of the cancer.

After the cancer is found and staged, the cancer care team discusses the treatment options with the patient. In choosing a treatment plan, the most significant factors to consider are the type of lung cancer (small cell or non-small cell) and the stage of the cancer. It is very important that the doctor order all the tests needed to determine the stage of the cancer. Other factors to consider include the patient's overall physical health; the likely side effects of the treatment; and the probability of curing the disease, extending the patient's life, or relieving his or her symptoms.

Chronic obstructive pulmonary disease

Although surgery is rarely used to treat COPD, it may be considered for people who have severe symptoms that have not improved with medication therapy. A significant number of patients with advanced COPD face a miserable existence and are at high risk of death, despite advances in medical technology. This group includes patients who remain symptomatic despite the following:

• smoking cessation

• use of inhaled bronchodilators

• treatment with **antibiotics** for acute bacterial infections, and inhaled or oral corticosteroids

• use of supplemental oxygen with rest or exertion

• pulmonary rehabilitation

After the severity of the patient's airflow obstruction has been evaluated, and the foregoing interventions implemented, a pulmonary disease specialist should examine him or her, with consideration given to surgical treatment.

Surgical options for treating COPD include laser therapy or the following procedures:

• Bullectomy. This procedure removes the part of the lung that has been damaged by the formation of large air-filled sacs called bullae.

> ## KEY TERMS
>
> **Bronchodilator**—A drug that relaxes the bronchial muscles, resulting in expansion of the bronchial air passages.
>
> **Corticosteroids**—Any of various adrenal-cortex steroids used as anti-inflammatory agents.
>
> **Emphysema**—A chronic disease characterized by loss of elasticity and abnormal accumulation of air in lung tissue.
>
> **Mycobacterium**—Any of a genus of nonmotile, aerobic, acid-fast bacteria that include numerous saprophytes and the pathogens causing tuberculosis and leprosy.
>
> **Perfusion scan**—A lung scan in which a tracer is injected into a vein in the arm. It travels through the bloodstream and into the lungs to show areas of the lungs that are not receiving enough air or that retain too much air.
>
> **Pulmonary rehabilitation**—A program to treat COPD, which generally includes education and counseling, exercise, nutritional guidance, techniques to improve breathing, and emotional support.
>
> **Ventilation scan**—A lung scan in which a tracer gas is inhaled into the lungs to show the quantity of air that different areas of the lungs are receiving.
>
> **V/Q scan**—A test in which both a perfusion scan and ventilation scan are done (separately or together) to show the quantity of air that different areas of the lungs are receiving.

• Lung volume reduction surgery. In this procedure, the surgeon removes a portion of one or both lungs, making room for the remaining lung tissue to work more efficiently. Its use is considered experimental, although it has been used in selected patients with severe emphysema.

• Lung transplant. In this procedure a healthy lung from a donor who has recently died is given to a person with COPD.

Resources

BOOKS

Braunwald, Eugene, M. D., Anthony S. Fauci, M. D., Dennis L. Kasper, M. D., et al., eds. *Harrison's Principles of Internal Medicine*, 15th ed. New York: McGraw-Hill Professional, 2001.

Henschke, Claudia I., Peggy McCarthy, and Sarah Wernick. *Lung Cancer: Myths, Facts, Choices—And Hope*, 1st ed. New York, NY: W. W. Norton & Company, Inc., 2002.

Johnston, Lorraine. *Lung Cancer: Making Sense of Diagnosis, Treatment, and Options*. Sebastopol, CA: O'Reilly & Associates, 2001.

Pass, H., M. D., D. Johnson, M. D., James B. Mitchell, PhD., et al., eds. *Lung Cancer: Principles and Practice*, 2nd ed. Philadelphia, PA: Lippincott Williams & Wilkins, 2000.

Tierney, Lawrence M., Stephen J. McPhee, and Maxine A. Papadakis, eds. *Current Medical Diagnosis & Treatment 2003*, 42nd ed. New York, NY: McGraw-Hill/Appleton & Lange, 2002.

PERIODICALS

Crystal, Ronald G. "Research Opportunities and Advances in Lung Disease." *Journal of the American Medical Association* 285 (2001): 612-618.

Grann, Victor R., and Alfred I. Neugut. "Lung Cancer Screening at Any Price?" *Journal of the American Medical Association* 289 (2003): 357-358.

Mahadevia, Parthiv J., Lee A. Fleisher, Kevin D. Frick, et al. "Lung Cancer Screening with Helical Computed Tomography in Older Adult Smokers: A Decision and Cost-Effectiveness Analysis." *Journal of the American Medical Association* 289 (2003): 313-322.

Pope III, C. Arden, Richard T. Burnett, Michael J. Thun, et al. "Lung Cancer, Cardiopulmonary Mortality, and Long-Term Exposure to Fine Particulate Air pollution." *Journal of the American Medical Association* 287 (2002): 1132-1141.

ORGANIZATIONS

American Cancer Society. 1599 Clifton Road, N.E., Atlanta, GA 30329-4251. (800) 227-2345. <www.cancer.org>.

American Lung Association, National Office. 1740 Broadway, New York, NY 10019. (800) LUNG-USA. <www.lung usa.org>.

National Cancer Institute (NCI), Building 31, Room 10A03, 31 Center Drive, Bethesda, MD 20892-2580. Phone: (800) 4-CANCER. (301) 435-3848. <www.nci.nih.gov>.

National Comprehensive Cancer Network. 50 Huntingdon Pike, Suite 200, Rockledge, PA 19046. (215) 728-4788. Fax: (215) 728-3877. <www.nccn.org/>.

National Heart, Lung and Blood Institute (NHLBI). 6701 Rockledge Drive, P.O. Box 30105, Bethesda, MD 20824-0105. (301) 592-8573. <www.nhlhi.nih.gov/>.

OTHER

Aetna InteliHealth Inc. *Lung Cancer*. [cited May 17, 2003]. <www.intelihealth.com.>.

American Cancer Society (ACS). *Cancer Reference Information* [cited May 17, 2003]. <www3.cancer.org/cancer info>.

Michael Zuck, Ph.D.
Crystal H. Kaczkowski, M.Sc.

Local anesthetic *see* **Anesthesia, local**

Long-term care insurance

Definition

Long-term care (LTC) insurance provides for a person's care in cases of chronic illness or disability. Policies for LTC provide insurance coverage for times when an individual cannot independently manage the essential activities of daily living (ADLs). These are universally known as feeding, dressing, bathing, toileting, and walking, as well as moving oneself from a bed to a chair (transferring). However, disabilities are not confined to these physical situations; they can be mental as well. The key element is that they limit the individual's ability to perform any of these functions.

Purpose

The purpose of LTC insurance is to provide coverage for a succession of caregiving services for the elderly, the chronically ill, the disabled, or the seriously injured. This care may be provided in a skilled nursing facility (SNF); a nursing home; a mental hospital; in a person's home with a registered nurse (RN), a licensed practical nurse (LPN), or nurse's aide; or even in an assisted living facility (ALF). It is important to note the societal changes responsible for the increased need for professional services to care for our loved ones. Although today's families are smaller and a number of women are working outside the home, the majority of LTC continues to be provided by unpaid, informal caregivers—family members and friends.

In 2003, more than 24 million households in the United States included a caregiver who was 50 years of age or older. About 73% of unpaid caregivers were women—and one-third of them are more than 65 years old. Many caregivers, especially women, balance multiple roles by providing care for both their parents and their children. Caring for a loved one full-time can overwhelm even the most devoted family member. As a result, more caregivers than ever are turning to outside resources to help with the care of a family member.

Demographics

In 2030, it is anticipated that people aged 65 and over will comprise 20% of the population. The United States Census Bureau is projecting that the population aged 65 and over will be 39.7 million in 2010, 53.7 million in 2020, and 70.3 million in 2030. As of 2003, at least 6.4 million people aged 65 and over require LTC; one in two people over the age of 85 require this kind of care now, and at least half of the population who are over the age of 85 will need help with ADLs.

Although the elderly rely on LTC most frequently, younger persons who have chronic illnesses, severe disabilities, or have experienced a serious injury may also benefit from having LTC insurance.

Advantages to purchasing LTC insurance

The financial risks of illness and injury are rarely considered when one is healthy and able, but that is also when the greatest choice of products with the best flexibility in cost is available for those considering LTC insurance. Having a LTC insurance policy enables access to quality care and choice of care provider when the need is greatest. Purchasing a policy when a person does not need it gives them the opportunity to investigate the company's financial stability (whether it is solid and how it is rated), operating performance, insurance industry rating, and its claims ratio. Rates should be guaranteed renewable, and coverage shouldn't be canceled because of age or a change in a person's health nor should premiums be increased on a class-wide basis.

There are several government organizations that can be of assistance in the purchase, evaluation, and monitoring of LTC insurance. One is the state health insurance assistance program—SHIP—that can review the policy before the actual purchase. Another excellent organization is the Health Insurance Association of America (HIAA), which protects consumers from the financial risks of injury and illness by providing affordable and flexible services that represent a choice. In the United States, HIAA focuses on managed care, and, specifically, advocates on issues such as disability income and LTC insurance.

The mission of the Health Insurance Association of America is to preserve financial security, freedom of choice, and dignity in LTC insurance. Because of its mission, HIAA seeks to:

• Provide access to quality care and let a person choose where care is obtained.

• Eliminate out-of-pocket costs and avoid reliance on government programs for the poor.

• Ensure quality of life for a patient's caregivers.

Description

Advantages

Having a LTC insurance policy cuts out-of-pocket costs and keeps the patient from having to rely on government assistance programs. Studies from the United States Department of Health and Human Services estimate that people with LTC insurance save between $60,000 and $75,000 in nursing home costs, more than $100,000 for assisted living, and actually ensure a higher quality of life for their caregiver. By having LTC at home, spouses and other family members are able to continue working or run errands while their loved one is being care for.

People of all ages usually prefer to receive LTC in their own homes, or in homelike assisted-living facilities. More than three-quarters of older Americans in need of LTC live in their communities. Most receive no paid services. The majority of LTC is provided by unpaid, informal caregivers, such as family members and friends.

Government assistance

Long-term care options can be uncoordinated and expensive for individuals, their families, and public programs. According to AARP (formerly known as American Association of Retired Persons) millions of Americans have no access to LTC services. They are caught in the trap of having too much money to qualify for government assistance, but not enough money to afford the types of services they need.

Recent changes in the United States federal tax law allow for a portion of a long-term insurance premium to be tax-deductible. The amount of the deduction increases with the insured person's age.

Medicare may cover a month or two of home health care after a stay in the hospital, but benefits are then usually capped. This government program, administered by the Social Security Administration, is well known for providing financial assistance to seniors 65 years of age and older and to the disabled—for medical and hospital expenses—but it does not cover LTC expenses. Medicare Supplement Insurance does not cover LTC either.

The federal/state **Medicaid** program is available, but the criteria to qualify for assistance is strict. Those who meet the guidelines for Medicaid must demonstrate financial need to receive assistance; most individuals must deplete most or all of their savings and assets before becoming eligible for any benefits. Still, in 2003, approximately two-thirds of nursing home residents were dependent on Medicaid to finance at least some of their care. For the majority of residents, LTC insurance is cost-prohibitive. To make matters worse, preexisting conditions often prevent them from obtaining coverage for which they might qualify.

Personal policies

Long-term care insurance policies are often complex. People who purchase them may not read the fine print and are later forced to cancel their policies because they do not fit their needs. Increasing rates factored into some long-term policies, known as climbing premiums,

QUESTIONS TO ASK BEFORE PURCHASING LTC INSURANCE

- Will the policy meet my needs?
- Is the policy affordable?
- What restrictions or exemptions exist?
- Under what conditions, if any, can this plan be canceled?
- Are there any laws to protect me from insurance companies or LTC facilities that provide substandard conditions and/or services?

may also become prohibitively expensive. However, long-term care insurance can benefit consumers, provided that such items as affordability, coverage gaps, and timing of purchase are carefully considered.

It is advisable to check the financial stability and the claims ratio of an insurance company. Long-term insurance is a serious financial investment and should be considered a part of estate planning. A qualified, independent professional should be consulted to review the policy before purchase. The state health insurance assistance program (SHIP) is also available to answer questions.

The type of care that an individual seeks or requires is an important consideration before purchasing a policy. Currently, there is no universal standard for defining long-term care facilities. A placement that is covered under one company's policy may not be covered by another. Physicians can also play a part in denial of a placement by stating that the facility of choice is either not adequate or too advanced for an individual's needs.

When to purchase a policy is another important consideration. Individuals with a preexisting diagnosis for a debilitating condition or illness may not be eligible for coverage. This clause is common in most insurance policies of any type. However, purchasing a policy too far in advance of an anticipated need can work against a buyer. The health care industry is currently in a state of flux, and technological advances are rapid. The benefits provided in a policy that is purchased at one point in time may not match the care available in the distant future, giving the company reason to deny benefits.

Generally, LTC insurance operates as an indemnity program for potential nursing home and home health care costs. Additionally, many policies provide coverage for adult daycare, for care delivered in an assisted living facility, and for hospice care. Rarely are all costs cov-

ered. Some LTC policies are pure indemnity programs, which pay the insured a daily benefit contracted for by the insured. The pure indemnity program pays the full daily benefit regardless of the amount of care that the insured receives each day.

Other LTC policies pay for covered losses, or the cost of care actually received each day, up to the selected daily benefit level. This type of policy is referred to as a pool-of-money contract.

Insurance for LTC is available either as part of a group or as individual coverage, although most policies are currently purchased by individuals. Most policies cover skilled, custodial, and intermediate LTC services. A purchaser would be wise to consider a contract that covers all of these levels.

Benefits under a LTC contract are triggered in a tax-qualified policy when an insured person becomes unable to perform a number of activities associated with normal daily living or develops a cognitive impairment that requires supervision. Non–tax-qualified policies usually offer more liberal eligibility criteria. This includes long-term benefits required due to medical necessity.

Risks

Long-term care insurance policies can be expensive and may be restrictive in what they provide. Before purchasing the policy, persons should be certain that the cost is within their means and that the plan will meet their anticipated needs. Some policies allow policy holders to use survivor death benefits for health care needs. It is advisable for several different policies to be compared in detail. Policies that seem too inexpensive when compared against the competition should be carefully evaluated. There may be hidden clauses in the contracts that limit coverage.

Organizations that can help consumers

The Health Insurance Association of America (HIAA) protects consumers from the financial risks of illness and injury by providing flexible and affordable products and services that embody freedom of choice, and advocates on a number of issues—including LTC insurance.

The United States Department of Health and Human Services oversees the Administration on Aging's Ombudsmen Program. Established in 1972 by the Older Americans Act, the Program operates throughout the country on behalf of aging residents. Its purpose is to investigate over 260,000 complaints annually regarding various topics, including selection and payment of LTC insurance policies. The ombudsmen advocate for residents of **nursing homes**, LTC homes, assisted living facilities, and similar adult care facilities, they have made dramatic differences in the lives of LTC residents. On behalf of individuals and groups of residents, they provide information to residents and their families about the LTC system and work to improve local, state and national level programs. Ombudsmen also provide an ongoing presence in LTC facilities, monitoring care and conditions and providing a voice for those who are unable to speak for themselves.

Alternatives

The only alternative to LTC insurance for individuals is to pay for all expenses themselves when the need for LTC arises.

See also Private insurance plans.

Resources

BOOKS

Abromovitz, L. *Long-Term Care Insurance Made Simple.* Los Angeles, CA: Health Information Press, 1999.
Lipson, B. *J. K. Lasser's Choosing the Right Long-Term Care Insurance.* New York, Wiley, 2002.
McCall, N. *Who Will Pay for Long-Term Care: Insights from the Partnership Programs.* Chicago, IL: Health Administration Press, 2001.
Stevens, W. S. *Health Insurance: Current Issues and Background.* Hauppauge, NY: Nova Science Publishers, 2003.

PERIODICALS

Cohen, M. A. "Private Long-term Care Insurance: A Look Ahead." *Journal of Aging and Health* 15, no. 1 (2003): 74–98.
Cubanski J., and J. Kline. "Medicaid: Focusing on State Innovation." *Commonwealth Fund Issue Brief* 617 (2003): 1–8.
Luecke R. W., and D. T. Blair. "Designing Long-term Disability Plans: Tax Efficiency vs. Maximizing Wage Replacement." *Benefits Quarterly* 19, no. 1 (2003): 51–60.
Polivka, L., et al. "The Nursing Home Problem in Florida." *Gerontologist* 43, no. 2 (2003): 7–18.
Schwartz, M. "Dentistry for the Long-term Care Patient." *Dentistry Today* 22, no. 1 (2003): 52–57.

ORGANIZATIONS

AARP. 601 E. Street NW, Washington, DC 20049. (800) 424-3410. <http://www.aarp.org>.
American College of Healthcare Executives. One North Franklin, Suite 1700, Chicago, IL 60606-4425. (312) 424-2800. <http://www.ache.org>.
American Medical Association. 515 N. State Street, Chicago, IL 60610. (312) 464-5000. <http://www.ama-assn.org>.
Health Insurance Association of America. 1201 F Street, NW, Suite 500, Washington, DC 20004-1204. (202) 824-1600. <http://www.hiaa.org>.
U.S. Administration on Aging (AOA), United States Department of Health and Human Services. 330 Independence Avenue, SW, Washington, DC 20201. (202) 619-0724. <http://www.aoa.gov>.

United States Department of Health and Human Services, 200 Independence Avenue, SW, Washington, DC 20201. (877) 696-6775. <http://www.hhs.gov>.

OTHER

American Health Care Association, National Center for Assisted Living. Cited May 6, 2003. <http://www.longtermcareliving.com>.
The Federal Long Term Care Insurance Program. July 1, 2003 (cited July 7, 2003). <http://www.ltcfeds.com>.
The National Council on the Aging. Cited July 7, 2003. <http://www.unitedseniorshealth.org>.

KEY TERMS

Chronic illness—A condition that lasts a year or longer, limits activity, and may require ongoing care.

Estate planning—Preparation of a plan of administration and disposition of one's property before or after death, including will, trusts, gifts, and power of attorney.

Indemnity—Protection, as by insurance, against damage or loss.

Long-term care (LTC)—The type of care one may need if one can no longer perform activities of daily living (ADLs) alone, such as eating, bathing or getting dressed. It also includes the kind of care one would need with a severe cognitive impairment, such as Alzheimer's disease. Care can be received in a variety of settings, including the home, assisted living facilities, adult day care centers, or hospice facilities.

Medicaid—Public assistance funded through the state to individuals unable to pay for health care. Medicaid can be accessed only when all prior assets and funds are depleted.

Medicare—A government program, administered by the Social Security Administration, which provides financial assistance to individuals over the age of 65 for hospital and medical expenses. Medicare does not cover long-term care expenses.

Skilled nursing facility (SNF)—A facility equipped to handle individuals with 24-hour nursing needs, postoperative recuperation, or complex medical care demands, as well as chronically-ill individuals who can no longer live independently. These facilities must be licensed by the state in which they operate to meet standards of safety, staffing, and care procedures.

"Planning for Long-Term Care." Booklet. United Seniors Health Council, Washington, DC. New York: McGraw-Hill, 2002.

Teachers Insurance Annuity Association of America (TIAA-CREF). (Cited May 6, 2003.) <http://www.tiaa-cref.org/ltc>.

L. Fleming Fallon, Jr., MD, DrPH
Randi B. Jenkins, BA

Lower GI exam *see* **Barium enema**

LTC insurance *see* **Long-term care insurance**

Lumbar laminectomy *see* **Laminectomy**

Lumbar puncture *see* **Cerebrospinal fluid (CSF) analysis**

Lumpectomy

Definition

Lumpectomy is a type of surgery for breast cancer. It is considered "breast-conserving" surgery because only the malignant tumor and a surrounding margin of normal breast tissue are removed. Lymph nodes in the armpit (axilla) may also be removed. This procedure is also called lymph node dissection.

Purpose

Lumpectomy is a surgical treatment for newly diagnosed breast cancer. It is estimated that at least 50% of women with breast cancer are good candidates for this procedure. The location, size, and type of tumor are of primary importance when considering breast cancer surgery options. The size of the breast is another factor the surgeon considers when recommending surgery. The patient's psychological outlook, as well as her lifestyle and preferences, should also be taken into account when treatment decisions are being made.

The extent and severity of a cancer is evaluated, or "staged," according to a fairly complex system. Staging considers the size of the tumor and whether the cancer has spread (metastasized) to adjacent tissues, such as the chest wall, the lymph nodes, and/or to distant parts of the body. Women with early stage breast cancers are usually better candidates for lumpectomy. In most cases, a

course of radiation therapy after surgery is part of the treatment. Chemotherapy or hormone treatment may also be prescribed.

In some instances, women with later stage breast cancer may be able to have lumpectomies. Chemotherapy may be administered before surgery to decrease tumor size and the chance of metastasis in selected cases.

Contraindications to lumpectomy

There are a number of factors that may prevent or prohibit a breast cancer patient from having a lumpectomy. The tumor itself may be too large or located in an area where it would be difficult to remove with good cosmetic results. Sometimes several areas of cancer are found in one breast, so the tumor cannot be removed as a single lump. A cancer that has already attached itself to nearby structures, such as the skin or the chest wall, needs more extensive surgery.

Certain medical or physical circumstances may also eliminate lumpectomy as a treatment option. Sometimes lumpectomy may be attempted, but the surgeon is unable to remove the tumor with a sufficient amount of surrounding normal tissue. This may be termed "persistently positive margins," or "lack of clear margins." Lumpectomy is suitable for women who have had previous lumpectomies and have a recurrence of breast cancer.

Because of the need for radiation therapy after lumpectomy, this surgery may be medically unacceptable. A breast cancer discovered during pregnancy is not amenable to lumpectomy because radiation therapy is part of the treatment. Radiation therapy cannot be administered to pregnant women because it may injure the fetus. If, however, delivery would be completed prior to the need for radiation, pregnant women may

910

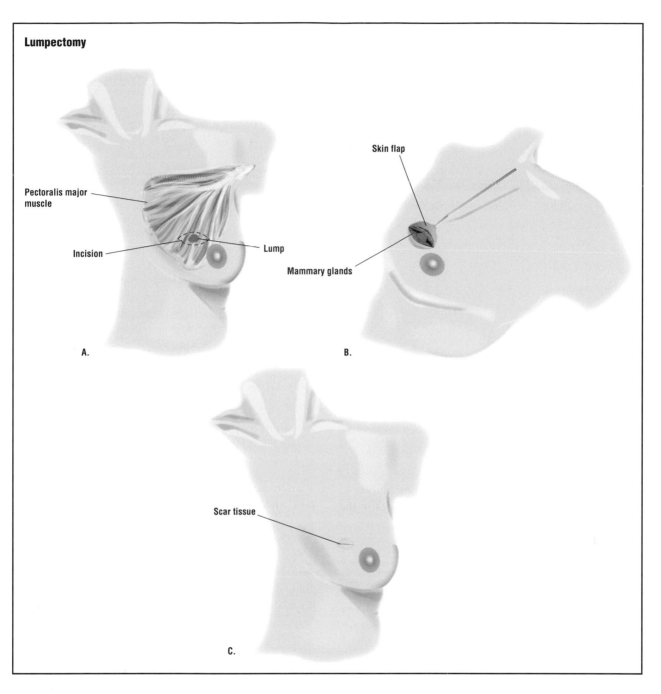

Lumpectomy

A.

Pectoralis major muscle

Incision

Lump

B.

Skin flap

Mammary glands

C.

Scar tissue

During a lumpectomy, a small incision is made around the area of the lump (A). The skin is pulled back, and the tumor removed (B). The incision is closed (C). *(Illustration by GGS Inc.)*

undergo lumpectomy. A woman who has already had therapeutic radiation to the chest area for other reasons cannot undergo additional exposure for breast cancer therapy.

The need for radiation therapy may also be a barrier due to nonmedical concerns. Some women simply fear this type of treatment and choose more extensive surgery so that radiation will not be required. The commitment of time, usually five days a week for six weeks, may not be acceptable for others. This may be due to financial, personal, or job-related constraints. Finally, in geographically isolated areas, a course of radiation therapy may require lengthy travel and perhaps unacceptable amounts of time away from family and other responsibilities.

Demographics

The American Cancer Society estimated that in 2003, 211,300 new cases of breast cancer would be diagnosed in the United States and 39,800 women would die as a result of the disease. Approximately one in eight women will develop breast cancer at some point in her life. The risk of developing breast cancer increases with age: women aged 30 to 40 have a one in 252 chance of developing breast cancer; women aged 40 to 50 have a one in 68 chance; women aged 50 to 60 have a one in 35 chance; and women aged 60 to 70 have a one in 27 chance—and these statistics do not even account for genetic and environmental factors.

In the 1990s, the incidence of breast cancer was higher among white women (113.1 cases per 100,000 women) than African-American women (100.3 per 100,000). The death rate associated with breast cancer, however, was higher among African American women (29.6 per 100,000) than white women (22.2 per 100,000). Rates were lower among Hispanic women (14.2 per 100,000), American Indian women (12.0), and Asian women (11.2 per 100,000).

Description

Any amount of tissue, from 1–50% of the breast, may be removed and called a lumpectomy. Breast conservation surgery is a frequently used synonym for lumpectomy. Partial mastectomy, **quadrantectomy**, segmental excision, wide excision, and tylectomy are other, less commonly used names for this procedure.

The surgery is usually done while the patient is under general anesthetic. Local anesthetic with additional sedation may be used for some patients. The tumor and surrounding margin of tissue is removed and sent to a pathologist for examination. The surgical site is then closed.

If axillary lymph nodes were not removed before, a second incision is made in the armpit. The fat pad that contains lymph nodes is removed from this area and is also sent to the pathologist for analysis. This portion of the procedure is called an axillary lymph node dissection; it is critical for determining the stage of the cancer. Typically, 10 to 15 nodes are removed, but the number may vary. Surgical drains may be left in place in either location to prevent fluid accumulation. The surgery may last from one to three hours.

Diagnosis/Preparation

Routine preoperative preparations, such as having nothing to eat or drink the night before surgery, are typically ordered for a lumpectomy. Information about expected outcomes and potential complications is also part of preparation for lumpectomy, as it is for any surgical procedure. It is especially important that women know about sensations they might experience after the operation, so the they are not misinterpreted as signs of further cancer or poor healing.

If the tumor is not able to be felt (not palpable), a pre-operative localization procedure is needed. A fine wire, or other device, is placed at the tumor site, using x ray or ultrasound for guidance. This is usually done in the radiology department of a hospital. The woman is most often sitting up and awake, although some sedation may be administered.

Aftercare

The patient may stay in the hospital one or two days, or return home the same day. This generally depends on the extent of the surgery, the medical condition of the patient, and physician and patient preferences. A woman usually goes home with a small bandage. The inner part of the surgical site usually has dissolvable stitches. The skin may be sutured or stitched; or the skin edges may be held together with steristrips, which are special thin, clear pieces of tape.

After a lumpectomy, patients are usually cautioned against lifting anything which weighs over five pounds for several days. Other activities may be restricted (especially if the axillary lymph nodes were removed) according to individual needs. Pain is often enough to limit inappropriate motion. Women are often instructed to wear a well-fitting support bra both day and night for approximately one week after surgery.

Pain is usually well controlled with prescribed medication. If it is not, the patient should contact the surgeon, as severe pain may be a sign of a complication, which needs medical attention. A return visit to the surgeon is normally scheduled approximately ten days to two weeks after the operation.

Radiation therapy is usually started as soon as possible after lumpectomy. Other additional treatments, such as chemotherapy or hormone therapy, may also be prescribed. The timing of these is specific to each individual patient.

Risks

The risks are similar to those associated with any surgical procedure. Risks include bleeding, infection, breast asymmetry, anesthesia reaction, or unexpected scarring. A lumpectomy may also cause loss of sensation in the breast. The size and shape of the breast will be affected by the operation. Fluid can accumulate in the area where tissue was removed, requiring drainage.

If lymph node dissection is performed, there are several potential complications. A woman may experience decreased feeling in the back of her armpit. She may also experience other sensations, including numbness, tingling, or increased skin sensitivity. An inflammation of the arm vein, called phlebitis, can occur. There may be injury to the nerves controlling arm motion.

There is a risk of developing lymphedema (swelling of the arm) after axillary lymph node dissection. This swelling can range from mild to very severe. It can be treated with elastic bandages and specialized physical therapy, but it is a chronic condition, requiring continuing care. Lymphedema can arise at any time, even years after surgery.

Normal results

When lumpectomy is performed, it is anticipated that it will be the definitive surgical treatment for breast cancer. Other forms of therapy, especially radiation, are often prescribed as part of the total treatment plan. The expected outcome is no recurrence of the breast cancer.

Morbidity and mortality rates

Approximately 2–10% of patients develop lymphedema after axillary lymph node dissection. Five percent of women are unhappy with the cosmetic effects of the surgery. The rate of cancer recurrence after five years is about 5–10%, and 10–15% after 10 years.

Alternatives

A procedure in which the entire affected breast is removed, called a mastectomy, has been shown to be equally effective in treating breast cancer as lumpectomy, in terms of rates of recurrence and survival. Some women may choose to have a mastectomy because they strongly fear a recurrence of breast cancer, and may consider a

lumpectomy too risky. Others may feel uncomfortable with a breast that has had a cancer, and would experience more peace of mind with the entire breast removed.

A new technique that may eliminate the need for removing many axillary lymph nodes is being tested. Sentinel lymph node mapping and biopsy is based on the idea that the condition of the first lymph node in the network, which drains the affected area, can predict whether the cancer may have spread to the rest of the nodes. It is thought that if this first, or sentinel, node is cancer-free, then there is no need to look further. Many patients with early-stage breast cancers may be spared the risks and complications of axillary lymph node dissection as the use of this approach continues to increase.

Resources

BOOKS

Love, Susan M., with Karen Lindsey. *Dr. Susan Love's Breast Book,* 3rd ed. Cambridge: Perseus Publishing, 2000.

Robinson, Rebecca Y. and Jeanne A. Petrek. *A Step-by-Step Guide to Dealing With Your Breast Cancer.* New York: Carol Publishing Group, 1999.

PERIODICALS

Apantaku, Leila. "Breast-Conserving Surgery for Breast Cancer." *American Family Physician* 66, no. 12 (December 15, 2002): 2271–8.

Dershaw, D. David. "Breast imaging and the conservative treatment of breast cancer." *Radiologic Clinics of North America* 40, no. 3 (May 2002): 501–16.

ORGANIZATION

American Cancer Society. 1599 Clifton Rd. NE, Atlanta, GA 30329-4251. (800) 227-2345. <http://www.cancer.org>.

National Cancer Institute (NCI) <http://cancertrials.nci.nih.gov/types/breast/treatment/sentnode>.

National Lymphedema Network. 2211 Post St., Suite 404, San Francisco, CA 94115-3427. (800) 541-3259 or (415) 921-1306. <http://www.wenet.net/~lymphnet>.

Ellen S. Weber, MSN
Stephanie Dionne Sherk

Lung biopsy

Definition

Lung biopsy is a procedure for obtaining a small sample of lung tissue for examination. The tissue is usually examined under a microscope, and may be sent to a microbiological laboratory for culture. Microscopic examination is performed by a pathologist.

Purpose

A lung biopsy is usually performed to determine the cause of abnormalities, such as nodules that appear on chest x rays. It can confirm a diagnosis of cancer, especially if malignant cells are detected in the patient's sputum or bronchial washing. In addition to evaluating lung tumors and their associated symptoms, lung biopsies may be used to diagnose lung infections, especially tuberculosis and Pneumocystis pneumonia, drug reactions, and chronic diseases of the lungs such as sarcoidosis and pulmonary fibrosis.

A lung biopsy can be used for treatment as well as diagnosis. **Bronchoscopy**, a type of lung biopsy performed with a long, flexible slender instrument called a bronchoscope, can be used to clear a patient's air passages of secretions and to remove airway blockages.

Demographics

According to the American Cancer Society, approximately 77% of all cancers are diagnosed in people ages 55 and older. Lung cancer is the leading cause of cancer deaths in the United States. Each year, about 170,000 Americans are diagnosed with lung cancer. It is much more prevalent among African Americans than the general population. Nine out of 10 cases of lung cancer are caused by smoking cigarettes, pipes, or cigars.

Description

Overview

The right and left lungs are separated by the mediastinum, which contains the heart, trachea, lymph nodes, and esophagus. Lung biopsies sometimes involve **mediastinoscopy**.

Types of lung biopsies

Lung biopsies are performed using a variety of techniques, depending on where the abnormal tissue is located in the lung, the health and age of the patient, and the presence of lung disease. A bronchoscopy is ordered if a lesion identified on the x ray seems to be located on the wall (periphery) of the chest. If the suspicious area lies close to the chest wall, a needle biopsy can be done. If both methods fail to diagnose the problem, an open lung biopsy may be performed. When there is a question about whether the lung cancer or suspicious mass has spread to the lymph nodes in the mediastinum, a mediastinoscopy is performed.

BRONCHOSCOPIC BIOPSY. During the bronchoscopy, a thin, lighted tube (bronchoscope) is passed from the nose or mouth, down the windpipe (trachea) to the air passages (bronchi) leading to the lungs. Through the bronchoscope, the physician views the airways, and is able to clear mucus from blocked airways, and collect cells or tissue samples for laboratory analysis.

NEEDLE BIOPSY. The patient is mildly sedated, but awake during the needle biopsy procedure. He or she sits in a chair with arms folded in front on a table. An x ray technician uses a computerized axial tomography (CAT) scanner or a fluoroscope to identify the precise location of the suspicious areas. Markers are placed on the overlying skin to identify the biopsy site. The skin is thoroughly cleansed with an antiseptic solution, and a local anesthetic is injected to numb the area. The patient will feel a brief stinging sensation when the anesthetic is injected.

The physician makes a small incision, about half an inch (1.25 cm) in length. The patient is asked to take a deep breath and hold it while the physician inserts the biopsy needle through the incision into the lung tissue to be biopsied. The patient may feel pressure, and a brief sharp pain when the needle touches the lung tissue. Most patients do not experience severe pain. The patient should refrain from coughing during the procedure. The needle is withdrawn when enough tissue has been obtained. Pressure is applied at the biopsy site and a sterile bandage is placed over the incision. A **chest x ray** is performed immediately after the procedure to check for potential complications. The entire procedure takes 30 to 60 minutes.

OPEN BIOPSY. Open biopsies are performed in a hospital **operating room** under general anesthesia. Once the anesthesia has taken effect, the surgeon makes an incision over the lung area, a procedure called a **thoracotomy**. Some lung tissue is removed and the incision is closed with sutures. Chest tubes are placed with one end inside the lung and the other end protruding through the closed incision. Chest tubes are used to drain fluid and blood, and re-expand the lungs. They are usually removed the day after the procedure. The entire procedure normally takes about an hour. A chest x ray is performed immediately after the procedure to check for potential complications.

VIDEO-ASSISTED THORACOSCOPIC SURGERY. A minimally invasive technique, video-assisted thoracoscopic surgery (VATS) can be used to biopsy lung and mediastinal lesions. VATS may be performed on selected patients in place of open lung biopsy. While the patient is under general anesthetia, the surgeon makes several small incisions in the his or her chest wall. A thorascope, a thin, hollow, lighted tube with a tiny video camera mounted on it, is inserted through one of the small incisions. The other incisions allow the surgeon to insert special instruments to retrieve tissue for biopsy.

MEDIASTINOSCOPY. This procedure is performed under general anesthesia. A 2–3 in (5–8 cm) incision is made at the base of the neck. A thin, hollow, lighted tube, called a mediastinoscope, is inserted through the incision into the space between the right and the left lungs. The surgeon removes any lymph nodes or tissues that look abnormal. The mediastinoscope is then removed, and the incision is sutured and bandaged. A mediastinoscopy takes about an hour.

Diagnosis/Preparation

Diagnosis

Before scheduling a lung biopsy, the physician performs a careful evaluation of the patient's medical history and symptoms, and performs a **physical examination**. Chest x rays and sputum cytology (examination of cells obtained from a deep-cough mucus sample) are other diagnostic tests that may be performed. An electrocardiogram (EKG) and laboratory tests may be performed before the procedure to check for blood clotting problems, anemia, and blood type, should a **transfusion** become necessary.

Preparation

During a preoperative appointment, usually scheduled within one to two weeks before the procedure, the patient receives information about what to expect during the procedure and the recovery period. During this appointment or just before the procedure, the patient usually meets with the physician (or physicians) performing the procedure (the pulmonologist, interventional radiologist, or thoracic surgeon).

A chest x ray or CAT scan of the chest is used to identify the area to be biopsied.

About an hour before the biopsy procedure, the patient receives a sedative. Medication may also be given to dry up airway secretions. General anesthesia is not used for this procedure.

For at least 12 hours before the open biopsy, VATS, or mediastinoscopy procedures, the patient should not eat or drink anything. Prior to these procedures, an intravenous line is placed in a vein in the patient's arm to deliver medications or fluids as necessary. A hollow tube, called an endotracheal tube, is passed through the patient's mouth into the airway leading to the lungs. Its

---

---

purpose is to deliver the general anesthetic. The chest area is cleansed with an antiseptic solution. In the mediastinoscopy procedure, the neck is also cleansed to prepare for the incision.

Smoking cessation

Patients who will undergo surgical diagnostic and treatment procedures should be encouraged to stop smoking and stop using tobacco products. The patient needs to make the commitment to be a nonsmoker after the procedure. Patients able to stop smoking several weeks before surgical procedures have fewer postoperative complications. **Smoking cessation** programs are available in many communities. The patient should ask a health care provider for more information if he or she needs help with smoking cessation.

Informed consent

Informed consent is an educational process between health care providers and patients. Before any procedure is performed, the patient is asked to sign a consent form. Prior to signing the form, the patient should understand the nature and purpose of the diagnostic procedure or treatment, its risks and benefits, and alternatives, including the option of not proceeding with the test or treatment. During the discussions, the health care providers are available to answer the patient's questions about the consent form or procedure.

Aftercare

Needle biopsy

Following a needle biopsy, the patient is allowed to rest comfortably. He or she may be required to lie flat for

---

QUESTIONS TO ASK THE DOCTOR

- Why is this procedure being performed?
- Are there any alternative options to having this procedure?
- What type of lung biopsy procedure is recommended?
- Is minimally invasive surgery an option?
- Will the patient be awake during the procedure?
- Who will be performing the procedure? How many years of experience does this physician have? How many other lung biopsies has the physician performed?
- Can medications be taken the day of the procedure?
- Can the patient have food or drink before the procedure? If not, how long before the procedure should these activities be stopped?
- How long is the hospitalization?
- After discharge, how long will it take to recover from the procedure?
- How is pain or discomfort relieved after the procedure?
- What types of symptoms should be reported to the physician?
- When can normal activities be resumed?
- When cam driving be resumed?
- When can the patient return to work?
- When will the results of the procedure be given to the patient?
- How often are follow-up physician visits needed after the procedure?

two hours following the procedure to prevent the risk of bleeding. The nurse checks the patient's status at two-hour intervals. If there are no complications after four hours, the patient can go home once he or she has received instructions about resuming normal activities. The patient should rest at home for a day or two before returning to regular activities, and should avoid strenuous activities for one week after the biopsy.

Open biopsy, VATS, or mediastinoscopy

After an open biopsy, VATS, or mediastinoscopy, the patient is taken to the **recovery room** for observation.

The patient receives oxygen via a face mask or nasal cannula. If no complications develop, the patient is taken to a hospital room. Temperature, blood oxygen level, pulse, blood pressure, and respiration are monitored. Chest tubes remain in place after surgery to prevent the lungs from collapsing, and to remove blood and fluids. The tubes are usually removed the day after the procedure.

The patient may experience some grogginess for a few hours after the procedure. He or she may have a sore throat from the endotracheal tube. The patient may also have some pain or discomfort at the incision site, which can be relieved by pain medication. It is common for patients to require some pain medication for up to two weeks following the procedure.

After receiving instructions about resuming normal activities and caring for the incision, the patient usually goes home the day after surgery. The patient should not drive while taking narcotic pain medication.

Patients may experience fatigue and muscle aches for a day or two because of the general anesthesia. The patient can gradually increase activities, as tolerated. Walking is recommended. Sutures are usually removed after one to two weeks.

The physician should be notified immediately if the patient experiences extreme pain, light-headedness, or difficulty breathing after the procedure. Sputum may be slightly bloody for a day or two after the procedure. Heavy or persistent bleeding requires evaluation by the physician.

Risks

Lung biopsies should not be performed on patients who have a bleeding disorder or abnormal blood clotting because of low platelet counts, or prolonged prothrombin time (PT) or partial thromboplastin time (PTT). Platelets are small blood cells that play a role in the blood clotting process. PT and PTT measure how well blood is clotting. If clotting times are prolonged, it may be unsafe to perform a biopsy because of the risk of bleeding. If the platelet count is lower than 50,000/cubic mm, the patient may be given a platelet transfusion as a temporary relief measure, and a biopsy can then be performed.

In addition, lung biopsies should not be performed if other tests indicate the patient has enlarged alveoli associated with emphysema, pulmonary hypertension, or enlargement of the right ventricle of the heart (cor pulmonale).

The normal risks of any surgical procedure include bleeding, infection, or pneumonia. The risk of these complications is higher in patients undergoing open biopsy procedures, as is the risk of pneumothorax (lung collapse). In rare cases, the lung collapses because of air

KEY TERMS

Bronchoscopy—A medical test that enables the physician to see the breathing passages and the lungs through a hollow, lighted tube.

Chest x ray—Brief exposure of the chest to radiation to produce an image of the chest and its internal structures.

Endotracheal tube—A hollow tube that is inserted into the windpipe to administer anesthesia.

Lung nodule—See pulmonary nodule.

Lymph nodes—Small, bean-shaped structures that serve as filters, scattered along the lymphatic vessels. Lymph nodes trap bacteria or cancer cells that are traveling through the lymphatic system.

Malignant—Cancerous.

Mediastinoscopy—A procedure that allows the physician to see the organs in the mediastinal space using a thin, lighted, hollow tube (a mediastinoscope).

Mediastinum—The area between the lungs, bounded by the spine, breastbone, and diaphragm.

Pleural cavity—The space between the lungs and the chest wall.

Pneumothorax—A condition in which air or gas enters the pleura (area around the lungs) and causes a collapse of the lung.

Pulmonary nodule—A lesion surrounded by normal lung tissue. Nodules may be caused by bacteria, fungi, or a tumor (benign or cancerous).

Sputum—A mucus-rich secretion that is coughed up from the passageways (bronchial tubes) and the lungs.

Sputum cytology—A lab test in which a microscope is used to check for cancer cells in the sputum.

Thoracentesis—Removal of fluid from the pleural cavity.

that leaks in through the hole made by the biopsy needle. A chest x ray is done immediately after the biopsy to detect the development of this potential complication. If a pneumothorax occurs, a chest tube is inserted into the pleural cavity to re-expand the lung. Signs of pneumothorax include shortness of breath, rapid heart rate, or blueness of the skin (a late sign). If the patient has any of these symptoms after being discharged from the hospital, it is important to call the health care provider or emergency services immediately.

Bronchoscopic biopsy

Bronchoscopy is generally safe, and complications are rare. If they do occur, complications may include spasms of the bronchial tubes that can impair breathing, irregular heart rhythms, or infections such as pneumonia.

Needle biopsy

Needle biopsy is associated with fewer risks than open biopsy because it does not involve general anesthesia. Some hemoptysis (coughing up blood) occurs in 5% of needle biopsies. Prolonged bleeding or infection may also occur, although these are very rare complications.

Open biopsy

Possible complications of an open biopsy include infection or pneumothorax. If the patient has very severe breathing problems before the biopsy, breathing may be further impaired following the operation. Patients with normal lung function prior to the biopsy have a very small risk of respiratory problems resulting from or following the procedure.

Mediastinoscopy

Complications due to mediastinoscopy are rare. Possible complications include pneumothorax or bleeding caused by damage to the blood vessels near the heart. Mediastinitis, infection of the mediastinum, may develop. Injury to the esophagus or larynx may occur. If the nerves leading to the larynx are injured, the patient may be left with a permanently hoarse voice. All of these complications are rare.

Normal results

Normal results indicate no evidence of infection in the lungs, no detection of lumps or nodules, and cells that are free from cancerous abnormalities.

Abnormal results of needle biopsy, VATS, and open biopsy may be associated with diseases other than cancer. Nodules in the lungs may be due to active infections such as tuberculosis, or may be scars from a previous infection. In 33% of biopsies using a mediastinoscope, the biopsied lymph nodes prove to be cancerous. Abnormal results should always be considered in the context of the patient's medical history, physical examination, and other tests such as sputum examination, and chest x rays before a final diagnosis is made.

Morbidity and mortality rates

The risk of death from needle biopsy is rare. The risk of death from open biopsy is one in 3,000 cases. In mediastinoscopy, death occurs in fewer than one in 3,000 cases.

Alternatives

The type of alternative diagnostic procedures available depend upon each patient's diagnosis.

Some people may be eligible to participate in clinical trials, research programs conducted with patients to evaluate a new medical treatment, drug, or device. The purpose of clinical trials is to find new and improved methods of treating different diseases and special conditions. For more information on current clinical trials, visit the National Institutes of Health's ClinicalTrials.gov at <http://www.clinicaltrials.gov> or call (888) FIND-NLM [(888) 346-3656] or (301) 594- 5983.

The National Cancer Institute (NCI) has conducted a clinical trial to evaluate a technology—low-dose helical computed tomography—for its effectiveness in screening for lung cancer. One study concluded that this test is more sensitive in detecting specific conditions related to lung cancer than other screening tests.

Resources

BOOKS

"Bronchoscopy." In *The Merck Manual of Diagnosis and Therapy,* Seventeenth Edition. Edited by Beers, M.D., Mark H., and Robert Berkow, M.D. Whitehouse Station, NJ: Merck & Co., Inc., 1999.

Groenwald, S.L. et al. *Cancer Nursing Principles and Practice.* Fifth Edition. Sudbury, MA: Jones and Bartlett Publishers, 2000.

ORGANIZATIONS

American Association for Respiratory Care (AARC). 11030 Ables Lane, Dallas, TX 75229. E-mail: info@aarc.org. <http://www.aarc.org>.

American Cancer Society. 1599 Clifton Road, N.E., Atlanta, GA 30329. (800) 227-2345 or (404) 320-3333. <http://www.cancer.org>.

American College of Chest Physicians. 3300 Dundee Road, Northbrook, IL 60062-2348. (847) 498-1400. <http://www.chestnet.org>.

American Lung Association and American Thoracic Society. 1740 Broadway, New York, NY 10019-4374. (800) 586-4872 or (212) 315-8700. <http://www.lungusa.org> and <http://www.thoracic.org>.

Cancer Research Institute. 681 Fifth Avenue, New York, NY 10022. (800) 992-2623. <http://www.cancerresearch.org>.

Lung Line National Jewish Medical and Research Center. 14090 Jackson Street, Denver, CO 80206. (800) 222-5864. E-mail: lungline@njc.org. <http://www.national jewish.org>.

National Cancer Institute (National Institutes of Health). 9000 Rockville Pike, Bethesda, MD 20892. (800) 422-6237. <http://www.nci.nih.gov>.

National Heart, Lung and Blood Institute. Information Center. P.O. Box 30105, Bethesda, MD 20824-0105. (301) 251-2222. <http://www.nhlbi.nih.gov>.

OTHER

Dailylung.com <http://www.dailylung.com>.

Chest Medicine On-Line <http://www.priory.com/chest.htm>.

National Lung Health Education Program. <http://www.nlhep.com>.

Pulmonarypaper.org P.O. Box 877, Ormond Beach, FL 32175. (800) 950- 3698. <http://www.pulmonarypaper.org>.

Pulmonary Forum <http://www.pulmonarychannel.com>.

Barbara Wexler
Angela M. Costello

Lung surgery *see* **Lobectomy, pulmonary**

Lung transplantation

Definition

Lung transplantation involves removal of one or both diseased lungs from a patient and the replacement of the lungs with healthy organs from a donor. Lung transplantation may refer to single, double, or even **heart-lung transplantation**.

Purpose

The purpose of lung transplantation is to replace a lung that no longer functions with a healthy lung. To perform a lung transplantation, there should be potential for rehabilitated breathing function. Other medical treatments should be attempted before transplantion is considered. Many candidates for this procedure have end-stage fibrotic lung disease, are dependent on **oxygen therapy**, and are likely to die of their disease in 12 to 18 months.

Demographics

In order to qualify for lung transplantation, a patient must suffer from severe lung disease such as:

- emphysema
- cystic fibrosis

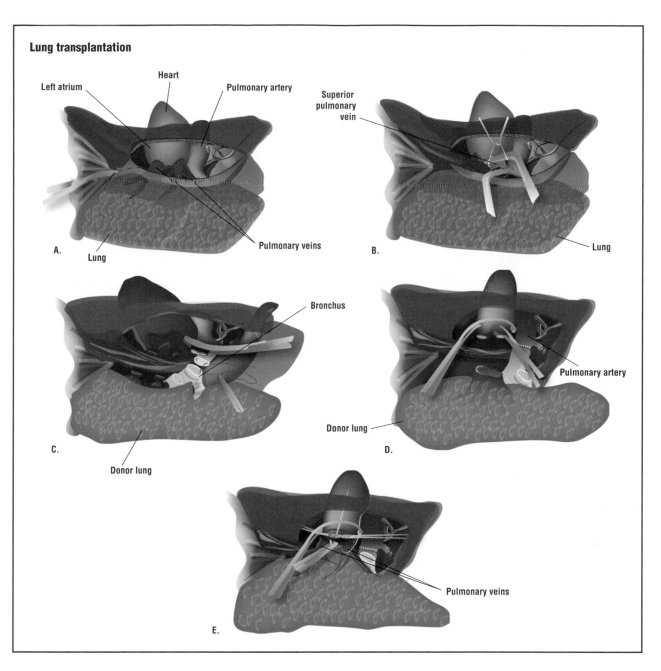

Lung transplantation

During a lung transplant, the chest is opened to reveal the heart, lungs, and major blood vessels (A). Inferior and superior pulmonary veins and pulmonary artery are separated, and lung is removed (B). The bronchus of the donor lung is connected to the patient's existing bronchus (C). The pulmonary artery is attached (D), and the pulmonary vein and other blood vessels are also connected (E). *(Illustration by GGS Inc.)*

- pulmonary fibrosis
- pulmonary hypertension
- bronchiectasis
- sarcoidosis
- silicosis

Patients with emphysema or chronic obstructive pulmonary disease (COPD) should be under 60 years of age, have a life expectancy without transplantation of two years or less, progressive deterioration, and emotional stability in order to be considered for lung transplantation. Young patients with end-stage silicosis may be candidates for lung or heart-lung transplantation. Patients with stage III or stage IV sarcoidosis with cor pulmonale (right-sided heart failure) should be considered as early as possible for lung transplantation.

WHO PERFORMS THE PROCEDURE AND WHERE IS IT PERFORMED?

Lung transplantations are performed in a specialized organ transplantation hospital. Every transplant hospital in the United States is a member of the United Network for Organ Sharing (UNOS) and must meet specific requirements.

Lung transplantations involve specialized transplant teams usually consisting of an anesthesiologist, an infectious disease specialist, a thoracic surgeon, an ear, nose, and throat (ENT) specialist, a cardiologist, and a transplant dietician who all perform with a high level of coordination.

Description

Once a patient has been selected as a possible organ recipient, the process of waiting for a donor organ match begins. The donor organ must meet specific requirements for tissue match in order to reduce the chance of organ rejection. It is estimated that it takes an average of one to two years to receive a suitable donor lung, and the wait is made less predictable by the necessity for tissue match. Patients on a recipient list must be available and ready to come to the hospital immediately when a donor match is found, since the life of the lungs outside the body is brief.

Single lung transplantation is performed via a standard **thoracotomy** (incision in the chest wall) with the patient under general anesthesia. Cardiopulmonary bypass (diversion of blood flow from the heart) is not always necessary for a single lung transplant. If bypass is necessary, it involves re-routing of the blood through tubes to a heart-lung bypass machine. Double lung transplantation involves implanting the lungs as two separate lungs, and cardiopulmonary bypass is usually required. The patient's lung or lungs are removed and the donor lungs are stitched into place. Drainage tubes are inserted into the chest area to help drain fluid, blood, and air out of the chest.

Heart-lung transplants always require the use of cardiopulmonary bypass. An incision is made through the middle of the sternum. The heart, lung, and supporting structures are transplanted into the recipient at the same time.

Diagnosis/Preparation

Patients who have diseases or conditions that may make them more susceptible to organ rejection are not selected for lung transplant. This includes patients who are acutely ill and unstable; have uncontrolled or untreatable pulmonary infection; significant dysfunction of other organs, particularly the liver, kidney, or central nervous system; and those with significant coronary disease or left ventricular dysfunction. Patients who actively smoke cigarettes or are dependent on drugs or alcohol may not be selected. There are a variety of protocols that are used to determine if a patient will be placed on a transplant recipient list, and criteria may vary depending on location.

The following diagnostic tests are usually performed to evaluate a patient for lung transplantation:

- Arterial blood gases (ABG) test, which measures the amount of oxygen that the blood is able to carry to body tissues.
- Pulmonary function tests (PFTs), which measure lung volume and the rate of air flow through the lungs; the results measure the progress of the lung disease.
- Radiographic studies (x rays). The most common is the **chest x ray** (CXR), which takes an internal picture of the chest including the lungs, ribs, heart, and the contours of the major vessels of the chest.
- Computerized tomography (CT) scan. A chest CT scan is taken of horizontal slices of the chest to provide detailed images of the structure of the chest.
- Ventilation perfusion scan (lung scan, V/Q scan) is a test that compares right and left lung function.
- Electrocardiogram (EKG) is performed by placing electrodes on the chest and one electrode on each of the four limbs. A recording of the electrical activity of the heart is obtained to provide information about the rate and rhythm of the heartbeat, and to assess any damage.
- Echocardiogram (ECHO) is an ultrasound of the heart, performed to evaluate the impact of lung disease on the heart. It examines the chambers, valves, aorta, and the wall motion of the heart. ECHO also provides information concerning the blood pressure in the pulmonary arteries. This information is required to plan the transplantation surgery.
- Blood tests. Blood samples are required for both routine and specialized testing.

In addition to tests and criteria for selection as a candidate for transplantation, patients are prepared by discussing at length the procedure, risks, and expected prognosis with the doctor. Patients should continue to follow all therapies and medications for treatment of the underlying disease, unless otherwise instructed by their physician. Since lung transplantation takes place under general anesthesia, patients are advised not to take food or drink from midnight before the surgery.

Aftercare

Transplantation requires a long hospital stay, and recovery can last up to six months. Careful monitoring will take place in a **recovery room** immediately following the surgery and in the patient's hospital room. Patients must take immunosuppressive, or anti-rejection, drugs to reduce the risk of rejection of the transplanted organ. The body considers the new organ an invader and will fight its presence. The anti-rejection drugs lower the body's immune function in order to improve acceptance of the new organs. This also makes the patient more susceptible to infection.

Frequent check-ups, including x ray and blood tests, will be necessary following surgery, probably for a period of several years.

Risks

Lung transplantation is a complicated and risky procedure, partly because of the organs and systems involved, and also because of the risk of rejection by the recipient's body. Acute rejection most often occurs within the first four months following surgery, but may occur years later. Infection is a substantial risk for organ recipients. An early complication of the surgery can be poor healing of the bronchial and tracheal openings created during the surgery. A late complication and risk is chronic rejection. This can result in inflammation of the bronchial tubes or in late infection from the prolonged use of immunosuppressive drugs to fight rejection.

Normal results

Demonstration of normal results for lung transplantation patients include adequate lung function and improved quality of life, as well as lack of infection and rejection.

Morbidity and mortality rates

According to the Scientific Registry of Transplant Recipients (SRTR), a total of 1,076 lung transplants and 31 heart-lungs transplants were performed in the United States in 2002. Of these transplants, 1,041 lungs were obtained from deceased donors and 35 from living donors. The survival rate at one year after transplant was 77% for lung transplants and 64% for heart-lung transplants.

See also Heart transplantation; Thoracotomy.

Resources

BOOKS

Couture, K. A. *The Lung Transplantation Handbook: A Guide For Patients,* 2nd edition. Victoria, BC: Trafford, 2001.

Hertz, M. I., R. M. Bolman, and J. M. Dunitz. *Manual of Lung Transplant Medical Care.* Minneapolis, MN: Fairview Press, 2001.

Maurer, Janet R., Ronald F. Grossman, and Noel Zamel. "Lung Transplantation." In *Textbook of Respiratory Medicine,* 2nd edition, edited by John F. Murray and Jay A. Nadel. Philadelphia: W. B. Saunders Co., 1994.

Schum, J. M. *Taking Flight: Inspirational Stories in Lung Transplanation.* Victoria, BC: Trafford, 2002.

PERIODICALS

Algar, F. J., et al. "Lung Transplantation in Patients under Mechanical Ventilation." *Transplantation Proceedings,* 35 (March 2003): 737–738.

Burns, K. E., B. A. Johnson, and A. T. Iacono. "Diagnostic Properties of Transbronchial Biopsy in Lung Transplant Recipients Who Require Mechanical Ventilation." *Journal of Heart and Lung Transplantation,* 22 (March 2003): 267–275.

Chan, K. M., and S. A. Allen. "Infectious Pulmonary Complications in Lung Transplant Recipients." *Seminars in Respiratory Infections,* 17 (December 2002): 291–302.

Helmi, M., R. B. Love, D. Welter, R. D. Cornwell, and K. C. Meyer. " *Aspergillus* Infection in Lung Transplant Recipients with Cystic Fibrosis: Risk Factors and Outcomes Comparison to Other Types of Transplant Recipients." *Chest,* 123 (March 2003): 800–808.

Kyle, U. G., L. Nicod, J. A. Romand, D. O. Slosman, A. Spiliopoulos, and C. Pichard. "Four-year Follow-up of Body Composition in Lung Transplant Patients." *Transplantation,* 75 (March 2003): 821–828.

Van Der Woude, B. T., et al. "Peripheral Muscle Force and Exercise Capacity in Lung Transplant Candidates." *International Journal of Rehabilitation Research,* 25 (December 2002): 351–355.

ORGANIZATIONS

American Society of Transplantation (AST). 17000 Commerce Parkway, Suite C, Mount Laurel, NJ 08054. (856) 439-9986. <http://www.a-s-t.org>.

Children's Organ Transplant Association, Inc. 2501 COTA Drive, Bloomington, IN 47403. (800) 366-2682. <http://www.cota.org>.

KEY TERMS

Anesthesia—The loss of feeling or sensation induced by use of drugs called anesthetics.

Bronchi—Any of the larger air passages of the lungs.

Bronchiectasis—Persistent and progressive dilation of bronchi or bronchioles as a consequence of inflammatory disease such as lung infections, obstructions, tumors, or congenital abnormality.

Bronchioles—The tiny branches of air tubes within the lungs that are the continuation of bronchi and connect to the lung air sacs (alveoli).

Cor pulmonale—Enlargement of the right ventricle of the heart caused by pulmonary hypertension that may result from emphysema or bronchiectasis; eventually, the condition leads to congestive heart failure.

Cystic fibrosis—A generalized disorder of infants, children, and young adults characterized by widespread dysfunction of the exocrine glands, and chronic pulmonary disease due to excess mucus production in the respiratory tract.

Emphysema—A pathological accumulation of air in tissues or organs, especially in the lungs.

Immunosuppressive—Relating to the weakening or reducing of the immune system's responses to foreign material; immunosuppressive drugs reduce the immune system's ability to reject a transplanted organ.

Pulmonary—Refers to the respiratory system, or breathing function and system.

Pulmonary fibrosis—Chronic inflammation and progressive formation of fibrous tissue in the pulmonary alveolar walls, with steadily progressive shortness of breath, resulting in death from lack of oxygen or heart failure.

Pulmonary hypertension—Abnormally high blood pressure within the pulmonary artery.

Rejection—Occurs when the body tries to attack a transplanted organ because it reacts to the organ or tissue as a foreign object and produces antibodies to destroy it. Anti-rejection (immunosuppressive) drugs help prevent rejection.

Sarcoidosis—A chronic disease with unknown cause that involves formation of nodules in bones, skin, lymph nodes, and lungs.

Silicosis—A progressive disease that results in impairment of lung function and is caused by inhalation of dust containing silica.

The National Heart, Lung, and Blood Institute (NHLBI). P.O. Box 30105, Bethesda, MD 20824-0105. (301) 592-8573. <http://www.nhlbi.nih.gov/index.htm>.

Second Wind Lung Transplant Association, Inc. 9030 West Lakeview Court, Crystal River, FL 34428. (888) 222-2690. <http://www.arthouse.com/secondwind>.

OTHER

"Lung Transplantation." The Brigham Women's Hospital. <http://www.cheshire-med.com/programs/pulrehab/transplant.html>.

"Lung Transplantation." *Medline Plus.* <http://www.nlm.nih.gov/medlineplus/lungtransplantation.html>.

Teresa Norris, RN
Monique Laberge, PhD

Luque rod *see* **Spinal instrumentation**

Lymph node biopsy *see* **Sentinel lymph node biopsy**

Lymph node removal *see* **Lymphadenectomy**

Lymphadenectomy

Definition

Lymphadenectomy, also called lymph node dissection, is a surgical procedure in which lymph glands are removed from the body and examined for the presence of cancerous cells. A limited or modified lymphadenectomy removes only some of the lymph nodes in the area around a tumor; a total or radical lymphadenectomy removes all of the lymph nodes in the area.

Purpose

The lymphatic system is responsible for returning excess fluid from body tissues to the circulatory system and for defending against foreign or harmful agents such as bacteria, viruses, or cancerous cells. The major components of the lymphatic system are lymph capillaries, lymph vessels, and lymph nodes. Lymph is a clear fluid found in tissues that originates from the circulatory system. Lymph capillaries are tiny vessels that carry excess lymph to larger lymph vessels; these in turn empty to the circulatory system. Lymph nodes are small, oval- or bean-shaped masses found throughout the lymphatic system that act as filters against foreign materials. They tend to group in clusters in such areas as the neck (cervical lymph nodes), under the arm (axillary lymph nodes), the pelvis (iliac lymph nodes), and the groin (inguinal lymph nodes).

The lymphatic system plays an important role in the spread of cancerous cells throughout the body. Cancer cells can break away from their primary site of growth and travel through the bloodstream or lymphatic system to other sites in body. They may then begin growing at these distant sites or in the lymph nodes themselves; this process is called metastasis. Removal of the lymph nodes, then, is a way that doctors can determine if a cancer has begun to metastasize. Lymphadenectomy may also be pursued as a cancer treatment to help prevent further spread of abnormal cells.

Demographics

The American Cancer Society estimates that approximately 1 million cases of cancer are diagnosed each year. Seventy-seven percent of cancers are diagnosed in men and women over the age of 55, although cancer may affect individuals of any age. Men are more often affected than women; during his lifetime, one in two men will be diagnosed with cancer, compared to one in three women. Cancer affects people of all races and ethnic backgrounds, although cancer type does vary somewhat depending upon these factors.

Description

Although the specific surgical procedure may differ according to which lymph nodes are to be removed, some steps are common among all lymphadenectomies. General anesthesia is usually administered for the duration of surgery; this ensures that the patient remain unconscious and relaxed, and awaken with no memory of the procedure.

First, an incision is made into the skin and through the subcutaneous layers in the area where the lymph nodes are to be removed. The lymph nodes are identified and isolated. They are then carefully taken out from surrounding tissues (that is, muscles, blood vessels, and nerves). In the case of axillary node dissection, the pad of fat under the skin of the armpit is removed; generally, about 10 to 20 lymph nodes are embedded in the fat and separately removed. The incision is sutured (stitched) closed with a drain left in place to remove excess fluid from the surgical site.

Alternatively, **laparoscopy** may be used as a less invasive method of removing lymph nodes. The laparo-

scope is a thin, lighted tube that is inserted into the abdominal cavity through a small incision. Images taken by the laparoscope may be seen on a video monitor connected to the scope. Certain lymph nodes, such as the pelvic and aortic lymph nodes, may be removed using this technology.

Diagnosis/Preparation

Lymph nodes may become swollen or enlarged as result of invasion by cancer cells. Swollen lymph nodes may be palpated (felt) during a physical exam. Before lymph nodes are removed, a small amount of tissue is usually removed. A biopsy will be performed on it to check for the presence of abnormal cells.

The patient will be asked to stop taking **aspirin** or aspirin-containing drugs for a period of time prior to surgery, as these can interfere with the blood's ability to clot. Such drugs may include prescription blood thinners (for example, Coumadin—generically known as warfarin and heparin). However, patients should discuss their medications with regard to their upcoming surgery with their doctors, and not make any adjustments or prescription changes on their own. No food or drink after midnight the night before surgery will be allowed.

Aftercare

Directly following surgery, the patient will be taken to the **recovery room** for constant monitoring and to recover from the effects of anesthesia. The patient may then be transferred to a regular room. If axillary nodes have been removed, the patient's arm will be elevated to help prevent postsurgical swelling. Likewise, the legs will be elevated if an inguinal lymphadenectomy had been performed. A drain placed during surgery to remove excess fluids from the surgical site will remain until the amount of fluid collected in the drain decreases significantly. The patient will generally remain in the hospital for one day.

Specific steps should be taken to minimize the risk of developing lymphedema, a condition in which excess

QUESTIONS TO ASK THE DOCTOR

- Why is lymphadenectomy recommended?
- How many lymph nodes will be removed?
- How long will the procedure take?
- When will I find out the results?
- Am I a candidate for sentinel node biopsy?
- What will happen if the results are positive for cancer?

fluid is not properly drained from body tissues, resulting in swelling. This swelling can sometimes become severe enough to interfere with daily activity. Common sites where lymphedema can develop are the arm or leg. Prior to being discharged, the patient will receive the following instructions for care of areas of the body that may be affected by lymph node removal:

- All cuts to the area should be properly cleaned, treated with an antibiotic ointment, and covered with a bandage.
- Heavy lifting should be avoided; bags should be carried on the unaffected arm.
- Tight jewelry and clothing with tight elastic bands should be avoided.
- Injections, blood draws, and blood pressure measurements should be done on the unaffected arm.
- Sunblock should be worn on the affected area to minimize the risk of sunburn.
- Steps should be taken to avoid cuts to the skin. For example, an electric razor should be used to shave the affected area; protective gloves should be worn when working with abrasive items.

Risks

Some of the risks associated with lymphadenectomy include excessive bleeding, infection, pain, excessive swelling, vein inflammation (phlebitis), and damage to nerves during surgery. Nerve damage may be temporary or permanent and may result in weakness, numbness, tingling, and/or drooping. Lymphedema is also a risk whenever lymph nodes have been removed; it may occur immediately following surgery or from months to years later.

Normal results

After removed lymph nodes have been examined microscopically for the presence of cancerous cells, they may be labeled node-negative (no presence of cancer cells) or node-positive (presence of cancer cells). These findings are the basis for deciding the next step in cancer treatment, if one is indicated.

Morbidity and mortality rates

The rate of complications following lymphadenectomy depends on the specific lymph nodes being removed. For example, following axillary lymphadenectomy, there is a 10% chance of chronic lymphedema and 20% chance of abnormal skin sensations. The overall rate of complications following inguinal lymphadenectomy is approximately 15%, and 5–7% following pelvic lymphadenectomy.

Alternatives

A technique designed to spare the unnecessary removal of normal lymph nodes is called sentinel node biopsy. When lymph fluid moves out of a region, the sentinel lymph node is the first node it reaches. The theory behind **sentinel lymph node biopsy** is that if cancer is not present in the sentinel node, it is unlikely to have spread to other nearby nodes. This procedure may allow individuals with early stage cancers to avoid the complications associated with partial or radical removal of lymph nodes if there is little or no chance that cancer has spread to them.

Resources

BOOKS

St. Louis, James D. and Richard L. McCann. "Lymphatic System" (Chapter 65). In *Sabiston Textbook of Surgery.* Philadelphia: W. B. Saunders Company, 2001.

PERIODICALS

Beneditti-Panici, Pierluigi, et al. "Pelvic and Aortic Lymphadenectomy." *Surgical Clinics of North America* 81, no. 4 (August 1, 2001): 841-58.

Colberg, John W. "Inguinal Lymph Node Dissection for Penile Carcinoma: Modified Verses Radical Lymphadenectomy." *Infections in Urology* 13, no. 5 (2000): 115-20.

Gervasoni, James E., et al. "Biological and Clinical Significance of Lymphadenectomy." *Surgical Clinics of North America* 80, no. 6 (December 1, 2000): 1631-73.

ORGANIZATIONS

American Cancer Society. 1599 Clifton Rd. NE, Atlanta, GA 30329-4251. (800) 227-2345. <http://www.cancer.org>.

Society of Surgical Oncology. 85 W. Algonquin Rd., Suite 550, Arlington Heights, IL 60005. (847) 427-1400. <http://www.surgonc.org>.

OTHER

"All About Cancer: Detailed Guide." *American Cancer Society.* 2003 [cited April 9, 2003]. <http://www.cancer.org/docroot/CRI/CRI_2_3.asp>.

Stephanie Dionne Sherk

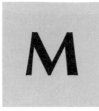

M

Magnetic resonance angiography *see*
Magnetic resonance imaging

Magnetic resonance imaging

Definition

Magnetic resonance imaging (MRI) is a unique and versatile medical imaging diagnostic tool. Using MRI, physicians obtain highly refined images of the body's interior. Strong magnetic fields and pulses of radio waves manipulate the body's natural magnetic, producing images not possible with other diagnostic imaging methods. MRI is particularly useful for imaging the brain and spine, as well as the soft tissues of joints and the interior structure of bones. The entire body can be imaged using MRI, and the technology poses few known health risks.

Purpose

MRI was developed in the 1980s. The latest additions to MRI technology are magnetic resonance **angiography** (MRA) and magnetic resonance spectroscopy (MRS). MRA studies blood flow, while MRS identifies the chemical composition of diseased tissue and produces color images of brain function. The many advantages of MRI include:

• Detail. MRI creates precise images of the body based on the varying proportions of magnetically polarizable elements in different tissues. Very minor fluctuations in chemical composition can be determined. MRI images have greater subject contrast than those produced with standard x rays, computed tomography (CT), or ultrasound, all of which depend on the differing physical properties of tissues. This contrast sensitivity lets MRI distinguish fine variations in tissues deep within the body. It is particularly useful for spotting and distinguishing diseased tissues (tumors and other lesions)

early in their development. Often, physicians prescribe an MRI scan to more fully investigate earlier findings from other imaging techniques.

• Scope. All body parts can be imaged using MRI. Moreover, MRI scans are not adversely affected by bone, gas, or body waste, which can hinder other imaging techniques. (The scans can, however, be degraded by motion such as breathing, heartbeat, and normal bowel activity.) A close series of two-dimensional images can provide a three-dimensional view of a targeted area. Unlike other techniques, MRI can provide images in multiple planes.

• Safety. MRI does not depend on potentially harmful ionizing radiation, as do standard x rays and **CT scans**. There are no known risks specific to the procedure, other than for people who have metal objects in their bodies.

Physicians sometimes choose other imaging techniques, such as ultrasound scanning, because the MRI process is complex, time-consuming, and costly. The process requires large, expensive, and complicated equipment; a highly trained operator; and a physician specializing in radiology. Generally, MRI is prescribed only when serious symptoms or negative results from other tests indicate a need. In many cases, an alternative imaging procedure is more appropriate for the type of diagnosis needed. However, some diseases such as multiple sclerosis are best imaged by MRI.

Physicians may prescribe an MRI scan of different areas of the body.

• Brain and head. MRI technology was developed because of the need for brain imaging. It is one of the few imaging tools that can see through bone (the skull) and deliver high quality pictures of the brain's delicate soft tissue structures. MRI may be needed for patients with symptoms of a brain tumor, stroke, or infection (such as meningitis). MRI also may be needed when cognitive or psychological symptoms suggest brain disease (such as Alzheimer's or Huntington's diseases, or multiple sclerosis), or when developmental retardation suggests a

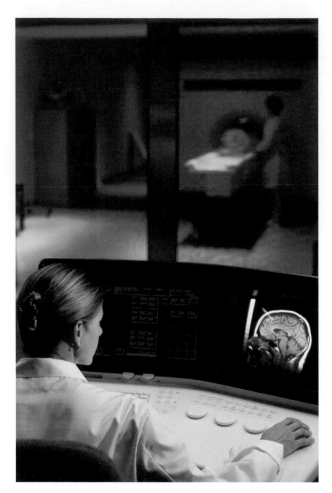

A patient receiving a magnetic resonance imaging (MRI) scan. A technologist monitors the equipment in an adjacent control room. *(Will & Deni McIntyre/Photo Researchers, Inc. Reproduced by permission.)*

birth defect. MRI can also provide pictures of the sinuses and other areas of the head beneath the face.

- Spine. Spinal problems can cause neck or back pain, or numbness or weakness in the arm or leg. MRI is particularly useful for identifying and evaluating degenerated or herniated intervertebral discs. It can also be used to determine the condition of nerve tissue within the spinal cord.

- Joints. MRI scanning is often used to diagnose and assess joint problems. MRI can provide clear images of the bone, cartilage, ligaments, and tendons that comprise a joint. MRI can be used to diagnose joint damage due to sports, advancing age, or arthritis. It can also be used to diagnose shoulder problems, such as a torn rotator cuff. MRI can detect the presence of an otherwise hidden tumor or infection in a joint, and can be used to diagnose the nature of developmental joint abnormalities in children.

- Skeleton. The properties of MRI that allow it to see though the skull also allow it to view the interior of bones. It can be used to detect bone cancer, inspect the marrow for leukemia and other diseases, assess bone loss (osteoporosis), and examine complex fractures.

- The rest of the body. While CT and ultrasound satisfy most chest, abdominal, and general body imaging needs, MRI may be required to provide more detailed images in certain circumstances, or when repeated scanning is necessary. MRI is also used in cases when the progress of therapy, such as liver cancer treatment, needs to be monitored, and the effect of repeated x ray exposure is a concern.

Description

Magnetic resonance imaging

MRI produces a map of hydrogen atoms distributed in the body. Hydrogen is the simplest element known, the most abundant in biological tissue, and one that can be magnetically polarized. It will align itself within a strong magnetic field, like the needle of a compass. The earth's magnetic field is not strong enough to polarize a person's hydrogen atoms, but the superconducting magnet of an MRI machine can do this. The strength of the earth's magnetic field is approximately 1 gauss. Typical field strength of an MRI unit, with a superconducting magnet, is 1,500 gauss, expressed as 1.5 kilogauss or 1.5 Tesla units. This comprises the "magnetic" part of MRI. There are also low field units with 0.5 Tesla strength, often with open MRI units.

Once a patient's hydrogen atoms have been aligned in the magnet, pulses of very specific radio wave frequencies jolt them out of alignment. The hydrogen atoms alternately absorb and emit radio wave energy, vibrating back and forth between their resting (polarized) state and their agitated (radio pulse) state. This comprises the "resonance" part of MRI. The patient does not detect this process.

The MRI equipment detects the duration, strength, and source location of the signals emitted by the atoms as they relax. This data is translated into an image on a television monitor. The amount of hydrogen in diseased tissue differs from the amount in healthy tissue of the same type, making MRI particularly effective at identifying tumors and other lesions. In some cases, chemical agents such as gadolinium can be injected to improve the contrast between healthy and diseased tissue.

A single MRI exposure produces a two-dimensional image of a slice through the entire target area. A series of these image slices closely spaced (usually less than half an inch [1.25 cm]) provides a virtual three-dimensional view of the area.

Magnetic resonance spectroscopy

Magnetic resonance spectroscopy (MRS) is different from MRI because MRS uses a continuous band of radio wave frequencies to excite hydrogen atoms in a variety of chemical compounds other than water. These compounds absorb and emit radio energy at characteristic frequencies, or spectra, that can be used to identify them. Generally, a color image is created by assigning a hue to each distinctive spectral emission. This comprises the "spectroscopy" part of MRS. MRS is still experimental, and is available in only a few research centers.

Physicians mainly use MRS to study the brain and disorders such as epilepsy, Alzheimer's disease, brain tumors, and the effects of drugs on brain growth and metabolism. The technique is also useful in evaluating metabolic disorders of the muscles and nervous system.

Magnetic resonance angiography

Magnetic resonance angiography (MRA) is a variation on standard MRI. MRA, like other types of angiography, looks specifically at blood flow within the vascular system, without the injection of contrast agents (dye) or radioactive tracers. Standard MRI cannot detect blood flow, but MRA uses specific radio pulse sequences to capture usable signals. The technique is generally used in combination with MRI to obtain images that show both the structure of blood vessels and flow within the brain and head in cases of stroke, suspected blood clot, or aneurysm. In general, MRA is performed without contrast when examining the brain. Intravenous contrast is usually administered when other blood vessels, such as those in the neck, chest, or abdomen are studied.

Procedure

Regardless of the type of MRI planned, or area of the body targeted, the procedure involved is basically the same, and occurs in a special MRI suite. The patient lies back on a narrow table and is made as comfortable as possible. Transmitters are positioned on the body and the cushioned table that the patient is lying on moves into a long tube that houses the magnet. The tube is the length of an average adult lying down, and the tube is narrow and open at both ends. Once the area to be examined has been properly positioned, a radio pulse is applied. Then a two-dimensional image corresponding to one slice through the area is made. The table then moves a fraction of an inch and the next image is made, and so on. Each image exposure takes several seconds, and the entire exam lasts 30–90 minutes. During this time, the patient is not allowed to move. Movement during the scan results in an unclear image.

Depending on the area to be imaged, the radio-wave transmitters are positioned in different locations.

- For the head and neck, a helmet-like hat is worn.
- For the spine, chest, and abdomen, the patient lies down on transmitters known as coils.
- For the knee, shoulder, or other joint, the transmitters are applied directly to the joint.

Additional probes will monitor such **vital signs** as pulse and respiration.

The process is very noisy and confining. The patient hears a thumping sound for the duration of the procedure. To increase comfort, music supplied via earphones is often provided. Some patients become anxious, or they may panic because they are inside a small, enclosed tube. This is why vital signs are monitored, and the patient and medical team communicate with each other. If a patient has claustrophobia, the physician may prescribe an anti-anxiety drug prior to the procedure. If the chest or abdomen is to be imaged, the patient is asked to hold his or her breath for each exposure. Other instructions may be given as needed.

In many cases, the entire examination will be performed by an MRI operator who is not a physician. However, the supervising radiologist should be available to consult as necessary during the exam, and will view and interpret the results at a later time.

Open MRI units

Many adult patients and, especially children, become extremely claustrophobic when placed inside the confines of a full strength (1.5 Tesla) superconducting magnet. This problem is often severe enough to prevent them from having an MRI scan. In an alternative design, the magnet is comprised of two opposed halves with a large space in between. These units are known as open MRI machines. The advantage is that they can be used for patients who are claustrophobic. The disadvantage is that the field strength of the magnets is lower (usually 0.2–0.5 Tesla) than with standard full-strength machines. Lower strength magnetic fields require more time for image acquisition, increasing the risk of image problems because patients may have difficulty remaining still for longer periods of time.

Preparation

In some cases (such as for MRI brain scanning or MRA), a chemical designed to increase image contrast may be given by the radiologist immediately before the exam. If a patient suffers from anxiety or claustrophobia, drugs may be given to help the patient relax.

The patient must remove all metal objects (i.e., watches, jewelry, eyeglasses, hair clips). Any magnetized objects, such as credit and bank machine cards or audio tapes, should be kept far away from the MRI equipment because they can be erased. The patient cannnot bring a wallet or keys into the MRI machine. He or she may be asked to wear clothing without metal snaps, buckles, or zippers, unless a medical gown is provided. The patient may also be asked to remove any hair spray, hair gel, or cosmetics that could interfere with the scan.

Side effects

The potential side effects of magnetic and electric fields on human health remain a source of debate. In particular, the possible effects on an unborn baby are not well known. Any woman who is, or may be, pregnant should carefully discuss this issue with her physician and radiologist before undergoing a scan.

Chemical agents may be injected to improve the image or allow for the imaging of blood or other fluid flow during MRA. In rare cases, patients may be allergic to or intolerant of these agents, and should not receive them. If chemical agents are to be used, patients should discuss any concerns they have with their physician and radiologist.

As in other medical imaging techniques, obesity greatly interferes with the quality of MRI.

Aftercare

No aftercare is necessary, unless the patient received medication or had a reaction to a contrast agent. Normally, patients can return to their daily activities immediately. If the exam reveals a serious condition that requires more testing or treatment, appropriate information and counseling will be needed.

Precautions

MRI scanning should not be used when there is the potential for an interaction between the strong MRI magnetic field and metal objects that might be imbedded in a patient's body. The force of magnetic attraction on certain types of metal objects (including surgical steel and clips used to pinch off blood vessels) could move them within the body and cause serious injury. The movement would occur when the patient is placed into and out of the magnetic field. Metal may be imbedded in a person's body for several reasons:

• Medical. People with implanted cardiac **pacemakers**, metal aneurysm clips, or who have had broken bones repaired with metal pins, screws, rods, or plates must inform their radiologist prior to having an MRI scan.

KEY TERMS

Angiography—Any of the different methods for investigating the condition of blood vessels, usually via a combination of radiological imaging and injections of chemical tracing and contrast agents.

Gadolinium—A very rare metallic element useful for its sensitivity to electromagnetic resonance, among other things. Traces of it can be injected into the body to enhance MRI images.

Hydrogen—The simplest, most common element known in the universe. It is composed of a single electron (negatively charged particle) circling a nucleus consisting of a single proton (positively charged particle). It is the nuclear proton of hydrogen that makes MRI possible by reacting resonantly to radio waves while aligned in a magnetic field.

Ionizing radiation—Electromagnetic radiation that can damage living tissue by disrupting and destroying individual cells. All types of nuclear decay radiation (including x rays) are potentially ionizing. Radio waves do not damage organic tissues through which they pass.

Magnetic field—The three-dimensional area surrounding a magnet, in which its force is active. During MRI, the patient's body is permeated by the force field of a superconducting magnet.

Radio waves—Electromagnetic energy of the frequency range corresponding to that used in radio communications, usually 10,000 cycles per second to 300 billion cycles per second. Radio waves are the same as visible light, x rays, and all other types of electromagnetic radiation, but are of a higher frequency.

Generally, a joint replacement or other orthopedic hardware is not a problem if another part of the body is being scanned.

• Injury. Patients must tell their physicians if they have bullet fragments or other metal pieces in their body from old wounds. The suspected presence of metal, whether from an old or recent wound, should be confirmed before scanning.

• Occupational. People with significant work exposure to metal particles (working with a metal grinder, for example) should discuss this with their physician and radiologist. The patient may need prescan testing—usually a single, standard x ray of the eyes to see if any metal is present.

Normal results

A normal MRI, MRA, or MRS result is one that shows that the patient's physical condition falls within the normal range for the target area scanned.

Generally, MRI is prescribed only when serious symptoms or negative results from other tests indicate a need. There often exists strong evidence of a condition that the scan is designed to detect and assess. Thus, the results will often be abnormal, confirming the earlier diagnosis. At that point, further testing and appropriate medical treatment are needed. For example, if the MRI indicates the presence of a brain tumor, an MRS may be prescribed to determine the type of tumor so that aggressive treatment can begin immediately without the need for a surgical biopsy.

Resources

BOOKS

Haaga, John R., et al., eds. *Computed Tomography and Magnetic Resonance Imaging of the Whole Body.* St. Louis, MO: Mosby, 1994.

Hornak, Ph.D., P. Joseph. *The Basics of MRI.* <http//www.cis.rit.edu/htbooks/mri/>.

Zaret, Barry L., et al., eds. *The Patient's Guide to Medical Tests.* Boston: Houghton Mifflin Company, 1997.

PERIODICALS

Jung, H. "Discrimination of Metastatic from Acute Osteoporotic Compression Spinal Fractures with MR Imaging." *Radiographics* 179 (January/February 2003).

Kevles, Bettyann "Body Imaging." *Newsweek* Extra Millennium Issue (Winter 97/98): 74–6.

ORGANIZATIONS

American College of Radiology. 1891 Preston White Dr., Reston, VA 22091. (703) 648-8900. <http://www.acr.org. >.

American Society of Radiologic Technologists. 15000 Central Ave. SE, Albuquerque, NM 87123-3917. (505) 298-4500. <http://www.asrt.org>.

Center for Devices and Radiological Health. United States Food and Drug Administration. 1901 Chapman Ave., Rockville, MD 20857. (301) 443-4109. <http://www.fda.gov/cdrh>.

OTHER

Smith, Steve. "Brief Introduction to FMRI." FMRIB. 1998. <http://www.fmrib.ox.ac.uk/fmri_intro/>.

Stephen John Hage, AAAS, RT-R, FAHRA
Lee A. Shratter, M.D.

Magnetic resonance spectroscopy *see* **Magnetic resonance imaging**

Mallet toe surgery *see* **Hammer, claw, and mallet toe surgery**

Mammography

Definition

Mammography is the study of the breast using x rays. The actual test is called a mammogram. It is an x ray of the breast which shows the fatty, fibrous, and glandular tissues. There are two types of mammograms. A screening mammogram is ordered for women who have no problems with their breasts. It consists of two x ray views of each breast: a craniocaudal (from above) and a mediolateral oblique (from the sides). A diagnostic mammogram is for evaluation of abnormalities in either men or women. Additional x rays from other angles, or special coned views of certain areas, are taken.

Purpose

The purpose of screening mammography is breast cancer detection. A screening test, by definition, is used for patients without any signs or symptoms, in order to detect disease as early as possible. Many studies have shown that having regular mammograms increases a woman's chances of finding breast cancer in an early stage, when it is more likely to be curable. It has been estimated that a mammogram may find a cancer as much as two or three years before it can be felt. The American Cancer Society (ACS) guidelines recommend an annual screening mammogram for every woman of average risk beginning at age 40. Radiologists look specifically for the presence of microcalcifications and other abnormalities that can be associated with malignancy. New digital mammography and computer-aided reporting can automatically enhance and magnify the mammograms for easier finding of these tiny calcifications.

The highest risk factor for developing cancer is age. Some women are at an increased risk for developing breast cancer, such as those with a positive family history of the disease. Beginning screening mammography at a younger age may be recommended for these women.

Diagnostic mammography is used to evaluate an existing problem, such as a lump, discharge from the nipple, or unusual tenderness in one area. It is also done to evaluate further abnormalities that have been seen on screening mammograms. The radiologist normally views the films immediately and may ask for additional views such as a magnification view of one specific area. Additional studies such as an ultrasound of the breast may be performed as well to determine if the lesion is cystic or solid. Breast-specific **positron emission tomography (PET)** scans as well as an MRI (**magnetic resonance imaging**) may be ordered to further evaluate a tumor, but mammography is still the first choice in detecting small tumors on a screening basis.

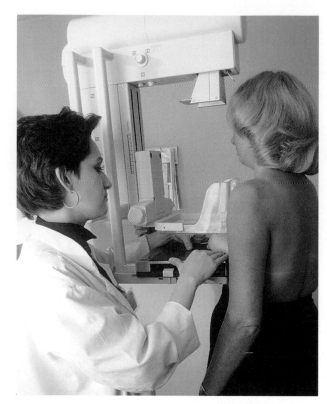

Mammography can detect breast cancer before it can be felt, increasing the chances that it can be treated successfully. *(D. Weinstein/Custom Medical Stock Photo. Reproduced by permission.)*

Description

A mammogram may be offered in a variety of settings. Hospitals, outpatient clinics, physician's offices, or other facilities may have mammography equipment. In the United States only places certified by the Food and Drug Administration (FDA) are legally permitted to perform, interpret, or develop mammograms. Mammograms are taken with dedicated machines using high frequency generators, low kvp, molybdenum targets and specialized x ray beam filtration. Sensitive high contrast film and screen combinations along with prolonged developing enable the visualization of minute breast detail.

In addition to the usual paperwork, a woman will be asked to fill out a questionnaire asking for information on her current medical history. Beyond her personal and family history of cancer, details about menstruation, previous breast surgeries, child bearing, birth control, and hormone replacement therapy are recorded. Information about breast self-examination (BSE) and other breast health issues are usually available at no charge.

At some centers, a technologist may perform a **physical examination** of the breasts before the mammogram. Whether or not this is done, it is essential for the technologist to record any lumps, nipple discharge, breast pain or other concerns of the patient. All visible scars, tattoos and nipple alterations must be carefully noted as well.

Clothing from the waist up is removed, along with necklaces and dangling earrings. A hospital gown or similar covering is put on. A small self-adhesive metal marker may be placed on each nipple by the x ray technologist. This allows the nipple to be viewed as a reference point on the film for concise tumor location and easier centering for additional views.

Patients are positioned for mammograms differently, depending on the type of mammogram being performed:

• Craniocaudal position (CC): The woman stands or sits facing the mammogram machine. One breast is exposed and raised to a level position while the height of the cassette holder is adjusted to the same level. The breast is placed mid-film with the nipple in profile and the head turned away from the side being x rayed. The shoulder is relaxed and pulled slightly backward while the breast is pulled as far forward as possible. The technologist holds the breast in place and slowly lowers the compression with a foot pedal. The breast is compressed between the film holder and a rectangle of plastic (called a paddle). The breast is compressed until the skin is taut and the breast tissue firm when touched on the lateral side. The exposure is taken immediately and the compression released. Good compression can be uncomfortable, but it is very necessary. Compression reduces the thickness of the breast, creates a uniform density and separates overlying tissues. This allows for a detailed image with a lower exposure time and decreased radiation dose to the patient. The same view is repeated on the opposite breast.

• Mediolateral oblique position (MLO): The woman is positioned with her side towards the mammography unit. The film holder is angled parallel to the pectoral muscle, anywhere from 30 to 60 degrees depending on the size and height of the patient. The taller and thinner the patient the higher the angle. The height of the machine is level with the axilla (armpit). The arm is placed at the top of the cassette holder with a corner touching the armpit. The breast is lifted forward and upward and compression is applied until the breast is held firmly in place by the paddle. The nipple should be in profile and the opposite breast held away if necessary by the patient. This procedure is repeated for the other breast. A total of four x rays, two of each breast, are taken for a screening mammogram. Additional x rays, using special paddles, different breast positions, or other techniques may be taken for a diagnostic mammogram.

The mammogram may be seen and interpreted by a radiologist right away, or it may not be reviewed until later. If there is any questionable area or abnormality, extra x rays may be recommended. These may be taken during the same appointment. More commonly, especially for screening mammograms, the woman is called back on another day for these additional films.

A screening mammogram usually takes approximately 15 to 30 minutes. A woman having a diagnostic mammogram can expect to spend up to an hour for the procedure.

The cost of mammography varies widely. Many mammography facilities accept "self referral." This means women can schedule themselves without a physician's referral. However, some insurance policies do require a doctor's prescription to ensure payment. **Medicare** will pay for annual screening mammograms for all women over age 39.

Preparation

The compression or squeezing of the breast necessary for a mammogram is a concern of many women. Mammograms should be scheduled when a woman's breasts are least likely to be tender. One to two weeks after the first day of the menstrual period is usually best, as the breasts may be tender during a menstrual period. Some women with sensitive breasts also find that stopping or decreasing caffeine intake from coffee, tea, colas, and chocolate for a week or two before the examination decreases any discomfort. Women receiving hormone therapy may also have sensitive breasts. Over-the-counter pain relievers are recommended an hour before the mammogram appointment when pain is a significant problem.

Women should not put deodorant, powder, or lotion on their upper body on the day the mammogram is performed. Particles from these products can get on the breast or film holder and may show up as abnormalities on the mammogram. Most facilities will have special wipes available for those patients who need to wash before the mammogram.

Aftercare

No special aftercare is required.

Risks

The risk of radiation exposure from a mammogram is considered minimal and not significant. Experts are unanimous that any negligible risk is by far outweighed by the potential benefits of mammography. Patients who have **breast implants** must be x rayed with caution and compression is minimally applied so that the sac is not ruptured. Special techniques and positioning skills must be learned before a technologist can x ray a patient with breast implants.

Some breast cancers do not show up on mammograms, or "hide" in dense breast tissue. A normal (or negative) study is not a guarantee that a woman is cancer-free. The false-negative rate is estimated to be 15–20%, higher in younger women and women with dense breasts.

False positive readings are also possible. Breast biopsies may be recommended on the basis of a mammogram, and find no cancer. It is estimated that 75–80% of all breast biopsies resulted in benign (no cancer present) findings. This is considered an acceptable rate, because recommending fewer biopsies would result in too many missed cancers.

Normal results

A mammography report describes details about the x ray appearance of the breasts. It also rates the mammogram according to standardized categories, as part of the Breast Imaging Reporting and Data System (BIRADS) created by the American College of Radiology (ACR). A normal mammogram may be rated as BIRADS 1 or negative, which means no abnormalities were seen. A normal mammogram may also be rated as BIRADS 2 or benign findings. This means there are one or more abnormalities but they are clearly benign (not cancerous), or variations of normal. Some kinds of calcifications, enlarged lymph nodes or obvious cysts might generate a BIRADS 2 rating.

Many mammograms are considered borderline or indeterminate in their findings. BIRADS 3 means either additional images are needed, or an abnormality is seen and is probably (but not definitely) benign. A follow-up mammogram within a short interval of six to 12 months is suggested. This helps to ensure that the abnormality is not changing, or is "stable." Only the affected side will be x rayed at this time. Some women are uncomfortable or anxious about waiting, and may want to consult with their doctor about having a biopsy. BIRADS 4 means suspicious for cancer. A biopsy is usually recommended in this case. BIRADS 5 means an abnormality is highly suggestive of cancer. A biopsy or other appropriate action should be taken.

Screening mammograms are not usually recommended for women under age 40 who have no special risk factors and a normal physical breast examination. A mammogram may be useful if a lump or other problem is discovered in a woman aged 30–40. Below age 30, breasts tend to be "radiographically dense," which means the breasts contain a large amount of glandular tissue which is difficult to image in fine detail. Mammograms for this age group are controversial. An ultrasound of the breasts is usually done instead.

Patient education

The mammography technologist must be empathetic to the patient's modesty and anxiety. He or she must explain that compression is necessary to improve the quality of the image but does not harm the breasts. Patients may be very anxious when additional films are requested. Explaining that an extra view gives the radiologist more information will help to ease the patient's tension. One in eight women in North America will develop breast cancer. Educating the public on monthly breast self-examinations and yearly mammograms will help in achieving an early diagnosis and therefore a better cure.

Resources

PERIODICALS

Carmen, Ricard, R. T. R. *Mammography: Techniques and Difficulties.* O.T.R.Q., 1999.

Gagnon, Gilbert. *Radioprotection in Mammography.* O.T.R.Q., 1999.

Ouimet, Guylaine, R. T. R. *Mammography: Quality Control.* O.T.R.Q., 1999.

ORGANIZATIONS

American Cancer Society (ACS), 1599 Clifton Rd., Atlanta, GA 30329. (800) ACS-2345. <http://www.cancer.org>.

Federal Drug Administration (FDA), 5600 Fishers Ln., Rockville, MD 20857. (800) 532-4440. <http://www.fda.gov>.

National Cancer Institute (NCI) and Cancer Information Service (CIS), Office of Cancer Communications, Bldg. 31, Room 10A16, Bethesda, MD 20892. (800) 4-CANCER (800) 422-6237. Fax: (800) 624-2511 or (301) 402-5874. <cancermail@cips.nci.nih.gov>. <http://cancernet.nci.nih.gov>.

Lorraine K. Ehresman
Lee A. Shratter, M.D.

Managed care plans

Definition

Managed care plans are health-care delivery systems that integrate the financing and delivery of health care. Managed care organizations generally negotiate agreements with providers to offer packaged health care benefits to covered individuals.

Purpose

The purpose for managed care plans is to reduce the cost of health care services by stimulating competition and streamlining administration.

Description

A majority of insured Americans belongs to a managed care plan, a health care delivery system that applies corporate business practices to medical care in order to reduce costs and streamline care. The managed care era began in the late 1980s in response to skyrocketing health care costs, which stemmed from a number of sources. Under the fee-for-service, or indemnity, model that preceded managed care, doctors and hospitals were financially rewarded for using a multitude of expensive tests and procedures to treat patients. Other contributors to the high cost of health care were the public health advances after World War II that lengthened the average lifespan of Americans. This put increased pressure on the health care system. In response, providers have adopted state-of-the-art diagnostic and treatment technologies as they have become available.

Managed care companies attempted to reduce costs by negotiating lower fees with clinicians and hospitals in exchange for a steady flow of patients, developing standards of treatment for specific diseases, requiring clinicians to get plan approval before hospitalizing a patient (except in the case of an emergency), and encouraging clinicians to prescribe less expensive medicines. Many plans offer financial incentives to clinicians who minimize referrals and diagnostic tests, and some even apply financial penalties, or disincentives, on those considered to have ordered unnecessary care. The primary watchdog and accreditation agency for managed care organizations is the National Committee for Quality Assurance (NCQA), a non-profit organization that also collects and disseminates health plan performance data.

Three basic types of managed care plans exist: health maintenance organizations (HMOs), preferred provider organizations (PPOs), and point-of-service (POS) plans.

- HMOs, in existence for more than 50 years, are the best known and oldest form of managed care. Participants in HMO plans must first see a primary care provider, who may be a physician or an advanced practice registered nurse (APRN), in order to be referred to a specialist. Four types of HMOs exist: the Staff Model, Group Model, Network Model, and the Independent Practice Association (IPA). The Staff Model hires clinicians to work onsite. The Group Model contracts with group practice physicians on an exclusive basis. The Network Model resembles the group model except participating physicians can treat patients who are not plan members. The Independent Practice Association (IPA) contracts with physicians in private practice to see HMO patients at a prepaid rate per visit as a part of their practice.

- PPOs are more flexible than HMOs. Like HMOs, they negotiate with networks of physicians and hospitals to get discounted rates for plan members. But, unlike HMOs, PPOs allow plan members to seek care from specialists without being referred by a primary care practitioner. These plans use financial incentives to encourage members to seek medical care from providers inside the network.

- POS plans are a blend of the other types of managed care plans. They encourage plan members to seek care from providers inside the network by charging low fees for their services, but they add the option of choosing an out-of-plan provider at any time and for any reason. POS plans carry a high premium, a high deductible, or a higher co-payment for choosing an out-of-plan provider.

Several managed care theories such as those stressing continuity of care, prevention, and early intervention are applauded by health care practitioners and patients alike. But managed care has come under fire by critics who feel patient care may be compromised by managed care cost-cutting strategies such as early hospital discharge and use of financial incentives to control referrals, which may make clinicians too cautious about sending patients to specialists. In general, the rise of managed care has shifted decision-making power away from plan members, who are limited in their choices of providers, and away from clinicians, who must concede to managed-care administrators regarding what is considered a medically necessary procedure. Many people would like to see managed care restructured to remedy this inequitable distribution of power. Such actions would maximize consumer choice and allow health care practitioners the freedom to provide the best care possible. According to the American Medical Association, rejection of care resulting from managed care stipulations should be subjected to an independent appeals process.

The health-care industry today is dominated by corporate values of managed care and is subject to corporate principles such as cost cutting, mergers and acquisitions, and layoffs. To thrive in such an environment, and to provide health care in accordance with professional values, health care practitioners must educate themselves on the business of health care, including hospital operations and administrative decision making, in order to influence institutional and regional health-care policies. A sampling of the roles available for registered nurses in a managed care environment include:

- Primary care provider. The individual responsible for determining a plan of care, including referrals to specialists.

- Case manager. The person who tracks patients through the health care system to maintain continuity of care.

- Triage nurse. In a managed care organization, these individuals help direct patients through the system by determining the urgency and level of care necessary and advising incoming patients on self-care when appropriate.

- Utilization/Resource reviewer. This individual helps manage costs by assessing the appropriateness of specialized treatments.

Normal results

It is difficult to predict the effect of the managed care revolution on the health care profession. All health care providers will benefit from building broad coalitions at the state and federal levels to publicize their views on patient care issues. These coalitions will also be useful to monitor developing trends in the industry, including the impact of proposed mergers and acquisitions of health care institutions on the provision of care.

See also Finding a surgeon; Long-term insurance; Medicare; Nursing homes.

Resources

BOOKS

Bondeson, W. B., and J. W. Jones. *Ethics of Managed Care: Professional Integrity and Patient Rights.* Amsterdam: Kluwer Academic Publishers, 2002.

Kongstvedt, P. R. *Essentials of Managed Health Care, 4th Edition.* Boston: Jones & Bartlett, 2003.

Kongstvedt, P. R., and W. Knight. *Managed Care: What It Is and How It Works, 2nd edition.* Boston: Jones & Bartlett, 2002.

Orin, Rhonda. *Making Them Pay: How to Get the Most from Health Insurance and Managed Care.* New York: St. Martin's Press, 2001.

PERIODICALS

Kirkman-Liff, B. "Restoring Trust to Managed Care, Part 1: A Focus on Patients." *American Journal of Managed Care* 9, no.2 (2003): 174–180.

Kirkman-Liff, B. "Restoring Trust to Managed Care, Part 2: A Focus on Physicians." *American Journal of Managed Care* 9, no.3 (2003): 249–252.

Rogoski, R. R. "Managed Care's Challenges. Health Plans Use New IT to Meet the Burgeoning Challenges of Costs and Consumerism." *Health Management Technology* 24, no.3 (2003): 20–25.

Sparer, M. S. "Managed Long-term Care: Limits and Lessons." *Journal of Aging and Health* 15, no.1 (2003): 269–291.

ORGANIZATIONS

Agency for Health Care Research and Quality. 2101 E. Jefferson St., Suite 501, Rockville, MD 20852. (301) 594-1364.

American Association of Managed Care Nurses. P.O. Box 4975, Glen Allen, VA 23058-4975. (804) 747-9698. <http://www.aamcn.org/joinaamcn.htm>.

American College of Physicians. 190 N. Independence Mall West, Philadelphia, PA 19106-1572. 800) 523-1546, x2600, or (215) 351-2600. <http://www.acponline.org>.

American College of Surgeons. 633 North St. Clair Street, Chicago, IL 60611-32311. (312) 202-5000; Fax: (312) 202-5001. E-mail: <postmaster@facs.org>. <http://www.facs.org>.

American Hospital Association. One North Franklin, Chicago, IL 60606-3421. (312) 422-3000. <http://www.aha.org/index.asp>.

American Medical Association. 515 N. State Street, Chicago, IL 60610. (312) 464-5000. <http://www.ama-assn.org>.

American Nurses Association. 600 Maryland Avenue, SW, Suite 100 West, Washington, DC 20024. (800) 274-4262. <http://www.nursingworld.org>.

Center for Bioethics at the University of Pennsylvania. Suite 320, 3401 Market Street, Philadelphia, PA 19104-3308. (215) 898-7136. <http://bioethics.org>.

National Committee for Quality Assurance. 2000 L St. NW, Washington, DC 20036. (202) 955-3500. <http://www.ncqa.org>.

OTHER

American Academy of Pediatrics. [cited March 24, 2003]. <http://www.aap.org/family/mancarbr.htm>.

Centers for Medicare & Medicaid Services. [cited March 24, 2003] <http://www.medicare.gov/choices/withdraws.asp>.

National Committee for Quality Assurance. [cited March 24, 2003] <http://www.ncqa.org>.

Pennsylvania Health Law Project. [cited March 24, 2003] <http://www.phlp.org/education/managedcareeast.html>.

L. Fleming Fallon, Jr, MD, DrPH

Marshall-Marchetti-Krantz procedure *see* **Retropubic suspension**

Mastectomy *see* **Lumpectomy; Modified radical mastectomy; Axillary dissection; Simple mastectomy; Quadrantectomy**

Mastoid tympanoplasty *see* **Mastoidectomy**

Mastoidectomy

Definition

A mastoidectomy is a surgical procedure that removes an infected portion of the mastoid bone when medical treatment is not effective.

Purpose

A mastoidectomy is performed to remove infected mastoid air cells resulting from ear infections, such as mastoiditis or chronic otitis, or by inflammatory disease of the middle ear (cholesteatoma). The mastoid air cells are open spaces containing air that are located throughout the mastoid bone, the prominent bone located behind the ear that projects from the temporal bone of the skull. The air cells are connected to a cavity in the upper part of the bone, which is in turn connected to the middle ear. Aggressive infections in the middle ear can thus sometimes spread through the mastoid bone. When **antibiotics** can't clear this infection, it may be necessary to remove the infected area by surgery. The primary goal of the surgery is to completely remove infection so as to produce an infection-free ear. Mastoidectomies are also performed sometimes to repair paralyzed facial nerves.

Demographics

According to the American Society for Microbiology, middle ear infections increased in the United States from approximately three million cases in 1975 to over nine million in 1997. Middle ear infections are now the second leading cause of office visits to physicians, and this diagnosis accounts for over 40% of all outpatient antibiotic use. Ear infections arc also very common in children between the ages of six months and two years. Most children have at least one ear infection before their eighth birthday.

Description

A mastoidectomy is performed with the patient fully asleep under general anesthesia. There are several different types of mastoidectomy procedures, depending on the amount of infection present:

- Simple (or closed) mastoidectomy. The operation is performed through the ear or through a cut (incision) behind the ear. The surgeon opens the mastoid bone and removes the infected air cells. The eardrum is incised to drain the middle ear. Topical antibiotics are then placed in the ear.

- Radical mastoidectomy. The procedure removes the most bone and is usually performed for extensive spread of a cholesteatoma. The eardrum and middle ear structures may be completely removed. Usually the stapes, the "stirrup" shaped bone, is spared if possible to help preserve some hearing.

- Modified radical mastoidectomy. In this procedure, some middle ear bones are left in place and the eardrum is rebuilt by tympanoplasty.

After surgery, the wound is stitched up around a drainage tube and a dressing is applied.

Diagnosis/Preparation

The treating physician gives the patient a thorough ear, nose, and throat examination and uses detailed diagnostic tests, including an audiogram and imaging studies of the mastoid bone using x rays or **CT scans** to evaluate the patient for surgery.

The patient is prepared for surgery by shaving the hair behind the ear on the mastoid bone. Mild soap and a water solution are commonly used to cleanse the outer ear and surrounding skin.

Aftercare

The drainage tube inserted during surgery is typically removed a day or two later.

Painkillers are usually needed for the first day or two after the operation. The patient should drink fluids freely. After the stitches are removed, the bulky mastoid dressing can be replaced with a smaller dressing if the ear is still draining. The patient is given antibiotics for several days.

WHO PERFORMS THE PROCEDURE AND WHERE IS IT PERFORMED?

An mastoidectomy is performed in a hospital by surgeons specialized in otolaryngology, the branch of medicine concerned with the diagnosis and treatment of disorders and diseases of the ears, nose and throat. The procedure usually takes between two and three hours. It is occasionally performed on an outpatient basis in adults but usually involves hospitalization.

The patient should inform the physician if any of the following symptoms occur:

- bright red blood on the dressing

- stiff neck or disorientation (These may be signs of meningitis.)

- facial paralysis, drooping mouth, or problems swallowing

Risks

Complications do not often occur, but they may include:

- persistent ear discharge

- infections, including meningitis or brain abscesses

- hearing loss

- facial nerve injury (This is a rare complication.)

- temporary dizziness

- temporary loss of taste on the side of the tongue

Normal results

The outcome of a mastoidectomy is a clean, healthy ear without infection. However, both a modified radical and a radical mastoidectomy usually result in less than normal hearing. After surgery, a hearing aid may be considered if the patient so chooses.

Morbidity and mortality rates

In the United States, death from intracranial complications of cholesteatoma is uncommon due to earlier recognition, timely surgical intervention, and supportive antibiotic therapy. Cholesteatoma remains a relatively common cause of permanent, moderate, and conductive hearing loss.

Alternatives

Alternatives to mastoidectomy include the use of medications and delaying surgery. However, these alternative methods carry their own risk of complications and a varying degree of success. Thus, most physicians are of the opinion that patients for whom mastoidectomy is indicated should best undergo the operation, as it provides the patient with the best chance of successful treatment and the lowest risk of complications.

See also Tympanoplasty.

Resources

BOOKS

Fisch, H. and J. May. *Tympanoplasty, Mastoidectomy, and Stapes Surgery.* New York: Thieme Medical Pub., 1994.

PERIODICALS

Cristobal, F., Gomez-Ullate, R., Cristobal, I., Arcocha, A., and R. Arroyo. "Hearing results in the second stage of open mastoidectomy: A comparison of the different techniques." *Otolaryngology - Head and Neck Surgery* 122 (May 2000): 350-351.

Garap, J. P., and S. P. Dubey. "Canal-down mastoidectomy: experience in 81 cases." *Otology & Neurotology* 22 (July 2001): 451-456.

Jang, C. H. "Changes in external ear resonance after mastoidectomy: open cavity mastoid versus obliterated mastoid cavity." *Clinical Otolaryngology* 27 (December 2002): 509-511.

Kronenberg, J., and L. Migirov. "The role of mastoidectomy in cochlear implant surgery." *Acta Otolaryngologica* 123 (January 2003): 219-222.

ORGANIZATIONS

American Academy of Otolaryngology-Head and Neck Surgery, Inc. One Prince St., Alexandria VA 22314-3357. (703) 836-4444. <http://www.entnet.org>.

American Hearing Research Foundation. 55 E. Washington St., Suite 2022, Chicago, IL 60602. (312) 726-9670. <http://www.american-hearing.org/>.

Better Hearing Institute. 515 King Street, Suite 420, Alexandria, VA 22314. (703) 684-3391.

OTHER

"Mastoidectomy series." *MedlinePlus.* <www.nlm.nih.gov/medlineplus/ency/presentations/100032_1.htm>.

Carol A. Turkington
Monique Laberge, Ph.D.

Maze procedure for atrial fibrillation

Definition

The Maze procedure, also known as the Cox-Maze procedure, is a surgical treatment for chronic atrial fibrillation. The procedure restores the heart's normal rhythm by surgically interrupting the conduction of abnormal impulses.

Purpose

When the heart beats too fast, blood no longer circulates effectively in the body. The Maze procedure is used to stop this abnormal beating so that the heart can begin its normal rhythm and pump more efficiently. The procedure is also intended to control heart rate and prevent blood clots and strokes.

Demographics

The Maze procedure has been performed since 1987 and was developed by Dr. James L. Cox. The average age of patients undergoing this procedure is about 52.

The Maze procedure is used to treat chronic or paroxysmal atrial fibrillation, a type of abnormal heart rhythm in which the upper chamber of the heart quivers instead of pumping in an organized way. In general, patients usually have atrial fibrillation for about eight years before undergoing the Maze procedure. The Maze procedure may be recommended for patients who need surgical treatment for coronary artery disease or valve disease. Therefore, the Maze procedure may be performed in combination with coronary artery bypass surgery (CABG), valve repair, valve replacement, or other cardiac surgery.

The Maze procedure may be recommended for patients whose atrial fibrillation has not been successfully treated with medications or other non-surgical interventional procedures. It may also be a treatment option for patients who have a history of stroke or cardiac thrombus.

Abnormal heart rhythms are slightly more common in men than in women, and the prevalence of abnormal heart rhythms, especially atrial fibrillation, increases with age. Atrial fibrillation is relatively uncommon in people under age 20.

Description

Elective Maze surgery is usually scheduled in advance. After arriving at the hospital, an intravenous (IV) catheter will be placed in the arm to deliver medications and fluids. General anesthesia is administered to put the patient to sleep.

In most cases, a traditional incision is made down the center of the patient's chest, cuts through the breastbone (sternum), and the rib cage is retracted open to expose the heart. The patient is connected to a heart-lung bypass machine, also called a cardiopulmonary bypass pump, which takes over for the heart and lungs during the surgery. The heart-lung machine removes carbon dioxide from the blood and replaces it with oxygen. A tube is inserted into the aorta to carry the oxygenated blood from the bypass machine to the aorta for circulation to the body. The heart-lung machine allows the heart's beating to be stopped so the surgeon can operate on a still heart.

Some patients may be candidates for off-pump surgery, in which the surgery is performed without the

use of a heart-lung bypass machine. This is also called beating heart surgery.

The Maze surgery may be an option for some patients. The minimally invasive technique enables the surgeon to work on the heart through small chest holes called ports and other small incisions. Advantages of minimally invasive surgery over the traditional method include smaller incisions, a shorter hospital stay, a shorter recovery period, and lower costs.

During the procedure, precise incisions, also called lesions, are made in the right and left atria to isolate and stop the unusual electrical impulses from forming. The incisions form a maze through which the impulses can travel in one direction from the top of the heart to the bottom. When the heart heals, scar tissue forms and the abnormal electrical impulses can no longer travel through the heart.

These energy sources may be used during the procedure:

• Radiofrequency: A radiofrequency energy catheter is used to create the incisions or lesions in the heart.

• Microwave: A wand-like catheter is used to direct microwave energy to create the lesions in the heart.

• Cryothermy (also called cryoablation): Very cold temperatures are transmitted through a probe (cryoprobe) to create the lesions.

When these energy sources are used, the procedure is called surgical pulmonary vein isolation.

Diagnosis/Preparation

Diagnosis of abnormal heart rhythms

A doctor may be able to detect an irregular heartbeat during a physical exam by taking the patient's pulse. In

QUESTIONS TO ASK THE DOCTOR

- Am I a candidate for minimally invasive surgery?

- Am I a candidate for the "off-pump" surgery technique?

- Who will be performing the surgery? How many years of experience does this surgeon have? How many other Maze procedures has this surgeon performed?

- Can I take my medications the day of the surgery?

- Can I or drink the day of the surgery? If not, how long before the surgery should I stop eating and/or drinking?

- How long will I have to stay in the hospital after the surgery?

- After I go home from the hospital, how long will it take me to recover from surgery?

- What should I do if I experience symptoms similar to those I felt before surgery?

- What types of symptoms should I report to my doctor?

- What types of medications will I have to take after surgery?

- When will I be able I resume my normal activities, including work and driving?

- When will I find out if the surgery was successful?

- What if the surgery was not successful?

- If I have had the surgery once, can I have it again to correct future blockages?

- Will I have any pain or discomfort after the surgery? If so, how can I relieve this pain or discomfort?

- Are there any medications, foods, or activities I should avoid to prevent my symptoms from recurring?

- How often do I need to see my doctor for follow-up visits after the surgery?

addition, the diagnosis may be based upon the presence of certain symptoms, including:

- palpitations (feeling of skipped heartbeats or fluttering in the chest)

- pounding in the chest

- shortness of breath

- chest discomfort

- fainting

- dizziness or feeling light-headed

- weakness, fatigue, or feeling tired

Not everyone with abnormal heart rhythms will experience symptoms, so the condition may be discovered upon examination for another medical condition.

DIAGNOSTIC TESTS. Tests used to diagnose an abnormal heart rhythm or determine its cause include:

- blood tests

- chest x rays

- electrocardiogram

- ambulatory monitors such as the Holter monitor, loop recorder, and trans-telephonic transmitter

- stress test

- echocardiogram

- cardiac catheterization

- electrophysiology study (EPS)

- head-upright tilt table test

- nuclear medicine test such as a **MUGA scan** (multiple-gated acquisition scanning)

Preparation

During a preoperative appointment, usually scheduled within one to two weeks before surgery, the patient will receive information about what to expect during the surgery and the recovery period. The patient will usually meet the cardiologist, anesthesiologist, nurse clinicians, and surgeon during this appointment or just before the procedure.

Medication to thin the blood (blood thinner or anticoagulant) is usually given for at least three weeks before the procedure.

If the patient develops a cold, fever, or sore throat within a few days before the surgery, he or she should notify the surgeon's office.

From midnight before the surgery, the patient should not eat or drink anything.

The morning of the procedure, the patient should take all usual medications as prescribed, with a small sip of water, unless other instructions have been given. Patients who take diabetes medications or anticoagulants should ask their doctor for specific instructions.

The patient is usually admitted to the hospital the same day the surgery is scheduled. The patient should bring a list of current medications, allergies, and appropriate medical records upon **admission to the hospital**.

The morning of surgery, the chest area is shaved and heart monitoring begins. The patient is given general anesthesia before the procedure, so he or she will be asleep during the procedure.

The traditional Maze procedure takes about an hour to perform, while the surgical pulmonary vein isolation procedure generally takes only a few minutes to perform. However, the preparation and recovery time add a few hours to both procedures. The total time in the **operating room** for each of these procedures is about three to four hours.

Aftercare

Recovery in the hospital

The patient recovers in a surgical **intensive care unit** for one to two days after the surgery. The patient will be connected to chest and breathing tubes, a mechanical ventilator, a heart monitor, and other monitoring equipment. A urinary catheter will be in place to drain urine. The breathing tube and ventilator are usually removed about six hours after surgery, but the other tubes usually remain in place as long as the patient is in the intensive care unit.

Drugs are prescribed to control pain and to prevent unwanted blood clotting. Daily doses of **aspirin** are started within six to 24 hours after the procedure.

The patient is closely monitored during the recovery period. **Vital signs** and other parameters such as heart sounds and oxygen and carbon dioxide levels in arterial blood are checked frequently. The chest tube is checked to ensure that it is draining properly. The patient may be fed intravenously for the first day or two.

Chest physiotherapy is started after the ventilator and breathing tube are removed. The therapy includes coughing, turning frequently, and taking deep breaths. Sometimes oxygen is delivered via a mask to help loosen and clear secretions from the lungs. Other exercises will be encouraged to improve the patient's circulation and prevent complications from prolonged bed rest.

If there are no complications, the patient begins to resume a normal routine around the second day. This includes eating regular food, sitting up, and walking around a bit. Before being discharged from the hospital, the patient usually spends a few days under observation in a non-surgical unit. During this time, counseling is usually provided on eating right and starting a light **exercise** program to keep the heart healthy.

The average hospital stay after the Maze surgery is five to seven days, depending on the patient's rate of recovery.

Recovery at home

MEDICATIONS. The doctor may prescribe anti-arrhythmic medications (such as beta-blockers, digitalis, or calcium channel blockers) to prevent the abnormal heart rhythm from returning. Some patients may need to take a diuretic for four to eight weeks after surgery to reduce fluid retention that may occur after surgery. Potassium supplements may be prescribed along with the diuretic medications. Some patients may be prescribed anticoagulant medication such as warfarin and aspirin to reduce the risk of blood clots. The medications prescribed may be adjusted over time to determine the best dosage and type of medication so the abnormal heart rhythm is adequately controlled.

INCISION AND SKIN CARE. The incision should be kept clean and dry. When the skin is healed, the incision should be washed with soapy water. The scar should not be bumped, scratched, or otherwise disturbed. Ointments, lotions, and dressings should not be applied to the incision unless specific instructions have been given.

DISCOMFORT. While the incision scar heals, which takes one to two months, it may be sore. Itching, tightness, or numbness along the incision is common. Muscle or incision discomfort may occur in the chest during activity.

LIFESTYLE CHANGES. The patient needs to make several lifestyle changes after surgery, including:

• Quitting smoking. Smoking causes damage to blood vessels, increases the patient's blood pressure and heart rate, and decreases the amount of oxygen available in the blood.

• Managing weight. Maintaining a healthy weight, by watching portion sizes and exercising, is important. Being overweight increases the work of the heart.

• Participating in an exercise program. The cardiac rehabilitation exercise program is usually tailored for the patient, who will be supervised by fitness professionals.

• Making dietary changes. Patients should eat a lot of fruits, vegetables, grains, and non-fat or low-fat dairy products, and reduce fats to less than 30% of all calories.

• Taking medications as prescribed. Aspirin and other heart medications may be prescribed, and the patient may need to take these medications for life.

• Following up with health-care providers. An exercise test is often scheduled during one of the first follow-up visits to determine how effective the surgery was and to confirm that progressive exercise is safe. The patient needs to regularly see the physician for follow-up visits to monitor his or her recovery and control risk factors.

Risks

The Maze procedure is major surgery and patients may experience any of the normal complications associated with major surgery and anesthesia, such as the risk of bleeding, pneumonia, or infection. The risk of stroke is 1%. One common complication that has occurred early after surgery is fluid retention. However, **diuretics** are now prescribed to reduce the risk of this complication. To date, minimal long-term adverse effects have been reported in patients undergoing the Maze procedure.

Normal results

Full recovery from the Maze procedure takes six to eight weeks. Upon release from the hospital, the patient will feel weak because of the extended bed rest in the hospital. Within a few weeks, the patient should begin to feel stronger.

Most patients are able to drive in about three to four weeks, after receiving approval from their physician. Sexual activity can generally be resumed in three to four weeks, depending on the patient's rate of recovery.

It takes about six to eight weeks for the sternum to heal. During this time, the patient should not perform activities that cause pressure or put weight on the breastbone or tension on the arms and chest. Pushing and pulling heavy objects (such as mowing the lawn) should be avoided and lifting objects more than 20 lb (9 kg) is not permitted. The patient should not hold his or her arms above shoulder level for a long period of time. The patient should try not to stand in one place for longer than 15 minutes. Stair climbing is permitted unless other instructions have been given.

Within four to six weeks, people with sedentary office jobs can return to work; people with physical jobs (such as construction work or jobs requiring heavy lifting) must wait longer (up to 12 weeks).

In about 30% of all patients, atrial fibrillation will recur temporarily right after surgery. This is common. Medications are usually prescribed to control atrial fibrillation after surgery. About three months after the surgery, medications are often reduced and then stopped.

In about 7–10% of patients, a permanent pacemaker is needed as a result of the procedure or sometimes due to underlying sinus node dysfunction.

About 90–95% of patients have a return of normal heart rhythm within one year after the surgery. Among U.S. surgeons reporting their data in the January 2000 issue of Seminars in Thoracic and Cardiovascular Surgery, the overall success rate of the Maze procedure is from 90–97%. Some hospitals report a 95–98% success rate in lone atrial fibrillation patients (those who do not have any other underlying heart conditions) undergoing the traditional Maze procedure. An 80–90% success rate has been reported for the surgical pulmonary vein isolation procedure.

Morbidity and mortality rates

The overall operative mortality for patients undergoing the Maze procedure is 3%. The mortality rate increases among patients over age 65.

Atrial fibrillation is not immediately life threatening, but it can lead to other heart rhythm problems. Follow-up data from the Framingham Heart Study and the Anti-arrhythmia Versus Implantable Defibrillators Trial have shown that atrial fibrillation is a predictor of increased mortality.

According to a 2002 study published in the *New England Journal of Medicine*, controlling a patient's heart rate is as important as controlling the patient's heart rhythm to prevent death and complications from cardiovascular causes. The study also concluded that anticoagulant therapy is important to reduce the risk of stroke and is appropriate therapy in patients who have recurring, persistent atrial fibrillation even after they received treatment.

Alternatives

Health care providers usually try to correct the heart rhythm with medication and recommend lifestyle changes and other interventional procedures such as **cardioversion** before recommending the Maze procedure.

Lifestyle changes often recommended to treat abnormal heart rhythms include:

- quitting smoking
- avoiding activities that prompt the symptoms of abnormal heart rhythms
- limiting alcohol intake
- limiting or not using caffeine, which may produce more symptoms in some people with abnormal heart rhythms
- avoiding medications containing stimulants such as some cough and cold remedies

If the Maze procedure is not successful in restoring the normal heart rhythm, other treatments for abnormal heart rhythms include:

KEY TERMS

Ablation—The removal or destruction of tissue.

Ablation therapy—A procedure used to treat arrhythmias, especially atrial fibrillation.

Ambulatory monitors—Small portable electrocardiograph machines that record the heart's rhythm, and include the Holter monitor, loop recorder, and trans-telephonic transmitter.

Anti-arrhythmic—Medication used to treat abnormal heart rhythms.

Anticoagulant—A medication, also called a blood thinner, that prevents blood from clotting.

Atria—The right and left upper chambers of the heart.

Cardiac catheterization—An invasive procedure used to create x rays of the coronary arteries, heart chambers and valves.

Cardioversion—A procedure used to restore the heart's normal rhythm by applying a controlled electric shock to the exterior of the chest.

Echocardiogram—An imaging procedure used to create a picture of the heart's movement, valves and chambers.

Electrocardiogram (ECG, EKG)—A test that records the electrical activity of the heart using small electrode patches attached to the skin on the chest.

Electrophysiology study (EPS)—A test that evaluates the electrical activity within the heart.

Head-upright tilt table test—A test used to determine the cause of fainting spells.

Implantable cardioverter-defibrillator (ICD)—An electronic device that is surgically placed to constantly monitor the patient's heart rate and rhythm. If a very fast, abnormal heart rate is detected, the device delivers electrical energy to the heart to resume beating in a normal rhythm.

Nuclear imaging—Method of producing images by detecting radiation from different parts of the body after a radioactive tracer material is administered.

Pacemaker—A small electronic device implanted under the skin that sends electrical impulses to the heart to maintain a suitable heart rate and prevent slow heart rates.

Pulmonary vein isolation—A surgical procedure used to treat atrial fibrillation.

Stress test—A test used to determine how the heart responds to stress.

Ventricles—The lower pumping chambers of the heart; the heart has two ventricles: the right and the left.

- permanent pacemakers
- implantable cardioverter-defibrillator
- ablation therapy

Resources

BOOKS

McGoon, Michael D., ed. and Bernard J. Gersh. *Mayo Clinic Heart Book: The Ultimate Guide to Heart Health, Second Edition.* New York: William Morrow and Co., Inc., 2000.

Topol, Eric J. *Cleveland Clinic Heart Book: The Definitive Guide for the Entire Family from the Nation's Leading Heart Center.* New York: Hyperion, 2000.

Trout, Darrell, and Ellen Welch. *Surviving with Heart: Taking Charge of Your Heart Care.* Golden, CO: Fulcrum Publishing, 2002.

PERIODICALS

Benjamin, E. J., P. A. Wolf, R. B. D'Agostino, H. Silbershatz, W. B. Kannel, and D. Levy. "Impact of Atrial Fibrillation on the Risk of Death: The Framingham Heart Study." *Circulation,* 98 (1998): 946–952.

Wyse, D. G., et al. "Atrial Fibrillation: A Risk Factor for Increased Mortality—An AVID Registry Analysis." *Journal of Interventional Cardiac Electrophysiology,* 5 (2001): 267–273.

ORGANIZATIONS

American College of Cardiology. Heart House. 9111 Old Georgetown Rd., Bethesda, MD 20814-1699. (800) 253-4636 ext. 694 or (301) 897-5400. <http://www.acc.org>.

American Heart Association. 7272 Greenville Ave., Dallas, TX 75231. (800) 242-8721 or (214) 373-6300. <http://www.americanheart.org>.

The Cleveland Clinic Heart Center, The Cleveland Clinic Foundation. 9500 Euclid Avenue, F25, Cleveland, OH 44195. (800) 223-2273 ext. 46697 or (216) 444-6697. <http://www.clevelandclinic.org/heartcenter>.

National Heart, Lung and Blood Institute. National Institutes of Health. Building 1. 1 Center Dr., Bethesda, MD 20892. E-mail: <NHLBIinfo@rover.nhlbi.>. <http://www.nhlbi.nih.gov>.

Texas Heart Institute. Heart Information Service. P.O. Box 20345, Houston, TX 77225-0345. <http://www.tmc.edu/thi>.

North American Society of Pacing and Electrophysiology. 6 Strathmore Rd., Natick, MA 01760-2499. (508) 647-0100. <http://www.naspe.org>.

OTHER

About Atrial Fibrillation. <http://www.aboutatrialfibrillation.com>.
HeartCenterOnline. <http://www.heartcenteronline.com>.
The Heart: An Online Exploration. The Franklin Institute Science Museum. 222 North 20th Street, Philadelphia, PA, 19103. (215) 448-1200. <http://sln2.fi.edu/biosci/heart.html>.
Heart Information Network. <http://www.heartinfo.org>.
Heart Surgeon.com. <http:www.heartsurgeon.com>.

Angela M. Costello

Mean corpuscular hemoglobin *see* **Red blood cell indices**

Mean corpuscular volume *see* **Red blood cell indices**

Mechanical circulation support

Definition

Mechanical circulatory support is used to treat patients with advanced heart failure. A mechanical pump is surgically implanted to provide pulsatile or non-pulsatile flow of blood to supplement or replace the blood flow generated by the native heart. Types of circulatory support pumps include pneumatic and electromagnetic pumps. Rotary pumps are also available.

Purpose

Heart failure causes low cardiac output, which results in inadequate blood pressure and reduced blood flow to the brain, kidneys, heart, and/or lungs. Pharmaceutical and surgical treatments (other than transplantation) are all typically exhausted before mechanical circulatory support is initiated. The extent of failure exhibited by one or both ventricles of the heart determines if univentricular or biventricular support is required. In either case, blood flow is supplemented or replaced by a mechanical circulatory support device. The device works by removing blood from the inlet of the ventricle(s) and reinjecting it at the outlet of the ventricle(s) in order to increase blood pressure and blood flow to the brain, kidneys, heart, and lungs.

Some devices, along with the intra-aortic balloon pump (IABP), centrifugal pump, and extracorporeal membrane oxygenation (ECMO), are systems that are meant to sustain the patient until the heart recovers. If recovery does not occur, or is not expected, then **heart transplantation** becomes the next desired course of treatment. In this case, intermediate- to long-term mechanical circulatory support devices are required.

Description

Short-, intermediate-, and long-term support requires bedside monitoring of the equipment and patient throughout treatment. The specialized nature of the equipment and the intensive patient care require dedicated staff who are able to provide continuous bedside treatment.

In most instances, patients receive anticoagulants, drugs that prevent clots in the blood. Frequent laboratory testing determines the proper amount of medication required to prevent blood clots. To mimic the lining of blood vessels, some surfaces of the device attract the body's cells, which stick to the device surface and eliminate the need for anticoagulation.

Blood flow generated by these devices is able to sustain blood pressure and flow to the heart, kidneys, liver, and brain. Temporary assist devices sustain vital organ tissues in situations where recovery of the heart function is anticipated. Long-term support devices sustain patients until a donor heart is available for transplantation.

Short- to intermediate-term support devices

ECMO circulatory support provides cardiopulmonary bypass. Both cardiac and pulmonary (lung) function can be supplemented with this device. The complexity of care and the need for highly trained staff with specialized equipment limit the availability of ECMO to specialty care facilities. Surgical cannulation (placement of tubes) is required. **Postoperative care** in the critical care unit requires dedicated bedside staffing.

Blood flow to the lungs is reduced as blood is drained from the venous circulation. Blood pumped by the left ventricle is also reduced as blood is returned directly to the systemic circulation. The heart is allowed to rest, pumping less blood than needed to maintain pressure and flow to the vital organs. As cardiac function improves, flow from ECMO support is reduced, allowing the heart to gradually resume normal function. The cannulae are surgically removed from the patient once the heart can maintain adequate cardiac output. Systemic anticoagulation is required throughout the length of support, and often leads to complications of stroke and coagulapathies. Long-term use of ECMO is limited since the patient is immobilized and sedated during treatment.

Ease of insertion for placement in the aorta makes the intra-aorta balloon pump (IABP) the most often used **ventricular assist device**. Specialty care centers provide this service in the **cardiac catheterization** laboratory, **operating room**, critical care unit, and emergency room. Secondary-care-level hospitals can also employ this technology. Well-trained staff are required to monitor equipment at regular intervals and troubleshoot problems.

Left ventricular (the lower left chamber of the heart) support with the IABP reduces the workload of the heart and increases blood flow to the vital organs. The balloon inflates during diastole (the filling phase of the heart) to deliver increased oxygen-saturated blood to the heart; blood flow is also increased to the arteries. Deflation of the balloon occurs prior to systole (the emptying phase of the heart).

With recovery of the heart, the IABP device is timed to inflate with every second or third heart beat. The catheter is removed, non-surgically, when the heart can sustain blood pressure and systemic blood flow. Anticoagulation is achieved with minimal drugs throughout the treatment. The device can be in place up to several weeks, but duration is limited because the patient must be immobilized during the treatment.

Centrifugal pumps are able to provide support to one or both ventricles. Blood is removed from the left or right atrium (upper chamber) and returned to the aorta or pulmonary artery, respectively; therefore, surgery is required to place the device. Specialty care facilities have the staff and equipment to provide treatment to heart failure patients with the use of mechanical circulatory support devices. Postoperative care in critical care units requires continuous monitoring by dedicated staff.

The cannulae are passed through the chest wall to attach to a pump that draws blood into the device and propels it to the arterial cannula. As the heart recovers, blood flow is decreased from the centrifugal pump until the device can be removed. An anticoagulant drug is delivered continuously during treatment with a centrifugal pump, and patient immobilization limits the length of support to several weeks.

Intermediate- to long-term support devices

When short-term support devices such as ECMO, IABP, and the centrifugal pump are ineffective to sustain the patient to recovery or organ transplantation, a medium- or long-term device is required. An advantage of treatment with a medium- to long-term device is that it allows the patient to be mobile. In some instances, patients have been able to leave the hospital for continued treat-ment at home with the implanted device. Complete recovery of the heart has been demonstrated in 5–15% of patients being supported as a bridge to organ transplantation.

Pulsatile paracorporeal mechanical circulatory support devices provide pulsatile support for the left or right ventricle, or both. Cannulation of the left or right atrium, along with the aorta or pulmonary artery, respectively, requires a surgical approach. The heart is emptied of blood by the assist device, so there is little ejection from the body's heart.

Removal of the device occurs at the time of cardiac transplant, unless the body's heart has healed during support. Anticoagulation is achieved by low doses of drugs. Some patients regain mobility while assisted by these devices.

Destination therapies

Destination therapies intended to supplement or permanently replace the body's heart are provided by chronic implantation of the mechanical circulatory support system. For example, total artificial hearts (TAH) replace the body's heart. Upon removal of the native heart, the TAH will be attached to the major blood vessels, thereby supplying blood pressure and flow to both the pulmonary and systemic circulation. Destination therapies are currently in clinical trials, offering those patients not eligible for organ transplantation a promising future.

Preparation

General anesthetic is given to the patient if a chest incision will be used to expose the heart or if blood vessels need to be exposed. Sedation with local anesthetic is sufficient if the vessels can be accessed with a needle stick. Cardiac monitoring will be performed, including electrocardiograph and cardiovascular pressures. Blood tests prior to surgery are used to measure blood elements and electrolytes. Once all sterile connections are complete, the physician will request that mechanical circulatory support be initiated. Adjustments may be frequent initially, but decrease as the patient stabilizes.

Normal results

Once stable following device implant, the patient is cared for in the **intensive care unit** (ICU). Any change in patient status is reported to the physician. Around-the-clock bedside care is provided by trained nursing staff.

These patients are very ill when they require device implant, often suffering from multi-system organ failure as a result of poor blood flow. The long-term survival is superior at one year when compared to medical treatment alone. Patients that continue to improve on inter-

KEY TERMS

Anticoagulant—Pharmaceutical to prevent clotting proteins and platelets in the blood to be activated to form a blood clot.

Cannulae—Tubes that provide access to the blood once inserted into the heart or blood vessels.

Cardiac—Of or relating to the heart.

Cardiac output—The liter per minute blood flow generated by contraction of the heart.

Cardiopulmonary bypass—Diversion of blood flow away from the right atrium and return of blood beyond the left ventricle to bypass the heart and lungs.

mediate-, long-term, and TAH increase in activity level and begin a regular **exercise** program. Eventually, with proper training about device maintenance, they are able to leave the hospital to live at home, returning to a normal lifestyle, until further medical treatment is required.

Resources

BOOKS

DeBakey, Michael, and Antonio M. Gotto. *The New Living Heart*. Holbrook: Adams Media Corporation, 1997.

Gravelee, Glenn P., Richard F. Davis, Mark Kurusz, and Joe R. Utley. *Cardiopulmonary Bypass: Principles and Practice, Second Edition*. Philadelphia: Lippincott Williams & Wilkins, 2000.

PERIODICALS

Stevenson, Lynne W., et al. "Mechanical Cardiac Support 2000: Current Applications and Future Trial Design." *The Journal of Heart and Lung Transplantation* (January 2001): 1–38.

ORGANIZATIONS

Commission on Accreditation of Allied Health Education Programs. 1740 Gilpin St., Denver, CO 80218. (303) 320-7701. <http://www.caahep.org>.

Extracorporeal Life Support Organization (ELSO). 1327 Jones Dr., Ste. 101, Ann Arbor, MI 48105. (734) 998-6600. <http://www.elso.med.umich.edu/>.

Joint Commission on Accreditation of Health Organizations. One Renaissance Boulevard, Oakbrook Terrace, IL 60181. (630) 792-5000. <http://www.jcaho.org/>.

OTHER

"Spare Hearts: A Houston Chronicle Four-Part Series." *The Houston Chronicle* October 1997. <http://www.chron.com/content/chronicle/metropolitan/heart/index.html>.

Allison Joan Spiwak, BS, CCP

Mechanical ventilation

Definition

Mechanical ventilation is the use of a mechanical device (machine) to inflate and deflate the lungs.

Purpose

Mechanical ventilation provides the force needed to deliver air to the lungs in a patient whose own ventilatory abilities are diminished or lost.

Description

Breathing requires the movement of air into and out of the lungs. This is normally accomplished by the diaphragm and chest muscles. A variety of medical conditions can impair the ability of these muscles to accomplish this task, including:

• muscular dystrophies

• motor neuron disease, including ALS

• damage to the brain's respiratory centers

• polio

• myasthenia gravis

• myopathies affecting the respiratory muscles

• scoliosis

Mechanical ventilation may also be used when the airway is obstructed, especially at night in sleep apnea.

Mechanical ventilation may be required only at night, during limited daytime hours, or around the clock, depending on the patient's condition. Some patients require mechanical ventilation only for a short period, during recovery from traumatic nerve injury, for instance. Others require it chronically, and may increase the number of hours required over time as their disease progresses.

Mechanical ventilation is not synonymous with the use of an oxygen tank. Supplemental oxygen is used in patients whose gas exchange capacity has diminished, either through lung damage or obstruction of a major airway. For these patients, the muscles that deliver air work well, but too little oxygen can be exchanged in the remaining lung, and so a higher concentration is supplied with each breath. By the same token, many patients who require mechanical ventilation do not need supplemental oxygen. Their gas exchange capacity is normal, but they cannot adequately move air into and out of the lungs. In fact, excess oxygen may be dangerous, since it can suppress the normal increased respiration response to excess carbon dioxide in the lungs.

Mechanical ventilation systems come in a variety of forms. Almost all systems use a machine called a ventilator that pushes air through a tube for delivery to the patient's airways. The air may be delivered through a nasal or face mask, or through an opening in the trachea (windpipe), called a tracheostomy. Much rarer are systems that rhythmically change the pressure around a patient's chest when the pressure is low, air flows into the lungs, and when it increases, air flows out.

Ventilators

Ventilators can either deliver a set volume with each cycle, or can be set to a specific pressure regimen. Both are in common use. Volume ventilator settings are adjustable for total volume delivered, timing of delivery, and whether the delivery is mandatory or determined by the patient's initial inspiratory effort.

Pressure ventilators deliver one of two major pressure regimens. Continuous positive airway pressure (CPAP) delivers a steady pressure of air, which assists the patient's inspiration (breathing in) and resists expiration (breathing out). The pressure of CPAP is not sufficient to completely inflate the lungs; instead its purpose is to maintain an open airway, and for this reason it is used in sleep apnea, in which a patient's airway closes frequently during sleep.

Bilevel positive airway pressure (BiPAP) delivers a higher pressure on inspiration, helping the patient obtain a full breath, and a low pressure on expiration, allowing the patient to exhale easily. BiPAP is a common choice for neuromuscular disease.

The choice of ventilator type is partly determined by the knowledge and preferences of the treating physician. Settings are adjusted to maintain patient comfort and appropriate levels of oxygen and carbon dioxide in the blood.

Masks vs. tracheostomy

Delivery of air from a ventilator may be either through a mask firmly held to the face, or through a tube inserted into the trachea toward the bottom of the throat. A mask interface is called noninvasive ventilation, while a tracheostomy tube is called invasive ventilation.

Until the mid-1990s, invasive ventilation was the option used by virtually all patients requiring long-term mechanical ventilation. For some patients, tracheostomy continues to be a preferred option. It is commonly used when 24-hour ventilation assistance is required, and may

be preferred by patients who find masks uncomfortable or unsightly. Some patients feel ventilation through a "trach tube" is more reassuring. Tracheostomy is also the preferred option for most patients with swallowing difficulties. The potential to choke and suffocate on improperly swallowed food is avoided with a tracheostomy.

Tracheostomies may require more frequent suctioning of airway secretions, produced in response to the presence of the tube and the inflatable cuff that some patients require to hold it in place. The risk of infection is higher, and air must be carefully humidified and cleaned, since these functions are not being served by the nasal passages. Tracheostomies do not prevent speech, despite misinformation to the contrary that even some doctors believe. Speech requires passage of air around the trach tube, which can occur either with an uncuffed tube, or with the presence of a special valve that allows air passage past the cuff.

Noninvasive interfaces come in a variety of forms. A simple mouthpiece may be used, which a patient bites down on to seal the lips around the tube as the pressure cycle delivers a breath. Most masks are individually fitted to the patient's face, and held in place with straps. A tight fit is essential, since the pressure must be delivered to the patient's lungs, and not be allowed to blow out the sides of the mask. Masks may be used around the clock. Nasal masks do not prevent speech, though the tone may change. Oral or full-face masks do interfere with speech, and are typically used at night or intermittently throughout the day, for patients who do not need continuous ventilation assistance.

Other alternatives

The iron lung was an early mechanical ventilation device, and is still in use in some hospitals. The patient's head remains outside of it, while the interior depressurizes. This allows air to push in to the lungs. Repressurizing deflates the lungs again.

A device that works on the same principle is the chest shell (something like a turtle's shell swung around to the front). The pneumobelt applies pressure to deflate, and relaxes it to allow inflation. A rocking bed is used for nighttime ventilation. Tilting the head of the bed down deflates the lungs by allowing the abdominal contents to press against the diaphragm. Reversing the angle reverses the process, allowing inflation.

Preparation

Patients with diseases in which mechanical ventilation may be required are advised to learn as much as possible about treatment options before they become necessary. In particular, it is important to learn about and make decisions about invasive vs. noninvasive ventilation before the time comes. Many patients who begin ventilation with emergency tracheostomy have a difficult time switching to noninvasive ventilation later on (though it is certainly possible).

It is often a good idea to try out different masks and other interfaces before their need arises, and to have these fitted in preparation for a planned transition to the ventilator. Patients can find support groups and other sources of information to learn more about the options and the features of each means of ventilation. Patients may have to help educate their doctors if they are not familiar with noninvasive options.

Patients with neuromuscular disease may have as much or more need for a deep cough as they do for ventilatory assistance, and many patients who undergo emergency tracheostomy do so because their airways have become clogged with mucus build up. Physical therapy cough assistance and a cough assist device are important options for full respiratory health.

Normal results

Mechanical ventilation is a life saver, and provides comfort and confidence to patients who require it. Proper ventilation restores levels of oxygen and carbon dioxide in the blood, improving sleep at night and increasing the ability to engage in activities during the day. When combined with proper respiratory hygiene, it can prolong life considerably. Patients with progressive diseases such as ALS may wish to consider end-of-life decisions before commencing mechanical ventilation, or before the ability to communicate is lost.

Resources

BOOKS

Bach, John R. *Noninvasive Mechanical Ventilation*. Hanley and Belfus, 2002.

Kinnear, W. J. M. *Assisted Ventilation at Home: A practical Guide*. Oxford: Oxford Medical Publications, 1994.

PERIODICALS

Robinson, R. "A Breath of Fresh Air." *Quest Magazine* 5 (October 1998) [cited July 1, 2003]. <http://www.mdausa.org/publications/Quest/q56freshair.html>.

Robinson, R. "Breathe Easy." *Quest Magazine* 5(October 1998) [cited July 1, 2003]. <http://www.mdausa.org/publica tions/Quest/q55breathe.html>.

ORGANIZATIONS

ALS Association. 27001 Agoura Road, Suite 150 Calabasas Hills, CA 91301-5104. (800) 782-4747. <http://www.alsa.org>.

Muscular Dystrophy Association. 3300 E. Sunrise Drive Tucson, AZ 85718. (800) 572-1717. <http://www.mdausa.org>.

Richard Robinson

Meckel's diverticulectomy

Definition

Meckel's diverticulectomy is a surgical procedure that isolates and removes an abnormal diverticulum (Meckel's diverticulum) or pouch, as well as surrounding tissue, in the lining of the small intestine. It is performed to remove an obstruction, adhesions, infection, or inflammation.

Purpose

Meckel's diverticulum is an intestinal diverticulum (pouch) that results from the inability of the vitteline (umbilical) duct to close at five weeks of embryonic development. The vitteline duct is lined with layers of intestinal tissue containing cells that can develop into many different forms, called pluripotent cells. Meckel's diverticulum is a benign congenital condition that has no symptoms for some people, and develops complications in others.

Ninety percent of diverticula are close to the ileocecal valve in the upper intestine, and tissue made up predominantly of gastric and pancreatic cells is thought to cause chemical changes in the mucosa, or lining of the intestines.

The most common cells found in the mucosa of diverticula are gastric cells (present in 50% of all Meckel's diverticulum cases). The highly acidic secretions of gastric tissue may cause the early symptoms of Meckel's diverticulum. The alkaline secretions of pancreatic tissue are also thought to be a source of diverticula inflammation in a small number—about 5%—of cases.

Inflammation of the diverticula or infection of the intestines around the diverticula results in a condition known as diverticulitis, which may be treated with **antibiotics**. However, when it is acute and causes obstructions and bleeding, surgery is the treatment of choice.

Demographics

Meckel's diverticulum is present in approximately 2% of the population. It is the most commonly encountered congenital anomaly of the small intestine. Although the abnormality occurs in both sexes, men have

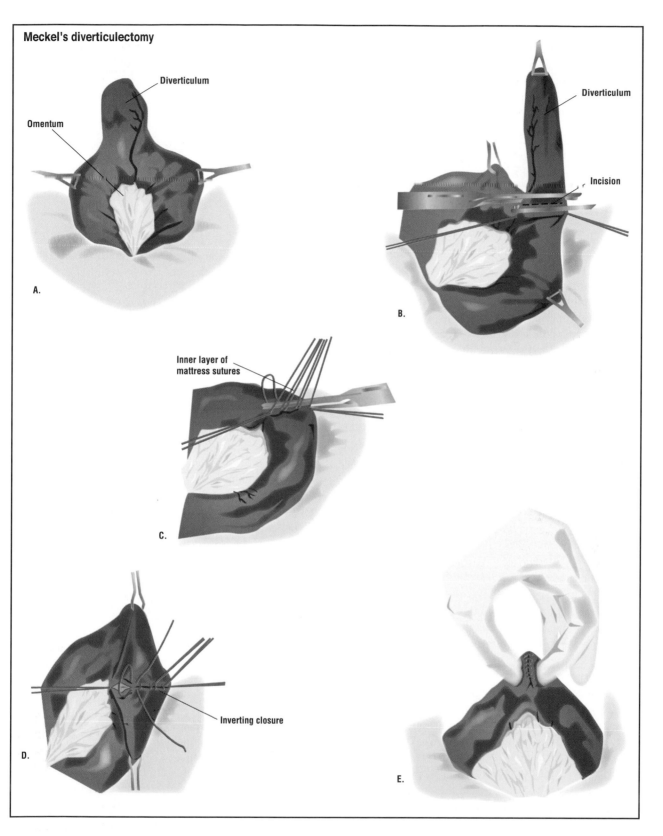

Meckel's diverticulectomy

During Meckel's diverticulectomy, the abdomen is opened above the area of the diverticulum, which is exposed along with the bowel (A). The diverticulum is clamped off at the base, and then cut off (B). Two layers of stitches are used to repair the bowel (C and D). *(Illustration by GGS Inc.)*

WHO PERFORMS THE PROCEDURE AND WHERE IS IT PERFORMED?

Surgery takes place in a hospital setting by a physician with advanced training in surgery and gastrointestinal surgery. If the surgery is minimally invasive, requiring only small incisions, it may be performed in an outpatient surgical area of the hospital.

QUESTIONS TO ASK THE DOCTOR

• Is this surgery necessary or can changing the diet and medical treatment be just as effective?

• Because this surgery was on an emergency basis, how extensive was the surgery and how much of the intestine was removed?

more frequent complications with the condition and are more often diagnosed with it. One 15-year study set the complication risk of the abnormality at 4.2%. A recent 10-year study done retrospectively reported an even age distribution for complications of the diverticulum. Malignancy is found in only 0.5–4.9% of patients with complications of Meckell's diverticulum.

Description

Open surgery of the intestines is indicated in acute cases. In the surgery, the intestinal segment containing the diverticulum, usually the ileum or upper intestines, is removed. After the diverticulum is removed, the healthy portions of the intestine are joined together. Some debate exists about whether surgery for asymptomatic Meckel's diverticulum found incidentally is recommended. Some researchers have shown that preventive removal of the diverticulum is less risky than surgical complications, and point to the fact that 6.4% of patients with Meckel's diverticulum develop complications of the condition over their lifetime.

Depending on the surgeon's decision, the operation may be minimal, isolating and then removing the pouch containing the inflammation, or it may be more extensive. In the latter cases, surrounding tissue is removed due to the presence of pervasive inflammation, obstruction, or incarceration in an inguinal hernia (Littre's hernia). Removing additional tissue is done to prevent recurrences. Recent studies have demonstrated the feasibility of laparoscopic, or minimally invasive diverticulectomy, utilizing small incisions and video imagery via tiny cameras. No long-term studies of this procedure have been conducted.

Surgery is performed under general anesthetic. The small intestine is isolated and the diverticulum is removed, sometimes with a small segment of the intestines. Operative techniques are used to conjoin the end sections of the intestines that have been severed.

Some surgeons prefer to perform two surgeries, and do not join together the intestinal sections until some healing of the segments has occurred. In this case, a stoma, or temporary outlet for tubal connection to the intestines, is created in the wall of the abdomen where an external appliance, called an ostomy, can receive waste until the intestinal sections are rejoined.

Diagnosis/Preparation

The vast majority of Meckel's diverticulum diagnoses are incidental, that is, discovered during barium studies, abdominal surgery for other conditions, or autopsy. The most common symptom of the condition is intestinal bleeding, which occurs in 25–50% of patients who have complications. Hemorrhage is the most significant symptom in children two years old and younger. Intestinal obstructions are common, resulting from complications of the tissue surrounding the diverticula. Symptomatic Meckel's diverticulum has symptoms similar to appendicitis. Lower abdominable pain or diverculitits accounts for 10–20% of cases, and requires careful diagnosis to distinguish it from appendicitis. Left untreated, diverticulitis can lead to perforation of the intestine and peritonitis.

Patients who have diverticulitis symptoms, such as acute abdominal pain are given various imaging tests, including a CT scan, **colonoscopy**, or a **sigmoidoscopy** (view of the lower colon through a tiny video instrument placed in the rectum). For children, a special chemical diagnostic test of sodium Tc-pertechnetate, a radioisotope that reacts to the mucosa in the diverticulum, allows inflammation or infection to be viewed radiographically. In adult patients, barium studies may help with diagnosis. When acute hemorrhaging is present, MR imaging of blood vessels is an effective diagnostic tool.

If surgery is indicated for Meckel's diverticulum, an enema is given (unless contraindicated by complications) to completely clear the bowel and avoid infection during surgery.

Aftercare

Intestinal surgery is a serious procedure, and recovery may take two weeks. The number of postoperative days spent in the hospital depends on the extent of the diverticulum surgery and complications of the condition prior to surgery. Barring complications, patients usually stay in the hospital for about one week. Immediately after surgery, the patient is observed carefully, and given intravenous fluids and antibiotics. Surgical catheters, or stents, are removed over the next two days, with food by mouth offered once bowel sounds are heard.

Risks

Intestinal surgery has the surgical complications associated with any open surgery. These include lung and heart complications, as well as reactions to medications, bleeding, and infection.

Normal results

The usual results of this surgery are an end to obstruction, pain, and infection. Highly successful results include the return of bowel function and daily activities.

Morbidity and mortality rates

Patients with complications of Meckel's diverticulum have a 10–12% incidence of early postoperative complications such as an intestinal leak, a suture line leak or intra-abdominal abscess. Later complications occur in about 7% of patients, and include bowel obstructions and intestinal adhesions. The reported mortality rate for surgery on patients with symptomatic diverticulum is 2–5%. With asymptomatic patients who undergo incidental diverticulectomy, both early and late complications occur in 2% of cases, and the mortality rate is 1%.

Alternatives

Diverticulitis is routinely treated with a change in diet that includes increasing bulk with high-fiber foods and bulk additives like Metamucil. Recurrent attacks, perforation, tissue adhesions, or infections are initially treated with antibiotics, a liquid diet, and bed rest. If medical treatment does not clear the complications, **emergency surgery** may be required.

Resources

BOOKS

Townsend, Courtney M. "Diverticular Disease" In *Sabiston Textbook of Surgery* 16th ed. W. B. Saunders Company, 2001.

KEY TERMS

Diverticulitis—Inflammation or infection of the diverticula of the intestines.

Diverticulum—Pouches or bulges of tissue in the lining of organs or canals that can become infected, especially in the intestines and esophagus.

Littre's hernia—A Meckel's diverticulum incarcerated in an inguinal hernia.

Merkel's diverticulum—Tissue faults in the lining of the intestines that are the result of a congenital abnormality originating in the umbilical duct's failure to close. Largely asymptomatic, the diverticula in some cases can become infected or obstructed.

Perforation—The rupture or penetration by injury or infection of the lining of an organ or canal that allows infection to spread into a body cavity, as in peritonitis, the infection of the lining of the stomach or intestines.

PERIODICALS

"Laparoscopy-assisted Resection of Complicated Meckel's Diverticulum in Adults." *Surgical Laparoscopy, Endoscopy and Percutaneous Techniques* 12(3) (June 1, 2000): 190-4.

"Meckel's Diverticulum." *American Family Physician* 61(4) (February 15, 2000).

ORGANIZATIONS

International Foundation for Functional Gastrointestinal Disorders (IFFGD).P.O. Box 170864, Milwaukee, WI 53217-8076. (888) 964-2001 or (414) 964-1799. fax: (414) 964-7176. <http://www.iffgd.org>.

National Digestive Diseases Information Clearinghouse. 2 Information Way, Bethesda, Maryland 20892-3570. <http://www.niddk.nih.gov>.

OTHER

"Meckel's diverticulectomy." *MedlinePlus* <http://www.nlm.nih/medlineplus.gov>.

Nancy McKenzie, Ph.D.

Mediastinoscopy

Definition

Mediastinoscopy is a surgical procedure that allows physicians to view areas of the mediastinum, the cavity behind the sternum (breastbone) that lies between the lungs. The organs in the mediastinum include the heart and its vessels, the lymph nodes, trachea, esophagus, and thymus.

Mediastinoscopy is most commonly used to detect or stage cancer. It is also ordered to detect infection, and to confirm diagnosis of certain conditions and diseases of the respiratory organs. The procedure involves insertion of an endotracheal (within the trachea) tube, followed by a small incision in the chest. A mediastinoscope is inserted through the incision. The purpose of this equipment is to allow the physician to directly see the organs inside the mediastinum, and to collect tissue samples for laboratory study.

Purpose

Mediastinoscopy is often the diagnostic method of choice for detecting lymphoma, including Hodgkin's disease. The diagnosis of sarcoidosis (a chronic lung disease) and the staging of lung cancer can also be accomplished through mediastinoscopy. Lung cancer staging involves a determination of the level or progression of the cancer into stages. These stages help a physician study cancer and provide consistent cancer definition levels and corresponding treatments. They also provide some guidance as to prognosis. The lymph nodes in the mediastinum are likely to reveal if lung cancer has spread beyond the lungs. Mediastinoscopy allows a physician to observe and extract a sample from the nodes for further study. Involvement of these lymph nodes indicates the diagnosis and stage of lung cancer.

Mediastinoscopy may also be ordered to verify a diagnosis that was not clearly confirmed by other methods, such as certain radiographic and laboratory studies. Mediastinoscopy may aid in some surgical biopsies of nodes or cancerous tissue in the mediastinum. In fact, a surgeon may immediately perform a surgical procedure if a malignant tumor is confirmed while the patient is undergoing mediastinoscopy. In these cases, the diagnostic exam and surgical procedure are combined into one operation.

Mediastinoscopy provides a diagnosis in 10–75% of cases, depending on histology, location, and size of cancer. The false positive rate, however can be as high as 20%.

Demographics

Approximately 130,000 new pulmonary nodules are diagnosed each year in the United States. Of those, half are malignant. The majority of pulmonary nodules are diagnosed via mediastinoscopy.

Description

Mediastinoscopy is usually performed in a hospital under general anesthesia. Before the general anesthesia is administered, local anesthesia is applied to the throat while an endotracheal tube is inserted. Once the patient is under general anesthesia, a small incision is made, usually just below the neck or at the notch at the top of the sternum. The surgeon may clear a path and feel the person's lymph nodes first to evaluate any abnormalities within the nodes. Next, the physician inserts the mediastinoscope through the incision. The scope is a narrow, hollow tube with an attached light that allows the surgeon to see inside the area. The surgeon can insert tools through the hollow tube to help perform biopsies. A tissue sample from the lymph nodes or a mass can be removed and sent for study under a microscope, or to a laboratory for further testing.

In some cases, tissue sample analysis that shows malignancy will suggest the need for immediate surgery while the person is already prepared and under anesthesia. In other cases, the surgeon will complete the visual study and tissue removal, and stitch the small incision closed. The person will remain in the surgerical recovery area until the effects of anesthesia have lessened and it is safe to leave the area. The entire procedure should require about an hour, not counting preparation and recovery time. Studies have shown that mediastinoscopy is a safe, thorough, and cost-effective diagnostic tool with less risk than some other procedures.

Diagnosis/Preparation

Because mediastinoscopy is a surgical procedure, it should only be performed when the benefits of the exam's findings outweigh the risks of surgery and anesthesia. Individuals who previously had mediastinoscopy should not receive it again if there is scarring from the first exam.

Several other medical conditions, such as impaired cerebral circulation, obstruction or distortion of the upper airway, or thoracic aortic aneurysm (abnormal dilation of the thoracic aorta) may also preclude mediastinoscopy. Certain structures in a person's anatomy that can be compressed by the mediastinoscope may complicate these pre-existing medical conditions.

Patients are asked to sign a consent form after reviewing the risks of mediastinoscopy and known risks and reactions to anesthesia. The physician will normally instruct the patient to fast from midnight before the test until after the procedure is completed. A physician may also prescribe a sedative the night before the exam and again before the procedure. Often a local anesthetic will be applied to the throat to prevent discomfort during placement of the endotracheal tube.

Aftercare

Following mediastinoscopy, patients will be carefully monitored and watched for changes in **vital signs**, or symptoms of complications from the procedure or anesthesia. The patient may have a sore throat from the endotracheal tube, experience temporary chest pain, and have soreness or tenderness at the incision site.

Risks

Complications from the actual mediastinoscopy procedure are relatively rare. The overall complication rates in various studies have been reported in the range of 1.3–3%. However, the following complications, in decreasing order of frequency, have been reported:

• hemorrhage

• pneumothorax (air in the pleural space)

• recurrent laryngeal nerve injury, causing hoarseness

• infection

• tumor implantation in the wound

• phrenic nerve injury (injury to a thoracic nerve)

• esophageal injury

• chylothorax (chyle is milky lymphatic fluid in the pleural space)

• air embolism (air bubble)

• transient hemiparesis (paralysis on one side of the body)

The usual risks associated with general anesthesia also apply to this procedure.

Normal results

In the majority of procedures performed to diagnose cancer, a normal result indicates the presence of small, smooth lymph nodes, and no abnormal tissue, growths, or signs of infection. In the case of lung cancer staging, results are related to the severity and progression of the cancer.

Morbidity and mortality rates

Abnormal findings may indicate lung cancer, tuberculosis, the spread of disease from one body part to another, sarcoidosis (a disease that causes nodules, usually affecting the lungs), lymphoma (abnormalities in the lymph tissues), and Hodgkin's disease.

Complications of mediastinoscopy include bleeding, pain, and post-procedure infection. These are relatively uncommon. Mortality is extremely rare.

Alternatives

A less invasive technique is ultrasound. However, it is not as specific as mediastinoscopy, and the information obtained is not as useful in making a diagnosis.

Although still performed, there is a decline in the use of mediastinoscopy as a result of advancements in computed tomography (CT), **magnetic resonance imaging** (MRI), and ultrasonography techniques. In addition, improved fine-needle aspiration (withdrawing fluid using suction) results of and core-needle biopsy (using a needle to obtain a small tissue sample) investigations, along with new techniques in thoracoscopy (examination of the thoracic cavity with a lighted instrument called a thoracoscope) offer additional options in examining masses in the mediastinum. Mediastinoscopy may be required when other methods cannot be used or when they provide inconclusive results.

See also Lung biopsy; Thoracic surgery.

Resources

BOOKS

Bland, K.I., W.G. Cioffi, M.G. Sarr, *Practice of General Surgery.* Philadelphia: Saunders, 2001.

Fischbach, F. and F. Talaska *A Manual of Laboratory and Diagnostic Tests* 6th ed. Philadelphia: Lippincott Williams and Wilkins, 2000.

KEY TERMS

Endotracheal—Placed within the trachea, also known as the windpipe.

Hodgkin's disease—A malignancy of lymphoid tissue found in the lymph nodes, spleen, liver, and bone marrow.

Lymph nodes—Small round structures located throughout the body; contain cells that fight infections.

Pleural space—Space between the layers of the pleura (membrane lining the lungs and thorax).

Sarcoidosis—A chronic disease characterized by nodules in the lungs, skin, lymph nodes, and bones; however, any tissue or organ in the body may be affected.

Thymus—An unpaired organ in the mediastinal cavity that is important in the body's immune response.

Grace, P.A., A. Cuschieri, D. Rowley, N. Borley, A. Darzi *Clinical Surgery* 2nd Edition. London: Blackwell Publishing, 2003.

Schwartz, S.I., J.E. Fischer, F.C. Spencer, G.T. Shires, J.M. Daly, J.M. *Principles of Surgery* 7th edition. New York: McGraw Hill, 1998.

Townsend, C., K.L. Mattox, R.D. Beauchamp, B.M. Evers, D.C. Sabiston *Sabiston's Review of Surgery* 3rd Edition. Philadelphia: Saunders, 2001.

PERIODICALS

Beadsmoore C.J., N.J. Screaton. "Classification, Ttaging and Prognosis of Lung Cancer." *European Journal of Radiology* 45(1) (2003): 8–17.

Choi, Y.S., Y.M. Shim, J. Kim, K. Kim. "Mediastinoscopy in Patients with Clinical Ctage I Non-small Cell Lung Cancer." *Annals of Thoracic Surgery* 75(2) (2003): 364–6.

Detterbeck, F.C., M.M. DeCamp, Jr., L.J. Kohman, G.A. Silvestri. "Lung cancer. Invasive staging: the guidelines." *Chest* 123(1 Suppl) (2003): 167S–175S.

Falcone F., F. Fois, D. Grosso. "Endobronchial Ultrasound." *Respiration* 70(2) (2003): 179–94.

Sterman, D.H., E. Sztejman, E. Rodriguez, J. Friedberg. "Diagnosis and Staging of 'Other Bronchial Tumors'." *Chest Surgery Clinics of North America* 13(1) (2003): 79–94.

ORGANIZATIONS

American Board of Surgery. 1617 John F. Kennedy Boulevard, Suite 860, Philadelphia, PA 19103. (215) 568-4000, fax: 215-563-5718. <http://www.absurgery.org>.

American Cancer Society. 1599 Clifton Rd. NE, Atlanta, GA 30329. (800) 227-2345, <http://www.cancer.org> .

American College of Surgeons. 633 North St. Clair Street, Chicago, IL 60611-32311. (312) 202-5000, fax: (312) 202-5001. <postmaster@facs.org>. <http://www.facs.org>.

American Lung Association. 1740 Broadway, New York, NY 10019-4374. (800) 586-4872. <http://www.lungusa.org>.

American Medical Association. 515 N. State Street, Chicago, IL 60610. (312) 464-5000, <http://www.ama-assn.org>.

Society of Thoracic Surgeons. 633 N. Saint Clair St., Suite 2320, Chicago, IL 60611-3658. (312) 202-5800, fax: 312-202-5801. <sts@sts.org>. <http://www.sts.org>.

OTHER

Creighton University School of Medicine [cited May 14, 2003]. <http://medicine.creighton.edu/forpatients/mediast/mediastin.html>.

Harvard University Medical School [cited May 14, 2003]. <http://www.health.harvard.edu/fhg/diagnostics/mediastinoscopy/mediastinoscopy.shtml>.

Merck Manual [cited May 14, 2003]. <http://www.merck.com/pubs/mmanual/section6/chapter65/65i.htm>.

University of Missouri [cited May 14, 2003]. <http://www.ellisfischel.org/thoracic/testing/mediastinoscopy.shtml>.

L. Fleming Fallon, Jr., M.D., Dr.PH.

Medicaid

Definition

Medicaid is a federal-state entitlement program for low-income citizens of the United States. The Medicaid program is part of Title XIX of the Social Security Act Amendment that became law in 1965. Medicaid offers federal matching funds to states for costs incurred in paying health care providers for serving covered individuals. State participation is voluntary, but since 1982, all 50 states have chosen to participate in Medicaid.

Description

Medicaid benefits

Medicaid benefits cover basic health care and long-term care services for eligible persons. About 58% of Medicaid spending covers hospital and other acute care services. The remaining 42% pays for nursing home and long-term care.

States that choose to participate in Medicaid must offer the following basic services:

• hospital care, both inpatient and outpatient

• nursing home care

• physician services

- laboratory and diagnostic x ray services

- immunizations and other screening, diagnostic, and treatment services for children

- family planning

- health center and rural health clinic services

- nurse midwife and nurse practitioner services

- physician assistant services

Participating states may offer the following optional services and receive federal matching funds for them:

- prescription medications

- institutional care for the mentally retarded

- home- or community-based care for the elderly, including case management

- personal care for the disabled

- dental and vision care for eligible adults

Because participating states are allowed to design their own benefits packages as long as they meet federal minimum requirements, Medicaid benefits vary considerably from state to state. About half of all Medicaid spending covers groups of people and services above the federal minimum.

Eligibility for Medicaid

Medicaid covers three major groups of low-income Americans:

- All recipients. In 2001, Medicaid covered 44 million low-income persons in the United States.

- Parents and children. In 2001, Medicaid covered 24 million low-income children, approximately one-fifth of all children in the United States. It provided coverage to an estimated 9.3 million low-income adults in families with children; most of these low-income adults were women.

- The elderly. In 2001, Medicaid covered five million adults over the age of 65. Medicaid is the largest single purchaser of long-term and nursing home care in the United States.

- The disabled. About 17% of Medicaid recipients are blind or disabled. Most of these persons are eligible for Medicaid because they receive assistance through the Supplemental Security Income (SSI) program.

All Medicaid recipients must have incomes and resources below specified eligibility levels. These levels vary from state to state depending on the local cost of living and other factors. For example, in 2001, the federal poverty level (FPL) was determined to be $14,630 for a family of three on the mainland of the United States, but $16,830 in Hawaii and $18,290 in Alaska.

In most cases, persons must be citizens of the United States to be eligible for Medicaid, although legal immigrants may qualify in some circumstances depending on their date of entry. Illegal aliens are not eligible for Medicaid, except for emergency care.

Persons must fit into an eligibility category to receive Medicaid, even if their income is low. Childless couples and single childless adults who are not disabled or elderly are not eligible for Medicaid.

Medicaid costs

Medicaid is by far the government's most expensive general welfare program. In 1966, Medicaid accounted for 1.4% of the federal budget, but by 2001, its share had risen to nearly 9%. Combined federal and state spending for Medicaid takes approximately 20 cents of every tax dollar. The federal government covers about 56% of costs associated with Medicaid. The states pay for the remaining 44%.

As of 2001, costs for Medicaid rose at an average annual rate of 7.9%. The federal government spent $107 billion on Medicaid in fiscal year (FY) 1999, a sum that is expected to rise to $159 billion in 2004. The states spent $81 billion to cover Medicaid costs in FY 1999. These costs are projected to increase to $120 billion by FY 2004.

Although more than half (54%) of all Medicaid beneficiaries are children, most of the money (more than 70%) goes for services for the elderly and disabled. The single largest portion of Medicaid money pays for long-term care for the elderly. Only 18% of Medicaid funds are spent on services for children.

There are several factors involved in the steep rise of Medicaid costs:

- The rise in the number of eligible individuals. As the lifespan of most Americans continues to increase, the number of elderly individuals eligible for Medicaid also rises. The fastest-growing age group in the United States is people over 85.

- The price of medical and long-term care. Advances in medical technology, including expensive diagnostic imaging tests, cause these costs to rise.

- The increased use of services covered by Medicaid.

- The expansion of state coverage from the minimum benefits package to include optional groups and optional services.

Normal results

The need to contain Medicaid costs is considered one of the most problematic policy issues facing legisla-

KEY TERMS

Categorically needy—A term that describes certain groups of Medicaid recipients who qualify for the basic mandatory package of Medicaid benefits. There are categorically needy groups that states participating in Medicaid are required to cover, and other groups that the states have the option to cover.

Department of Health and Human Service (DHHS)—It is a federal agency that houses the Centers for Medicare and Medicaid Services, and distributes funds for Medicaid.

Entitlement—A program that creates a legal obligation by the federal government to any person, business, or government entity that meets the legally defined criteria. Medicaid is an entitlement both for eligible individuals and for the states that decide to participate in it.

Federal poverty level (FPL)—The definition of poverty provided by the federal government, used

as the reference point to determine Medicaid eligibility for certain groups of beneficiaries. The FPL is adjusted every year to allow for inflation.

Health Care Financing Administration (HCFA)—A federal agency that provides guidelines for the Medicaid program.

Medically needy—A term that describes a group whose coverage is optional with the states because of high medical expenses. These persons meet category requirements of Medicaid (they are children or parents or elderly or disabled) but their income is too high to qualify them for coverage as categorically needy.

Supplemental Security Income (SSI)—A federal entitlement program that provides cash assistance to low-income blind, disabled, and elderly people. In most states, people receiving SSI benefits are eligible for Medicaid.

tors. In addition, the complexity of the Medicaid system, its vulnerability to billing fraud and other abuses, the confusing variety of the benefits packages available in different states, and the time-consuming paperwork are other problems that disturb both taxpayers and legislators.

Medicaid has increased the demand for health care services in the United States without greatly impacting or improving the quality of health care for low-income Americans. Medicaid is the largest health insurer in the United States. As such, it affects the employment of several hundred thousand health care workers, including health care providers, administrators, and support staff. Participation in Medicaid is optional for physicians and **nursing homes**. Many do not participate in the program because the reimbursement rates are low. As a result, many low-income people who are dependent on Medicaid must go to overcrowded facilities where they often receive substandard health care.

See also Medicare.

Resources

BOOKS

Albanese, Beverly H. and Heidi Macomber. *Medicaid EZ: A Guide to Get Those Nursing Home Bills Paid.* New York: iUniverse, 2000.

Conklin, Joan H. *Medicare for the Clueless: The Complete Guide to This Federal Program.* New York: Kensington Publishing, 2002.

Pratt, David A., and Sean K. Hornbeck. *Social Security and Medicare Answer Book* Gaithersburg, MD: Aspen, 2002.

Stevens, Robert, and Rosemary Stevens. *Welfare Medicine in America: A Case Study of Medicaid.* Somerset, NJ: Transaction Publishers, 2003.

PERIODICALS

Benko, L. B. "Health Hazard. Medicaid Cuts Could Endanger Patients." *Modern Healthcare* 33 (2003): 26–27.

Chaudry, R. V, W. P. Brandon, C. R. Thompson, R. S. Clayton, and N. B. Schoeps. "Caring for Patients under Medicaid Mandatory Managed Care: Perspectives of Primary Care Physicians." *Qualitative Health Research* 13 (2003): 37–56.

Lambert, D., J. Gale, D. Bird, and D. Hartley. "Medicaid Managed Behavioral Health in Rural Areas." *Journal of Rural Health* 19 (2003): 22–32.

Vastag, B. "Capitol Health Call: Proposal for State Medicaid Autonomy under Fire." *Journal of the American Medical Association,* 289 (2003): 1093–1094.

ORGANIZATIONS

Health Care Financing Administration. United States Department of Health and Human Services. 200 Independence Avenue SW, Washington, D.C. 20201. <http://www.hcfa.gov>.

Kaiser Commission on Medicaid and the Uninsured. 1450 G Street NW, Suite 250, Washington, DC 20005. (202) 347-5270; Fax: (202) 347-5274. <http://www.kff.org>.

National Center for Policy Analysis. 655 15th Street NW, Suite 375, Washington, DC 20005. (202) 628-6671; Fax: (202) 628-6474. <http://www.ncpa.org>.

United States Department of Health and Human Services. 200 Independence Avenue SW, Washington, DC 20201. <http://www.hhs.gov>.

OTHER

Centers for Medicare and Medicaid Services, US Department of Health and Human Services [cited March 14, 2003]. <http://cms.hhs.gov/>.

National Association of State Medicaid Directors [cited March 14, 2003]. <http://www.nasmd.org/>.

National Governor's Association [cited March 14, 2003]. <http://www.nga.org/>.

Social Security Administration [cited March 14, 2003]. <http://www.ssa.gov/>.

L. Fleming Fallon, Jr, MD, DrPH

Medical charts

Definition

A medical chart is a confidential document that contains detailed and comprehensive information on an individual and the care experience related to that person.

Purpose

The purpose of a medical chart is to serve as both a medical and legal record of an individual's clinical status, care, history, and caregiver involvement. The specific information contained in the chart is intended to provide a record of a person's clinical condition by detailing diagnoses, treatments, tests and responses to treatment, as well as any other factors that may affect the person's health or clinical state.

Demographics

Every person who has a professional relationship with a health-care provider has a medical record. Because most people have such relationships with more than one health professional or caregiver, most people actually have more than one medical chart.

Description

The terms medical chart or medical record are a general description of a collection of information on a person. However, different clinical settings and systems utilize different forms of documentation to achieve this purpose. As technology progresses, more institutions are adopting computerized systems that aid in clearer documentation, enhanced access and searching, and more efficient storage and retrieval of individual records.

New uses of technology have also raised concerns about confidentiality. Confidentiality, or personal privacy, is an important principle related to the chart. Whatever system may be in place, it is essential that the health care provider protect an individual's privacy by limiting access only to authorized individuals. Generally, physicians and nurses write most frequently in the chart. Documentation by the clinician who is leading treatment decisions (usually a physician) often focuses on diagnosis and prognosis, while the documentation by members of the nursing team generally focuses on individual responses to treatment and details of day-to-day progress. In many institutions, the medical and nursing staff may complete separate forms or areas of the chart specific to their disciplines.

Other health-care professionals that have access to the chart include physician assistants; social workers; psychologists; nutritionists; physical, occupational, speech, or respiratory therapists; and consultants. It is important that the various disciplines view the notes written by other specialties in order to form a complete picture of a person and provide continuity of care. Quality assurance and regulatory organizations, legal bodies, and insurance companies may also have access to the chart for specific purposes such as documentation, institutional audits, legal proceedings, or verification of information for care reimbursement. It is important to know about institutional policies regarding chart access in order to ensure the privacy of personal records.

The medical record should be stored in a pre-designated, secure area and discussed only in appropriate and private clinical areas. All individuals have a right to view and obtain copies of their own records. Special state statutes may cover especially sensitive information such as psychiatric, communicable disease (i.e., HIV), or substance abuse records. Institutional and government policies govern what is contained in the chart, how it is documented, who has access, and policies for regulating access to the chart and protecting its integrity and confidentiality. In those cases in which individuals outside of the immediate care system must access chart contents, an individual or personal representative is asked to provide permission before records can be released. Individuals are often asked to sign these releases so that caregivers in new clinical settings may review their charts.

Diagnosis/Preparation

Training

Thorough training is essential prior to independent use of the medical chart. Whenever possible, a new clinician should spend time reviewing the chart to get a sense of organization and documentation format and style.

Training programs for health care professionals often include practice in writing notes or flow charts in mock medical records. Notes by trainees are often initially cosigned by supervisors to ensure accurate and relevant documentation and document-appropriate supervision.

Operation

Documentation in the medical record begins when an individual enters the care system, which may be a specific place such as a hospital or professional office, or a program such as a home health-care service. Frequently, a facility will request permission to obtain copies of previous records so that they have complete information on the person. Although chart systems vary from institution to institution, there are many aspects of the chart that are universal. Frequently used chart sections include the following:

- Admission paperwork. Includes legal paperwork such as a **living will** or **health care proxy**, consents for admission to the facility or program, demographics, and contact information.

- History and physical. Contains comprehensive review of an individual's medical history and physical examinations.

- Orders. Contains medication and treatment orders by the doctor, nurse practitioner, physician assistant, or other qualified health care team members.

- Medication record. Documents all medications administered.

- Treatment record. Documents all treatments received such as dressing changes or respiratory therapy.

- Procedures. Summarizes diagnostic or therapeutic procedures, i.e., **colonoscopy** or open-heart surgery.

- Tests. Provides reports and results of diagnostic evaluations, such as laboratory tests and **electrocardiography** tracings or radiography images or summaries of test results.

- Progress notes. Includes regular notes on the individual's status by members of the interdisciplinary care team.

- Consultations. Contains notes from specialized diagnosticians or external care providers.

- Consents. Includes permissions signed by the individual for procedures, tests, or access to chart. May also contain releases such as the release signed by any person when leaving the facility against medical advice (AMA).

- Flow records. Tracks specific aspects of professional care that occur on a routine basis, using tables or in a chart format.

- Care plans. Documents treatment goals and plans for future care within a facility or following discharge.

- Discharge. Contains final instructions for the person and reports by the care team before the chart is closed and stored following discharge.

- Insurance information. Lists health-care benefit coverage and insurance provider contact information.

These general categories may be further divided by individual facilities for their own purposes. For example, a psychiatric facility may use a special section for psychometric testing, or a hospital may provide sections specifically for operations, x ray reports, or electrocardiograms. In addition, certain details such as allergies or do not resuscitate orders may be displayed prominently (for instance, with large colored stickers or special chart sections) on the chart in order to communicate uniquely important information. It is important for health care providers to become familiar with the charting systems in place at their specific facilities or programs.

It is important that the information in the chart be clear and concise, so that those utilizing the record can easily access accurate information. The medical chart can also aid in clinical problem solving by tracking an individual's baseline, or status on admission or entry into an office or health care system; orders and treatments provided in response to specific problems; and individual responses. Another reason for the standard of clear documentation is the possibility that the record may be used in legal proceedings, when documentation serves as evidence in exploring and evaluating a person's care experience. When medical care is being referred to or questioned by the legal system, chart contents are frequently cited in court. For all of these purposes, certain practices that protect the integrity of the chart and provide essential information are recommended for adding information and maintaining the chart. These practices include the following:

- Date and time should be included on all entries into the record.

- A person's full name and other identifiers (i.e., medical record number, date of birth) should be included on all records.

- Continued records should be marked clearly (i.e., if a note is continued on the reverse side of a page).

- Each page of documentation should be signed.

- Blue or black non-erasable ink should be used on handwritten records.

- Records should be maintained in chronological order.

- Disposal or obliteration of any records or portions of records should be prevented.

- Documentation errors and corrections should be noted clearly, i.e., by drawing one line through the error and noting the presence of an error, and then initialing the area.

- Excess empty space on the page should be avoided. A line should be drawn through any unused space, the initial, time, and date included.

- Only universally accepted abbreviations should be used.

- Unclear documentation such as illegible penmanship should be avoided.

- Contradictory information should be avoided. For example, if a nurse documents that a person has complained of abdominal pain throughout a shift, while a physician documents that the person is free of pain, these discrepancies should be discussed and clarified. The resolution should be entered into the chart and signed by all parties involved in the disagreement.

- Objective rather than subjective information should be included. For example, personality conflicts between staff should not enter into the notes. All events involving an individual should be described as objectively as possible, i.e., describe a hostile person by simply stating the facts such as what the person said or did and surrounding circumstances or response of staff, without using derogatory or judgmental language.

- Any occurrence that might affect the person should be documented. Documented information is considered credible in court. Undocumented information is considered questionable since there is no written record of its occurrence.

- Current date and time should be used in documentation. For example, if a note is added after the fact, it should be labeled as an addendum and inserted in correct chronological order, rather than trying to insert the information on the date of the actual occurrence.

- Actual statements of people should be recorded in quotes.

- The chart shouldn't be left in an unprotected environment where unauthorized individuals may read or alter the contents.

Several methods of documentation have arisen in response to the need to accurately summarize a person's experience. In the critical care setting, flow records are often used to track frequent personal evaluations, checks of equipment, and changes of equipment settings that are required. Flow records also offer the advantages of displaying a large amount of information in a relatively small space and allowing for quick comparisons. Flow records can also save time for a busy clinician by allowing for the completion of checklists versus requiring written narrative notes.

Narrative progress notes, while more time consuming, are often the best way to capture specific information about an individual. Some institutions require only charting by exception (CBE), which requires notes only for significant or unusual findings. While this method may decrease repetition and lower required documentation time, most institutions that use CBE notes also require a separate flow record that documents regular contact with a person. Many facilities or programs require notes at regular intervals even when there is no significant occurrence, i.e., every nursing shift. Frequently used formats in individual notes include SOAP (subjective, objective, assessment, plan) notes. SOAP notes use an individual's subjective statement to capture an important aspect of care, follow with a key objective statement regarding the person's status, a description of the clinical assessment, and a plan for how to address individual problems or concerns. Focus charting and PIE (problem-intervention-evaluation) charting use similar systems of notes that begin with a particular focus such as a nursing diagnosis or an individual concern. Nursing diagnoses are often used as guides to nursing care by focusing on individual care-recipient needs and responses to treatment. An example of a nursing diagnosis is fluid volume for someone who is dehydrated. The notes would then focus on assessment for dehydration, interventions to address the problem, and a plan for continued care such as measurement of input and output and intravenous therapy.

Aftercare

Current medical charts are maintained by members of the health care team and usually require clerical assistance such as a unit clerk in the hospital setting or records clerk in a professional office. No alterations should be made to the record unless they are required to clarify or correct information and are clearly marked as such. After discharge, the medical records department of a facility checks for completeness and retains the record. Similar checks may be made in professional office settings. Sometimes, the record will be made available in another format, i.e., recording paper charts on microfilm or computer imaging. Institutional policies and state laws govern storage of charts on- and off-site and length of storage time required.

Risks

A major potential risk associated with medical charts is breach of confidentiality. This must be safeguarded at all times. Other risks include loss of materials in a chart or incorrectly filing a chart so that subsequent retrieval is impeded or impossible.

Normal results

All members of a health-care team require thorough understanding of the medical chart and documentation guidelines in order to provide competent care and maintain a clear, concise, and pertinent record. Health-care systems often employ methods to guarantee thorough and continuous use and review of charts across disciplines. For example, nursing staff may be required to sign below every new physician order to indicate that this information has been communicated, or internal quality assurance teams may study groups of charts to determine trends in missing or unclear documentation. In legal settings, health care team members may be called upon to interpret or explain chart notations as they relate to a specific legal case.

Morbidity and mortality rates

Medical charts are made of paper or other materials. They are subject to deterioration or loss. Transporting them may cause lifting injuries, but not lead to disease or death.

Alternatives

There are no alternatives for medical charts. Alternative mediums exist for paper records. These include fixing images on plastic media (photographs or x rays) or electronic storage. The latter can include magnetic tape or computer disks.

See also Health history; Physical examination; Talking to the doctor.

Resources

BOOKS

Carter, Jerome H. *Electronic Medical Records: A Guide for Clinicians and Administrators.* Philadelphia: American College of Physicians, 2001.

Leiner, F., W. Gaus, R. Haux, and P. Knaup-Gregori. *Medical Data Management: A Practical Guide.* New York: Springer-Verlag, 2003.

Skurka, Margaret A. *Health Information Management: Principles and Organization for Health Record Services, 5th edition.* San Francisc0: Jossey-Bass, 2003.

Van De Velde, Rudi, Patrice Degoulet, and Daryl J. Daley. *Clinical Information Systems: A Component-Based Approach.* New York: Springer-Verlag, 2003.

PERIODICALS

Gomez, E. "Health Insurance Portability and Accountability Act Protects Privacy of Medical Records." *Oncology Nursing Society News,* 18(1) 2003: 13.

O'Connor, P. J. "Electronic Medical Records and Diabetes Care Improvement: Are We Waiting for Godot?" *Diabetes Care,* 26(3) 2003: 942–943.

Ross, S. E, and C. T. Lin. "The Effects of Promoting Patient Access to Medical Records: A Review." *Journal of the American Medical Informatics Association,* 10(2) 2003: 129–138.

Vaszar, L. T, M. K. Cho, and T. A. Raffin. "Privacy Issues in Personalized Medicine." *Pharmacogenomics,* 4(2) 2003: 107–112.

Willison, D. J., K. Keshavjee, K. Nair, C. Goldsmith, and A. M. Holbrook. "Patients' Consent Preferences for Research Uses of Information in Electronic Medical Records: Interview and Survey Data." *British Medical Journal,* 326(7385) 2003: 373–378.

ORGANIZATIONS

American Academy of Family Physicians. 11400 Tomahawk Creek Parkway, Leawood, KS 66211-2672. (913) 906-6000. <fp@aafp.org>. <http://www.aafp.org>.

American Academy of Pediatrics. 141 Northwest Point Boulevard, Elk Grove Village, IL 60007-1098. (847) 434-4000; Fax: (847) 434-8000. <kidsdoc@aap.org>. <http://www.aap.org/default.htm>.

American College of Physicians. 190 N Independence Mall West, Philadelphia, PA 19106-1572. (800) 523-1546, x2600, or (215) 351-2600. <http://www.acponline.org>.

American Hospital Association. One North Franklin, Chicago, IL 60606-3421. (312) 422-3000. <http://www.aha.org/index.asp>.

American Medical Association. 515 N. State Street, Chicago, IL 60610. (312) 464-5000. <http://www.ama-assn.org>.

American Medical Informatics Association. 4915 St. Elmo Avenue, Suite 401, Bethesda, MD 20814. 301) 657-1291; Fax: (301) 657-1296. <http://www.amia.org/contact/f contact.html>. <http://www.amia.org>.

Consultation—Evaluation by an outside expert or specialist, someone other than the primary care provider.

Continuity—Consistency or coordination of details.

Discipline—In health care, a specific area of preparation or training such as social work, nursing, or nutrition.

Documentation—The process of recording information in the medical chart, or the materials contained in a medical chart.

Interdisciplinary—Consisting of several interacting disciplines that work together to care for an individual.

Objective—Not biased by personal opinion; repeatable.

Prognosis—Expected resolution or outcome of an illness or injury.

Regulatory organization—Organization designed to maintain or control quality in health care.

Subjective—Influenced by personal opinion, bias, or experience; not reliably repeatable.

OTHER

Amyotrophic Lateral Sclerosis Disease Foundation [cited March 1, 2003]. <http://www.lougehrigsdisease.net/als_news/990106medical_charts.htm>.

Electronic Privacy Information Center [cited March 1, 2003]. <http://www.epic.org/privacy/medical/>.

Peking University Health Sciences Center [cited March 1, 2003]. <http://mededucation.bjmu.edu.cn/chapter%20one/major%20componentof%20medical%20charts.htm>.

Privacy Rights Clearinghouse [cited March 1, 2003]. <http://www.privacyrights.org/fs/fs8-med.htm>.

L. Fleming Fallon, Jr, MD, DrPH

Medical errors

Introduction and definitions

The subject of medical errors is not a new one. However, it did not come to widespread attention in the United States until the 1990s, when government-sponsored research about the problem was undertaken by two physicians, Lucian Leape and David Bates. In 1999, a report compiled by the Committee on Quality of Health Care in America and published by the Institute of Medicine (IOM) made headlines with its findings. As a result of the IOM report, President Clinton asked the Quality Interagency Coordination Task Force (QuIC) to analyze the problem of medical errors and patient safety, and make recommendations for improvement. The Report to the President on Medical Errors was published in February 2000.

It is important to understand the terms used by the government and health-care professionals in describing medical errors in order to distinguish between injury or death resulting from mistakes made by people on the one hand, and unfortunate results of treatment on the other. Some allergic reactions to medications or failures to respond to cancer treatment, for example, result from physical differences among patients or the known side effects of certain treatments, and not from prescribing the wrong drug or therapy for the patient's condition. This type of negative outcome is called an adverse event in official documents. Adverse events can be defined as undesirable and unintentional, though not necessarily unexpected, results of medical treatment. An example of an adverse event is discomfort in an artificial joint that continues after the expected recovery period, or a chronic headache following a spinal tap.

A medical error, on the other hand, is an adverse event that could be prevented given the current state of medical knowledge. The QuIC task force expanded the IOM's working definition of a medical error to cover as many types of errors as possible. Their definition of a medical error is as follows: "The failure of a planned action to be completed as intended or the use of a wrong plan to achieve an aim. Errors can include problems in practice, products, procedures, and systems." A useful, brief definition of a medical error is that it is a preventable adverse event.

Statistics

The statistics contained in the IOM report were startling. The authors of the report stated that between 45,000 and 98,000 Americans die each year as the result of medical errors. If the lower figure is used as an estimate, deaths in hospitals resulting from medical errors are the eighth leading cause of mortality in the United States, surpassing deaths attributable to motor vehicle accidents (43,458), breast cancer (42,297), and AIDS (16,516). Moreover, these figures refer only to hospitalized patients; they do not include people treated in outpatient clinics, **ambulatory surgery centers**, doctors' or dentists' offices, college or military health services, or **nursing homes**. Medical errors certainly occur outside hospitals; in 1999, the Massachusetts State Board of Registration in Pharmacy estimated that 2.4 million prescriptions are filled incorrectly each year in that state—which is only one of 50 states.

In terms of health-care costs, the IOM report estimated that medical errors cost the United States about $37.6 billion each year; about half this sum pays for direct health care.

The United States is not unique in having a high rate of medical errors. The United Kingdom, Australia, and Sweden are presently undertaking studies of their respective health care systems. British experts estimate that 40,000 patients die each year in the United Kingdom as the result of medical errors. Australia has been testing a new system for reporting errors since 1995.

Description

There is no single universally accepted method of classifying medical errors in order to describe them more fully. The 2000 QuIC report lists five different classification schemes that have been used:

• type of health care given (medication, surgery, diagnostic imaging, etc.)

• severity of the injury (minor discomfort, serious injury, death, etc.)

• legal definitions (negligence, malpractice, etc.)

• setting (hospital, emergency room, **intensive care unit**, nursing home, etc.)

• persons involved (physician, nurse, pharmacist, patient, etc.)

The importance of these different ways to classify medical errors is their indication that different types of errors require different approaches to prevention and problem solving. For example, medication errors are often related to such communication problems as misspelled words or illegible handwriting, whereas surgical errors are often related to unclear or misinterpreted diagnostic images.

Causes of medical errors

The causes of medical errors are complex and not yet completely understood. Some causes that have been identified include the following:

• Communication errors. One widely publicized case from 1994 involved the death of a Boston newspaper columnist from an overdose of chemotherapy for breast cancer due to misinterpretation of the doctor's prescrip-

tion; the patient was given four times the correct daily dose, when the doctor intended the dosage to be administered instead over a four-day period. Other cases involve medication mix-ups due to drugs with very similar names. The Food and Drug Administration (FDA) has identified no fewer than 600 pairs of look-alike or sound-alike drug names since 1992.

• The increasing specialization and fragmentation of health care. The more people involved in a patient's treatment, the greater the possibility that important information will be missing along the chain.

• Human errors resulting from overwork and burnout. For some years, hospital interns, residents, and nurses have attributed many of the errors made in patient care to the long hours they are expected to work, many times with inadequate sleep. With the coming of managed care, many hospitals have cut the size of their nursing staff and require those that remain to work mandatory overtime shifts. A study published in the *Journal of the American Medical Association* in October 2002 found a clear correlation between higher-than-average rates of patient mortality and higher-than-average ratios of patients to nurses.

• Manufacturing errors. Instances have been reported of blood products being mislabeled during the production process, resulting in patients being given transfusions of an incompatible blood type.

• Equipment failure. A typical example of equipment failure might be intravenous pump with a malfunctioning valve, which would allow too much of the patient's medication to be delivered over too short a time period.

• Diagnostic errors. A misdiagnosed illness can lead the doctor to prescribe an inappropriate type of treatment. Errors in interpreting diagnostic imaging have resulted in surgeons operating on the wrong side of the patient's body. Another common form of diagnostic error is failure to act on abnormal test results.

• Poorly designed buildings and facilities. Hallways that end in sharp right angles, for example, increase the likelihood of falls or collisions between people on foot and patients being wheeled to an operating room.

Ways of thinking about medical errors

One subject that has been emphasized in recent reports on medical errors is the need to move away from a search for individual culprits to blame for medical errors. This judgmental approach has sometimes been called the "name, shame, and blame game." It is characterized by the belief that medical errors result from inadequate training or from a few "bad apples" in the system. It is then assumed that medical errors can be reduced or eliminated by identifying the individuals, and firing or disciplining them. The major drawback of this judgmental attitude is that it makes health care workers hesitate to report errors for fear of losing their own jobs or fear of some other form of reprisal. As a result of underreporting, hospital managers and others concerned with patient safety often do not have an accurate picture of the frequency of occurrence of some types of medical errors.

Both the IOM report and the QuIC report urge the adoption of a model borrowed from industry that incorporates systems analysis. This model emphasizes making an entire system safer rather than punishing individuals; it assumes that most errors result from problems with procedures and work processes rather than bad or incompetent people; and it analyzes all parts of the system in order to improve them. The industrial model is sometimes referred to as the continuous quality improvement model (CQI). Hospitals that are implementing error-reduction programs based on the CQI model have found that a non-punitive procedure for reporting medical errors has improved morale among the staff as well as significantly reduced the number of medical errors. At Columbia-Presbyterian Hospital, for example, patients as well as staff can report medical errors via the Internet, a telephone hotline, or paper forms.

Proposals for improvement

Current proposals for reducing the rate of medical errors in the American health care system include the following:

• Adopt stricter standards of acceptable error rates. One reason that industrial manufacturers have made great strides in product safety and error reduction is their commitment to improving the quality of the work process itself.

• Standardize medical equipment and build in mechanical safeguards against human error. Anesthesiology is the outstanding example of a medical specialty that has cut its error rate dramatically by asking medical equipment manufacturers to design ventilators with standardized controls and valves to prevent the oxygen content from falling below that of room air. These changes were the result of studies that showed that many medical errors resulted from doctors having to use unfamiliar ventilators and accidentally turning off the oxygen flow to the patient.

• Improve the working conditions for nurses and other hospital staff. Recommendations in this area include redesigning hospital facilities to improve efficiency and minimize falls and other accidents, as well as reducing the length of nursing shifts.

• Make use of new technology to improve accuracy in medication dosages and recording patients' **vital signs**. Innovations in this field include giving nurses and residents handheld computers for recording patient data so that they do not have to rely on human memory for so many details. Another innovation that helped Veterans Administration (VA) hospitals cut the rate of medication errors was the introduction of a handheld wireless bar-coding system. After the system went into operation at the end of 1998, the number of medication errors in VA hospitals dropped by 70%.

• Develop a nationwide database for error reporting and analysis. At present, there is no unified system for tracking different types of medical errors. An error in **liver transplantation** in August 2002 that cost the life of a baby led several researchers to recognize that there is still no national registry recording transplant mismatches. As a result, no one knows how many cases occur each year, let alone find ways to improve the present system.

• Encourage patients to become more active participants in their own health care. This recommendation includes asking more questions and requesting adequate explanations from health care professionals, as well as reporting medical errors.

• Address the fact that both patients and physicians have emotional as well as knowledge-related needs around the issue of medical errors. A report published in the *Journal of the American Medical Association* in February 2003 stated that patients clearly want emotional support from their doctors following an error, including an apology. The researchers also found, however, that doctors are as upset when an error occurs and, additionally, are unsure where to turn for emotional support.

What patients can do

Patients are an important resource in lowering the rate of medical errors. The QuIC task force has put together some fact sheets to help patients improve the safety of their health care. One of these fact sheets, entitled "Five Steps to Safer Health Care," gives the following tips:

• Do not hesitate to ask questions of your health-care provider, and ask him or her for explanations that you can understand.

• Keep lists of all medications, including over-the-counter items as well as prescribed drugs.

• Ask for the results of all tests and procedures, and find out what the results mean for you.

• Find out what choices are available to you if your doctor recommends hospital care.

• If your doctor suggests surgery, ask for information about the procedure itself, the reasons for it, and exactly what will happen during the operation.

This fact sheet, as well as a longer and more detailed patient fact sheet on medical errors, is available for free download from the Agency for Health Research and Quality (AHRQ) Website or by telephone order from the AHRQ Publications Clearinghouse at (800) 358-9295.

See also Managed care plans; Patient rights; Talking to the doctor.

Resources

BOOKS

Committee on Quality of Health Care in America, Institute of Medicine. *To Err Is Human: Building a Safer Health System.* Washington, DC: National Academy Press, 2000.

PERIODICALS

Aiken, Linda H., et al. "Hospital Nurse Staffing and Patient Mortality, Nurse Burnout, and Job Dissatisfaction." *Journal of the American Medical Association* 288 (October 23-30, 2002): 1987–1993.

Cottrill, Ken. "Mistaken Identity: Barcoding Recommended to Combat Medical Errors." *Traffic World* (July 2, 2001).

Dougherty, Matthew. "Preventing Errors: New Initiative Aims to Catch Mistakes before They Happen." *In Vivo: News from Columbia Health Sciences* 1 (February 11, 2002).

Dovey, S. M., R. L. Phillips, L. A. Green, and G. E. Fryer. "Types of Medical Errors Commonly Reported by Family Physicians." *American Family Physician* 67 (February 15, 2003): 697.

Friedman, Richard A. "Do Spelling and Penmanship Count? In Medicine, You Bet." *New York Times,* March 11, 2003.

Gallagher, T. H., et al. "Patients' and Physicians' Attitudes Regarding the Disclosure of Medical Errors." *Journal of the American Medical Association* 289 (February 26, 2003): 1001–1007.

Grady, Denise, and Lawrence K. Altman. "Suit Says Transplant Error Was Cause in Baby's Death in August." *New York Times,* March 12, 2003.

Hsia, David C. "Medicare Quality Improvement: Bad Apples or Bad Systems?" *Journal of the American Medical Association* 289 (January 15, 2003): 354–356.

Nordenberg, Tamar. "Make No Mistake: Medical Errors Can Be Deadly Serious." *FDA Consumer Magazine* (September-October 2000).

Pyzdek, Thomas. "Motorola's Six Sigma Program." *Quality Digest* (December, 1997).

ORGANIZATIONS

Agency for Healthcare Research and Quality (AHRQ). 2101 East Jefferson St., Suite 501, Rockville, MD 20852. (301) 594-1364. <www.ahcpr.gov>.

Institute of Medicine (IOM). The National Academies. 500 Fifth Street, NW, Washington, DC 20001. <www.iom. edu>.

United States Food and Drug Administration (FDA). 5600 Fishers Lane, Rockville, MD 20857-0001. (888) 463-6332. <www.fda.gov>.

KEY TERMS

Adverse event—An undesirable and unintended result of a medical treatment or intervention.

Medical error—A preventable adverse event.

Systems analysis—An approach to medical errors and other management issues that looks for problems in the work process rather than singling out individuals as bad or incompetent.

OTHER

Agency for Healthcare Research and Quality (AHRQ) Fact Sheet. *Medical Errors: The Scope of the Problem.* Publication No. AHRQ 00-PO37.

Agency for Healthcare Research and Quality (AHRQ) Patient Fact Sheet. *20 Tips to Help Prevent Medical Errors.* Publication No. AHRQ 00-PO38.

Burton, Susan. "The Biggest Mistake of Their Lives." *New York Times,* March 16, 2003. <www.nytimes.com/2003/03/16/magazine/16MISTAKE.html>.

Quality Interagency Coordination Task Force (QuIC)) Patient Fact Sheet. *Five Steps to Safer Health Care,* January 2001 [cited March 17, 2003]. <www.ahrq.gov/consumer/5steps.htm>.

Report of the Quality Interagency Coordination Task Force (QuIC) to the President. *Doing What Counts for Patient Safety: Federal Actions to Reduce Medical Errors and Their Impact,* 2000.

Rebecca Frey, PhD

Medical history *see* **Health history**

Medicare

Definition

Medicare is a national health insurance program created and administered by the federal government in the United States to address the medical needs of older American citizens. Medicare is available to U.S. citizens 65 years of age and older and some people with disabilities under age 65.

Description

Medicare is the largest health insurance program in the United States. The program was created as part of the

Social Security Act Amendment in 1965 and was put into effect in 1966. At the end of 1966, Medicare served approximately 3.9 million individuals. As of 2003, it serves about 41 million people. There are 5.6 million Medicare beneficiaries enrolled in managed care programs.

In 1973, the Medicare program was expanded to include people who have permanent kidney failure and need dialysis or transplants and people under the age of 65 who have specific types of disabilities. Medicare was originally administered by the Social Security Administration, but in 1977, the program was transferred to the Health Care Financing Administration (HCFA), which is part of the United States Department of Health and Human Services (DHHS). The Centers for Medicare and Medicaid Services, an agency of the DHHS, is the administrative agency. This agency also administers **Medicaid** programs.

Medicare is an entitlement program similar to Social Security and is not based on financial need. Medicare benefits are available to all American citizens over the age of 65 because they or their spouses have paid Social Security taxes through their working years. Since Medicare is a federal program, the rules for eligibility remain constant throughout the nation and coverage remains constant regardless of where an individual receives treatment in the United States.

Medicare benefits are divided into two different categories referred to as Part A and Part B. Medicare Part A is hospital insurance that provides basic coverage for hospital stays and post-hospital nursing facilities, home health care, and hospice care for terminally ill patients. Most people automatically receive Part A when they turn 65 and do not have to pay a premium because they or their spouse paid Medicare taxes while they were working.

Medicare Part B is medical insurance. It covers most fees associated with basic doctor visits and laboratory testing. It also pays for some outpatient medical services such as medical equipment, supplies, and home health care and physical therapy. However, these services and supplies are only covered by Part B when medically necessary and prescribed by a doctor. Enrollment in Part B is optional and the Medicare recipient pays a premium of approximately $65 per month for these added benefits. The amount of the premium is periodically adjusted. Not every person who receives Medicare Part A enrolls in Part B.

Although Medicare provides fairly broad coverage of medical treatment, neither Part A nor B pays for the cost of prescription drugs or other medications.

Medicare is funded solely by the federal government. States do not make matching contributions to the Medicare fund. Social Security contributions, monthly premiums paid by program participants, and general government revenues generate the money used to support the Medicare program. Insurance coverage provided by Medicare is similar to that provided by private health insurance carriers. Medicare usually pays 50–80% of the medical bill, while the recipient pays the remaining balance for services provided.

Normal results

As the population of the United States ages, concerns about health care and the financing of quality health care for all members of the elderly population grow. One concern is that health insurance provided by the Medicare program will become obsolete or will be cut from the federal budget in an attempt to save money. Another concern is that money provided by the Social Security Administration for Medicare will be depleted before the aging population of the United States can actually benefit from the taxes they are now paying. A third concern is coverage for prescription medications.

During the Clinton administration, several initiatives were started that saved funds for Medicare. The DHHS also supports several initiatives to save and improve the program. However, continuance of the federal health insurance program is still a problem that American citizens expect legislators to resolve.

During the George W. Bush administration, there has been debate concerning coverage for prescription drugs. Health care reformers suggest that prescription drugs be made available through the Medicare program due to the high cost of such medications. This debate has not been resolved as of early 2003, and legislation has not been enacted.

Some of the successful initiatives undertaken since 1992 include:

• Fighting fraud and abuse. Much attention has focused on Medicare abuse, fraud, and waste. As a result, overpayments were stopped, fraud was decreased, and abuse was investigated. This has saved the Medicare program approximately $500 million per year.

• Preserving the Medicare benefit. Due to aggressive action by the federal government, it is estimated that funds have been appropriated to keep Medicare viable through 2026.

• Supporting Preventive Medicine and the Healthy Aging Project. Medicare programs are supporting preventive medicine and diagnostic treatments in anticipation that preventive measures will improve the health of older Americans and thereby reduce health care costs.

Medicare benefits and health care financing are major issues in the United States. Legislators and federal agencies continue to work on initiatives that will keep

KEY TERMS

DHHS—The Department of Health and Human Service. This federal agency houses the Centers for Medicare and Medicaid Services and distributes funds for Medicaid.

Entitlement—A program that creates a legal obligation by the federal government to any person, business, or government entity that meets the legally defined criteria. Medicare is an entitlement for eligible individuals.

HCFA—Health Care Financing Administration. A federal agency that provides guidelines for the Medicaid program.

Medicare Part A—Hospital insurance provided by Medicare, provided free to persons aged 65 and older.

Medicare Part B—Medical insurance provided by Medicare that requires recipients to pay a monthly premium. Part B pays for some medical services Part A does not.

health-care programs in place and working for the good of American citizens.

See also Medicaid.

Resources

BOOKS

Blumenthal, David and Jon Erickson. *Long-Term Care and Medicare Policy: Can We Improve the Continuity of Care?* Washington, DC: Brookings Institution Press, 2003.

Marmor, Theodore R. *The Politics of Medicare.* Second edition. Hawthorne, NY: Aldine de Gruyter, 2000.

Oberlander, Jonathan. *Political Life of Medicare.* Chicago: University of Chicago Press, 2003.

Pratt, David A. and Sean K. Hornbeck. *Social Security and Medicare Answer Book.* Gaithersburg, MD: Aspen, 2002.

Stevens, Robert and Rosemary Stevens. *Welfare Medicine in America: A Case Study of Medicaid.* Somerset, NJ: Transaction Publishers, 2003.

PERIODICALS

Charatan, Fred. "Bush proposes Medicare reform." *British Medical Journal* 326, no. 7389 (March 15, 2003): 570–572.

Hyman, David A. "Does Medicare care about quality? " *Perspectives in Biology and Medicine* 46, no. 1 (Winter 2003): 55–68.

Pulec, Jack L. "Medicare: all or nothing." *Ear Nose and Throat Journal* 82, no. 1 (January 2003): 7–8.

Smith, John J., and Leonard Berlin. "Medicare fraud and abuse." *American Journal of Roentgenology* 180, no. 3 (2003): 591–595.

ORGANIZATIONS

American College of Physicians, 190 North Independence Mall West, Philadelphia, PA 19106-1572. (800) 523-1546 x2600 or (215) 351-2600. <http://www.acponline.org>.

American College of Surgeons, 633 North St. Clair Street, Chicago, IL 60611-32311. (312) 202-5000 fax: (312) 202-5001. <http://www.facs.org>.

American Hospital Association, One North Franklin, Chicago, IL 60606-3421. (312) 422-3000 fax: (312) 422-4796. <http://www.aha.org>.

American Medical Association, 515 North State Street, Chicago, IL 60610. (312) 464-5000. <http://www.ama-assn.org>.

Center for Medicare Advocacy, P.O. Box 350, Willimantic, CT 06226. (860) 456-7790 or (202) 216-0028. <http://www.medicareadvocacy.org>.

OTHER

Centers for Medicare and Medicaid Services, U.S. Department of Health and Human Services. <http://cms.hhs.gov>.

Medicare Information Center, <http://www.medicare.org>.

Medicare Rights Center, <http://www.medicarerights.org>.

United States Government Medicare Information, <http://www.medicare.gov>.

L. Fleming Fallon, Jr., MD, DrPH

Meningocele repair

Definition

A meningocele repair is a surgical procedure performed to repair an abnormal opening in the spinal column (called spina bifida) by draining excess fluid and closing the opening.

Purpose

The surgery is necessary to close this abnormal opening to decrease the risk of infection and protect the integrity of the spinal column and the tissue inside.

Demographics

According to the Spina Bifida Association of America, spina bifida is both the most common neural tube defect and the most common birth defect resulting in permanent disability. It is estimated that about 40% of Americans have spina bifida occulta. However, some people who have it may have no symptoms and may therefore be unaware of their condition, so the percentage is an approximation. Meningocele and myelomeningocele are noticeable at birth and are paired together as spina bifida manifesta. Spina bifida manifesta occurs in about one in 1,000 births, with 4–5% being meningocele and 95–96% being myelomeningocele.

Description

The term meningocele may be used to refer to more than one condition. Spina bifida is a neural tube birth defect involving an abnormal opening in the spine. It occurs when the fetus's spine does not close properly during the first month of fetal development. In spina bifida occulta an opening in the spinal bones exists, but the neural tissue and membrane covering the spine (the meninges) are not exposed. Because there is no opening, the defect may appear as a dimple, or depression, at the base of the spine (the sacrum). Another sign of spina bifida occulta is the presence of tufts of hair at the sacrum. It is possible that while there is no opening, vertebrae are missing and there is damage to nerve tissue.

A meningocele is a sac protruding from the spinal column, which contains some of the spinal fluid and meninges. The sac may be covered with skin or with the meninges, and does not contain neural tissue. It may be located near the brain or along the spinal column. Hydrocephalus is rarely present, and the neurological examination may be normal. Because the neural tissue remains intact, it can be repaired by the experienced neurosurgeon, with excellent results.

A myelomeningocele is the most severe type of spina bifida because the spinal cord has herniated into the protruding sac. Neural tissue and nerves may be exposed. About 80% of myelomeningoceles occur at the lower back, where the lumbar and sacral regions join. Some people refer to myelomeningocele as spina bifida. Because of the exposed neural tissue, significant symptoms may be present. These symptoms may include:

- muscle weakness or paralysis in the hips and lower limbs

- no sensation in the part of the body below the defect

- lack of bowel and bladder function

- fluid build-up in the brain, known as hydrocephalus

Because of the risk of neural tissue damage, swelling, and infection into the spinal fluid and brain with an opening in the spinal column, surgery to repair the meningocele or myelomeningocele is usually done within 24 hours of birth. However, although the opening is closed, whatever damage has already been done to the neural tissue is permanent. If hydrocephalus is developing, the meningocele repair may be done first. Then, a few days later, a shunt can be inserted to resolve the hydrocephalus. If the hydrocephalus is present at birth, the two surgeries may be done at the same time to decrease

---

WHO PERFORMS THE PROCEDURE AND WHERE IS IT PERFORMED?

Surgery on the spine is a very delicate procedure and needs to be done by a surgeon specializing in pediatric **neurosurgery**. It is best performed in a hospital with a pediatric intensive care unit available to closely monitor the infant after the surgery.

---

the risks associated with increasing pressure on the brain. To prevent drying of the sac, it may be kept moist with sterile dressings until surgery is begun. Once the anesthesia has put the baby to sleep and the surgery is pain-free, a surgical incision is made into the sac. Excess fluid is drained, and the meninges is wrapped around the spine to protect it. The opening is then closed with sutures.

Diagnosis/Preparation

If an individual has spina bifida occulta, with no outward signs of a neural tube defect and no symptoms, the condition may go undetected. The protruding sacs associated with meningocele and myelomeningocele are quite noticeable at birth. To understand the extent of the defect x rays, ultrasound, computed tomography (CT) scans, or **magnetic resonance imaging** (MRI) of the spine may be taken.

Spina bifida may be diagnosed while the mother is still pregnant, through prenatal screening. If spina bifida is indicated, a blood test will show an elevated alpha fetoprotein. However, elevated levels can be present without spina bifida, so further testing should be done if the test is positive. There is an elevated alpha fetoprotein level in about 85% of women with a fetus with spina bifida. An ultrasound can reliable reveal the spinal structure of the fetus. An **amniocentesis** may be done to check for chromosomal abnormalities. In amniocentesis, a long syringe is used to draw amniotic fluid out from the uterus through the mother's abdomen. Because the protruding sac of the meningocele and myelomeningocele can look the same on the outside, it is important to have a clear diagnosis, as the anticipated outcome of the two conditions is very different.

Aftercare

The infant will first spend some time in the **recovery room**, and then be transferred to an **intensive care unit**. The infant will be monitored for signs of excess bleeding

---

QUESTIONS TO ASK THE DOCTOR

- What is the extent of the neurological damage?
- Is my child likely to walk?
- What experience do you have with this procedure?
- What complications have your patients experienced with this procedure?
- How long is my child likely to stay in the hospital?

and infection. Temperature will be closely monitored. **Antibiotics** will be given to decrease the risk of infection, and the infant will be positioned to lie flat on the stomach to avoid pressure on the surgical wound. Extreme care is taken to keep the wound clean of urine and stool.

Risks

Surgical risks include infection and bleeding. Anesthesia risks include a reaction to the medications used, including difficulty breathing. During meningocele and myelomeningocele repair, there are additional risks of damage to the spinal column and infection of the spinal fluid surrounding the spine and brain. Damage to the neural tissue could result in paralysis, or loss of nerve function (for example, loss of bowel and bladder control). There may also be an increased risk of an urinary tract infection. An infection of the meninges is called meningitis. However, further damage would be expected if surgery were not done, and serious infection would be likely. As in all surgery, one must weigh the potential risks against the expected benefits.

Normal results

Results depend greatly on the extent of involvement of exposed neural tissue and the condition of the infant prior to surgery. A meningocele repair can have excellent results, as neural tissue does not extend into the protruding sac. In myelomeningocele, the amount of exposed neural tissue will determine the extent of lower limb weakness, or paralysis. The infant will usually spend a few weeks in the hospital after surgery before being able to be discharged home. As the child grows, it may be necessary to use braces, crutches, or a wheelchair for mobility. If surgery for hydrocephalus is successful, the prognosis is better. Children with a repaired myelomeningocele

KEY TERMS

Folic acid—A water-soluable vitamin belonging to the B-complex group of vitamins.

Meninges—The membrane covering neural tissue.

Shunt—A shunt is a tube than is used to drain excess fluid. It is surgically implanted. The shunt drains the fluid from around the brain and sends it into the abdomen.

may be able to go to school, but will benefit from special education and associated services. There may be varying degrees of learning problems, and difficulties with the child's attention span. An effective bowel and bladder-training program can help make attending school easier. Because of muscle weakness or paralysis, a child with spina bifida will need physical therapy and may require future surgeries.

Morbidity and mortality rates

With current medical and surgical treatments, about 85% of infants survive, and about 50% will be able to walk. Bowel and bladder disorders contribute significantly to morbidity and mortality in those with spina bifida who survive past the age of two years.

Alternatives

There is no alternative to surgical repair. Risk of infection and damage to the spine and brain is high with an opening to the spine, so surgery is necessary to close the opening and drain the excess fluid that could put pressure on the brain. The Spina Bifida Association of America recommends that all women of childbearing age take 0.4 mg of folic acid daily, as this amount has been shown to decrease the likelihood of neural tube defects. Once a woman is aware of being pregnant, the critical first month of neural tube development has already past, and folic acid cannot cure any damage that has been done.

Resources

BOOKS

Senisi, Ellen B. *All Kinds of Friends, Even Green!* Woodbine House, November 2002.

ORGANIZATIONS

March of Dimes Birth Defects Foundation. 1275 Mamaroneck Avenue; White Plains, NY. Telephone (914) 428-7100. <http://wwwmodimes.org>.

National Library of Medicine. <http://www.nlm.nih.gov>.

Spina Bifida Association of America. 4590 MacArthur Boulevard, NW, Suite 250; Washington, DC 20007-4226. Telephone (800) 621-3141, (202)944-3285. sbaa@sbaa.org. <http://www.sbaa.org>.

Esther Csapo Rastegari, R.N., B.S.N., Ed.M.

Mentoplasty

Definition

Mentoplasty is a term that refers to plastic surgery procedures for the chin. It comes from the Latin word *mentum*, which means chin, and the Greek verb *plassein*, which means "to form" or "to shape." Mentoplasty is also known as genioplasty or chinplasty.

Purpose

Mentoplasty may be done for several reasons:

• To correct malformations of the chin resulting from developmental abnormalities of the bones in the jaw. Sometimes the jawbones continue to grow on one side of the face but not the other, leading to facial asymmetry. In other instances a part of the jawbone is missing; this condition is known as congenital agenesis of the jaw.

• To reshape a chin that is out of proportion to other facial features.

• As part of gender reassignment surgery. The size and shape of the chin and lower jawline are somewhat different in men and women. Some people choose to have mentoplasty as part of their gender transition.

• As part of **craniofacial reconstruction** following trauma or cancer surgery.

• As part of orthognathic surgery. Orthognathic surgery involves repositioning the facial bones in order to correct deformities that affect the patient's ability to speak or chew normally.

Insurance coverage for mentoplasty depends on its purpose. Chin reshaping that is done to improve personal appearance is not usually covered by insurance. Mentoplasty that is performed as a reconstructive procedure after trauma, genetic deformity, or orthognathic surgery may be covered by insurance.

The cost of mentoplasty varies considerably according to the complexity of the procedure. The average surgeon's fee for a chin implant was $1,612 in 2002. The average fee for a sliding genioplasty, however, was $4,000–$6,000.

**WHO PERFORMS
THE PROCEDURE AND
WHERE IS IT PERFORMED?**

Mentoplasties may be performed by plastic surgeons, oral surgeons, or maxillofacial surgeons. Fat injections and facial liposuction are usually performed by plastic surgeons.

Chin implant insertions or direct reductions are usually performed as outpatient procedures in the surgeon's office or an ambulatory surgery center. The patient may be given either general or local anesthesia. Sliding genioplasties can be done as outpatient procedures; however, they are usually performed in hospitals under general anesthesia, particularly if the patient is having orthognathic surgery at the same time.

Demographics

In spite of the fact that chin deformities are the most common facial abnormality, mentoplasty is not one of the more frequently performed procedures in plastic surgery. In 2002, there were 18,352 mentoplasties performed in the United States, compared to 117,831 face lifts and 282,876 liposuctions. Most mentoplasties are done in combination with rhinoplasties.

Mentoplasty is primarily performed in adult patients; it is not usually done in children until all permanent teeth have come in and the jaw is close to its adult size. According to the American Society of Plastic Surgeons, 7% of patients who had mentoplasties in the United States in 2002 were 18 or younger; 35% were between the ages of 19 and 34; 40% were between the ages of 35 and 50, while another 15% were between 51 and 64. Only 3% were over 65.

With respect to sex, women account for 69% of mentoplasty patients; only 31% are men.

Description

Mentoplasties fall into two large categories: procedures that augment (increase) small or receding chins; and those that reduce large or protruding chins. Chin augmentation is done more frequently than chin reduction, reflecting the fact that microgenia (small chin) is the most common abnormality of the chin.

Chin augmentation

Chin augmentation can be performed by inserting an implant under the skin of the chin or by performing a sliding genioplasty. Insertion of an implant takes 30–60 minutes, while a sliding genioplasty takes slightly longer, 45–90 minutes. If the mentoplasty is done together with orthognathic surgery, the operation may take as long as three hours.

Chin implants are used in patients with mild or moderate microgenia. At one time they were made of cartilage taken from donors or from other sites on the patient's body, but as of 2003 alloplastic implants (made from inert foreign materials) are used more often because they reduce the risk of infection. To insert the implant, the surgeon can choose to make the incision under the chin (submental) or inside the mouth (intraoral). In either case, the surgeon cuts through several layers of tissue, taking care to avoid damaging the major nerve in the chin. The surgeon makes a pocket in the connective tissue inside the chin and washes it out with an antiseptic solution. The sterile implant is then inserted in the pocket and positioned properly. The incision is closed and the wound covered with Steri-Strips.

A sliding genioplasty may be performed if the patient's chin is too small for augmentation with an implant, or if the deformity is more complex. In this procedure, the surgeon cuts through the jawbone with an oscillating saw and removes part of the bone. He or she then moves the bone segment forward, holding it in place with metal plates and screws. After the bone segment has been fixed in place, the incision is closed and the patient's head is wrapped with a pressure dressing.

Chin reduction

Reduction of an overly large or protruding chin may be done either by direct reduction or a sliding genioplasty. In a direct reduction, the surgeon makes either a submental or an intraoral incision and removes excess bone from the chin with a burr. A sliding genioplasty reduction is similar to a genioplasty to augment the chin, except that the bone segment is moved backward rather than forward.

Diagnosis/Preparation

Diagnosis

Diagnostic evaluation consists of a facial analysis as well as a complete dental and medical history. The chin is one of the three most significant parts of the face from an aesthetic standpoint, the others being the forehead and the nose. Many patients who are concerned about the size of their nose, for example, can be helped by having a too-small chin augmented as well as having the nose reshaped. In the facial analysis, the face is divided into thirds, with the mouth and chin in the lowest third. The surgeon compares the proportions of the features in each third in order to determine the most suitable procedure for restoring balance. The patient will be photographed from several angles to document the condition of the chin before surgery.

The dental history and x ray studies of the head and jaw are necessary in order to determine whether the facial disproportion can be corrected by an implant or simple reduction, or whether orthognathic surgery is required. Patients who have severe malocclusion (irregular contact between the teeth in the upper and lower jaws) or deformities of the facial bones are usually referred to a maxillofacial specialist for reconstructive surgery.

Lastly, the surgeon will evaluate the patient for any signs of psychological instability, including unrealistic expectations of the results of surgery.

Preparation

Patients should stop smoking and discontinue all medications containing **aspirin** or NSAIDs for two weeks prior to mentoplasty. If the surgeon is planning to make a submental incision, the patient should use an antibacterial facial cleanser for two days before surgery. Patients scheduled for an intraoral approach should rinse the mouth with mouthwash three times a day for two days before surgery. They should not eat or drink anything for eight hours prior to the procedure.

Aftercare

Patients should have someone drive them home after the procedure. They are given medication for discomfort and a one-week course of antibiotic medication to reduce the risk of infection. Most patients can return to work in seven to 10 days.

Other aspects of aftercare include the following:

• a soft or liquid diet for four to five days

• raising the head of the bed or using two to three pillows

• rinsing the mouth with a solution of hydrogen peroxide and warm water two to three times daily

- avoiding sleeping on the face and unnecessary touching of the chin area
- avoiding vigorous physical **exercise** for about two weeks

Risks

In addition to infection, bleeding, and an allergic reaction to the anesthetic, the risks of insertion of a chin implant include:

- deformity of the chin following an infection
- injury to the major nerve in the chin, leading to loss of feeling or paralysis of the chin muscles
- erosion of the bone beneath the implant
- moving around or dislocation of the implant
- extrusion (pushing out) of the implant

Specific risks associated with sliding genioplasties include:

- under- or over-correction of the defect
- injury to the major nerve in the chin
- failure of the bone segment to reunite properly with the other parts of the jaw
- damage to the roots of the teeth
- hematoma (a collection of blood within a body organ or tissue caused by leakage from broken blood vessels; it can damage the results of a mentoplasty by causing pressure that distorts the final shape of the chin)

Normal results

Normal results of either augmentation or reduction mentoplasty include correction of facial asymmetry and disproportion. The functioning of the jaw is also often improved. Patients who have had a mentoplasty are usually very satisfied with the results.

Morbidity and mortality rates

The rate of complications with chin implants as well as sliding genioplasties is about 5%.

Alternatives

Fat injections

In some cases, fat may be injected into the area below the chin to plump up the skin and minimize the apparent size of the chin. This technique, however, is limited to minor disproportions of chin size. In addition, fat injections must be repeated periodically as the fat is gradually absorbed by the body.

Liposuction

Facial **liposuction** can be used together with or instead of mentoplasty to improve the patient's profile. In particular, removal of fatty tissue below the chin can make a receding chin look larger or more prominent.

See also Face lift; Rhinoplasty.

Resources

BOOKS

Sargent, Larry, MD. *The Craniofacial Surgery Book*. Chattanooga, TN: Erlanger Health System, 2000.

"Temporomandibular Disorders." In *The Merck Manual of Diagnosis and Therapy*, edited by Mark H. Beers, MD, and Robert Berkow, MD. Whitehouse Station, NJ: Merck Research Laboratories, 1999.

PERIODICALS

Abraham, Manoj T., MD, and Thomas Romo III, MD. "Liposuction of the Face and Neck." *eMedicine*. January 8, 2003 [cited April 22, 2003]. <http://www.emedicine.com/ent/topic581.htm>.

Chang, Edward, MD, DDS, Samuel M. Lam, MD, and Edward Farrior, MD. "Genioplasty." *eMedicine*. June 7, 2002 [cited April 20, 2003]. <http://www.emedicine.com/ent/topic106.htm>.

Chang, E. W., S. M. Lam, M. Karen, and J. L. Donlevy. "Sliding Genioplasty for Correction of Chin Abnormalities." *Archives of Facial Plastic Surgery* 3 (January-March 2001): 8–15.

Danahey, D. G., S. H. Dayan, A. G. Benson, and J. A. Ness. "Importance of Chin Evaluation and Treatment to Optimizing Neck Rejuvenation Surgery." *Facial Plastic Surgery* 17 (May 2001): 91–97.

Galli, Suzanne K. D., MD, and Philip J. Miller, MD. "Chin Implants." *eMedicine*. May 15, 2002 [cited April 22, 2003]. <http://www.emedicine.com/ent/topic628.htm>.

Grossman, John A., MD. "Facial Alloplastic Implants, Chin." *eMedicine*. July 5, 2001 [cited April 21, 2003]. <http://www.emedicine.com/plastic/topic56.htm>.

Jafar, M., and R. A. Younger. "Screw Fixation Mentoplasty." *Journal of Otolaryngology* 29 (October 2000): 274–278.

Meszaros, Liz. "Sliding Genioplasty Successful in Correcting Chin Abnormalities." *Cosmetic Surgery Times*, September 1, 2001.

Patel, Pravin K., MD, Hongshik Han, MD, and Nak-Heon Kang, MD. "Craniofacial, Orthognathic Surgery." *eMedicine*. December 27, 2001 [cited April 21, 2003]. <http://www.emedicine.com/plastic/topic177.htm>.

Siwolop, Sana. "Beyond Botox: An Industry's Quest for Smooth Skin." *New York Times,* March 9, 2003 [cited March 9, 2003]. <http://www.nytimes.com/2003/03/09/business/09FACE.html>.

ORGANIZATIONS

American Academy of Facial Plastic and Reconstructive Surgery (AAFPRS). 310 South Henry Street, Alexandria, VA 22314. (703) 299-9291. <http://www.facemd.org>.

American Society of Plastic Surgeons (ASPS). 444 East Algonquin Road, Arlington Heights, IL 60005. (847) 228-9900. <http://www.plasticsurgery.org>.

KEY TERMS

Aesthetic—Pertaining to beauty. Plastic surgery done to improve the patient's appearance is sometimes called aesthetic surgery.

Agenesis—The absence of an organ or body part due to developmental failure.

Alloplast—An implant made of an inert foreign material such as silicone or hydroxyapatite.

Congenital—Present at the time of birth.

Extrusion—Pushing out or expulsion. Extrusion of a chin implant is one possible complication of mentoplasty.

Genioplasty—Another word for mentoplasty. It comes from the Greek word for "chin."

Hematoma—A localized collection of blood in an organ or tissue due to broken blood vessels.

Intraoral—Inside the mouth.

Malocclusion—Malpositioning and defective contact between opposing teeth in the upper and lower jaws.

Microgenia—An extremely small chin. It is the most common deformity of the chin.

Orthognathic surgery—Surgery that corrects deformities or malpositioning of the bones in the jaw. The term comes from two Greek words meaning straight and jaw.

Sliding genioplasty—A complex plastic surgery procedure in which the patient's jawbone is cut, moved forward or backward, and repositioned with metal plates and screws.

Submental—Underneath the chin.

FACES: The National Craniofacial Association. P. O. Box 11082, Chattanooga, TN 37401. (800) 332-2373. <http://www.faces-cranio.org>.

OTHER

American Academy of Facial Plastic and Reconstructive Surgery. *2001 Membership Survey: Trends in Facial Plastic Surgery.* Alexandria, VA: AAFPRS, 2002.

American Academy of Facial Plastic and Reconstructive Surgery. *Procedures: Understanding Mentoplasty Surgery.* [cited April 20, 2003]. <http://www.facial-plastic-surgery.org/patient/procedures/mentoplasty.html>.

American Society of Plastic Surgeons. *Procedures: Facial Implants.* [cited April 20, 2003]. <http://www.plasticsurgery.org/public_education/procedures/FacialImplants.cfm>.

Rebecca Frey, Ph.D.

Microalbumin test *see* **Urinalysis**

Microsurgery

Definition

Microsurgery is surgery that is performed on very small structures, such as blood vessels and nerves, with specialized instruments under a microscope.

Purpose

Microsurgical procedures are performed on parts of the body that are best visualized under a microscope. Examples of such structures are small blood vessels, nerves, and tubes. Microsurgery uses techniques that have been performed by surgeons since the early twentieth century, such as blood vessel repair and organ transplantation, but under conditions that make traditional **vascular surgery** difficult or impossible.

The first microvascular surgery, using a microscope to aid in the repair of blood vessels, was described by Jules Jacobson of the University of Vermont in 1960. The first successful replantation (reattachment of an amputated body part) was reported in 1964 by Harry Bunke. This replantation of a rabbit's ear was significant because blood vessels smaller than 0.04 in (0.1 cm)—similar in size to the blood vessels found in a human hand—were successfully attached. Two years later, the successful replantation of a toe to the hand of a monkey was made possible using microsurgical techniques. Soon thereafter, microsurgery began being used in a number of clinical settings.

Numerous surgical specialties utilize the techniques of microsurgery. Otolaryngologists (ear, nose, and throat doctors) perform microsurgery on the small, delicate structures of the inner ear or the vocal cords. Cataracts are removed by ophthalmologists (eye doctors), who also perform corneal transplants and treat eye conditions like glaucoma. Urologists can reverse vasectomies (male sterilization), and gynecologists can reverse tubal ligations (female sterilization), giving people new choices about having children. Microsurgical techniques are used by plastic surgeons to reconstruct damaged or disfigured skin, muscles, or other tissues, or to transplant tissues from other parts of the body. And, importantly, a number of specialties can collaborate to treat patients who have limbs or other body parts; under certain circumstances, amputated parts can be reattached, or another body part can be replanted in the

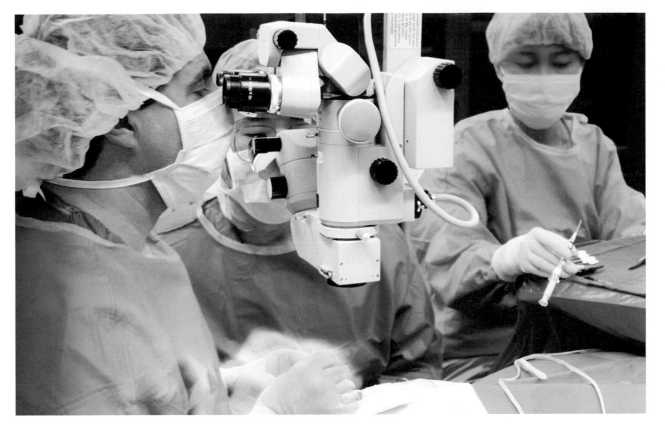

Surgeon performing microsurgery using specialized instruments and a microscope. *(Custom Medical Stock Photo. Reproduced by permission.)*

place of one lost (for example, a great toe replacing a lost or damaged thumb).

Today, microsurgery can be lifesaving. Neurosurgeons can treat vascular abnormalities found in the brain, and cancerous tumors can be removed.

Description

Equipment

Microsurgical equipment magnifies the operating field, provide instrumentation precise enough to maneuver under high magnification, and allow the surgeon to operate on structures barely visible to the human eye. The most important tools used by the microsurgeon are the microscope, microsurgical instruments, and microsuture materials.

MICROSCOPE. While operating microscopes may differ according to their specific use, certain features are standard. The microscope may be floor- or ceiling-mounted, with a moveable arm that allows the surgeon to manipulate the microscope's position. A view of the surgical site is afforded by a set of lenses and a high-intensity light source. This lighting is enhanced by maintaining

a low level of light in the rest of the **operating room**. Two or more sets of lenses allow a surgeon and an assistant to view the operating field and focus and zoom independently. A video camera allows the rest of the **surgical team** to view the operating field on a display screen. Features that come on some microscopes include foot and/or mouth switch controls and motorized zoom and focus.

A magnification of five to forty times (5–40x) is generally required for microsurgery. A lower magnification may be used to identify and expose structures, while a higher magnification is most often used for microsurgical repair. Alternatively, surgical loupes (magnifying lenses mounted on a pair of eyeglasses) may be used for lower magnifications (2–6x).

INSTRUMENTS. Microsurgical instruments differ from conventional instruments in a number of ways. They must be capable of delicately manipulating structures barely visible to the naked eye, but with handles large enough to hold comfortably and securely. They must also take into account the tremor of the surgeon's hand, greatly amplified under magnification.

Some of the various instruments that are used in microsurgery include:

- forceps

- needle holders (for suturing)

- scissors

- vascular clamps (for controlling bleeding) and clamp applicators

- irrigators (for washing structures in the surgical field)

- vessel dilators (for opening up the cut end of a blood vessel)

- various standard surgical tools

SUTURE MATERIALS. Suturing, or stitching, is done by means of specialized thread and needles. The diameter (gauge) of suture thread ranges in size and depends on the procedure and tissue to be sutured. Conventional suturing usually requires gauges of 2-0 (0.3 mm) to 6-0 (0.07 mm). Conversely, gauges of 9-0 (0.03 mm) to 12-0 (0.001 mm) are generally used for microsurgery. Suture thread may be absorbable (able to be broken down in the body after a definite amount of time) or non-absorbable (retaining its strength indefinitely), natural (made of silk, gut, linen, or other natural material) or synthetic (made of nylon, polyester, wire, or other man-made material). The type of suture thread used depends on the procedure and tissue to be sutured.

The suture needle comes in various sizes (diameters and length) and shapes (straight or curved), and also with different point types (rounded, cutting, or blunt). It comes with suture thread preattached to one end; this is called the swage. As in the case of suture thread, the type of needle used depends on the procedure and tissue to be sutured; generally, needles with a diameter of less than 0.15 mm are used for microsurgery.

Training

For a surgeon to perform microsurgery in a clinical setting, extensive training and practice are required. A basic knowledge of anatomy and surgical techniques is essential. After a thorough introduction to the operating microscope and other microsurgical equipment, basic techniques are introduced using small animals as the experimental model. Specifically, surgeons must be taught how to maintain correct posture and to maintain constant visual contact with the microscope during surgery, how to properly hold and use the instruments, how to minimize the amount of hand tremor, and how to perform basic techniques, such as suturing. After becoming proficient at these skills, more advanced techniques can be taught, including procedures regarding how to treat specific conditions.

Extensive and ongoing practice is necessary for a surgeon to maintain adequate proficiency at microsur-

gical techniques. For this reason, a microsurgical laboratory is made available to surgeons for training and practice.

Techniques

Most microsurgical procedures utilize a set of basic techniques that must be mastered by the surgeon. These include blood vessel repair, vein grafting, and nerve repair and grafting.

BLOOD VESSEL REPAIR. Blood vessel, or vascular anastomosis, is the connection of two cut or separate blood vessels to form a continuous channel. Anastomoses may be end-to-end (between two cut ends of a blood vessel) or end-to-side (a connection of one cut end of a blood vessel to the wall of another vessel).

The first step of creating an anastomosis is to identify and expose the blood vessel by isolating it from surrounding tissues. Each end of the vessel is irrigated (washed) and secured with clamps for the duration of the procedure. A piece of contrast material is placed behind the surgical site so that the tiny vessel can be more easily visualized. The magnification is then increased for the next segment of surgery. The first suture is placed through the full thickness of the vessel wall; the second and third sutures are then placed at 120° from the first. Subsequent sutures are placed evenly in the remaining spaces. Arteries 1 millimeter in diameter generally require between five and eight stitches around the perimeter, and veins of the same size between seven and 10. Once the last suture has been placed, the clamps are released and blood is allowed to flow through the anastomosis. If excessive bleeding occurs between the stitches, the vessel is reclamped and additional sutures are placed.

The procedure for an end-to-side anastomosis is similar, except that an oval-shaped hole is cut in the wall of the recipient vessel. Sutures are first placed at each of the oval to connect the attaching vessel to the recipient vessel, and then placed evenly to fill in the remaining spaces.

VEIN GRAFTING. Vein grafting is an alternative procedure to end-to-end anastomosis and may be pursued if cut ends of a blood vessel cannot be attached without tension. Nonessential veins similar in diameter to the recipient blood vessel can be removed from the hand, arm, or foot. If the graft is to be used to reconstruct an artery, its direction is reversed so that the venous valves do not interfere with blood flow. End-to-end anastomosis is then performed on each end of the graft, using the suture techniques described above.

NERVE REPAIR. The process of connecting two cut ends of a nerve is called neurorrhaphy, or nerve anastomosis. Peripheral nerves are composed of bunches of nerve fibers called fascicles that are enclosed by a layer called the perineurium; the epineurium is the outer layer of the nerve that encases the fascicles. Nerve repair may involve suturing of the epineurium only, the perineurium only, or through both layers.

Many of the techniques used for blood vessel anastomoses are also used for nerves. The cut ends of the nerve are exposed, then isolated from surrounding tissues. The ends are trimmed so that healthy nerve tissue is exposed, and a piece of contrast material placed behind the nerve for better visualization. Each nerve end is examined to determine the pattern of fascicles; the nerve ends are then rotated so that the fascicle patterns align. Sutures may be placed around the circumference of the epineurium; this is called epineurial neurorrhaphy. The perineurium of each cut fascicle end may be stitched with excess epineurium removed (perineurial neurorrhaphy), or both layers may be sutured (epiperineurial neurorrhaphy).

NERVE GRAFTING. If there is a large gap between the cut ends of a nerve, neurorrhaphy cannot be performed without creating tension in the nerve that can interfere with postsurgical function. A piece of nerve from another part of body may be used to create a nerve graft that is stitched into place using anastomosis techniques. A disadvantage to nerve grafting is that a loss of function or sensation is experienced from the donor nerve site. A common nerve used for grafting is the sural nerve, which innervates parts of the lower leg.

Diagnosis/Preparation

In an emergency situation, such as an **amputation** or crushing injury, a number of steps must be taken immediately to improve the odds that replantation or reconstruction will be successful. An IV line is placed so that fluids and **antibiotics** can be administered. The injured area is x rayed so that the extent of the injury can be determined, and the amputated body part is wrapped in sterile gauze and placed on ice, so that the tissues are preserved. To prevent freezing, the body part must not be packed below the ice. The patient is transported by ambulance or helicopter to the nearest surgical center capable of microsurgical repair.

In other cases, a patient may suffer from a chronic condition or wound, and microsurgery can be scheduled as an elective procedure. Prior to surgery, the patient will be instructed to refrain from tobacco use because it interferes with healing. In addition, the patient will be told not to eat after midnight the day of surgery. It is important that the patient inform the doctor completely about any prior surgeries, medical conditions, or medications

taken on a regular basis, including **nonsteroidal anti-inflammatory drugs** (NSAIDs), such as **aspirin**. Patients taking blood thinners, such as Coumadin or Heparin (generic name: warfarin), should not adjust their medication themselves, but should speak with their prescribing doctors regarding their upcoming surgery). Patients should never adjust dosage without their doctors' approval. This is especially important for elderly patients, asthmatics, those with hypertension, or those who are on ACE inhibitors.

The patient will be placed under general anesthesia for the duration of the procedure. The advantages to general anesthesia are that the patient remains unconscious and completely relaxed during the procedure, imperative because of the precise nature and extended duration of the surgery. The patient must be able to tolerate the long surgery and therefore must be relatively stable condition; complex surgeries may take up to 12 hours or more.

Microsurgery makes possible a number of reconstructive procedures that would be more difficult or impossible with conventional surgery. Some of the more frequently performed microsurgical procedures include:

• Replantation. This **emergency surgery** is performed to reattach an amputated body part such as a finger, arm, or foot. Replantation surgery requires a series of time- and energy-intensive steps to reattach all of the structures while the amputated part is still viable. The cut bone must be shortened slightly so that blood vessels and nerves can be reattached without tension. Anastomoses are created between cut arteries and veins and blood flow is reestablished to the amputated part. Tendons (if present) are then repaired, followed by nerves and soft tissues. Further procedures may be necessary to completely the reconstruction depending on the extent of the injury.

• Transplantation. In some cases an amputated part cannot be reattached, or tissue is deformed because of a congenital defect or an injury. Transplantation may then be an option. The great toe or second toe may be removed from a patient's foot and transplanted to the hand to replace a missing finger. A segment of rib along with its blood supply can be used to reconstruct bones in the face and jaw.

• Free-tissue transfers. Also called free flaps, free-tissue transfers may be used to reconstruct damaged tissues that cannot be treated with skin grafts, closed by traditional methods such as suturing, or allowed to heal without intervention. This includes tissues that have constricted after a burn, injuries in which there is not sufficient skin to properly close the wound, or tissues that have been removed as a result of treatment for cancer. Examples of tissues that may be transferred with

KEY TERMS

Capillaries—Tiny blood vessels that deliver oxygen to tissues.

Peripheral nerves—The nerves outside of the brain and spinal cord.

Vascular surgery—A branch of medicine that deals with the surgical repair of disorders of or injuries to the blood vessels.

Venous valves—Folds on the inner lining of the veins that prevent the backflow of blood.

microsurgical techniques are skin, muscle, fat, bone, and intestine.

Aftercare

Following surgery, the patient is given intravenous fluids and usually progresses to a liquid diet within 12 to 24 hours, and a regular diet soon thereafter. The patient must be kept warm and adequately hydrated, and the surgical site is elevated if possible to help drain excess fluids. Medications are administered to help manage pain. The color, temperature, quality of capillary refill, and tissue turgor (fullness) of the surgical site are closely monitored. Skin should be pink, warm, and have one- to two-second capillary refill. Conversely, tissue that is pale or blue, cool, with no refill or rapid refill may indicate a problem with blood flow.

Certain tests may be recommended to further evaluate the surgical site. These include:

• Doppler ultrasound. This technology uses high-frequency sound waves to evaluate the flow of blood to and from the surgical site.

• Intravenous fluorescein. After a chemical dye called fluorescein is administered to the patient, a specialized machine called a fluorimeter is used to determine how much blood is flowing through the surgical site.

• Pulse oximetry. A **pulse oximeter** measures the amount of oxygen in the blood and tracks the patient's pulse.

• Arteriography. X rays are taken of the surgical site after a contrast dye has been injected into the bloodstream to determine the condition of vascular anastomoses.

When the patient is discharged from the hospital, he or she will receive instructions for aftercare. Exposure to tobacco must be limited for at least six weeks following the surgery, as nicotine interferes with circulation. The patient must remain warm as body temperature also af-

fects circulation. Bed rest may be prescribed for a period of days to weeks after surgery, depending on the procedure. Patients who have had a hand, finger, or multiple fingers replanted must keep the part elevated at heart level to help blood flow and decrease swelling.

Some form of rehabilitation is often recommended after microsurgery. This includes a program of individualized exercises used to restore function to a replanted or transplanted body part. In some cases where problems with circulation occur after surgery, leech therapy may be recommended. Leeches are worms that attach to the skin and draw blood while also injecting substances into the skin that act as a local anesthetic and an anticoagulant (preventing the formation of blood clots). Therapy involves attaching a leech to the replanted part or tissue flap and allow it to feed for 15 to 30 minutes, several times a day, until blood flow is established.

Resources

BOOKS

Jobe, Mark T. "Microsurgery" (Chapter 60). In *Campbell's Operative Orthopedics,* 10th ed. Philadelphia: Mosby, Inc., 2003.

ORGANIZATIONS

American Society for Reconstructive Microsurgery. 20 North Michigan Ave., Suite 700, Chicago, IL 60602. (312) 456-9579. <http://www.microsurg.org>.

OTHER

Buncke, Harry J. *Microsurgery: Transplantation-Replantation.* 2002 [cited April 25, 2003]. <http://buncke.org/book/contents.html>.

Chang, James. "Principles of Microsurgery." *eMedicine.* August 5, 2002 [cited April 25, 2003]. <http://www.emedicine.com/plastic/topic262.htm>.

"Microsurgery." *California Pacific Medical Center.* [cited April 25, 2003]. <http://www.cpmc.org/advanced/microsurg/>.

"Online Atlas of Microsurgery." *Microsurgeon.org.* March 20, 2003 [cited April 25, 2003]. <http://www.microsurgeon.org>.

Stephanie Dionne Sherk

Minimally invasive heart surgery

Definition

Minimally invasive heart surgery refers to surgery performed on the beating heart to provide coronary artery bypass grafting. This technique is often referred to as MIDCAB, minimally invasive direct coronary artery bypass; or OPCAB, off-pump CABG.

Purpose

Minimally invasive heart surgery is performed on the diseased heart to reroute blood around clogged arteries and improve the blood and oxygen supply to the heart. This approach provides patients some benefit in that cardiopulmonary bypass (use of a heart-lung machine) may be avoided, and smaller incisions can be used instead of the standard sternotomy (incision through the sternum, or breast bone) approach. Faster recovery time, decreased procedure costs, and reduced morbidity and mortality are the goals of this technique.

Minimally invasive technique is not new to the field of cardiac surgery. It was performed as early as the 1950s, although the technology associated with stabilizing the cardiac structure during the procedure has become more sophisticated. Also, the anesthesiologist and perfusionist (person monitoring blood flow) have developed better techniques to preserve cardiac function during the procedure to help the surgeon achieve the desired outcome. During the 1990s these new techniques were named: off-pump CABG (OPCAB) and minimally invasive direct coronary artery bypass (MIDCAB). The MIDCAB procedure includes procedures done both with and without cardiopulmonary bypass, the later being referred to as off-pump MIDCAB. Unless otherwise specified, MIDCAB refers to both types of procedures.

Minimally invasive valve surgery has been an outgrowth of the success with minimally invasive coronary artery bypass grafting. Incisions other then the traditional sternotomy allow access to the heart. Minimally invasive valve surgery still requires cardiopulmonary bypass, since this is a true open-heart procedure, (i.e. this is not surgery that is done while the heart is beating). New tools in managing cardioplegic cardiac arrest allow for the smaller incision unobstructed by the required instrumentation. Cannulation of the femoral vessels instead of the larger vessels of the heart also improves visualization.

Demographics

Patients under the age of 70, but not limited by age, with a history of coronary artery disease can be evaluated for this procedure. High risk patients with advanced age, at risk for stroke, or suffering peripheral vascular disease, renal disease, or with poor lung function may benefit from OPCAB and MIDCAB.

Typically disease of the left anterior descending coronary artery is treated with the technique called off-

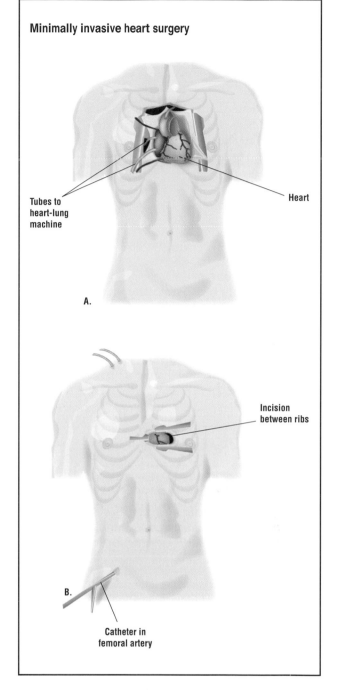

Minimally invasive heart surgery

Tubes to heart-lung machine

Heart

A.

Incision between ribs

B.

Catheter in femoral artery

In traditional open heart surgery, a large incision is made in the chest, and the sternum must be broken (A). Minimally invasive surgery uses a much smaller incision between the ribs to access the heart (B). *(Illustration by GGS Inc.)*

pump MIDCAB. With sternotomy, disease of the right and left coronary arteries can also be addressed by OPCAB. The significance and location of the coronary artery lesions may limit the success of the MIDCAB or OPCAB procedure. Most practices have at least one surgeon skilled in performing revascularizations without cardiopulmonary bypass. Of all coronary artery bypass grafting procedures, approximately 10–20% are performed in this manner.

Description

The patient receives cardiac monitoring during general anesthesia. Systemic anticoagulation is given to avoid clot formation from foreign surfaces and any periods of artery blockage (occlusion).

MIDCAB

If cardiopulmonary bypass is not employed, the procedure is called an off-pump MIDCAB. The surgeon performs an alternative incision (rather than a midline sternotomy), typically a left anterior **thoracotomy**. The left internal mammary artery is dissected from the left chest wall. A stabilizer device is placed on the heart to provide support of the left anterior descending artery as the heart continues to beat. This device applies gentle pressure or suction, mildly limiting cardiac function. The left internal mammary artery is sutured to the left anterior descending artery to bypass the blockage (anastomosis).

If cardiopulmonary bypass is indicated, the surgeon inserts cannulae (small, flexible tubes) into the femoral vessels. Aortic occlusion and cardioplegia are administered through a catheter advanced through the contralateral femoral artery into the aortic root (ascending aorta). This catheter has a balloon tip that stops blood flow to the coronary arteries when inflated, but allows selective administration of cardioplegia (a solution that stops the heart) to the coronary arteries. **Angiography** is performed to provide visualization of catheter placement.

The surgeon performs an alternative incision (rather than a midline sternotomy), typically a left anterior thoracotomy. The left internal mammary artery is dissected from the left chest wall. Cardiopulmonary bypass can be instituted with or without cardioplegic arrest. Cardioplegic arrest requires cardiopulmonary bypass. The use of cardioplegic arrest makes this a non-beating heart procedure, but it is still considered MIDCAB. Cardioplegic arrest of the heart occurs as the balloon tip of the catheter is inflated. The left internal mammary artery is sutured to the left anterior descending artery to bypass the blockage (anastomosis). Once the anastomosis is complete the balloon is deflated, allowing the heart to begin to beat. Cardiopulmonary bypass is discontinued once cardiac function is stabilized. The cannulae and catheter are removed, and the groin wounds are closed with sutures.

OPCAB

The OPCAB procedure does not use cardiopulmonary bypass. The incision of choice can be a midline sternotomy or a left anterior thoracotomy (incision into the side). The midline sternotomy allows access to both the right and left internal mammary arteries. Additional vascular bypass conduits may be acquired by harvesting the saphenous vein (in the leg), gastroepiploic artery (near the stomach), or radial artery (in the arm). A stabilizing device is used to secure the coronary artery of choice. This device applies gentle pressure or suction, mildly limiting cardiac function, but providing better access to posterior and inferior vessels of the heart. The surgeon makes the necessary anastomosis to the targeted coronary arteries. If conduits other then the mammary arteries are used they are connected to the ascending aorta to provide systemic blood flow.

If an anticoagulant was administered, drugs are given to reverse the anticoagulant. Upon completion of the off-pump MIDCAB, MIDCAB, or OPCAB procedure, the chest is closed. If a midline sternotomy was performed, stainless steel wires are implanted to hold the sternal bone together. Sutures are used to close the skin wound, and sterile bandages are applied as a wound dressing.

Diagnosis/Preparation

An electrocardiogram detects the presence of acute coronary blockage (occlusion). A history of myocardial infarction can also be detected by electrocardiogram. Patients with a history of angina also are evaluated for coronary artery disease. Coronary angiography provides the best diagnostic information about the extent and location of the coronary artery disease.

Aftercare

The patient receives continued cardiac monitoring in the **intensive care unit**. Once the patient is able to breathe on his/her own, the breathing tube is removed (extubation), if it is not removed immediately post-operatively. Any medications to treat poor cardiac function or manage blood pressure are discontinued as cardiac function improves and blood pressure stabilizes. Blood drainage tubes protruding from the chest cavity are removed once internal bleeding decreases. The patient also may be equipped with external cardiac pacing to maintain heart rate. The pacing is terminated once the heart is beating at an adequate rate free of arrhythmia. A warming blanket may be used to warm the patient's core temperature that was decreased by the surgical exposure.

The duration of the post-operative hospital stay is reduced by one to two days in these procedures. Pain also should be reduced. Homecare for the wound is described prior to discharge, and instructions for responding to adverse events after discharge also are given. Patients who have undergone these procedures should expect to return to normal activities sooner than those who have undergone traditional coronary artery bypass grafting.

Risks

MIDCAB can result in a higher rate of restenosis (recurrence of narrowing of the arteries) then traditional coronary artery bypass grafting, but these numbers continue to decrease as experience with the procedure improves. Some patients may have to have the procedure converted to a standard sternotomy with cardiopulmonary bypass, if the anastomosis can not be completed from the MIDCAB approach. Rib fracture is the most common adverse event. Pericarditis also is a possible complication. Supraventricular arrhythmias and ST segment elevation also may develop.

In the event of systemic blood pressure abnormalities, arrhythmia, poor surgical anastomosis, or poor exposure of the coronary blood vessels, OPCAB patients may require conversion to cardiopulmonary bypass for completion of the anastomosis. Post-operatively some patients may need additional surgery to control bleeding or to address poor sternal healing. This is related to the increased use of both internal mammary arteries for these procedures. Cerebral complications and atrial fibrillation also may be experienced. These post-operative complications are comparable to those seen in patients who have undergone traditional coronary artery bypass grafting.

Normal results

Patency (openess) of the grafted vessels is expected to be the same as what is seen in traditional coronary

---

QUESTIONS TO ASK THE DOCTOR

- Is there a surgeon associated with this practice skilled with OPCAB or MIDCAB procedures?
- Can the surgeon skilled in these procedures evaluate the patient for an OPCAB or MIDCAB procedure?
- How many procedures has the surgeon performed in the last year? In the last five years?
- What is the surgeon's reoperation rate in regards to length of graft patency?

---

artery bypass grafting. When compared to traditional coronary artery bypass grafting, minimally invasive heart surgery also is expected to result in a shorter hospital stay, less pain, fewer blood transfusions, and quicker return to normal activity.

Morbidity and mortality rates

MIDCAB

Conversion to a full sternotomy or sternotomy with cardiopulmonary bypass is expected in 1–2% of patients. Redo procedures and **reoperation** can occur in over 5% of patients, which is still lower than the risk of a second procedure associated with balloon **angioplasty** and stent placement. Over 90% of all patients are expected to be free of adverse events. Complications most frequently involve rib fracture (over 10% of patients). Mortality associated with MICAB is low and is not seen during the surgical procedure in most instances, but is associated with post-operative complications.

OPCAB

Conversion to cardiopulmonary bypass may be required in patients if anastomosis cannot be completed due to unstable blood pressure, arrhythmia, ischemia, poor anastomosis, or poor surgical access. The same operative mortality is expected when compared to cardiopulmonary bypass patients. The expected decrease in neurological events, renal dysfunction, pulmonary complications, or arrhythmias has not yet been shown to be a consistent benefit, therefore all of these complications can still occur.

Alternatives

Percutaneous balloon angioplasty and **coronary stenting** of the left anterior descending artery are successful alternative procedures. MIDCAB may be a preferred treatment when compared to balloon angioplasty and stenting because fewer repeat interventions are required. An additional alternative is traditional on-pump, cardiopulmonary bypass; coronary artery bypass grafting is a powerful technique with a long record of safety and effectiveness since the 1960s.

Resources

BOOKS

Hensley, Frederick A., Donald E. Martin, and Glenn P. Gravlee, eds. *A Practical Approach to Cardiac Anesthesia.* 3rd ed. Philadelphia: Lippincott Williams & Wilkins 2003.

PERIODICALS

Borst, H. G. and F. W. Mohr. "The History of Coronary Artery Surgery—A Brief Review." *The Thoracic and Cardiovascular Surgeon* 49 (2001): 195–198.

Holubkov, R., et al. "MIDCAB Characteristics and Results: the CardioThoracic Systems (CTS) Registry." *European Journal of Cardio-Thoracic Surgery* 14, suppl.1 (1998): S25–S30.

Lund, O., et al. "On-pump Versus Off-pump Coronary Artery Bypass: Independent Risk Factors and Off-Pump Graft Patency." *European Journal of Cardio-Thoracic Surgery* 20 (2001): 901–907.

Moussa, I., et al. "Frequency of Early Occlusion and Stenosis in Bypass Grafts After Minimally Invasive Direct Coronary Arterial Bypass Surgery." *The American Journal of Cardiology* 88 (2001): 311–313.

Allison Joan Spiwak, MSBME

Minor tranquilizers *see* **Antianxiety drugs**

Mitral valve repair

Definition

Mitral valve repair is a surgical procedure used to improve the function of a stenotic (narrowed), prolapsed, or insufficient mitral valve of the heart.

Purpose

The mitral valve can become diseased, preventing it from adequately controlling the direction of the blood flow between the left atrium and left ventricle. It also can become insufficient (regurgitant), letting blood flow backwards into the left atrium (upper chamber) from the left ventricle (lower chamber) during ventricular contraction (systole). The mitral valve also can become stenotic (narrowed), preventing the flow of blood from the left atrium into the left ventricle during ventricular filling (diastole). In mitral valve prolapse, one or more of the mitral valve's cusps protrude back into the left atrium during ventricular contraction. Mitral valve repair is performed to improve the function of the diseased valve so that it correctly controls the direction of blood flow.

Demographics

Approximately 65,000 valve repairs and replacements are performed in the United States annually.

Twice as many women as men are affected by mitral valve stenosis. About 60% of patients with mitral valve stenosis have had rheumatic fever. After rheumatic fever there is usually a latency period of 10–20 years before symptoms of mitral valve stenosis appear. The prevalence of mitral valve stenosis has declined in the United States because there has been a decline in the number of cases of rheumatic fever. Mitral valve stenosis may be present at birth (congenital); however, it rarely occurs alone but rather in conjunction with other heart defects.

Mitral valve prolapse is the most common condition of the heart valves, and is present in about 2% of the general population. Recent studies indicate that similar numbers of men and women have mitral valve prolapse. Having this condition does not guarantee that mitral insufficiency will develop. Patients with a history of rheumatic fever, coronary artery disease, infective endocarditis, or collagen vascular disease also may develop mitral insufficiency.

Description

Cardiac monitoring is instituted and general anesthesia is provided. The surgeon uses a sternotomy to access the heart and great blood vessels. Anticoagulation is given as cannulae are inserted into the great vessels, femoral vessels, or a combination. Cardiopulmonary bypass is instituted. The heart is arrested as the cross clamp is applied to the ascending aorta to stop blood flow through the organ. The surgeon opens the heart to visualize the mitral valve. He/she may expose the mitral valve by opening the right atrium and then opening the atrial septum. Another approach requires a large left atrium that can be opened directly, making the mitral valve visible.

Mitral commissurotomy

Mitral commissurotomy is used to repair mitral stenosis associated with rheumatic disease. The commissures—openings between the valve leaflets—are manually separated by the surgeon. Fused chordae tendineae (cords of connective tissue that connect the mitral valve to the papillary muscle of the heart's left ventricle) are separated, along with papillary muscles. Calcium deposits may be removed from the valve leaflets. The left atrial appendage is removed to reduce the risk of future thromboemboli (blood clot) generation.

Chordae tendineae repair

The chordae tendineae can become lengthened or rupture, resulting in mitral valve prolapse. A skilled surgeon repairs the mitral valve structure by placing sutures in the valve leaflets to stabilize the valve structure. Typically the posterior leaflet requires this type of repair.

Annuloplasty

A flexible fabric ring is sutured to the valve annulus to provide support and reconstruction for the patient's valve annulus. The size of the ring is selected to match the patient's own valve size. This repair allows the valve to function normally.

The heart is closed with sutures. Deairing of the heart is performed prior to removal of the cross clamp. When the cross clamp is removed, deairing continues to ensure that no air is delivered to the systemic circulation. At this time a transesophageal echocardiogram (TEE) may be used to test that the valve is functioning correctly and that the heart is free of air. If the surgeon is not satisfied with the repair, **mitral valve replacement** is performed. Once the surgeon is satisfied that the valve is working correctly, cardiopulmonary bypass is terminated, anticoagulation is reversed, and the cannulae are removed from the vessels. The sternotomy is closed. Permanent stainless steel wires are used to hold the sternum bone together. The skin incision is closed with sutures, and sterile bandages are applied to the wound.

Diagnosis/Preparation

Mitral valve stenosis is diagnosed by history, **physical examination**, listening to the sounds of the heart (cardiac auscultation), **chest x ray**, and ECG. Patients may have no symptoms of a valve disorder or may have shortness of breath (dyspnea), fatigue, or pulmonary edema (fluid in the lungs). Other patients present with atrial fibrillation (a cardiac arrhythmia) or an embolic event (result of a blood clot). Doppler **echocardiography** is the preferred diagnostic tool for evaluation of mitral valve stenosis, and can be performed in conjunction with non-invasive **exercise** testing by treadmill or bicycle. **Cardiac catheterization** is reserved for patients who demonstrate discrepancies in Doppler testing. Both left- and right-heart catheterization should be performed in the presence of elevated pulmonary artery pressures.

A diagnosis of mitral insufficiency requires a detailed patient history. Listening to the heart (auscultation) reveals the presence of a third heart sound. Chest x ray and ECG provide additional information. Again, Doppler echocardiography provides valuable information. Exercise testing with Doppler echocardiography can show the true severity of the disease.

After initial findings, patients may be followed with repeat visits and testing to monitor disease progress. If the patient has reached NYHA Class III or IV, replace-

ment is considered. Severe pulmonary hypertension with pulmonary artery systolic pressures greater than 60 mm Hg is considered an indication for surgery. Left ventricular ejection fraction less than 60% also is an indication for surgery.

Aftercare

The patient receives continued cardiac monitoring in the **intensive care unit** and usually remains in intensive care for 24–48 hours after surgery. Ventilation support is discontinued when the patient is able to breathe on his/her own. If mechanical circulatory support and inotropic agents (a substance that influences the force of muscle contractions, e.g. digitalis) were needed during the surgical procedure, they are discontinued as cardiac function recovers. Tubes draining blood from the chest cavity are removed as bleeding from the surgical procedure decreases. Prophylactic **antibiotics** are given to prevent infective endocarditis and prevent the recurrence of rheumatic carditis.

If the patient recovers normally, **discharge from the hospital** occurs within a week of surgery. At discharge, the patient is given specific instructions about **wound care** and infection recognition, as well as contact information for the physician and guidelines about when a visit to the emergency room is indicated. Within three to four weeks after discharge, the patient is seen for follow-up office visit with the physician, at which time physical status will have improved for evaluation. Thereafter, asymptomatic, uncomplicated patients are seen at yearly intervals. Few limitations are placed on patient activity once recovery is complete.

Risks

There are always risks associated with general anesthesia and cardiopulmonary bypass. Risks specifically associated with mitral valve repair include embolism, bleeding, or operative valvular endocarditis. When valve repair does not produce adequate results, then increased operative time is required to replace the mitral valve. If the patient's mitral valve is replaced with a mechanical valve, the patient must take an anticoagulation drug, such as Coumadin, for the rest of his/her life. An inadequately repaired valve, if left untreated, results in continued myocardial dysfunction resulting in pulmonary edema, congestive heart failure, and systemic thromboemboli generation.

Normal results

Patients treated by mitral valve repair for mitral insufficiency can expect improved myocardial function and relief of symptoms. Oxygen consumption by skele-

Mitral valve repair

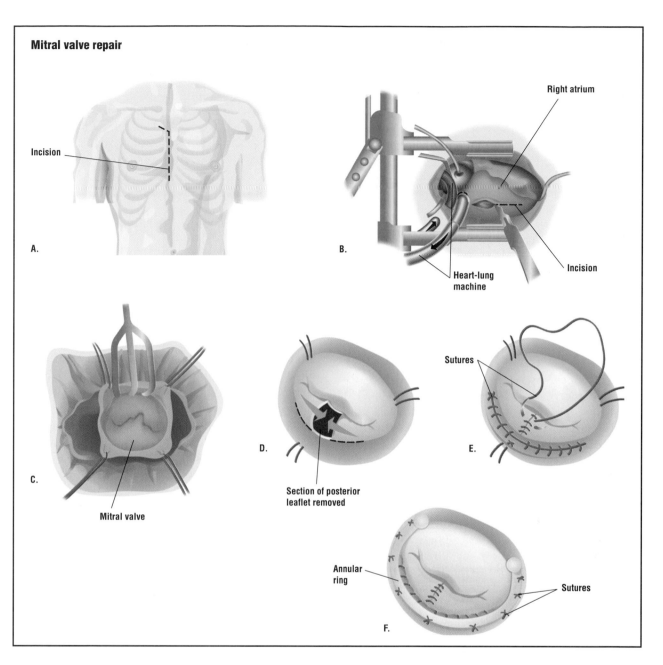

During a mitral valve repair, the patient's chest is opened along the sternum (A). The heart is connected to a heart-lung machine, and an incision is made into the right atrium, or upper chamber of the heart (B), exposing the mitral valve (C). A section of the valve is removed, and the area is repaired with sutures (D and E). A flexible fabric ring may be stitched to the outside of the valve to strengthen it, in a procedure called an annuloplasty (F). *(Illustration by GGS Inc.)*

tal muscle continues to improve. Cardiac output improves and pulmonary hypertension resolves over several months after the initial decrease in left atrial pressure, pulmonary artery pressure, and pulmonary arteriolar resistance.

Excellent results in terms of improved cardiac function and symptom relief also are expected for patients that undergo mitral valve repair for mitral stenosis.

Morbidity and mortality rates

Operative mortality associated with mitral valve repair for stenosis is 1–3%. The prognosis for restenosis (re-narrowing) is 30% at five years and 60% at nine years; additional surgery is required in 4–7% of patients at five years. Eighty to 90% of patients whose mitral valve stenosis was repaired by commissurotomy are complication free at five years after surgery.

KEY TERMS

Acute—Rapid onset.

Annulus—A ring-shaped structure.

Anticoagulants—Drugs that are given to slow blood clot formation.

Cannula—A small, flexible tube.

Cardiac catheterization—A diagnostic procedure (using a catheter inserted through a vein and threaded through the circulatory system to the heart) which does a comprehensive examination of how the heart and its blood vessels function.

Cardiopulmonary bypass—Use of the heart-lung machine to provide systemic circulation cardiac output and ventilation of the blood.

Chordae tendineae—The strands of connective tissue that connect the mitral valve to the papillary muscle of the heart's left ventricle.

Chronic—Long-term.

Commissures—The normal separations between the valve leaflets.

Doppler echocardiography—A testing technique that uses Doppler ultrasound technology to evaluate the pattern and direction of blood flow in the heart.

Endocarditis—Infection of the heart endocardium tissue, the inner most tissue and structures of the heart.

NYHA heart failure classification—A classification system for heart failure developed by the New York Heart Association. It includes the following four categories: I, symptoms with more than ordinary activity; II, symptoms with ordinary activity; III, symptoms with minimal activity; IV, symptoms at rest.

Oxygen consumption—Oxygen utilization for energy production.

Rheumatic carditis—Inflammation of the heart muscle associated with acute rheumatic fever.

Rheumatic fever—An inflammatory disease that arises as a complication of untreated or inadequately treated strep throat infection. Rheumatic fever can seriously damage the heart valves.

Sternotomy—A surgical opening into the thoracic cavity through the sternum (breastbone).

Systemic circulation—Circulation supplied by the aorta including all tissue and organ beds, except the alveolar sacs of the lungs used for gas exchange and respiration.

Thromboemboli—Blood clots that develop in the circulation and lodge in capillary beds of tissues and organs.

Transesophageal echocardiography—A diagnostic test using an ultrasound device that is passed into the esophagus of the patient to create a clear image of the heart muscle and other parts of the heart.

Mitral valve repair for mitral insufficiency is the preferred approach because it preserves the valvular apparatus and left ventricular function. It also eliminates the risk of mechanical valve failure and the need for lifelong anticoagulation.

Alternatives

The asymptomatic patient with a history of rheumatic fever can be treated with prophylactic antibiotics and followed until symptoms are appear. If atrial fibrillation develops antiarrhythmic medications can be used for treatment. Atrial **defibrillation** may relieve atrial fibrillation. Anticoagulants may be prescribed to prevent the occurrence of systemic embolization.

Mitral valve repair for mitral regurgitation is not as successful if the anterior leaflet is involved. Rheumatic, ischemic, or calcific diseases decrease the likelihood of repair in even the most skilled hands. In the absence of mitral valve replacement, mitral valve repair is indicated.

Resources

BOOKS

Hensley, Frederick A., Donald E. Martin, and Glenn P. Gravlee, eds. *A Practical Approach to Cardiac Anesthesia*. 3rd ed. Philadelphia: Lippincott Williams & Wilkins, 2003.

Topol, Eric J., ed. *Textbook of Interventional Cardiology*. Philadelphia: W. B. Saunders, 2002.

PERIODICALS

Bonow, R., et al. "ACC/AHA Guidelines for the Management of Patients with Valvular Heart Disease." *Journal of the American College of Cardiology* 32 (November 1998): 1486–1582.

Brown, Katherine Kay. "Minimally Invasive Valve Surgery" *Critical Care Nursing Quarterly* 20 (February 1998): 40–52.

Wiegand, Debra Lynn-McHale. "Advances in Cardiac Surgery: Valve Repair" *Critical Care Nurse* 23 (April 2003): 72–90.

Allison Joan Spiwak, MSBME

Mitral valve replacement

Definition

Mitral valve replacement is a surgical procedure in which the diseased mitral valve of the heart is replaced by a mechanical or biological tissue valve.

Purpose

The mitral valve can become diseased, preventing it from adequately controlling the direction of the flow of blood between the left atrium and left ventricle. It also can become insufficient (regurgitant) and allow blood to flow backwards into the left atrium from the left ventricle during ventricular contraction (systole). In addition, the mitral valve can become stenotic (narrowed), preventing the flow of blood from the left atrium into the left ventricle during ventricular filling (diastole). In mitral valve prolapse, one or more of the mitral valve's cusps protrude back into the left atrium during ventricular contraction. Mitral valve replacement is performed to remove the diseased valve and provide a new mechanical valve or biological tissue valve that correctly controls the direction of blood flow.

Demographics

Approximately 65,000 valve repairs and replacements are performed in the United States each year.

Twice as many women as men are affected by mitral valve stenosis. About 60% of patients with mitral valve stenosis have had rheumatic fever. After rheumatic fever there is usually a latency period of 10–20 years before symptoms of mitral valve stenosis appear. The prevalence of mitral valve stenosis has declined in the United States because there has been a decline in the number of cases of rheumatic fever. Mitral valve stenosis may be present at birth (congenital); however, it rarely occurs alone but rather in conjunction with other heart defects.

Mitral valve prolapse is the most common condition of the heart valves, and is present in about 2% of the general population. Recent studies indicate that similar numbers of men and women have mitral valve prolapse. Having this condition does not guarantee that mitral insufficiency will develop. Patients with a history of rheumatic fever, coronary artery disease, infective endocarditis, or collagen vascular disease also may develop mitral insufficiency.

> ## WHO PERFORMS THE PROCEDURE AND WHERE IS IT PERFORMED?
>
> Cardiothoracic and cardiovascular surgeons provide surgical treatment. Surgeons are trained during the residency to perform these procedures. Medical centers that perform cardiac surgery are able to provide mitral valve replacement.

Description

Cardiac monitoring is instituted and general anesthesia is provided. The surgeon uses a sternotomy to access the heart and great blood vessels. Anticoagulation is given as cannulae are inserted into the large vessels of the heart, femoral vessels, or a combination. Cardiopulmonary bypass is instituted. The heart is arrested as the cross clamp is applied to the ascending aorta to stop blood flow through the organ. The surgeon opens the heart to visualize the mitral valve. He/she may expose the mitral valve by opening the right atrium and then opening the atrial septum. Another approach requires a large left atrium that can be opened directly, making the mitral valve visible.

Next, the surgeon cuts the diseased valve away from the valve annulus (outer ring). The annulus is sized so that the proper size of valve can be selected for the patient's anatomy. Sutures are applied around the valve annulus, the valve is sutured into place, and tied into position. The atrial septum is closed with suture or left to heal naturally, and the heart is closed with sutures.

Deairing of the heart is performed prior to removal of the cross clamp. When the cross clamp is removed, deairing continues to ensure that no air is delivered to the systemic circulation. At this time a transesophageal echocardiogram (TEE) may be used to test that the valve is functioning correctly and that the heart is free of air. Once the surgeon is satisfied that the valve is working correctly, cardiopulmonary bypass is terminated, anticoagulation is reversed, and the cannulae are removed from the vessels. The sternotomy is closed. Permanent stainless steel wires are used to hold the sternum bone together. The skin incision is closed with sutures, and sterile bandages are applied to the wound.

A heart valve is a structure within the heart that prevents the backflow of blood by opening and closing with each heartbeat. Replacement heart valves are either mechanical or biological tissue valves. For patients under the age of 65, the mechanical valve offers superior longevity, but the use of this type of valve requires that the patient take an anticoagulation drug for the rest of his/her life. The biological tissue valve does not require anticoagulation therapy, but this type of valve is prone to deterioration leading to **reoperation**, particularly in those under the age of 50. Women who may want to have children after a valve replacement should usually receive a biological tissue valve, because the anticoagulant (Coumadin/warfarin) most often prescribed for patients with mechanical valves is associated with fetal birth defects. **Aspirin** can be substituted for warfarin in certain circumstances.

Diagnosis/Preparation

Mitral valve stenosis is diagnosed by history, **physical examination**, listening to the sounds of the heart (cardiac auscultation), **chest x ray**, and ECG. Patients may have no symptoms of a valve disorder or may have shortness of breath (dyspnea), fatigue, or frank pulmonary edema. Other patients present with atrial fibrillation (a cardiac arrhythmia) or an embolic event. Doppler **echocardiography** is the preferred diagnostic tool for evaluation of mitral valve stenosis, and it can be performed in conjunction with non-invasive **exercise** testing by treadmill or bicycle. **Cardiac catheterization** is reserved for patients who demonstrate discrepancies in Doppler testing. Both left- and right-heart catheterization should be performed in the presence of elevated pulmonary artery pressures.

A diagnosis of mitral insufficiency requires a detailed patient history. Listening to the heart (auscultation) reveals the presence of a third heart sound. Chest x ray and ECG provide additional information. Again, Doppler echocardiography provides valuable information. Exercise testing with Doppler echocardiography can show the true severity of the disease.

After initial findings, patients may be followed with repeat visits and testing to monitor disease progress. If the patient has reached NYHA Class III or IV, replacement is considered. Severe pulmonary hypertension with pulmonary artery systolic pressures greater than 60 mm Hg is considered an indication for surgery. Left ventricular ejection fraction (a measure of output) less than 60% also is an indication for surgery.

Aftercare

The patient receives continued cardiac monitoring in the **intensive care unit** and usually remains in intensive care for 24–48 hours after surgery. Ventilation support is discontinued when the patient is able to breathe on his/her own. If mechanical circulatory support and inotropic agents (a substance that influences the force of muscle contractions, e.g. digitalis) were needed during the surgical procedure, they are discontinued as cardiac function recovers. Tubes draining blood from the chest cavity are removed as bleeding from the surgical procedure decreases. Prophylactic **antibiotics** are given to prevent infective endocarditis and the recurrence of rheumatic carditis.

Both mechanical and biological tissue valves require anticoagulation therapy after surgery, and while patients are hospitalized their anticoagulant status is monitored and dosages are adjusted accordingly. Patients with biological tissue valves can discontinue anticoagulation therapy within three months of implantation, but those with mechanical valves must take an anticoagulant (aspirin, warfarin, or a combination of the two) for the rest of their lives. These patients are regularly monitored for INR values, which are maintained between 2.0 and 4.5.

If the patient recovers normally, **discharge from the hospital** occurs within a week of surgery. At discharge, the patient is given specific instructions about **wound care** and infection recognition, as well as contact information for the physician and guidelines about when a visit to the emergency room is indicated. Within three or

KEY TERMS

Annulus—A ring-shaped structure.

Anticoagulants—Drugs that are given to slow blood clot formation.

Biological tissue valve—An autograft is a valve that comes from the patient, usually the pulmonary valve. An autologous pericardial valve is constructed from the patient's pericardium (the fibrous sac that surrounds the heart and the roots of the great vessels and also forms the outer layer of the heart wall) at the time of surgery. A homograft (or allograft) valve is a valve harvested from a human cadaver. A porcine (pig) heterograft is a porcine tissue valve that is rendered bioacceptable by destroying antigenicity with glutaraldehyde sterilization.

Cardiac catheterization—A diagnostic procedure (using a catheter inserted through a vein and threaded through the circulatory system to the heart) which does a comprehensive examination of how the heart and its blood vessels function.

Cardiopulmonary bypass—Use of the heart-lung machine to provide systemic circulation cardiac output and ventilation of the blood.

Commissures—The normal separations between the valve leaflets.

Doppler echocardiography—A testing technique that uses Doppler ultrasound technology to evaluate the pattern and direction of blood flow in the heart.

Endocarditis—Infection of the heart endocardium tissue, the inner most tissue and structures of the heart.

Mechanical valve—There are three types of mechanical valve: ball valve, disk valve, and bileaflet valve.

NYHA heart failure classification—A classification system for heart failure developed by the New York Heart Association. It includes the following four categories: I, symptoms with more than ordinary activity; II, symptoms with ordinary activity; III, symptoms with minimal activity; IV, symptoms at rest.

Rheumatic carditis—Inflammation of the heart muscle associated with acute rheumatic fever.

Rheumatic fever—An inflammatory disease that arises as a complication of untreated or inadequately treated strep throat infection. Rheumatic fever can seriously damage the heart valves.

Sternotomy—A surgical opening into the thoracic cavity through the sternum (breastbone).

Systemic circulation—Circulation supplied by the aorta including all tissue and organ beds, except the alveolar sacs of the lungs used for gas exchange and respiration.

Thromboemboli—Blood clots that develop in the circulation and lodge in capillary beds of tissues and organs.

Transesophageal echocardiography—A diagnostic test using an ultrasound device that is passed into the esophagus of the patient to create a clear image of the heart muscle and other parts of the heart.

---

four weeks after discharge, the patient is seen for follow-up office visit with the physician, at which time physical status will have improved for evaluation. Thereafter, asymptomatic, uncomplicated patients are seen at yearly intervals. Few limitations are placed on patient activity once recovery is complete.

Risks

There are always risks associated with general anesthesia and cardiopulmonary bypass. Risks specifically associated with mitral valve replacement include embolism, bleeding, and operative valvular endocarditis. Hemolysis (the breakdown of red blood cells) is associated with certain types of mechanical valves, but is not a contraindication for implantation.

Normal results

Patients treated by mitral valve replacement for mitral insufficiency can expect relief of symptoms. Improvement in myocardial function is not likely, but the current status is preserved. For patients who received mechanical valves, anticoagulation therapy is continued lifelong to elevate the INR to between 2.0 and 4.5, depending on the type of mechanical valve implanted. Since thromboembolic complications are associated with initial implant of biological tissue valves, patients who received this type of valve take an anticoagulant for three months after surgery to maintain an INR of 2.0–3.0. If non-cardiac surgery or dental care is needed, the anticoagulation therapy is adjusted to prevent bleeding complications.

Patients who undergo mitral valve replacement for mitral stenosis can expect excellent improvement of symptoms. Those patients with symptoms consistent with NYHA class IV before surgery have better outcome after mitral valve replacement compared to no treatment.

Morbidity and mortality rates

Mitral valve replacement carries a less than 5% risk of death in young, healthy patients. With increased age, additional medical problems, or pulmonary hypertension the risk of death increases to 10–20%. Post-replacement the five year survival is 80%. Patients over the age of 75 have poorer outcomes when mitral valve replacement is used to treat mitral insufficiency.

Alternatives

The asymptomatic patient with a history of rheumatic fever can be treated with prophylactic antibiotics and followed until symptoms are appear. If atrial fibrillation develops, antiarrhythmic medications can be used for treatment. Atrial **defibrillation** may relieve atrial fibrillation. Anticoagulants may be prescribed to prevent the occurrence of systemic embolization. The patient with symptoms may benefit from percutaneous mitral balloon valvotomy. Surgery to perform a commissurotomy may be used instead of valve replacement.

Mitral valve insufficiency or prolapse that develops atrial fibrillation should be treated with drugs to regulate the heart rhythm or atrial defibrillation. Anticoagulation therapy is employed to avoid systemic emboli during periods of atrial fibrillation. **Mitral valve repair** maybe beneficial instead of mitral valve replacement.

Resources

BOOKS

Hensley, Frederick A., Donald E. Martin, and Glenn P. Gravlee, eds. *A Practical Approach to Cardiac Anesthesia.* 3rd ed. Philadelphia: Lippincott Williams & Wilkins, 2003.

Topol, Eric J., ed. *Textbook of Interventional Cardiology.* Philadelphia: W. B. Saunders, 2002.

PERIODICALS

Bonow, R., et al. "ACC/AHA Guidelines for the Management of Patients with Valvular Heart Disease." *Journal of the American Collge of Cardiology* 32 (November 1998): 1486–1582.

Brown, Katherine Kay. "Minimally Invasive Valve Surgery." *Critical Care Nursing Quarterly* 20 (February 1998): 40–52.

Sadovsky, Richard. "Using Warfarin After Heart Valve Replacement." *American Family Physician* 61 (April 1, 2000): 2219.

Allison Joan Spiwak, MSBME

Modified radical mastectomy

Definition

A surgical procedure that removes the breast, surrounding tissue, and nearby lymph nodes that are affected by cancer.

Purpose

The purpose for modified radical mastectomy is the removal of breast cancer (abnormal cells in the breast that grow rapidly and replace normal healthy tissue). Modified radical mastectomy is the most widely used surgical procedure to treat operable breast cancer. This procedure leaves a chest muscle called the pectoralis major intact. Leaving this muscle in place will provide a soft tissue covering over the chest wall and a normal-appearing junction of the shoulder with the anterior (front) chest wall. This sparing of the pectoralis major muscle will avoid a disfiguring hollow defect below the clavicle. Additionally, the purpose of modified radical mastectomy is to allow for the option of **breast reconstruction**, a procedure that is possible, if desired, due to intact muscles around the shoulder of the affected side. The modified radical mastectomy procedure involves removal of large multiple tumor growths located underneath the nipple and cancer cells on the breast margins.

Demographics

The highest rates of breast cancer occur in Western countries (more than 100 cases per 100,000 women) and the lowest among Asian countries (10–15 cases per 100,000 women). Men can also have breast cancer, but the incidence is much less when compared to women. There is a strong genetic correlation since breast cancer is more prevalent in females who had a close relative (mother, sister, maternal aunt, or maternal grandmother) with previous breast cancer. Increased susceptibility for development of breast cancer can occur in females who never breastfed a baby, had a child after age 30, started menstrual periods very early, or experienced menopause very late.

In the United States, there were approximately 175,000 cases of breast cancer in 1999 with more than 43,000 deaths. Breast cancer accounts for 30% of all cancer diagnosed in American women and for 16% of all cancer deaths. Breast cancer is a worldwide public health problem since there are approximately one million new cases diagnosed annually. A woman's lifetime risk of developing breast cancer is one in eight. The incidence rose

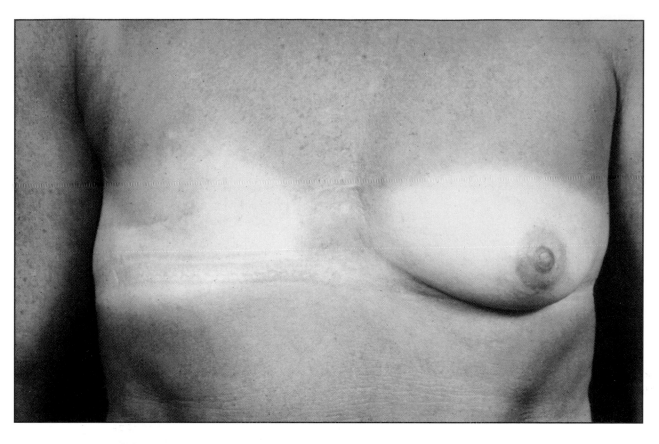

Woman with scars from a modified radical mastectomy. *(Biophoto Associates/Science Source. Reproduced by permission.)*

21% from 1973 to 1990, but in recent years there has been a decline.

Description

The surgeon's goal during this procedure is to minimize any chance of local/regional recurrence; avoid any loss of function; and maximize options for breast reconstruction. Incisions are made to avoid visibility in a low neckline dress or bathing suit. An incision in the shape of an ellipse is made. The surgeon removes the minimum amount of skin and tissue so that remaining healthy tissue can be used for possible reconstruction. Skin flaps are made carefully and as thinly as possible to maximize removal of diseased breast tissues. The skin over a neighboring muscle (pectoralis major fascia) is removed, after which the surgeon focuses in the armpit (axilla, axillary) region. In this region, the surgeon carefully identifies vital anatomical structures such as blood vessels (veins, arteries) and nerves. Accidental injury to specific nerves like the medial pectoral neurovascular bundle will result in destruction of the muscles that this surgery attempts to preserve, such as the pectoralis major muscle. In the armpit region, the surgeon carefully protects the vital structures while removing cancerous tissues. After

axillary surgery, breast reconstruction can be performed, if desired by the patient.

Diagnosis/Preparation

Modified radical mastectomy is a surgical procedure to treat breast cancer. In order for this procedure to be an operable option, a definitive diagnosis of breast cancer must be established. The first clinical sign for approximately 80% of women with breast cancer is a mass (lump) located in the breast. A lump can be discovered by monthly self-examination or by a health professional who can find 10–25% of breast cancers that are missed by yearly mammograms (a low radiation x ray of the breasts). A biopsy can be performed to examine the cells from a lump that is suspicious for cancer. The diagnosis of the extent of cancer and spread to regional lymph nodes determines the treatment course (i.e., whether surgery, chemotherapy, or radiation therapy, either singly or in combinations). Staging the cancer can estimate the amount of tumor, which is important not only for diagnosis but for prognosis (statistical outcome of the disease process). Patients with a type of breast cancer called ductal carcinoma in situ (DCIS), which is a stage 0 cancer, have the best out-

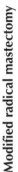

Modified radical mastectomy

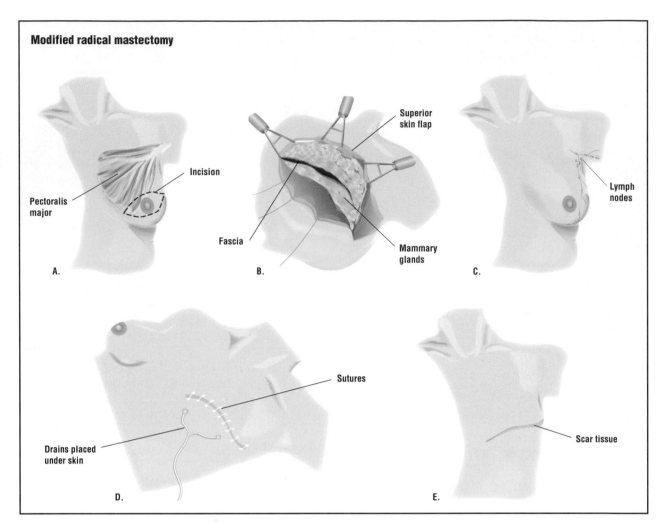

In a modified radical mastectomy, the skin on the breast is cut open (A). The skin is pulled back, and the tumor, lymph nodes, and breast tissue are removed (B and C). The incision is closed (D). *(Illustration by GGS Inc.)*

come (nearly all these patients are cured of breast cancer). Persons who have cancerous spread to other distant places within the body (metastases) have stage IV cancer and the worst prognosis (potential for survival). Persons affected with stage IV breast cancer have essentially no chance for cure.

Persons affected with breast cancer must undergo the staging of the cancer to determine the extent of cancerous growth and possible spread (metastasis) to distant organs. Patients with stage 0 disease have noninvasive cancer with a very good outcome. Stages I and II are early breast cancer, without lymph node involvement (stage I) and with node positive results (stage II). Persons with stage III disease have locally advanced disease and about a 50% chance for five-year survival. Stage IV disease is the most severe since the breast cancer cells have spread through lymph nodes to distant areas and/or other organs in the body. It is very unlikely that persons

with stage IV metastatic breast cancer survive 10 years after diagnosis.

It is also imperative to assess the degree of cancerous spread to lymph nodes within the armpit region. Of primary importance to stage determination and regional lymph node involvement is identification and analysis of the sentinel lymph node. The sentinel lymph node is the first lymph node to which any cancer would spread. The procedure for sentinel node biopsy involves injecting a radioactively labeled tracer (technetium 99) or a blue dye (isosulphan blue) into the tumor site. The tracer or dye will spread through the lymphatic system to the sentinel node, which should be surgically removed and examined for the presence of cancer cells. If the sentinel node and one or two other neighboring lymph nodes are negative, it is very likely that the remaining lymph nodes will not contain cancerous cells, and further surgery may not be necessary.

Once a breast lump (mass) has been identified by **mammography** or **physical examination**, the patient should undergo further evaluation to histologically (studying the cells) identify or rule out the presence of cancer cells. A procedure called fine-needle aspiration allows the clinician to extract cells directly from the lump for further evaluation. If a diagnosis cannot be established by fine-needle biopsy, the surgeon should perform an open biopsy (surgical removal of the suspicious mass). Preparation for surgery is imperative. The patient should plan for both direct care and recovery time after modified radical mastectomy. Preparation immediately prior to surgery should include no food or drink after midnight before the procedure. Post-surgical preparation should include caregivers to help with daily tasks for several days.

Aftercare

After breast cancer surgery, women should undergo frequent testing to ensure early detection of cancer recurrence. It is recommended that annual mammograms, physical examination, or additional tests (biopsy) be performed annually. Aftercare can also include psychotherapy since mastectomy is emotionally traumatic. Affected women may be worried or have concerns about appearance, the relationship with their sexual partner, and possible physical limitations. Community-centered support groups usually made up of former breast cancer surgery patients can be a source of emotional support after surgery. Patients may stay in the hospital for one to two days. For about five to seven days after surgery, there will be one or two drains left inside to remove any extra fluid from the area after surgery. Usually, the surgeon will prescribe medication to prevent pain. Movement restriction should be specifically discussed with the surgeon.

Risks

There are several risks associated with modified radical mastectomy. The procedure is performed under general anesthesia, which itself carries risk. Women may have short-term pain and tenderness. The most frequent risk of breast cancer surgery (with extensive lymph node removal) is edema, or swelling of the arm, which is usually mild, but the presence of fluid can increase the risk of infection. Leaving some lymph nodes intact instead of removing all of them may help lessen the likelihood of swelling. Nerves in the area may be damaged. There may be numbness in the arm or difficulty moving shoulder muscles. There is also the risk of developing a lump scar (keloid) after surgery. Another risk is that surgery did not remove all the cancer cells and that further treatment may be necessary (with chemotherapy and/or radiotherapy). By far, the worst risk is recurrence of cancer. However,

immediate signs of risk following surgery include fever, redness in the incision area, unusual drainage from the incision, and increasing pain. If any of these signs develop, it is imperative to call the surgeon immediately.

Normal results

If no complications develop, the surgical area should completely heal within three to four weeks. After mastectomy, some women may undergo breast reconstruction (which can be done during mastectomy). Recent studies have indicated that women who desire cosmetic reconstructive surgery have a higher quality of life and better sense of well-being than those who do not utilize this option.

Morbidity and mortality rates

The outcome of breast cancer is very dependent of the stage at the time of diagnosis. For stage 0 disease (5–10% of the cases), the five-year survival is 99%. For stage I (early/lymph node negative), which comprises 40–45% of total cases, the five-year survival is 85–95%. For stage II (early/lymph node positive), which comprises 35–40% of total cases, the five-year survival decreases to 65–75%. For stage III disease (locally advanced), which accounts for 10–15% of total cases, the five-year survival is 45–50%. Women with stage IV (metastatic) breast cancer account for about 7% of total cases; the five-year survival is 20–30%. Less than 1% of these women survive past 10 years.

Alternatives

There are no real alternatives to mastectomy. Surgical requirement is clear since mastectomy is recommended for tumors with dimensions over 2 in (5 cm). Additional treatment (adjuvant) is typically recommended with chemotherapy and/or radiation therapy to destroy any remaining cancer during surgery. Modified radical mastectomy is one of the standard treatment recommendations for stage III breast cancer.

Resources

BOOKS

Noble, John. *Textbook of Primary Care Medicine,* 3rd edition. St. Louis: Mosby, Inc., 2001.

Townsend, Courtney. *Sabiston Textbook of Surgery,* 16th edition. St. Louis: W. B. Saunders Company, 2001.

PERIODICALS

Fiorica, James. "Prevention and Treatment of Breast Cancer." *Obstetrics and Gynecology Clinics* 28 no. 4 (December 2001).

ORGANIZATIONS

American Cancer Society. (800) ACS-2345. <http://www.cancer.org.>.

KEY TERMS

Lymphatic system—A system that filters excess tissue fluids through lymph nodes to return to the bloodstream.

Cancer support groups. <http://www.cancernews.com>.
Y-ME National Breast Cancer Organization. <http://www.y-me.org.>.

Laith Farid Gulli, MD
Nicole Mallory, MS, PA-C

Mohs surgery

Definition

Mohs surgery, also called Mohs micrographic surgery, is a precise surgical technique that is used to remove all parts of cancerous skin tumors, while preserving as much healthy tissue as possible.

Purpose

Mohs surgery is used to treat such cancers of the skin as basal cell carcinoma, squamous cell carcinoma, and melanoma.

Malignant skin tumors may occur in strange, asymmetrical shapes. The tumor may have long finger-like projections that extend across the skin (laterally) or down into the skin. Because these extensions may be composed of only a few cells, they cannot be seen or felt. Standard surgical removal (excision) may miss these cancerous cells leading to recurrence of the tumor. To assure removal of all cancerous tissue, a large piece of skin needs to be removed. This causes a cosmetically unacceptable result, especially if the cancer is located on the face. Mohs surgery enables the surgeon to precisely excise the entire tumor without removing excessive amounts of the surrounding healthy tissue.

Mohs surgery is performed when:

• The cancer was treated previously and recurred.

• Scar tissue exists in the area of the cancer.

• The cancer is in at least one area where it is important to preserve healthy tissue for maximum functional and cosmetic result, such as on the eyelids, the nose, the ears, and the lips.

• The edges of the cancer cannot be clearly defined.

• The cancer grows rapidly or uncontrollably.

Demographics

According to the National Cancer Institute (NCI), about one million people in the United States are diagnosed with skin cancer every year. The two most common types of skin cancer are basal cell carcinoma and squamous cell carcinoma, with basal cell carcinoma accounting for more than 90% of all of skin cancers.

Melanoma is the most serious type of skin cancer. Each year in the United States more than 53,600 people are diagnosed with melanoma, and it is becoming more and more common, especially among Western countries. In the United States, the percentage of people who develop melanoma has more than doubled in the past 30 years.

Description

There are two types of Mohs surgery: fresh-tissue technique and fixed-tissue technique. Of the surgeons who perform Mohs surgery, 72% use only the fresh-tissue technique. The remaining surgeons (18%) use both techniques. However, the fixed-tissue technique is used in fewer than 5% of patients. The main difference between the two techniques is in the preparatory steps.

Fresh-tissue technique

Fresh-tissue Mohs surgery is performed under local anesthesia for tumors of the skin. The area to be excised is cleaned with a disinfectant solution and a sterile drape is placed over the site. The surgeon may outline the tumor using a surgical marking pen, or a dye. A local anesthetic (lidocaine plus epinephrine) is injected into the area. Once the local anesthetic has taken effect, the main portion of the tumor is excised (debulked) using a spoon-shaped tool (curette). To define the area to be excised and to allow for accurate mapping of the tumor, the surgeon makes identifying marks around the lesion. These marks may be made with stitches, staples, fine cuts with a scalpel, or temporary tattoos. One layer of tissue is carefully excised (first Mohs excision), cut into smaller sections, and taken to the laboratory for analysis.

If cancerous cells are found in any of the tissue sections, a second layer of tissue is removed (second Mohs excision). Because only the sections that have cancerous cells are removed, healthy tissue can be spared. The entire procedure, including surgical repair of the wound, is performed in one day. Surgical repair may be performed by the Mohs surgeon, a plastic surgeon, or another specialist. In certain cases, wounds may be allowed to heal naturally.

Fixed-tissue technique

With fixed-tissue Mohs surgery, the tumor is de-bulked, as described previously. Trichloracetic acid is applied to the wound to control bleeding, followed by a preservative (fixative) called zinc chloride. The wound is dressed and the tissue is allowed to fix for six to 24 hours, depending on the depth of the tissue involved. This period, called the fixation period, can be painful to the patient. The first Mohs excision is performed as described; however, anesthesia is not required because the tissue is dead. If cancerous cells are found, fixative is applied to the affected area for an additional six to 24 hours. Excisions are performed in this sequential process until all cancerous tissue is removed. Surgical repair of the wound may be performed once all fixed tissue has sloughed off—usually a few days after the last excision.

Diagnosis/Preparation

An oncologist will have diagnosed the skin cancer of the patient using such standard cancer diagnostic tools as biopsy of the tumor.

To prepare for surgery, and under certain conditions (such as the location of the skin tumor or health status of the patient), **antibiotics** may be given to the patient prior to the procedure; this is known as prophylactic antibiotic treatment. Patients are encouraged to eat prior to surgery and also to bring along snacks in case the procedure become lengthy. To reduce the risk of bleeding, the use of **nonsteroidal anti-inflammatory drugs** (NSAIDs), al-

cohol, vitamin E, and fish oil tablets should be avoided prior to the procedure. The patient who uses over-the-counter **aspirin** or the prescription blood-thinners, brands Coumadin (warfarin, generically) and heparin should consult with the prescribing physician before adjusting the dosage of any drug.

Aftercare

Patients should expect to receive specific **wound care** instructions from their physician or surgeon. Generally, however, wounds that have been repaired with absorbable stitches or skin grafts should be kept covered with a bandage for one week. Wounds that have been repaired using nonabsorbable stitches should also be covered with a bandage that should be replaced daily until the stitches are removed one to two weeks later. Signs of infection (e.g., redness, pain, drainage) should be reported to the physician immediately.

Risks

Using the fresh-tissue technique on a large tumor requires large amounts of local anesthetic that can be toxic. Complications of Mohs surgery include infection, bleeding, scarring, and nerve damage.

Tumors spread in unpredictable patterns. Sometimes a seemingly small tumor is found to be quite large and widespread, resulting in a much larger excision than was anticipated.

KEY TERMS

Carcinoma—Cancer that begins in the cells that cover or line an organ.

Fixative—A chemical that preserves tissue without destroying or altering the structure of the cells.

Fixed—A term used to describe chemically preserved tissue. Fixed tissue is dead so it does not bleed or sense pain.

Mohs excision—Referring to the excision of one layer of tissue during Mohs surgery. Also called stage.

Normal results

Most skin cancers treated by Mohs surgery are completely removed with minimal loss of normal skin.

Morbidity and mortality rates

Mohs surgery provides high cure rates for malignant skin tumors. For instance, the five-year cure rate for basal cell carcinoma treated by Mohs surgery is higher than 99%. The frequency of recurrence is much lower with Mohs surgery is much lower than with conventional surgical excision—less than 1%.

Alternatives

Mohs surgery is a specialized technique that is not indicated for the treatment of every type of skin cancer, and is most appropriately used under specific, well-defined circumstances. The majority of basal cell carcinomas can be treated with very high cure rates by standard methods, including electrodesiccation and curettage (ED&C), local excision, cryosurgery (freezing), and irradiation.

See also Cryotherapy.

Resources

BOOKS

PERIODICALS

Cook, J. L., and J. B. Perone. "A prospective evaluation of the incidence of complications associated with Mohs micrographic surgery." *Archives of Dermatology* 139 (February 2003): 143-152.

Jackson, E. M., and J. Cook. "Mohs micrographic surgery of a papillary cccrine adenoma." *Dermatologic Surgery* 28 (December 2002): 1168-1172.

Smeets, N. W., Stavast-Kooy, A. J., Krekels, G. A., Daemen, M. J., and H. A. Neumann. "Adjuvant Cytokeratin Staining in Mohs Micrographic Surgery for Basal Cell Carcinoma." *Dermatologic Surgery* 29 (April 2003): 375-377.

ORGANIZATIONS

American Society for Mohs Surgery. Private Mail Box 391, 5901 Warner Avenue, Huntington Beach, CA 92649-4659. (714) 840-3065. (800) 616-ASMS (2767). <www.mohssurgery.org>.

OTHER

"About Mohs Micrographic Surgery." *Mohs College.* <www.mohscollege.org/AboutMMS.html>.

Belinda Rowland, Ph.D.
Monique Laberge, Ph.D.

Mometasone *see* **Corticosteroids**

MR *see* **Magnetic resonance imaging**

MRA *see* **Magnetic resonance imaging**

MRI *see* **Magnetic resonance imaging**

MRS *see* **Magnetic resonance imaging**

MUGA scan **see Multiple-gated acquisition (MUGA) scan**

Multiple-gated acquisition (MUGA) scan

Definition

The multiple-gated acquisition (MUGA) scan, also called a cardiac blood pool study, is a non-invasive nuclear medicine test that enables clinicians to obtain information about heart muscle activity. The scan displays the distribution of a radioactive tracer in the heart. The images of the heart are obtained at intervals throughout the cardiac cycle, and are used to calculate ejection fraction (an important measure of heart performance) and evaluate regional myocardial wall motion.

Purpose

A MUGA scan may be done while the patient is at rest and again with stress. The resting study is usually performed to obtain the ejection fraction of the right and left ventricles, evaluate the left ventricular regional wall motion, assess the effects of cardiotoxic drugs (i.e., chemotherapy), and differentiate the cause of shortness of breath (pulmonary vs. cardiac). Ejection fraction and wall motion are also important measurements made during a stress study, but the stress study is performed primarily to detect coronary artery disease and evaluate angina.

Description

The MUGA scan is a series of images that demonstrate the flow of blood through the heart, providing information about heart muscle activity. Before images are taken, a radionuclide is injected into the bloodstream, a process that requires two injections in most health care facilities. The first injection contains a chemical that adheres to red blood cells, and the second contains a radioactive tracer (Tc99m) that attaches to that chemical. Alternatively, the two chemicals can be mixed together first and then injected, but the material tends to accumulate in bone and may obscure the heart.

The pictures are taken via gamma camera driven by a computer program that times the images, processes the information, and performs the mathematical calculations to provide ejection fraction and demonstrate wall motion. Images are obtained at various intervals during the cardiac cycle. Electrodes are placed on the patient so that a time frame can be established, for example, the time period between each "wave" (a part of the cardiac cycle seen on an EKG). The time frame is divided into several intervals, or "multiple gates." The result is a series of pictures showing the left and right ventricles at end-diastole (when the heart is dilated and filled with blood) and end-systole (when the heart is contracted and blood is being pumped out), and a number of stages in between.

A MUGA scan is performed in a hospital nuclear medicine department or in an outpatient facility. It takes approximately 30 minutes to one hour. The patient lies down on a bed alongside the gamma camera, receives the radionuclide injections, and multiple images are taken. If a stress study is indicated, the rest study is performed first. In a stress study, the patient usually lies on a special bed fitted with a bicycle apparatus. While an image is being recorded, the patient is asked to cycle for about two minutes, then the resistance of the wheels is increased. After two more minutes of **exercise**, another image is obtained and the resistance is increased again. Blood pressure and ECG are monitored during the procedure. After the stress portion is finished, one more resting, or recovery, study is obtained.

Preparation

Standard preparation for an ECG is required. Special handling of nuclear materials by a nuclear medicine technologist may be required for the injections.

Aftercare

The patient may resume normal activities immediately following the test.

Normal results

A normal MUGA scan should not demonstrate areas of akinesis (lack of movement), or hypokinesis (decreased movement) of the heart muscle walls. Abnormal motion, especially in the left ventricle, is suggestive of an infarct or other myocardial defect. The ejection fraction is a measure of heart function, and should be within the normal limits established by the testing facility.

Resources

BOOKS

DeBakey, Michael E. and Gotto, Antonio M., Jr. "Noninvasive Diagnostic Procedures." In *The New Living Heart.* Holbrook, MA: Adams Media Corporation, 1997, pp. 59–70.

Klingensmith III, M.D., Wm. C., Dennis Eshima, Ph.D., John Goddard, Ph.D. *Nuclear Medicine Procedure Manual 2000-2001.*

"Radionuclide Angiography." In *Cardiac Stress Testing & Imaging,* edited by Thomas H. Marwick. New York: Churchill Livingstone, 1996, pp. 517–21.

Raizner, Albert E. "Nuclear Cardiology Testing." In: *Indications for Diagnostic Procedures: Topics in Clinical Cardiology.* New York, Tokyo: Igaku-Shon, 1997, pp. 44–47.

Texas Heart Institute. "Diagnosing Heart Diseases." In *Texas Heart Institute Heart Owner's Handbook.* New York: John Wiley & Sons, 1996, p. 333.

Ziessman, Harvey, ed. *The Radiologic Clinics of North America, Update on Nuclear Medicine.* Philadelphia: W.B. Saunders Company, 2001.

ORGANIZATIONS

American Heart Association. National Center. 7272 Greenville Avenue, Dallas, TX 75231-4596. (214) 373-6300. <http://www.medsearch.com/pf/profiles/amerh/>.

Texas Heart Institute Heart Information Service. P.O. Box 20345, Houston, TX 77225-0345. (800) 292-2221. <http://www.tmc.edu/thi/his.html>.

Christine Miner Minderovic, B.S., R.T., R.D.M.S.
Lee A. Shratter, M.D.

Muscle relaxants

Definition

Skeletal muscle relaxants are drugs that relax striated muscles (those that control the skeleton). They are a separate class of drugs from the muscle relaxant drugs used during intubations and surgery to reduce the need for anesthesia and facilitate intubation.

Purpose

Skeletal muscle relaxants may be used for relief of spasticity in neuromuscular diseases such as multiple sclerosis, as well as for spinal cord injury and stroke. They may also be used for pain relief in minor strain injuries and control of the muscle symptoms of tetanus. Dantrolene (Dantrium) has been used to prevent or treat malignant hyperthermia in surgery.

Description

The muscle relaxants are divided into two groups: centrally acting and peripherally acting. The centrally acting group appears to act on the central nervous system (CNS), and contains 10 drugs that are chemically different. Only dantrolene has a direct action at the level of the nerve-muscle connection.

Baclofen (Lioresal) may be administered orally or intrathecally (introduced into the space under the arachnoid membrane that covers the brain and spinal cord) for control of spasticity due to neuromuscular disease.

Several drugs, including carisoprodol (Soma), chlorphenesin (Maolate), chlorzoxazone (Paraflex), cyclobenzaprine (Flexeril), diazepam (Valium), metaxalone (Skelaxin), methocarbamol (Robaxin), and orphenadrine (Norflex), are used primarily as an adjunct for rest in management of acute muscle spasms associated with sprains. Muscle relaxation may also be an adjunct to physical therapy in rehabilitation following stroke, spinal cord injury, or other musculoskeletal conditions.

Diazepam and methocarbamol are also used by injection for relief of tetanus.

Recommended dosage

Dose varies with the drug, route of administration, and purpose. There may be individual variations in absorption that require doses higher than those usually recommended (particularly with methocarbamol). The consumer is advised to consult specific references or ask a doctor for further information.

Precautions

All drugs in the muscle relaxant class may cause sedation. Baclofen, when administered intrathecally, may cause severe CNS depression with cardiovascular collapse and respiratory failure.

Diazepam may be addictive, and is a controlled substance under federal law.

Dantrolene has a potential for hepatotoxicity. The incidence of symptomatic hepatitis is dose related, but may occur even with a short period of doses at or above 800 mg per day, which greatly increases the risk of serious liver injury. Overt hepatitis has been most frequently observed between the third and twelfth months of therapy. Risk of liver injury appears to be greater in women, in patients over 35 years of age, and in patients taking other medications in addition to dantrolene.

Tizanidine may cause low blood pressure, but this may be controlled by starting with a low dose and increasing it gradually. Rarely, the drug may cause liver damage.

Methocarbamol and chlorzoxazone may cause harmless color changes in urine—orange or reddish purple with chlorzoxazone; and purple, brown, or green with methocarbamol. The urine will return to its normal color when the patient stops taking the medicine.

Most drugs in the muscle relaxant class are well tolerated, but not all of these drugs have been evaluated for safety in pregnancy and breastfeeding.

Baclofen is pregnancy category C. It has caused fetal abnormalities in rats at doses 13 times above the human dose. Baclofen passes into breast milk, so breastfeeding while taking baclofen is not recommended.

Diazepam is category D. All benzodiazepines cross the placenta. Although the drugs appear to be safe for use during the first trimester of pregnancy, use later in pregnancy may be associated with cleft lip and palate. Diazepam should not be taken while breastfeeding. It was found that infants who were breastfed while their mothers took diazepam were excessively sleepy and lethargic.

Dantrolene is category C. In animal studies, it has reduced the rate of survival of the newborn when given in doses seven times the normal human dose. Mothers should not breastfeed while receiving dantrolene.

Central nervous system (CNS)—The brain and spinal cord.

Intrathecal—Introduced into or occurring in the space under the arachnoid membrane that covers the brain and spinal cord.

Pregnancy category—A system of classifying drugs according to their established risks for use during pregnancy: category A: controlled human studies have demonstrated no fetal risk; category B: animal studies indicate no fetal risk, and there are no adequate and well-controlled studies in pregnant women; category C: no adequate human or animal studies, or adverse fetal effects in animal studies, but no available human data; category D: evidence of fetal risk, but benefits outweigh risks; category X: evidence of fetal risk that outweigh any benefits.

Sedative—Medicine used to treat nervousness or restlessness.

Spasm—Sudden, involuntary tensing of a muscle or a group of muscles.

Tranquilizer (minor)—A drug that has a calming effect and is used to treat anxiety and emotional tension.

Interactions

Skeletal muscle relaxants have many potential drug interactions. It is recommended that individual references be consulted.

Because these drugs cause sedation, they should be used with caution when taken with other drugs that may also cause drowsiness.

The activity of diazepam may be increased by drugs that inhibit its metabolism in the liver. These include cimetidine, oral contraceptives, disulfiram, fluoxetine, isoniazid, ketoconazole, metoprolol, propoxyphene, propranolol, and valproic acid.

Dantrolene may have an interaction with estrogens. Although no interaction has been demonstrated, the rate of liver damage in women over the age of 35 who were taking estrogens is higher than in other groups.

Resources

BOOKS

AHFS: Drug Information. Washington, DC: Amer Soc Health-systems Pharm, 2002.
Brody, T. M., J. Larner, K. P. Minneman, and H. C. Neu. *Human Pharmacology: Molecular to Clinical,* 2nd Edition. St. Louis: Mosby Year-Book, 1995.
Fukushima, K. *Muscle Relaxants: Physiologic and Pharmacologic Aspects,* 1st Edition, Heidelberg: Springer Verlang, 1995.
Karch, A. M. *Lippincott's Nursing Drug Guide.* Springhouse, PA: Lippincott Williams & Wilkins, 2003.
Reynolds, J. E. F. (ed). *Martindale. The Extra Pharmacopoeia,* 31st Edition. London: The Pharmaceutical Press, 1996.

OTHER

<http://www.anaesthesia.org.nz/Files/Help41A.pdf>.
<http://www.hendrickhealth.org/healthy/000923.htm>.

Samuel D. Uretsky, PharmD

Myelography

Definition

Myelography is an x-ray examination of the spinal canal. A contrast agent is injected through a needle into the space around the spinal cord to display the spinal cord, spinal canal, and nerve roots on an x ray.

Purpose

The purpose of a myelogram is to evaluate the spinal cord and nerve roots for suspected compression. Pressure on these delicate structures causes pain or other symptoms. A myelogram is performed when precise detail about the spinal cord is needed to make a definitive diagnosis. In most cases, myelography is used after other studies, such as **magnetic resonance imaging** (MRI) or a computed tomography scan (CT), have not provided enough information to be certain of the diagnosis. Sometimes myelography followed by CT scan is an alternative for patients who cannot have an MRI scan, because they have a pacemaker or other implanted metallic device.

A herniated or ruptured intervertebral disc, or related condition such as disc bulge or protrusion, popularly known as a slipped disc, is one of the most common causes for pressure on the spinal cord or nerve roots. The condition is popularly known as a pinched nerve. Discs are pads of fiber and cartilage that contain rubbery tissue. They lie between the vertebrae, or individual bones, which make up the spine.

Discs act as cushions, accommodating strains, shocks, and position changes. A disc may rupture suddenly, due to injury or a sudden strain with the spine in an unnatural position. In other cases, the problem may come on gradually as a result of progressive deterioration of the discs with aging. The lower back is the most common area for this problem, but it sometimes occurs in the neck, and rarely in the upper back. A myelogram can help accurately locate the disc or discs involved.

Myelography may be used when a tumor is suspected. Tumors can originate in the spinal cord or in tissues surrounding the cord. Cancers that have started in other parts of the body may spread or metastasize in the spine. It is important to precisely locate the mass causing pressure so effective treatment can be undertaken. Patients with known cancer who develop back pain may require a myelogram for evaluation.

Other conditions that may be diagnosed using myelography include arthritic bony growths (spurs), narrowing of the spinal canal (spinal stenosis), or malformations of the spine.

Description

Myelograms can be performed in a hospital x ray department or in an outpatient radiology facility. The patient lies face down on the x ray table. The radiologist first looks at the spine under fluoroscopy, and the images appear on a monitor screen. This is done to find the best location to position the needle. The skin is cleaned, numbed with local anesthetic, and then the needle is inserted. Occasionally, a small amount of cerebrospinal fluid, the clear fluid that surrounds the spinal cord and brain, may be withdrawn through the needle and sent for laboratory studies. Contrast material (dye that shows up on x rays) is then injected.

The x-ray table is tilted slowly, allowing the contrast material to reach different levels in the spinal canal. The flow is observed under fluoroscopy, and x rays are taken with the table tilted at various angles. A footrest and shoulder straps or supports keep the patient from sliding.

In many instances, a CT scan of the spine is performed immediately after a myelogram, while the contrast material is still in the spinal canal. This helps outline internal structures more clearly.

A myelogram takes approximately 30 to 60 minutes. A CT scan adds about another hour to the examination. If the procedure is done as an outpatient exam, some facilities prefer the patient to stay in a recovery area up to four hours.

Patients who are unable to lie still or cooperate with positioning should not have this examination. Severe congenital spinal abnormalities may make the examination technically difficult to carry out. Patients with a history of severe allergic reaction to contrast material (x-ray dye) should report this to their physician prior to having myelography. Medications to minimize the risk of severe reaction may be recommended before the procedure. Given the invasive nature and risks of myelograms and increased anatomic detail provided by MRI or CT, myelograms are generally not used as the first imaging test.

Preparation

Patients should be well-hydrated at the time they are undergoing a myelogram. Increasing fluids the day before the study is usually recommended. All food and fluid intake should be stopped approximately four hours before the procedure.

Certain medications may need to be stopped for one to two days before myelography is performed. These include some antipsychotics, antidepressants, blood thinners, and diabetic medications. Patients should discuss this with their physician or the staff at the facility where the study is to be done.

Patients who smoke may be asked to stop the day before the test. This helps decrease the chance of nausea or headaches after the myelogram. Immediately before the examination, patients should empty their bowels and bladder.

Aftercare

After the examination is complete, the patient usually rests for several hours, with the head elevated. Extra fluids are encouraged, to help eliminate the contrast material and prevent headaches. A regular diet and routine medications may be resumed. Strenuous physical activities, especially those that involve bending over, may be discouraged for one or two days. The physician should be notified if the patient develops a fever, excessive nausea and vomiting, severe headache, or a stiff neck.

Risks

Headache is a common complication of myelography. It may begin several hours to several days after the examination. The cause is thought to be changes in cerebrospinal fluid pressure, not a reaction to the dye. The headache may be mild and easily alleviated with rest and increased fluids. Sometimes, nonprescription medicines are recommended. In some instances, the headache may be more severe and require stronger medication or other measures for relief. Many factors influence whether the patient develops this problem, including the type of the needle used and his or her age and gender. Patients with a history of chronic or recurrent headaches are more likely to develop a headache after a myelogram.

The chance of a reaction to the contrast material is a very small, but potentially significant risk. It is estimated that only 5–10% of patients experience any effect from contrast exposure. The vast majority of reactions are mild, such as sneezing, nausea, or anxiety. These usually resolve by themselves. A moderate reaction, like wheezing or hives, may be treated with medication, but is not considered life threatening. Severe reactions, such as heart or respiratory failure, occur very infrequently, and require emergency medical treatment.

Rare complications of myelography include injury to the nerve roots from the needle or from bleeding into the spaces around the roots. Inflammation of the delicate covering of the spinal cord, called arachnoiditis, or infections, can also occur. Seizures are another very uncommon complication reported after myelography.

Normal results

A normal myelogram shows nerves that appear normal, and a spinal canal of normal width, with no areas of constriction or obstruction.

Abnormal results

A myelogram may reveal a herniated disk, tumor, bone spurs, or narrowing of the spinal canal (spinal stenosis).

Resources

BOOKS

Daffner, Richard. *Clinical Radiology, The Essentials.* Baltimore: Williams and Wilkins, 1993.

Pagana, Kathleen Deska. *Mosby's Manual of Diagnostic and Laboratory Tests.* St. Louis: Mosby, Inc., 1998.

Torres, Lillian. *Basic Medical Techniques and Patient Care in Imaging Technology.* Philadelphia: Lippincott, 1997.

ORGANIZATIONS

Spine Center. 1911 Arch St., Philadelphia, PA 19103. (215) 665-8300. <http://www.thespinecenter.com>

Ellen S. Weber, M.S.N.
Lee A. Shratter, M.D.

Myocardial resection

Definition

Myocardial resection is a surgical procedure in which a portion of the heart muscle is removed.

Purpose

Myocardial resection is done to improve the stability of the heart function or rhythm. Also known as endocardial resection, this open-heart surgery is done to destroy or remove damaged areas. These areas can generate life-threatening heart rhythms. Conditions resulting in abnormal heart rhythms caused by re-entry pathways or aberrant cells are corrected with this treatment.

Areas of the heart involved in a myocardial infarction change in contractility and function, becoming scar tissue

that thins and hinders its ability to contract. Removing this diseased area can improve myocardial contractility reversing the severity of chronic heart failure. This procedure has shown promise for patients with chronic heart failure, in order to improve cardiac output and quality of life.

Demographics

Patients are not limited by age, race or sex when being evaluated for myocardial resection surgery. Patients who experience angina, congestive heart failure, arrhythmias, and pulmonary edema (fluid on the lungs) are candidates for this procedure. Contraindications—conditions in which the surgery is not recommended—include right heart failure, elevated left ventricular end-diastolic pressures, and pulmonary hypertension (high blood pressure in the circulation around the lungs).

Description

After receiving a general anesthetic, an incision will be made in the chest to expose the heart. Cardiopulmonary bypass (to a heart-lung machine) will be instituted since this procedure requires direct visualization of the heart muscle. Since this is a true open heart procedure, the heart will be unable to pump blood during the surgery.

Arrhythmias

When the exact source of the abnormal rhythm is identified, it is removed. If there are areas around the source that may contribute to the problem, they can be frozen with a special probe to further insure against dangerous heart rates. The amount of tissue removed is so small, usually only 2–3 mm, that there is no damage to the structure of the heart.

Ventricular reconstruction

Weakened myocardium (cardiac muscle) allows the heart to remodel and become less efficient at pumping blood. The goal is to remove the damaged region of the free wall of the left ventricle along with any involved septum. The heart is then reconstructed to provide a more elliptical structure that pumps blood more efficiently. In some instances a Dacron graft is used to replace the removed myocardium to aid in the reconstruction.

Diagnosis/Preparation

Diagnosis of arrhythmias begins with a Holter monitor that can identify the type of arrhythmia. This is followed by a **cardiac catheterization** to find the aberrant cells generating the arrhythmia. The patient is then recommended for open-heart surgery to remove the cells generating the arrhythmia.

Diagnosis of chronic heart failure is demonstrated by a cardiac catheterization or nuclear medicine study. During cardiac catheterization, the patient's cardiac function will be measured by cardiac output, ejection fraction and cardiovascular pressures. A nuclear medicine study can demonstrate areas of myocardium that are damaged. Muscle that is akinetic (does not move) will be identified. This information allows the surgeon to identify candidates for myocardial resection.

This is major surgery and should be the treatment of choice only after medications have failed and the use of an **implantable cardioverter-defibrillator** (a device that delivers electrical shock to control heart rhythm) has been ruled out along with medical therapy.

Prior to surgery, the physician will explain the procedure and order blood tests of the formed blood elements and electrolytes.

Aftercare

Immediately after surgery, the patient will be transferred to the **intensive care unit** for further cardiac monitoring. Any medications to improve cardiac performance will be weaned as necessary to allow the native heart function to return. The patient will be able to leave the hospital within five days, assuming there are no complications. Complications may include the need for intra-aortic balloon pump **ventricular assist device**, surgical bleeding, and infection.

Risks

The risks of myocardial resection are based in large part on the patient's underlying heart condition and, therefore, vary greatly. The procedure involves opening the heart, so the person is at risk for the complications associated with major heart surgery, such as stroke, shock, infection, and hemorrhage. Since the amount of myocardium to remove is not precise, a patient may demonstrate little benefit in cardiac performance. If not enough or too much tissue is removed, the patient will continue to have heart problems.

General anesthetic with inhalation gases should be avoided as they can promote arrhythmias. Therefore, anesthesia should be limited to intravenous medications.

Normal results

Post-operative treatment for arrhythmias demonstrates 90% of patients are arrhythmia-free at the end of one year. A study of 245 patients published in 2001, demonstrated a 98% event free survival rate for patients after one year. After five years, 80% of patients had remained event free.

Morbidity and mortality rates

Cardiopulmonary bypass has an associated risk of complications separate from myocardial resection, with age greater than 70 years of age being a predictor for increased morbidity and mortality. In 1999, over 350,000 total procedures were performed using cardiopulmonary bypass.

KEY TERMS

Arrhythmia—An abnormal heart rhythm. Examples are a slow, fast, or irregular heart rate.

Cardiac catheterization—A diagnostic procedure in which a thin tube is inserted into an artery or vein and guided to the heart using x rays. The function of the heart and blood vessels can be evaluated using this technique.

Dacron graft—A synthetic material used in the repair or replacement of blood vessels.

Ejection fraction—The amount of blood pumped out at each heartbeat, usually referred to as a percentage.

Implantable cardioverter-defibrillator—A device placed in the body to deliver an electrical shock to the heart in response to a serious abnormal rhythm.

Infarction—Tissue death resulting from a lack of oxygen to the area.

Intra-aortic balloon pump—A temporary device inserted into the femoral artery and guided up to the aorta. The small balloon helps strengthen heart contractions by maintaining improved blood pressure.

Radiofrequency ablation—A procedure in which a catheter is guided to an area of heart where abnormal heart rhythms originate. The cells in that area are killed using a mild radiofrequency energy to restore normal heart contractions.

Wolff-Parkinson-White syndrome—An abnormal, rapid heart rhythm, due to an extra pathway for the electrical impulses to travel from the atria to the ventricles.

In the study of 245 patients, ventricular reconstruction by myocardial resection was found to have an associated in-hospital mortality rate of 78.1%.

Alternatives

If myocardial resection is being performed to prevent arrhythmia generation, new techniques allow for minimally invasive procedures to be performed, including radiofrequency ablation performed in an electrophysiology laboratory with mild sedation, instead of general anesthetic.

If ventricular restoration is contraindicated, medical treatment will be continued. Mechanical circulatory assist with a ventricular assist device may be a suitable op-

tion. Heart transplant and total artificial heart should also be explored as alternative therapies.

See also Heart transplantation; Mechanical circulation support.

Resources

BOOKS

Hensley, Frederick Jr., et al. *A Practical Approach to Cardiac Anesthesia*, 3rd ed. Philadelphia: Lippincott Williams & Wilkins, 2003.

McGoon, Michael D., ed. *Mayo Clinic Heart Book: The Ultimate Guide to Heart Health.* New York: William Morrow and Co., Inc., 1993.

PERIODICALS

Dor, Vincent, et al. "Intermediate survival and predictors of death after surgical restoration." *Seminars in Thoracic and Cardiovascular Surgery* 13, no. 4 (October 2001): 468–475.

ORGANIZATIONS

American Heart Association. 7320 Greenville Avenue, Dallas, TX 75231. (800) 242-8721 or (888) 478-7653. <http://www.americanheart.org>.

Dorothy Elinor Stonely
Allison J. Spiwak, MSBME

Myoglobin test *see* **Cardiac marker tests**

Myomectomy

Definition

Myomectomy is the removal of fibroids (non-cancerous tumors) from the wall of the uterus. Myomectomy is the preferred treatment for symptomatic fibroids in women who want to keep their uterus. Larger fibroids must be removed with an abdominal incision, but small fibroids can be taken out by **laparoscopy** or **hysteroscopy**.

Purpose

A myomectomy can remove uterine fibroids that are causing such symptoms as abnormal bleeding or pain. It is an alternative to surgical removal of the whole uterus (**hysterectomy**). The procedure can relieve fibroid-induced menstrual symptoms that have not responded to medication. Myomectomy also may be an effective treatment for infertility caused by the presence of fibroids.

Demographics

Uterine fibroids are more common among African-American women than among women of other ethnici-

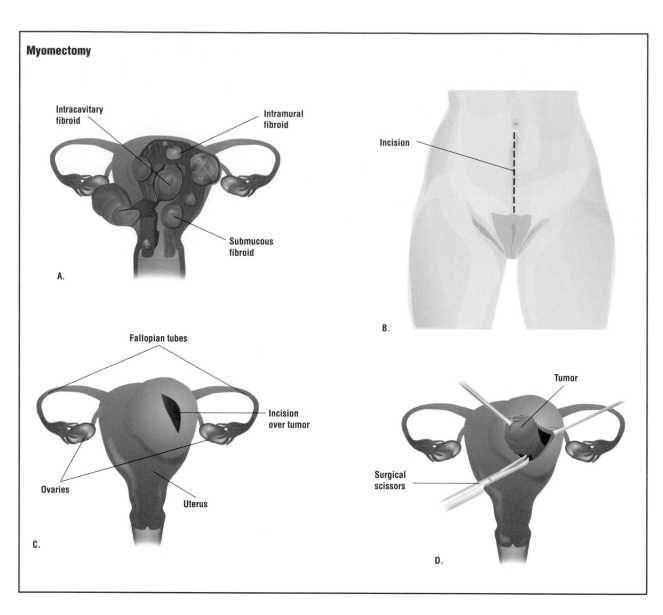

Myomectomy

Uterine fibroids can occur within the uterine cavity, in the mucous layer, or in the muscle (A). To remove them by myomectomy, an incision is made into the woman's lower abdomen (B). An incision is made in the uterus over the tumor (C), and it is removed (D). *(Illustration by GGS Inc.)*

ties. Fibroids affect 20–40% of all women over the age of 35, and 50% of African-American women. A 2001 study by the National Institute of Environmental Health Sciences found that the incidence of fibroids among African-American women in their late 40s was as high as 80%, while approximately 70% of white women of that age were diagnosed as having fibroids. Women who are obese, are older, or started menstruating at an early age are also at an increased risk of developing uterine fibroids. Another study published in 2003 indicated that women with less education were more likely to have a hysterectomy performed to treat fibroids, instead of a less-invasive procedure such as myomectomy.

Description

Usually, fibroids are buried in the outer wall of the uterus, and abdominal surgery is required. If they are on the inner wall of the uterus, uterine fibroids can be removed using hysteroscopy. If they are on a stalk (pedunculated) on the outer surface of the uterus, laparoscopy can be performed.

Removing fibroids through abdominal surgery is a more difficult and slightly more risky operation than a hysterectomy. This is because the uterus bleeds from the sites where the fibroids were removed, and it may be difficult or impossible to stop the bleeding. This surgery is usually performed under general anesthesia, although some patients may be given a spinal or epidural anesthesia.

The incision may be horizontal (the "bikini" incision) or a vertical incision from the navel downward. After separating the muscle layers underneath the skin, the surgeon makes an opening in the abdominal wall. Next, the surgeon makes an incision over each fibroid, grasping and pulling out each growth.

Every opening in the uterine wall is then stitched with sutures. The uterus must be meticulously repaired in order to eliminate potential sites of bleeding or infection. The surgeon then sutures the abdominal wall and muscle layers above it with absorbable stitches, and closes the skin with clips or non-absorbable stitches.

When appropriate, a laparoscopic myomectomy may be performed. In this procedure, the surgeon removes fibroids with the help of a viewing tube (laparoscope) inserted into the pelvic cavity through an incision in the navel. The fibroids are removed through a tiny incision under the navel that is much smaller than the 4–5 in (10–13 cm) opening required for a standard myomectomy.

If the fibroids are small and located on the inner surface of the uterus, they can be removed with a thin, telescope-like device called a hysteroscope. The hysteroscope is inserted into the vagina through the cervix and into the uterus. This procedure does not require any abdominal incision, so hospitalization is shorter.

Diagnosis/Preparation

Surgeons often recommend hormone treatment with a drug called leuprolide (Lupron) two to six months before surgery in order to shrink the fibroids. This makes the fibroids easier to remove. In addition, Lupron stops menstruation, so women who are anemic have an opportunity to build up their blood count. While the drug treatment may reduce the risk of excess blood loss during surgery, there is a small risk that smaller fibroids might be missed during myomectomy, only to enlarge later after the surgery is completed.

Aftercare

Patients may need four to six weeks of recovery following a standard myomectomy before they can return to normal activities. Women who have had laparoscopic or hysteroscopic myomectomies, however, can usually recover completely within one to three weeks.

Risks

The risks of a myomectomy performed by a skilled surgeon are about the same as hysterectomy (one of the most common and safest surgeries). Removing multiple

---

WHO PERFORMS THE PROCEDURE AND WHERE IS IT PERFORMED?

Myomectomies are usually performed in a hospital **operating room** or an outpatient setting by a gynecologist, a medical doctor who has specialized in the areas of women's general health, pregnancy, labor and childbirth, prenatal testing, and genetics.

---

fibroids is more difficult and slightly more risky. Possible complications include:

- infection
- blood loss
- weakening of the uterine wall to the degree that future deliveries need to be performed via **cesarean section**
- adverse reactions to anesthesia
- internal scarring (and possible infertility)
- reappearance of new fibroids

There is a risk that removal of the fibroids may lead to such severe bleeding that the uterus itself will have to be removed. Because of the risk of blood loss during a myomectomy, patients may want to consider banking their own blood before surgery (**autologous blood donation**).

Normal results

Removal of uterine fibroids will usually improve any side effects that the patient may have been suffering from, including abnormal bleeding and pain. Under normal circumstances, a woman who has had a myomectomy will be able to become pregnant, although she may have to deliver via cesarean section if the uterine wall has been weakened.

Morbidity and mortality rates

Depending on the surgical approach, the rate of complications for myomectomy is about the same as those for hysterectomy (anywhere between 3% and 9%). The rate of fibroid reoccurrence is approximately 15%. Adhesions (bands of scar tissue between organs that can form after surgery or trauma) occur in 15–53% of women postoperatively.

Alternatives

Hysterectomy (partial or full removal of the uterus) is a common alternative to myomectomy. The most frequent reason for hysterectomy in the United States is to remove fibroid tumors, accounting for 30% of all hysterectomies. A subtotal (or partial) hysterectomy is the preferable procedure because it removes the least amount of tissue (i.e., the opening to the cervix is left in place).

Fibroid embolization is a relatively new, less-invasive procedure in which blood vessels that feed the fibroids are blocked, causing the growths to shrink. The blood vessels are accessed via a catheter inserted into the femoral artery (in the upper thigh) and injected with tiny particles that block the flow of blood. The fibroids subsequently decrease in size and the patient's symptoms improve.

Resources

BOOKS

Connolly, Anne Marie and William Droegemueller. "Leiomyomas" In *Conn's Current Therapy 2003*. Philadelphia: Elsevier Science, 2003.

Ludmir, Jack and Phillip G. Stubblefield. "Surgical Procedures in Pregnancy: Myomectomy" (Chapter 19). In *Obstetrics: Normal & Problem Pregnancies*. Philadelphia: Churchill Livingstone, 2002.

ORGANIZATIONS

American College of Obstetricians and Gynecologists. 409 12th St., SW, P.O. Box 96920, Washington, DC 20090-6920. <http://www.acog.org>.

Center for Uterine Fibroids, Brigham and Women's Hospital. 623 Thorn Building, 20 Shattuck Street, Boston, MA 02115. (800) 722-5520. <http://www.fibroids.net>.

OTHER

de Candolle, G., and D. M. Walker. "Myomectomy." *Practical Training and Research in Gynecologic Endoscopy*. February 17, 2003 [cited March 13, 2003]. <http://www.gfmer.ch/Books/Endoscopy_book/Ch14_Myomectomy.html>.

"High Efficacy Rate Shown in Minimally Invasive Treatment of Uterine Fibroids." *Doctor's Guide*. January 13, 2003 [cited March 14, 2003]. <http://www.pslgroup.com/dg/2271BA.htm>.

Indman, Paul D. "Myomectomy: Removal of Uterine Fibroids." *All About Myomectomy*. 2002 [cited March 14, 2003]. <http://www.myomectomy.net>.

Toaff, Michael E. "Myomectomy." *Alternatives to Hysterectomy Page* [cited March 14, 2003]. <http://www.netreach.net/~hysterectomyedu/myomecto.htm>.

"Uterine Fibroids: Disproportionate Number of Black Women with More, Larger Tumors." National Institute of Environmental Sciences. March 2001 [cited March 14, 2003]. <http://www.niehs.nih.gov/oc/crntnws/2001mar/fibroids.htm>.

Carol A. Turkington
Stephanie Dionne Sherk

Myringotomy and ear tubes

Definition

Myringotomy is a surgical procedure in which a small incision is made in the eardrum (the tympanic membrane), usually in both ears. The English word is derived from *myringa,* modern Latin for drum membrane, and *tome,* Greek for cutting. It is also called myringocentesis, tympanotomy, tympanostomy, or **paracentesis** of the tympanic membrane. Fluid in the middle ear can be drawn out through the incision.

Ear tubes, or tympanostomy tubes, are small tubes open at both ends that are inserted into the incisions in the eardrums during myringotomy. They come in various shapes and sizes and are made of plastic, metal, or both. They are left in place until they fall out by themselves or until they are removed by a doctor.

Purpose

Myringotomy with the insertion of ear tubes is an optional treatment for inflammation of the middle ear

Myringotomy and ear tubes

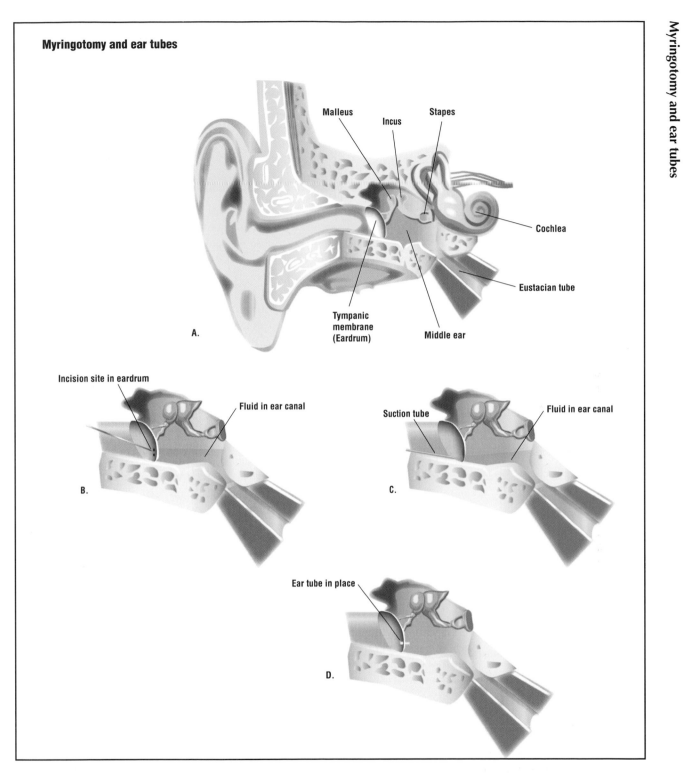

A.

Malleus

Incus

Stapes

Cochlea

Eustacian tube

Tympanic membrane (Eardrum)

Middle ear

Incision site in eardrum

Fluid in ear canal

B.

Suction tube

Fluid in ear canal

C.

Ear tube in place

D.

During a myringotomy, an incision is made into the ear drum, or tympanic membrane (B). The fluid in the ear canal is suctioned out (C), and a small tube is put in place to allow future drainage in the event of an infection (D). *(Illustration by GGS Inc.)*

with fluid collection (effusion) that lasts longer than three months (chronic otitis media with effusion) and does not respond to drug treatment. This condition is also called glue ear. Myringotomy is the recommended treatment if the condition lasts four to six months. Effusion refers to the collection of fluid that escapes from blood vessels or the lymphatic system. In this case, the effusion collects in the middle ear.

Initially, acute inflammation of the middle ear with effusion is treated with one or two courses of **antibiotics**. Antihistamines and decongestants have been used, but they have not been proven effective unless there is also hay fever or some other allergic inflammation that contributes to the problem. Myringotomy with or without the insertion of ear tubes is *not* recommended for initial treatment of otherwise healthy children with middle ear inflammation with effusion.

In about 10% of children, the effusion lasts for three months or longer, when the disease is considered chronic. In children with chronic disease, systemic steroids may help, but the evidence is not clear, and there are risks.

When medical treatment doesn't stop the effusion after three months in a child who is one to three years old, is otherwise healthy, and has hearing loss in both ears, myringotomy with insertion of ear tubes becomes an option. If the effusion lasts for four to six months, myringotomy with insertion of ear tubes is recommended.

The purpose of myringotomy is to relieve symptoms, to restore hearing, to take a sample of the fluid to examine in the laboratory in order to identify any microorganisms present, or to insert ear tubes.

Ear tubes can be inserted into the incision during myringotomy and left there. The eardrum heals around them, securing them in place. They usually fall out on their own in six to 12 months or are removed by a doctor.

While the tubes are in place, they keep the incision from closing, keeping a channel open between the middle ear and the outer ear. This allows fresh air to reach the middle ear, allowing fluid to drain out, and preventing pressure from building up in the middle ear. The patient's hearing returns to normal immediately and the risk of recurrence diminishes.

Demographics

In the United States, myringotomy and tube placement have become a mainstay of treatment for recurrent otitis media in children. An article published in the March 1998 *Consumer Reports* stated that the " ... number of myringotomies has risen nearly 250 percent in recent years, making the operation the sixth most common operation in the United States." According to the New York University School of Medicine, myringotomy and tube placement is the most common surgical procedure performed in children as of 2003, largely because otitis media is the most common reason for children to be taken to a doctor's office.

Myringotomy in adults is a less common procedure than in children, primarily because adults benefit from certain changes in the anatomy of the middle ear that occur after childhood. In particular, the adult ear is less likely to accumulate fluid because the Eustachian tube, which connects the middle ear to the throat area, lies at about a 45-degree angle from the horizontal. This relatively steep angle means that the force of gravity helps to keep fluids from the throat containing disease organisms out of the middle ear. In children, however, the Eustachian tube is only about 10 degrees above the horizontal, which makes it relatively easy for disease organisms to migrate from the nose and throat into the inner ear. Myringotomies in adults are usually performed as a result of barotrauma that is also known as pressure-related ear pain or barotitis media. Barotrauma refers to earache caused by unequal air pressure on the inside and outside of the eardrum. Adults with very narrow Eustachian tubes may experience barotrauma in relation to scuba diving, using elevators, or frequent flying. A myringotomy with tube insertion may be performed if the condition is not helped by decongestants or antibiotics.

Most myringotomies in children are performed in children between one and two years of age. One Canadian study found that the number of myringotomies performed was 12.8 per thousand for children 11 months old or younger; 54.2 per thousand for children between 12 and 23 months old; and 11.1 per thousand for children between three and 15 years old. Sex and race do not appear to affect the number of myringotomies in any age group, although boys are reported to have a slightly higher rate of ear infections than girls.

Description

When a conventional myringotomy is performed, the ear is washed, a small incision made in the eardrum, the fluid sucked out, a tube inserted, and the ear packed with cotton to control bleeding.

Recent developments include the use of medical acupuncture to control pain during the procedure, and the use of carbon dioxide lasers to perform the myringotomy itself. Laser-assisted myringotomy can be performed in a doctor's office with only a local anesthetic. It has several advantages over the older technique: it is less painful; less frightening to children; and minimizes the need for tube insertion because the hole in the eardrum produced by the laser remains open longer than an incision done with a scalpel.

Another technique to keep the incision in the eardrum open without the need for tube insertion is application of a medication called mitomycin C, which was originally developed to treat bladder cancer. The mitomycin prevents the incision from sealing over. As of 2003, however, this approach is still in its experimental stages.

There has also been an effort to design ear tubes that are easier to insert or to remove, and to design tubes that stay in place longer. As of 2003, ear tubes come in various shapes and sizes.

Diagnosis/Preparation

The diagnosis of otitis media is based on the doctor's visual examination of the patient's ear and the patient's symptoms. Patients with otitis media complain of earache and usually have a fever, sometimes as high as 105°F (40.5°C). There may or may not be loss of hearing. Small children may have nausea and vomiting. When the doctor looks in the ear with an otoscope, the patient's eardrum will look swollen and may bulge outward. The doctor can evaluate the presence of fluid in the middle ear either by blowing air into the ear, known as insufflation, or by tympanometry, which is an indirect measurement of the mobility of the eardrum. If the eardrum has already ruptured, there may be a watery, bloody, or pus-streaked discharge.

Fluid removed from the ear can be taken to a laboratory for culture. The most common bacteria that cause otitis media are *Pneumococcus, Haemophilus influenzae,* and *Moraxella catarrhalis.* Some cases are caused by viruses, particularly respiratory syncytial virus (RSV).

A child scheduled for a myringotomy should not have food or water for four to six hours before anesthesia. Antibiotics are usually not needed.

If local anesthesia is used, a cream containing lidocaine and prilocaine is applied to the ear canal about 30

QUESTIONS TO ASK THE DOCTOR

- What alternatives to myringotomy might work for my child?
- How can I lower my child's risk of recurrent ear infections?
- Do you perform laser-assisted myringotomies?
- What is your opinion of removing my child's adenoids to lower the risk of future hospitalizations?

minutes before the myringotomy. If medical acupuncture is used for pain control, the acupuncture begins about 40 minutes before surgery and is continued during the procedure.

Aftercare

The use of antimicrobial drops is controversial. Water should be kept out of the ear canal until the eardrum is intact. A doctor should be notified if the tubes fall out.

Risks

The risks include:

- cutting the outer ear
- formation at the myringotomy site of granular nodes due to inflammation
- formation of a mass of skin cells and cholesterol in the middle ear that can grow and damage surrounding bone (cholesteatoma)
- permanent perforation of the eardrum

It is also possible that the incision won't heal properly, leaving a permanent hole in the eardrum. This result can cause some hearing loss and increases the risk of infection.

The ear tube may move inward and get trapped in the middle ear, rather than move out into the external ear, where it either falls out on its own or can be retrieved by a doctor. The exact incidence of tubes moving inward is not known, but it could increase the risk of further episodes of middle-ear inflammation, inflammation of the eardrum or the part of the skull directly behind the ear, formation of a mass in the middle ear, or infection due to the presence of a foreign body.

The surgery may not be a permanent cure. As many as 30% of children undergoing myringotomy with insertion of ear tubes need to undergo another procedure within five years.

The other risks include those associated with sedatives or general anesthesia. Some patients may prefer acupuncture for pain control in order to minimize these risks.

An additional element of **postoperative care** is the recommendation of many doctors that the child use ear plugs to keep water out of the ear during bathing or swimming to reduce the risk of infection and discharge.

Normal results

Parents often report that children talk better, hear better, are less irritable, sleep better, and behave better after myringotomy with the insertion of ear tubes. Normal results in adults include relief of ear pain and ability to resume flying or deep-sea diving without barotrauma.

Morbidity and mortality rates

Morbidity following myringotomy usually takes the form of either otorrhea, which is a persistent discharge from the ear, or changes in the size or texture of the eardrum. The risk of otorrhea is about 13%. If the procedure is repeated, the eardrum may shrink, retract, or become flaccid. The eardrum may also develop an area of hardened tissue. This condition is known as tympanosclerosis. The risk of hardening is 51%; its effects on hearing aren't known, but they appear to be insignificant.

A report published in 2002 indicates that morbidity following myringotomy in the United States is highest among children from families of low socioeconomic status. The study found that children from poor urban families had more episodes of otorrhea following tube insertion then children from suburban families. In addition, the episodes of otorrhea in the urban children lasted longer.

Mortality rates are extremely low; case studies of fatalities following myringotomy are rare in the medical literature, and most involve adults.

Alternatives

Preventive measures

There are several lifestyle issues related to high rates of middle ear infection. One of the most serious is parental smoking. One study of the effects of passive smoking on children's health estimated that as many as 165,000 of the myringotomies performed each year on American children are related to the use of tobacco in the household.

Another risk factor is daycare placement. A 1997 study at the University of North Carolina found that 31% of the children in a sample of 346 children in daycare required myringotomy with tube insertion as compared to 11% of 63 children cared for at home. In addition, the children in daycare who had ventilation tubes had to have the tubes reinserted three times as often as the children in home care with ventilation tubes.

A third factor that affects a child's risk of recurrent middle ear infection is breastfeeding. Researchers at the University of Arizona reported in 1993 that infants who had been breastfed exclusively for at least four months had significantly fewer middle ear infections as toddlers.

Other surgical approaches

There is some controversy among doctors as to whether removal of the adenoids helps to lower the risk of recurrent ear infections. A 2001 Canadian study reported that removing the child's adenoids at the time of the first insertion of ventilation tubes significantly reduced the likelihood of additional ear operations in children two years of age and older. Other doctors think that **adenoidectomy** at the time of tube placement should be performed only on children with a large number of risk factors for recurrent otitis media. Most agree that further study of this question is needed.

Alternative medicine

According to Dr. Kenneth Pelletier, former director of the program in complementary and alternative medicine at Stanford University, there is some evidence that homeopathic treatment is effective in reducing the pain of otitis media in children and lowering the risk of recurrence.

Resources

BOOKS

"Acute Otitis Media." Section 7, Chapter 84 in *The Merck Manual of Diagnosis and Therapy*, edited by Mark H. Beers, MD, and Robert Berkow, MD. Whitehouse Station, NJ: Merck Research Laboratories, 2001.

Lanternier, Matthew L., MD. "Otolaryngology: Ear Pathology," Chapter 20 in *The University of Iowa Family Practice Handbook*, 4th edition, edited by Mark Graber, MD, and Matthew L. Lanternier, MD. St. Louis, MO: Mosby, 2001.

Pelletier, Kenneth R., MD. *The Best Alternative Medicine*, Part II: CAM Therapies for Specific Conditions: Otitis Media. New York: Simon & Schuster, 2002.

PERIODICALS

Ah-Tye, C., J. L. Paradise, and D. K. Colborn. "Otorrhea in Young Children After Tympanostomy-Tube Placement for Persistent Middle-Ear Effusion: Prevalence, Incidence, and Duration." *Pediatrics* 107 (June 2001): 1251–1258.

Coyte, P. C., R. Croxford, W. McIsaac, et al. "The Role of Adjuvant Adenoidectomy and Tonsillectomy in the Outcome

KEY TERMS

Acute otitis media—Inflammation of the middle ear with signs of infection lasting less than three months.

Adenoids—Clusters of lymphoid tissue located in the upper throat above the roof of the mouth. Some doctors think that removal of the adenoids may lower the rate of recurrent otitis media in high-risk children.

Barotrauma—Ear pain caused by unequal air pressure on the inside and outside of the ear drum. Barotrauma, which is also called pressure-related ear pain or barotitis media, is the most common reason for myringotomies in adults.

Chronic otitis media—Inflammation of the middle ear with signs of infection lasting three months or longer.

Effusion—The escape of fluid from blood vessels or the lymphatic system and its collection in a cavity, in this case, the middle ear.

Eustachian tube—A canal that extends from the middle ear to the pharynx.

Insufflation—Blowing air into the ear as a test for the presence of fluid in the middle ear.

Middle ear—The cavity or space between the eardrum and the inner ear. It includes the eardrum, the three little bones (hammer, anvil, and stirrup) that transmit sound to the inner ear, and the Eustachian tube, which connects the inner ear to the nasopharynx (the back of the nose).

Otolaryngologist—A surgeon who specializes in treating disorders of the ears, nose, and throat.

Tympanic membrane—The eardrum. A thin disc of tissue that separates the outer ear from the middle ear.

Tympanostomy tube—Ear tube. A small tube made of metal or plastic that is inserted during myringotomy to ventilate the middle ear.

of the Insertion of Tympanostomy Tubes." *New England Journal of Medicine* 344 (April 19, 2001): 1188–1195.

Desai, S. N., J. D. Kellner, and D. Drummond. "Population-Based, Age-Specific Myringotomy with Tympanostomy Tube Insertion Rates in Calgary, Canada." *Pediatric Infectious Disease Journal* 21 (April 2002): 348–350.

Gates, George A., MD. "Otitis Media—The Pharyngeal Connection." *Journal of the American Medical Association* 282 (September 8, 1999): 987–999.

Jassir, D., C. A. Buchman, and O. Gomez-Marin. "Safety and Efficacy of Topical Mitomycin C in Myringotomy Patency." *Otolaryngology—Head and Neck Surgery* 124 (April 2001): 368–373.

Lin, Yuan-Chi, MD. "Acupuncture Anesthesia for a Patient with Complex Congenital Anomalies." *Medical Acupuncture* 13 (Fall/Winter 2002) [cited February 22, 2003]. <http://www.medicalacupuncture.org/aama_marf/journal/vol13_2/poster3.html>.

Perkins, J. A. "Medical and Surgical Management of Otitis Media in Children." *Otolaryngology Clinics of North America* 35 (August 2002): 811-825.

Siegel, G. J., and R. K. Chandra. "Laser Office Ventilation of Ears with Insertion of Tubes." *Otolaryngology—Head and Neck Surgery* 127 (July 2002): 60–66.

ORGANIZATIONS

American Academy of Medical Acupuncture (AAMA). 4929 Wilshire Boulevard, Suite 428, Los Angeles, CA 90010. (323) 937-5514. <http://www.medicalacupuncture.org>.

American Academy of Otolaryngology, Head and Neck Surgery, Inc. One Prince Street, Alexandria, VA 22314-3357. (703) 836-4444. <http://www.entnet.org>.

American Academy of Pediatrics (AAP). 141 Northwest Point Boulevard, Elk Grove Village, IL 60007. (847) 434-4000. <http://www.aap.org>.

Mary Zoll, PhD
Rebecca Frey, PhD

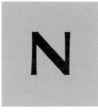

Narcotics *see* **Analgesics, opioid**

Nasal septum surgery *see* **Septoplasty**

Necessary surgery

Definition

Necessary surgery is a term that refers both to a medical requirement for the surgery determined by a physician and to an insurance plan's inclusion of the surgery in the covered conditions. For the most part, these two ways of talking about required surgery coincide. When they do not, the physician is asked to demonstrate to the insurance plan that the surgery is necessary by reference to the medical condition to be treated and the customary medical practice that deems it required as opposed to optional or elective.

Purpose

More than 40 million surgeries were performed in the United States in 2000, with an average of 4.6 days in hospital. Not all surgery is an emergency. Not all surgery is medically required. Some surgeries are for cosmetic or for aesthetic enhancements and are deemed optional or elective, both by physicians and by insurance plans.

Necessary surgery refers to surgical procedures that pertain to a condition that cannot be treated by other methods and, if left untreated, would threaten the life of the patient, fail to repair or improve a body function, increase the patient's pain, or prevent the diagnosis of a serious or painful condition. The emphasis here is that, according to medical judgment, surgery is mandated.

Not all necessary surgery is absolutely required until the patient is satisfied that he or she has all the information needed to opt for surgery. All surgery has risks and the decision to have surgery is one that needs to be made by both the physician and the patient.

Description

The decision to have surgery should be made by the patient after:

- complete evaluation by a physician to determine if the surgery is medically indicated

- discussion with the physician about alternative treatments

- discussion that allows the patient to understand why the surgery is necessary, what the surgery involves, and why the particular procedure has been chosen by the surgeon

- discussion of the complete risks and benefits of the procedure

- **second opinion** has been enlisted about the surgery and its components and/or alternatives (Many health insurance plans require this step and will pay for the second opinion.)

Only after a physician has taken the condition and symptoms into account with a complete evaluation of alternatives, will surgery be judged to be necessary. During the course of this evaluation, and after non-surgical treatments have failed, the patient needs to be actively involved in understanding the actual procedure that might mitigate the condition, the full array of risks and benefits of the surgery, and why the surgeon has arrived at the particular procedure. The patient should understand the likelihood of danger or risk if he or she foregoes the surgery and the patient needs to understand that there may be a possibility of improvement, given sufficient time, without the surgery. Before choosing to undergo a particular surgical procedure, the patient should get a second opinion about the wisdom, efficacy, risk, and benefits of the procedure.

Diagnosis/Preparation

Preparation for surgery should include knowing:

- Where surgery will take place and the length of stay in the hospital. Some insurance companies may press for shorter hospital stays.

KEY TERMS

Alternatives to surgery —Other treatments for the condition or illness that do not involve surgery; these are usually tried before surgery is an option.

Elective surgery—Surgery chosen by someone over 18 and/or a guardian for a patient that is not medically required for an illness, condition, or pain relief.

Surgical alternatives—Surgical options within a range of surgical procedures used to treat a specific condition.

• What pain medication will be used, and how medications for home use will be ordered for discharge. The physician should know all medications that are currently being taken.

• Who will make decisions on the patient's behalf and with what legal authority, should the patient be unable to make a decision in the hospital. The physician and the nursing team need to know who this "patient advocate" is.

• What the visiting hours, rules, and limits on children are.

• That the hospital plans to accommodate any dietary restrictions the patient may have.

• That there is sufficient at-home assistance and resources for the patient upon discharge.

• The dietary and behavioral requirements for the days just preceding surgery.

Resources

PERIODICALS

Lewis, C. "Sizing Up Surgery." *FDA Consumer Magazine,* (November–December 1998). <http://www.fda.gov/fdac/features/1998/698_surg.html.>.

ORGANIZATIONS

Patient Rights and Responsibilities. Agency for Health Care Research and Quality. <http://www.consumer.gov/qualityhealth/rights.htm/>.
Questions To Ask Your Doctor Before You Have Surgery. Agency for Health Care Research and Quality. <http://www.ahcpr.gov/consumer/surgery.htm#head2/>.

OTHER

Wax, C. M. "Preparation for Surgery." <http://www/HealthIsNumberOne.com>.

Nancy McKenzie, PhD

Neck dissection *see* **Radical neck dissection**

Needle bladder neck suspension

Definition

Needle bladder neck suspension, also known as needle suspension, or paravaginal surgery, is performed to support the hypermobile, or moveable urethra using sutures to attach it to tissues covering the pelvic floor. Of the three popular surgical procedures for urethral instability and its results in urinary stress incontinence, needle bladder neck suspension is the quickest and easiest to perform. It has many variants, such as the Raz, Stamey, modified Pereyra, or Gattes procedures, but its long-term results are less impressive than other, more extensive, anti-incontinent surgeries.

Purpose

Fifty years of surgical attempts to treat incontinence, especially in women, has resulted in three types of surgery tied to essentially three causes of a particular type of incontinence related to muscle weakening of the urethra and the "gate-keeping" sphincter muscles. Stress urinary incontinence, the uncontrollable leakage of urine when pressure is put on the bladder during sneezing, coughing, laughing, or exercising, is very common in women, and is estimated to affect 50% of elderly women in long-term care facilities. The inability to hold urine has two causes. One has to do with support for the urethra and bladder, known as genuine stress incontinence (GSI), and the other is related to the inability of sphincter muscles, or intrinsic sphincter deficiency (ISD), to keep the opening of the bladder closed.

In GSI, weak muscles supporting the urethra allow it to be displaced and/or descend into the pelvic-floor fascia (connective tissues) and create cystoceles, or pockets. The goal of surgery for GSI is to stabilize the suburethral fascia to prevent the urethra from being overly mobile during increased abdominal pressure.

The other major source of stress incontinence is due to weakening of the internal muscles of the sphincter, as they affect closure of the bladder. These muscles, called the intrinsic sphincter muscles, regulate the opening and closing of the bladder when a decision is made to urinate. Deficiency of the intrinsic sphincter muscles causes the opening to remain open and thus leads to chronic incontinence. ISD is a source of severe stress incontinence and may be combined with urethral hypermobility.

The challenge of surgery for stress incontinence is to adequately evaluate the actual source of incontinence, whether GSI or ISD, and also to determine the likelihood of cystoceles that may need repair. Under good diagnostic conditions, surgery for stress incontinence will utilize a suprapubic (above the pubic area) procedure, or Burch procedure, to secure the hypermobile urethra and stabilize it in a neutral position. Surgery for ISD uses what is known as a **sling procedure**, or "hammock" effect, that uses auxiliary tissue to undergird the urethra and provide contractive pressure to the sphincter. Most stress incontinence surgeries fall into one of these two procedures and their variants.

Needle neck bladder suspension, the third most utilized procedure for stress incontinence, simply attempts to attach the urethra neck to the posterior pelvic wall through the vagina or abdomen in order to stabilize the urethra. It is, however, considered a poor choice in comparison to the other two procedures because of its lack of long-term efficacy and its high incidence of urinary retention as an operative complication.

Demographics

More than 13 million people in the United States, both males and females, have urinary incontinence. Women experience it twice as often as men due to pregnancy, childbirth, menopause, and the structure of the female urinary and gynecological systems. Anyone can become incontinent due to neurological injury, birth defects, cardiac conditions, multiple sclerosis, and chronic conditions in later life. Incontinence does not naturally accompany old age but is associated with many chronic conditions that occur as age increases. Incontinence is highly associated with obesity and lack of **exercise**. As many as 15–30% of adults over 60 have some form of urinary incontinence. Stress incontinence is, by far, the most frequent form of incontinence and is the most com-

mon type of bladder control problem in younger and middle-age women.

Description

Needle bladder neck suspension surgery can be performed as open abdominal or vaginal surgery, or laproscopically, which allows for small incisions, video magnification of the operative field, and precise placement of sutures. Under a general anesthetic, the patient is placed in a position on her back with legs in stirrups allowing access to the suprapubic area. A Foley catheter is inserted into the bladder. The open procedure involves the passage of a needle from the suprapubic area to the vagina with multiple sutures through looping. Cytoscopic monitoring (using an endoscope passed into the urethra) prevents passage of the needle through the bladder or the urethra. The laproscopic method allows visualization of the needle pass made from the suprapubic area to the vagina and the looping technique. The vagina and the surrounding areas are thoroughly irrigated with an antibiotic solution throughout the procedure. The patient is discharged the same evening or the next morning with the catheter in place. She is kept on **antibiotics** and examined on the fourth day after surgery with the removal of the catheter. The follow-up examination includes wound inspection and a evaluation of residual urine. A pelvic examination is performed to check for bleeding or injury.

Diagnosis/Preparation

Stress urinary incontinence can have a number of causes. It is important that patients confer with their physicians to rule out medication-related, psychological, and/or behavioral sources of incontinence as well as physical and neurological causes. This involves complete medical history, as well as medication, clinical, neurological, and radiographic evaluations. Once these are completed, urodynamic tests that evaluate the urethra, bladder, flow, urine retention, and leakage, are performed and allow the physician to determine the primary source of the stress incontinence. Patients who are obese and/or engage in high-impact exercise are not good candidates for this surgery. Patients with ISD may not be cured with this procedure, since it is primarily intended to treat the hypermobile urethra.

Morbidity and mortality rates

Urologic surgery has inherent morbidity and mortality risks related primarily to **general surgery**, with lung conditions, blood clots, infections, and cardiac events occurring in a small percentage of surgeries, independent of the type of procedure. In addition, the American Urological Association (AUA) has concluded that needle suspension surgery has a number of complications related directly to suturing in the suprapulic area. These complications include:

• a 5% incidence of bladder injury

• urethral injury, although rare, in a small percentage of cases

• bleeding, with an incidence of 3–5%, primarily from the area below the pubic area

• nerve entrapment (8–16% of cases) due to lateral placement of the sutures into the fascia at the back of the suprapubic area (This has improved with a change in the placement of sutures.)

• wound infections in about 7% of cases, with higher rates among those with diabetes or obesity

These operative complications, coupled with the procedure's high rate (10%) of reported pain after surgery, and its relatively high rate (5%) of urinary retention lasting longer than four weeks, have resulted in needle neck suspension having a limited role in the management of stress urinary incontinence.

Normal results

Despite modifications in the needle suspension procedure, the long-term outcome of the procedure does not indicate its lasting efficacy. According to a recent report by the AUA, a study of the effects of needle suspension found only a 67% cure, or "dry rate," after 48 months, with delayed failures of sutures in a very high percentage (33-80%) of cases.

See also Sling procedure.

KEY TERMS

Genuine stress incontinence (GSI)—A specific term for a type of incontinence that has to do with the instability of the urethra due to weakened support muscles.

Hypermobile urethra—A term that denotes the movement of the urethra that allows for leakage or spillage of urine.

Intrinsic sphincter defiency—A type of incontinence caused by the inability of the aphincter muscles to keep the bladder closed.

Urinary stress incontinence—The involuntary release of urine due to pressure on the abdominal muscles during exercise or laughing or coughing.

Resources

BOOKS

"Urologic Surgery." In *Campbell's Urology.* 8th edition, edited by P. Walsh, et al. Philadelphia: W. B. Saunders, 2000.

PERIODICALS

Bodell, D. M. and G. E. Leach. "Needle Suspension Procedures for Female Incontinence." *Urologic Clinics* 29 (August 2002).

Liu, C. Y. "Laproscopic Treatment of Stress Urinary Incontinence." *Obstetrics and Gynecology Clinics* 26 (March 1999).

Takahashi, S., et al. "Complications of Stamey Needle Suspension for Female Stress Urinary Incontinence." *Urology International* 86 (January 2002): 148–151.

ORGANIZATIONS

American Foundation for Urologic Diseases. The Bladder Health Council. 300 West Pratt Street, Suite 401, Baltimore, MD 21201.

American Urological Association. 1120 North Charles Street, Baltimore, MD 21201.(410) 727-1100. Fax: 410-223-4370. <http://www.urologyhealth.org.>.

The Simon Foundation for Continence. P.O. Box 835, Wilmette, IL 60091. (800) 237-simon or (800) 237-4666. Voice - Toll-free: (847) 864-3913. Voice: (847) 864-9758.

OTHER

"Urinary Incontinence." MD Consult Patient Handout. January 2, 2003 [cited July 7, 2003]. <http://www.MDConsult.com.>.

Nancy McKenzie, PhD

Needle suspension *see* **Needle bladder neck suspension**

Needles *see* **Syringe and needle**

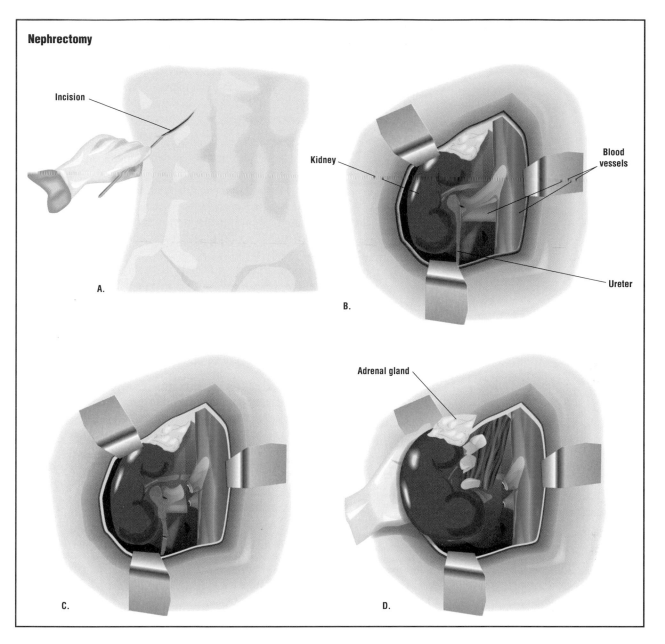

Nephrectomy

Incision

A.

Kidney

Blood vessels

Ureter

B.

C.

Adrenal gland

D.

To remove a kidney in an open procedure, an incision is made below the ribcage (A). The kidney is exposed (B) and connections to blood vessels and the ureter are severed (C). The kidney is removed in one piece (D). *(Illustration by GGS Inc.)*

Nephrectomy

Definition

A nephrectomy is a surgical procedure for the removal of a kidney or section of a kidney.

Purpose

Nephrectomy, or kidney removal, is performed on patients with severe kidney damage from disease, injury, or congenital conditions. These include cancer of the kidney (renal cell carcinoma); polycystic kidney disease (a disease in which cysts, or sac-like structures, displace healthy kidney tissue); and serious kidney infections. It is also used to remove a healthy kidney from a donor for the purposes of **kidney transplantation**.

Demographics

The HCUP Nationwide Inpatient Sample from the Agency for Healthcare Research and Quality (AHRQ)

WHO PERFORMS THE PROCEDURE AND WHERE IS IT PERFORMED?

If nephrectomy is required for the purpose of kidney donation, it will be performed by a transplant surgeon in one of over 200 UNOS-approved hospitals nationwide. For patients with renal cell carcinoma, nephrectomy surgery is typically performed in a hospital setting by a surgeon specializing in urologic oncology.

reports that 46,130 patients underwent partial or radical nephrectomy surgery for non-transplant-related indications in the United States in 2000. Patients with kidney cancer accounted for over half of those procedures. The American Cancer Society projects that an estimated 31,900 new cases of renal cell carcinoma will occur in the United States in 2003.

According to the United Network for Organ Sharing (UNOS), 5,974 people underwent nephrectomy to become living kidney donors in 2001. The majority of these donors—43.9%—were between the ages of 35 and 49, and 58.8% were female. Related donors were more common than non-related donors, with full siblings being the most common relationship between living donor and kidney recipients (28.5% of living donors).

Description

Nephrectomy may involve removing a small portion of the kidney or the entire organ and surrounding tissues. In partial nephrectomy, only the diseased or infected portion of the kidney is removed. Radical nephrectomy involves removing the entire kidney, a section of the tube leading to the bladder (ureter), the gland that sits atop the kidney (adrenal gland), and the fatty tissue surrounding the kidney. A simple nephrectomy performed for living donor transplant purposes requires removal of the kidney and a section of the attached ureter.

Open nephrectomy

In a traditional, open nephrectomy, the kidney donor is administered general anesthesia and a 6–10 in (15.2–25.4 cm) incision through several layers of muscle is made on the side or front of the abdomen. The blood vessels connecting the kidney to the donor are cut and clamped, and the ureter is also cut between the bladder and kidney and clamped. Depending on the type of nephrectomy procedure being performed, the ureter, adrenal gland, and/or surrounding tissue may also be cut. The kidney is removed and the vessels and ureter are then tied off and the incision is sutured (sewn up). The surgical procedure can take up to three hours, depending on the type of nephrectomy being performed.

Laparoscopic nephrectomy

Laparoscopic nephrectomy is a form of minimally invasive surgery that utilizes instruments on long, narrow rods to view, cut, and remove the kidney. The surgeon views the kidney and surrounding tissue with a flexible videoscope. The videoscope and **surgical instruments** are maneuvered through four small incisions in the abdomen, and carbon dioxide is pumped into the abdominal cavity to inflate it and improve visualization of the kidney. Once the kidney is isolated, it is secured in a bag and pulled through a fifth incision, approximately 3 in (7.6 cm) wide, in the front of the abdominal wall below the navel. Although this surgical technique takes slightly longer than a traditional nephrectomy, preliminary studies have shown that it promotes a faster recovery time, shorter hospital stays, and less post-operative pain.

A modified laparoscopic technique called hand-assisted laparoscopic nephrectomy may also be used to remove the kidney. In the hand-assisted surgery, a small incision of 3–5 in (7.6–12.7 cm) is made in the patient's abdomen. The incision allows the surgeon to place his hand in the abdominal cavity using a special surgical glove that also maintains a seal for the inflation of the abdominal cavity with carbon dioxide. This technique gives the surgeon the benefit of using his hands to feel the kidney and related structures. The kidney is then removed by hand through the incision instead of with a bag.

Diagnosis/Preparation

Prior to surgery, blood samples will be taken from the patient to type and crossmatch in case **transfusion** is required during surgery. A catheter will also be inserted into the patient's bladder. The surgical procedure will be described to the patient, along with the possible risks.

Aftercare

Nephrectomy patients may experience considerable discomfort in the area of the incision. Patients may also experience numbness, caused by severed nerves, near or on the incision. Pain relievers are administered following the surgical procedure and during the recovery period on an as-needed basis. Although deep breathing and coughing may be painful due to the proximity of the incision to the diaphragm, breathing exercises are encouraged to prevent pneumonia. Patients should not drive an automobile for a minimum of two weeks.

QUESTIONS TO ASK THE DOCTOR

- How many procedures of this type have you performed, and what are your success rates?
- Will my nephrectomy surgery be performed with a laparoscopic or an open technique?
- Will my nephrectomy be partial or radical, and what are the risks involved with my particular surgery?
- What will my recovery time be after the procedure?
- What are the chances that the transplant will be successful? (For those undergoing a nephrectomy to donate a kidney.)
- What are the odds of success, and will I require adjunctive treatment such as chemotherapy or immunotherapy? (For those undergoing a nephrectomy to treat kidney cancer.)

Risks

Possible complications of a nephrectomy procedure include infection, bleeding (hemorrhage), and post-operative pneumonia. There is also the risk of kidney failure in a patient with impaired function or disease in the remaining kidney.

Normal results

Normal results of a nephrectomy are dependent on the purpose of the procedure and the type of nephrectomy performed. Immediately following the procedure, it is normal for patients to experience pain near the incision site, particularly when coughing or breathing deeply. Renal function of the patient is monitored carefully after surgery. If the remaining kidney is healthy, it will increase its functioning over time to compensate for the loss of the removed kidney.

Length of hospitalization depends on the type of nephrectomy procedure. Patients who have undergone a laparoscopic radical nephrectomy may be discharged two to four days after surgery. Traditional open nephrectomy patients are typically hospitalized for about a week. Recovery time will also vary, on average from three to six weeks.

Morbidity and mortality rates

Survival rates for living kidney donors undergoing nephrectomy are excellent; mortality rates are only 0.03%—or three deaths for every 10,000 donors. Many

KEY TERMS

Cadaver kidney—A kidney from a brain-dead organ donor used for purposes of kidney transplantation.

Polycystic kidney disease—A hereditary kidney disease that causes fluid- or blood-filled pouches of tissue called cysts to form on the tubules of the kidneys. These cysts impair normal kidney function.

Renal cell carcinoma—Cancer of the kidney.

of the risks involved are the same as for any surgical procedure: risk of infection, hemorrhage, blood clot, or allergic reaction to anesthesia.

For patients undergoing nephrectomy as a treatment for renal cell carcinoma, survival rates depend on several factors, including the stage of the cancer and the patient's overall **health history**. According to the American Cancer Society, the five-year survival rate for patients with stage I renal cell carcinoma is 90–100%, while the five-year survival rate for stage II kidney cancer is 65–75%. Stage III and IV cancers have metastasized, or spread, beyond the kidney and have a lower survival rate, 40–70% for stage III and less than 10% for stage IV. Chemotherapy, radiation, and/or immunotherapy may also be required for these patients.

Alternatives

Because the kidney is responsible for filtering wastes and fluid from the bloodstream, kidney function is critical to life. Nephrectomy candidates diagnosed with serious kidney disease, cancer, or infection usually have few treatment choices aside from this procedure. However, if kidney function is lost in the remaining kidney, the patient will require chronic dialysis treatments or transplantation of a healthy kidney to sustain life.

Resources

BOOKS

Cameron, J. S. *Kidney Failure: The Facts.* New York: Oxford University Press, 1999.

Parker, James and Philip Parker, eds. *The 2002 Official Patient Sourcebook on Renal Cell Cancer.* San Diego: Icon Health Publications, 2002.

PERIODICALS

Johnson, Kate. "Laparoscopy is Big Hit With Living Donors." *Family Practice News* 31 (January 2001): 12.

ORGANIZATIONS

American Cancer Society. (800) 227-2345. <http://www.cancer.org>.

National Kidney Foundation. 30 East 33rd St., Suite 1100, New York, NY 10016. (800) 622-9010. <http://www.kidney.org>.

United Network for Organ Sharing (UNOS). 700 North 4th St., Richmond, VA 23219. (888) 894-6361. UNOS Transplant Connection: <http://www.transplantliving.org>.

OTHER

Living Donors Online. <http://www.livingdonorsonline.org>.

Paula Anne Ford-Martin

Nephrolithotomy, percutaneous

Definition

Percutaneous nephrolithotomy, or PCNL, is a procedure for removing medium-sized or larger renal calculi (kidney stones) from the patient's urinary tract by means of an nephroscope passed into the kidney through a track created in the patient's back. PCNL was first performed in Sweden in 1973 as a less invasive alternative to open surgery on the kidneys. The term "percutaneous" means that the procedure is done through the skin. Nephrolithotomy is a term formed from two Greek words that mean "kidney" and "removing stones by cutting."

Purpose

The purpose of PCNL is the removal of renal calculi in order to relieve pain, bleeding into or obstruction of the urinary tract, and/or urinary tract infections resulting from blockages. Kidney stones range in size from microscopic groups of crystals to objects as large as golf balls. Most calculi, however, pass through the urinary tract without causing problems.

Renal calculi are formed when the urine becomes supersaturated (overloaded) with mineral compounds that can form stones. This supersaturation may occur because the patient has low urinary output, is excreting too much salt, or has very acid urine. Urolithiasis is the medical term for the formation of kidney stones; the word is also sometimes used to refer to disease conditions associated with kidney stones.

There are several different types of kidney stones, in terms of chemical composition:

- Calcium oxalate calculi. About 80% of calculi found in patients in the United States are formed from calcium combined with oxalate, which is a salt formed from oxalic acid. Some foods, such as rhubarb and spinach, are high in oxalic acid. Oxalic acid is also formed in the body when vitamin C is broken down. Oxalic acid is ordinarily excreted through the urine but may be absorbed in large amounts due to chronic pancreatic disease or surgery involving the small intestine.

- Uric acid calculi. These stones develop from crystals of uric acid that form in highly acidic urine. Uric acid calculi account for about 5% of kidney stones. In addition, some kidney stones are a combination of calcium oxalate and uric acid crystals.

- Cystine calculi. Cystine calculi represent about 2% of kidney stones. Cystine is an amino acid found in proteins that may form hexagonal crystals in the urine when it is excreted in excessive amounts. Kidney stones made of cystine indicate that the patient has cystinuria, a hereditary condition in which the kidneys do not reabsorb this amino acid.

- Struvite calculi. Struvite is a hard crystalline form of magnesium aluminum phosphate. Kidney stones made of this substance are formed in patients with urinary tract infections caused by certain types of bacteria. Struvite calculi are also known as infection calculi for this reason.

- Staghorn calculi. Staghorn calculi are large branched calculi composed of struvite. They are often discussed separately because their size and shape complicate their removal from the urinary tract.

Some people are more likely than others to develop renal calculi. Risk factors for kidney stones include:

- Male sex.

- Family history. Having a first-degree relative with urolithiasis increases a person's risk of developing kidney stones.

- Age over 30.

- Diet. People whose diet is high in protein or who eat foods rich in oxalate are more likely to develop kidney stones.

- Dehydration. People who do not drink enough fluid each day to replace what is lost through perspiration and excretion produce very concentrated urine. It is easier for crystals to form in concentrated than in dilute urine, and to grow into kidney stones.

- Metabolic disorders affecting the body's excretion of salt or its absorption of calcium or oxalate. Most cases of urolithiasis in children are related to metabolic disorders.

- Intestinal bypass surgery and ostomies. People who have had these surgical procedures lose larger than average amounts of water from the digestive tract.

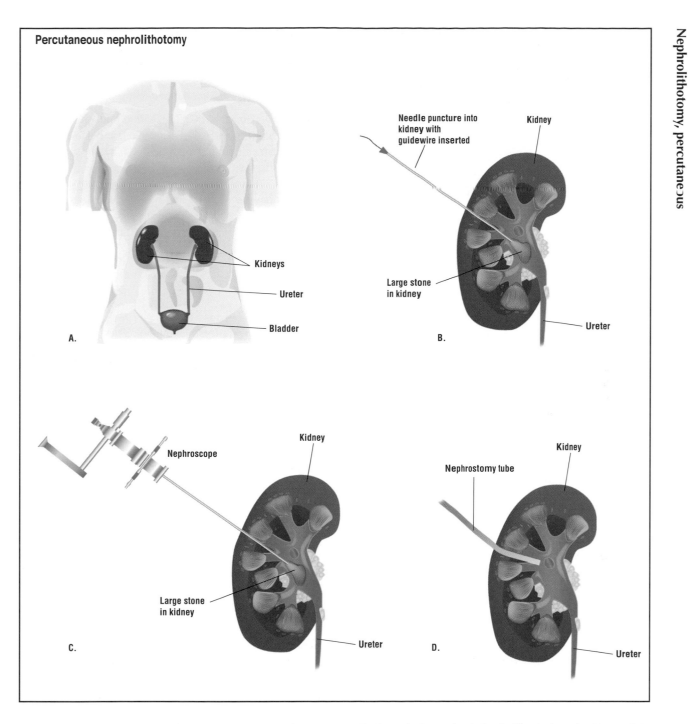

Percutaneous nephrolithotomy

A.
Kidneys
Ureter
Bladder

B.
Needle puncture into kidney with guidewire inserted
Kidney
Large stone in kidney
Ureter

C.
Nephroscope
Kidney
Large stone in kidney
Ureter

D.
Nephrostomy tube
Kidney
Ureter

During a percutaneous nephrolithotomy, the surgeon inserts a needle through the patient's back directly into the kidney (B). A nephroscope uses an ultrasonic or laser probe to break up large kidney stones (C). Pieces of the stones are suctioned out with the scope, and a nephrostomy tube drains the kidney of urine (D). *(Illustration by GGS Inc.)*

Demographics

Calculi in the urinary tract are common in the general United States population. Between seven and 10 in every 1,000 adults are hospitalized each year for treatment of urolithiasis; in addition, kidney stones are found in about 1% of bodies at autopsy. An estimated 10% of the population will suffer from kidney stones at some point in life. For reasons that are not yet known, the percentage of people with kidney stones has been rising in North America since 1980. In addition, the gender ratio is changing as more women are developing kidney stones. In 1980, the male:female ratio was 4:1; as of 2002, it was 3:1. Although more men develop renal calculi in general than women, more women develop infection calculi than men.

In terms of age groups, most people with urolithiasis are between the ages of 20 and 40; kidney stones are rare in children. A person who develops one kidney stone has a 50% chance of developing another.

With regard to race, Caucasians are more likely to develop kidney stones than African Americans.

Description

Standard PCNL

A standard percutaneous nephrolithotomy is performed under general anesthesia and usually takes about three to four hours to complete. After the patient has been anesthetized, the surgeon makes a small incision, about 0.5 in (1.3 cm) in length in the patient's back on the side overlying the affected kidney. The surgeon then creates a track from the skin surface into the kidney and enlarges the track using a series of Teflon dilators or bougies. A sheath is passed over the last dilator to hold the track open.

After the track has been enlarged, the surgeon inserts a nephroscope, which is an instrument with a fiberoptic light source and two additional channels for viewing the inside of the kidney and irrigating (washing out) the area. The surgeon may use a device with a basket on the end to grasp and remove smaller kidney stones directly. Larger stones are broken up with an ultrasonic or electrohydraulic probe, or a holmium laser lithotriptor. The holmium laser has the advantage of being usable on all types of calculi.

A catheter is placed to drain the urinary system through the bladder and a **nephrostomy** tube is placed in the incision in the back to carry fluid from the kidney into a drainage bag. The catheter is removed after 24 hours. The nephrostomy tube is usually removed while the patient is still in the hospital but may be left in after the patient is discharged.

Mini-percutaneous nephrolithotomy

A newer form of PCNL is called mini-percutaneous nephrolithotomy (MPCNL) because it is performed with a miniaturized nephroscope. MPCNL has been found to be 99% effective in removing calculi between 0.4 and 1 in (1 and 2.5 cm) in size. Although it cannot be used for larger kidney stones, MPCNL has the advantage of fewer complications, a shorter operating time (about one and a half hours), and a shorter recovery time for the patient.

Diagnosis/Preparation

Diagnosis

Kidney stones may be discovered during a routine x ray study of the patient's abdomen. These stones, which would ordinarily pass through the urinary tract unnoticed, are sometimes referred to as silent stones. In most cases, however, the patient seeks medical help for sudden intense pain in the lower back, usually on the side of the affected kidney. The pain is caused by the movement of the stone in the urinary tract as it irritates the tissues or blocks the passage of urine. If the stone moves further downward into the ureter (the tube that carries urine from the kidney to the bladder), pain may spread to the abdomen and groin area. The patient may also have nausea and vomiting, blood in the urine, pain on urination, or a need to urinate frequently. If the stone is associated with a UTI, the patient may also have chills and fever. The doctor will order both laboratory studies and imaging tests in order to rule out such other possible causes of the patient's symptoms as appendicitis, pancreatitis, peptic ulcer, and dissecting aneurysm.

The imaging studies most commonly performed are x ray and ultrasound. Pure uric acid and cystine calculi, however, do not show up well on a standard x ray, so the doctor may also order an intravenous pyelogram, or IVP. In an IVP, the radiologist injects a radioactive contrast material into a vein in the patient's arm, and records its passage through the urinary system in a series of x ray images. Blood and urine samples will be taken to test for indications of a urinary tract infection. If the patient passes the kidney stone, it is saved and sent to a laboratory for analysis.

Preparation

Most hospitals require patients to have the following tests before a PCNL: a complete **physical examination**; **complete blood count**; an electrocardiogram (EKG); a comprehensive set of metabolic tests; a urine test; and tests that measure the speed of blood clotting.

Aspirin and arthritis medications should be discontinued seven to 10 days before a PCNL because they thin the blood and affect clotting time. Some surgeons ask patients to take a laxative the day before surgery to minimize the risk of constipation during the first few days of recovery.

The patient is asked to drink only clear fluids (chicken or beef broth, clear fruit juices, or water) for 24 hours prior to surgery, with nothing by mouth after midnight before the procedure.

Aftercare

A standard PCNL usually requires hospitalization for five to six days after the procedure. The urologist may order additional imaging studies to determine whether any fragments of stones are still present. These can be removed with a nephroscope if necessary. The nephrostomy tube is then removed and the incision covered with a bandage. The patient will be given instructions for changing the bandage at home.

The patient is given fluids intravenously for one to two days after surgery. Later, he or she is encouraged to drink large quantities of fluid in order to produce about 2 qt (1.2 l) of urine per day. Some blood in the urine is normal for several days after PCNL. Blood and urine samples may be taken for laboratory analysis of specific risk factors for calculus formation.

Risks

There are a number of risks associated with PCNL:

• Inability to make a large enough track to insert the nephroscope. In this case, the procedure will be converted to open kidney surgery.

• Bleeding. Bleeding may result from injury to blood vessels within the kidney as well as from blood vessels in the area of the incision.

• Infection.

• Fever. Running a slight temperature (101.5°F; 38.5°C) is common for one or two days after the procedure. A high fever or a fever lasting longer than two days may indicate infection, however, and should be reported to the doctor at once.

• Fluid accumulation in the area around the incision. This complication usually results from irrigation of the affected area of the kidney during the procedure.

• Formation of an **arteriovenous fistula**. An arteriovenous fistula is a connection between an artery and a

QUESTIONS
TO ASK THE DOCTOR

• Am I a candidate for a mini-PCNL?

• Do you consider the higher success rate of a PCNL a greater advantage than the lower rate of complications with ESWL?

• What can I do to prevent recurrence of kidney stones?

• What are the chances of my needing another operation?

vein in which blood flows directly from the artery into the vein.

• Need for retreatment. In general, PCNL has a higher success rate of stone removal than extracorporeal shock wave **lithotripsy** (ESWL), which is described below. PCNL is considered particularly effective for removing stones larger than 1 in (0.5 cm); staghorn calculi; and stones that have remained in the body longer than four weeks. Retreatment is occasionally necessary, however, in cases involving very large stones.

• Injury to surrounding organs. In rare cases, PCNL has resulted in damage to the spleen, liver, lung, pancreas, or gallbladder.

Normal results

PCNL has a high rate of success for stone removal, over 98% for stones that remain in the kidney and 88% for stones that pass into the ureter.

Morbidity and mortality rates

Standard PCNL has a higher rate of complications than extracorporeal shock wave lithotripsy; however, it is more successful in removing calculi. The overall rate of complications following PCNL is reported as 5.6% in one recent study and 6.5% in a second article. About 20% of patients scheduled for PCNL require a blood **transfusion** during the procedure, with 2.8% needing treatment for bleeding after the procedure. The rate of fistula formation is about 2.5%.

Alternatives

Patients with kidney stones may be treated with one or more of the following procedures in addition to PCNL, depending on the size of their renal calculi and possible complications. One frequently used combina-

KEY TERMS

Bougie—A slender, flexible tube or rod inserted into the urethra in order to dilate it.

Calculus (plural, calculi)—The medical term for a kidney or gallbladder stone.

Cystine—An amino acid found in protein molecules that may form kidney stones when excreted in excessive amounts in the urine.

Cystinuria—A hereditary condition characterized by chronic excessive excretion of cystine and three other amino acids.

Infection calculi—Another name for struvite calculi.

Lithotripsy—A technique for breaking up kidney stones within the urinary tract, followed by flushing out the fragments.

Nephrolithotomy—The removal of renal calculi by an incision through the kidney. The term by itself usually refers to the standard open procedure for the surgical removal of kidney stones.

Nephroscope—An instrument used to view the inside of the kidney during PCNL. A nephroscope has channels for a fiberoptic light, a telescope, and an irrigation system for washing out the affected part of the kidney.

Percutaneous—Through the skin.

Staghorn calculus—A kidney stone that develops a branched shape resembling the antlers of a stag. Staghorn calculi are composed of struvite.

Struvite—A crystalline form of magnesium ammonium phosphate. Kidney stones made of struvite form in urine with a pH above 7.2.

Ureter—The tubelike structure that carries urine from the kidney to the bladder.

Ureteroscope—A special type of endoscope that allows a surgeon to remove kidney stones from the lower urinary tract without the need for an incision.

Urolithiasis—The medical term for the formation of kidney stones. It is also used to refer to disease conditions related to kidney stones.

---

tion, known as sandwich therapy, is extracorporeal shock wave lithotripsy for smaller stones followed by PCNL to remove larger calculi.

Conservative approaches

Conservative forms of treatment include the following:

• Watchful waiting.

• Hydration. Increasing the patient's fluid intake (to seven or more glasses of fluid each day) is a major component of treatment intended to prevent the formation of kidney stones. At least half of the fluid should be water.

• Dietary modification. Depending on the type of stone that has formed, the patient may benefit from eating less animal protein, avoiding vegetables with high oxalate content, cutting down on table salt and vitamin C intake, etc.

• Medications. Patients who tend to form uric acid stones may be given allopurinol, which decreases the formation of uric acid; those who form calcium oxalate stones may be given thiazide **diuretics**; and those who develop infection stones can be treated with oral antibiotics.

Open surgery

Open surgery is the most invasive form of treatment for urolithiasis. As of 2003, it is performed primarily to re-move very large and complex staghorn calculi or extremely hard stones that cannot be broken down by lithotripsy. Other indications for open surgery are extreme obesity, an anatomically abnormal kidney, or an infected and nonfunctioning kidney requiring complete removal. Patients are usually hospitalized for a week after open kidney surgery and take about six weeks to recover at home.

Extracorporeal shock wave lithotripsy (ESWL)

ESWL is a noninvasive procedure that was developed in the 1980s as a less invasive alternative to PCNL. It is presently used more often than PCNL to treat smaller renal calculi. In ESWL, the patient is given a local anesthetic and placed in a water bath or on a soft cushion while shock waves are transmitted through the tissues of the back to the stones inside the kidney. The shock waves cause the calculi to break up into smaller pieces that can be passed easily in the urine.

Although patients need less time to recuperate from ESWL, it has several disadvantages. It has lower success rates (50–90%) than PCNL. Moreover, it cannot be used to treat cystine calculi or calculi larger than 1.2 in (3 cm). An additional concern with shock wave lithotripsy is its safety in treating small or anatomically abnormal kidneys; it has been reported to cause temporary damage to kidney tubules in smaller-than-average kidneys.

Ureteroscopy

Ureteroscopy refers to removal of calculi that have moved downward into the ureter with the help of a special instrument. A ureteroscope is a small fiberoptic endoscope that can be passed through the patient's urethra and bladder into the ureter. The ureteroscope allows the surgeon to locate and remove stones in the lower urinary tract without the need for an incision.

Complementary and alternative (CAM) approaches

Vegetarian and other low-protein diets have been found helpful in preventing kidney stone formation. In addition, recent ethnobotanical studies of ammi visnaga (toothpick weed), a plant belonging to the parsley family, and *Phyllanthus niruri*, a traditional Brazilian folk remedy for kidney stones, indicate that extracts from these plants are effective in increasing urinary output and inhibiting the development of calcium oxalate calculi.

See also Urologic surgery.

Resources

BOOKS

Pelletier, Kenneth R., MD. "CAM Therapies for Specific Conditions: Kidney Stones." In *The Best Alternative Medicine.* New York: Simon & Schuster, 2002.

"Urinary Calculi." In *The Merck Manual of Diagnosis and Therapy*, edited by Mark H. Beers, MD, and Robert Berkow, MD. Whitehouse Station, NJ: Merck Research Laboratories, 1999.

PERIODICALS

Battino, B. S., W. DeFoor, F. Coe, et al. "Metabolic Evaluation of Children with Urolithiasis: Are Adult References for Supersaturation Appropriate?" *Journal of Urology* 168 (December 2002): 2568–2571.

Chan, D. Y., and T. W. Jarrett. "Mini-Percutaneous Nephrolithotomy." *Journal of Endourology* 14 (April 2000): 269–272.

Freitas, A. M., N. Schor, and M. A. Boim. "The Effect of *Phyllanthus niruri* on Urinary Inhibitors of Calcium Oxalate Crystallization and Other Factors Associated with Renal Stone Formation." *BJU International* 89 (June 2002): 829–834.

Jin, Chua Wei, and Chin Chong Min. "Management of Staghorn Calculus." *Medical Progress* (February 2003): 1–6.

Khan, Z. A., A. M. Assiri, H. M. Al-Afghani, and T. M. Maghrabi. "Inhibition of Oxalate Nephrolithiasis with Ammi Visnaga (Al-Khillah)." *International Urology and Nephrology* 33 (2001): 605–608.

Kim, S. C., R. L. Kuo, and J. E. Lingeman. "Percutaneous Nephrolithotomy: An Update." *Current Opinion in Urology* 13 (May 2003): 235–241.

Kinn, A. C., I. Fernstrom, B. Johansson, and H. Ohlsen. "Percutaneous Nephrolithotomy— The Birth of a New Technique." *Scandinavian Journal of Urology and Nephrology Supplement* 138 (1991): 11–14.

Lahme, S., K. H. Bichler, W. L. Strohmaier, and T. Gotz. "Minimally Invasive PCNL in Patients with Renal Pelvic and Calyceal Stones." *European Urology* 40 (December 2001): 619–624.

Parsons, J. K., T. W. Jarrett, V. Lancini, and L. R. Kavoussi. "Infundibular Stenosis After Percutaneous Nephrolithotomy." *Journal of Urology* 167 (January 2002): 35–38.

Ugras, M., A. Gunes, and C. Baydinc. "Severe Renal Bleeding Caused by a Ruptured Renal Sheath: Case Report of a Rare Complication of Percutaneous Nephrolithotomy." *BMC Urology* 2 (September 18, 2002): 10.

ORGANIZATIONS

American Foundation for Urologic Disease (AFUD). 1128 North Charles Street, Baltimore, MD 21201. (800) 242-2383. <http://www.afud.org>.

American Urological Association (AUA). 1120 North Charles Street, Baltimore, MD 21201. (410) 727-1100. <http://www.auanet.org>.

National Kidney Foundation. 30 East 33rd Street, Suite 1100, New York, NY 10016. (800) 622-9010 or (212) 889-2210. <http://www.kidney.org>.

National Kidney and Urologic Diseases Information Clearinghouse (NKUDIC). 3 Information Way, Bethesda, MD 20892-3580.

OTHER

National Kidney and Urologic Diseases Information Clearinghouse (NKUDIC). *Kidney Stones in Adults.* February 1998 [cited April 30, 2003]. NIH Publication No. 94-2495. <http://www.niddk.nih.gov/health/urolog/pubs/stonadul/stonadul.htm>.

Rebecca Frey, Ph.D.

Nephrostomy

Definition

A nephrostomy is a surgical procedure by which a tube, stent, or catheter is inserted through the skin and into the kidney.

Purpose

The ureter is the fibromuscular tube that carries urine from the kidney to the bladder. When this tube is blocked, urine backs up into the kidney. Serious, irreversible kidney damage can occur because of this backflow of urine. Infection is also a common consequence in this stagnant urine.

Nephrostomy is performed in several different circumstances:

- The ureter is blocked by a kidney stone.
- The ureter is blocked by a tumor.
- There is a hole in the ureter or bladder and urine is leaking into the body.
- As a diagnostic procedure to assess kidney anatomy.
- As a diagnostic procedure to assess kidney function.

Demographics

For unknown reasons, the number of people in the United States with kidney and ureter stones has been increasing over the past 20 years. White Americans are more prone to develop kidney stones than African Americans. Stones occur more frequently in men. The condition strikes most typically between the ages of 20 and 40. Once a person gets more than one stone, others are likely to develop.

Upper tract tumors develop in the renal pelvis (tissue in the kidneys that collects urine) and in the ureters. These cancers account for less than 1% of cancers of the reproductive and urinary systems. Upper tract tumors are often associated with bladder cancer.

Description

First, the patient is given an anesthetic to numb the area where the catheter will be inserted. The doctor then inserts a needle into the kidney. There are several imaging technologies such as ultrasound and computed tomography (CT) that are used to help the doctor guide the needle into the correct place.

Next, a fine guide wire follows the needle. The catheter, which is about the same diameter as IV (intravenous) tubing, follows the guide wire to its proper loca-

tion. The catheter is then connected to a bag outside the body that collects the urine. The catheter and bag are secured so that the catheter will not pull out. The procedure usually takes one to two hours.

Diagnosis/Preparation

Either the day before or the day of the nephrostomy, blood samples are taken. Other diagnostic tests done before the procedure may vary, depending on why the nephrostomy is being done, but the patient may have a CT scan or ultrasound to help the treating physician locate the blockage.

Patients should not eat for eight hours before a nephrostomy. On the day of the procedure, the patient will have an IV line placed in a vein in the arm. Through this line, the patient will receive **antibiotics** to prevent infection, medication for pain, and fluids. The IV line will remain in place after the procedure for at least several hours, and often longer.

People preparing for a nephrostomy should review with their doctor all the medications they are taking. People taking anticoagulants (blood thinners such as Coumadin) may need to stop their medication. People taking metformin (Glucophage) may need to stop taking the medication for several days before and after nephrostomy. Diabetics should discuss modifying their insulin dose because fasting is required before the procedure.

Aftercare

Outpatients are usually expected to stay in the clinic or hospital for eight to 12 hours after the procedure to make sure the nephrostomy tube is functioning properly. They should plan to have someone drive them home and stay with them for at least the first 24 hours after the procedure. Inpatients may stay in the hospital several days. Generally, people feel sore where the catheter is inserted for about a week to 10 days.

Care of the nephrostomy tube is important. It is located on the patient's back, so it may be necessary to have someone help with its care. The nephrostomy tube should be kept dry and protected from water when taking showers. The skin around it should be kept clean, and the dressing over the area changed frequently. It is the main part of the urine drainage system, and it should be treated very carefully to prevent bacteria and other germs from entering the system. If any germs get into the tubing, they can easily cause a kidney infection. The drainage bag should not be allowed to drag on the floor. If the bag should accidentally be cut or begin to leak, it must be changed immediately. It is not recommended to place the drainage bag in a plastic bag if it leaks.

Risks

A nephrostomy is an established and generally safe procedure. As with all operations, there is always a risk of allergic reaction to anesthesia, bleeding, and infection.

Bruising at the catheter insertion site occurs in about half of people who have a nephrostomy. This is a minor complication. Major complications include the following:

- injury to surrounding organs, including bowel perforation, splenic injury, and liver injury
- infection, leading to septicemia
- significant loss of functioning kidney tissue (<1%)
- delayed bleeding, or hemorrhage (<0.5%)
- blocking of a kidney artery (<0.5%)

Normal results

In a successful nephrostomy, the catheter is inserted, and urine drains into the collection bag. How long the catheter stays in place depends on the reason for its insertion. In people with pelvic cancer or bladder cancer where the ureter is blocked by a tumor, the catheter will stay in place until the tumor is surgically removed. If the cancer is inoperable, the catheter may have to stay in place for the rest of the patient's life.

Morbidity and mortality rates

The mortality rate of nephrostomies is of the order of less than 0.05% and the incidence of the specific complications listed above ranges between less than 0.05% (hemorrhage, kidney arterial blocking, and loss of kidney tissue) to less than 1% (injury to surrounding organs and septicemia).

Alternatives

In the treatment of ureter stones, extracorporeal shock wave **lithotripsy** (ESWL) has been most widely performed and has become the preferred treatment for this condition. ESWL is a new technique that offers an alternative to surgery for patients with kidney or ureter stones. ESWL works by pulverizing the stones into sand-like particles that can be excreted with little or no pain. This is achieved by the ESWL procedure approximately 90% of the time. The shock waves are a form of high-energy pressure that can travel in air or water. When generated outside the body, they pass through the tissues of the body without damaging them, but can destroy a stone inside a kidney or urethra. The shock waves pass through both without injury. A stone has a greater density and, when the shock wave hits it, the waves scatter and break it up.

QUESTIONS TO ASK THE DOCTOR

- Why am I having a nephrostomy?
- How do I prepare for surgery?
- How long will I have to stay in the hospital?
- How long do you expect the nephrostomy tube to stay in?
- How much help will I need in caring for the nephrostomy tube?

Resources

BOOKS

Rodman, J. S. and C. Seidman. *No More Kidney Stones.* New York: John Wiley & Sons, 1996.

PERIODICALS

Cozens, N. J. "How Should We Deliver an Out of Hours Nephrostomy Service?" *Clinical Radiology* 58 (May 2003): 410.

Dyer, R. B., J. D. Regan, P. V. Kavanagh, E. G. Khatod, M. Y. Chen, and R. J. Zagoria. "Percutaneous Nephrostomy with Extensions of the Technique: Step by Step." *Radiographics* 22 (May–June 2002): 503–524.

Koral, K., M. C. Saker, F. P. Morello, C. K. Rigsby, and J. S. Donaldson. "Conventional versus Modified Technique for Percutaneous Nephrostomy in Newborns and Young Infants." *Journal of Vascular and Interventional Radiology* 14 (January 2003): 113–116.

Little, B., K. J. Ho, S. Gawley, and M. Young. "Use of Nephrostomy Tubes in Ureteric Obstruction from Incurable Malignancy." *International Journal of Clinical Practice* 57 (April 2003): 180–0181.

ORGANIZATIONS

American Cancer Society. National Headquarters. 1599 Clifton Road NE, Atlanta, GA 30329. (800) ACS-2345. <http://www.cancer.org>.

American College of Radiology (ACR). 1891 Preston White Drive, Reston, VA 20191-4397. (800) 227-5463. <http://www.acr.org>.

American Urological Association (AUA). 1120 North Charles Street, Baltimore, MD 21201. (410) 727-1100. <http://www.auanet.org>.

United Ostomy Association (UOA). 19772 MacArthur Blvd., #200, Irvine, CA 92612-2405. (800) 826-0826. <http://www.uoa.org>.

OTHER

"Extracorporeal Shock Wave Lithotripsy (ESWL)." *Family Practice Notebook* May 28, 2003 [cited July 7, 2003]. <http://www.fpnotebook.com/SUR46.htm>.

"Nephrostomy." Mid-South Imaging and Therapeutics [cited July 7, 2003]. <http://www.msit.com>.

KEY TERMS

Catheter—A tubular, flexible, surgical instrument for withdrawing fluids from a cavity of the body, especially one for introduction into the bladder through the urethra for the withdraw of urine.

Ostomy—General term meaning a surgical procedure in which an artificial opening is formed to either allow waste (stool or urine) to pass from the body, or to allow food into the GI tract. An ostomy can be permanent or temporary, as well as single-barreled, double-barreled, or a loop.

Septicemia—Systemic disease associated with the presence and persistence of pathogenic microorganisms or their toxins in the blood.

Stent—A tube made of metal or plastic that is inserted into a vessel or passage to keep it open and prevent closure.

Ureter—The fibromuscular tube that conveys the urine from the kidney to the bladder.

"Percutaneous Nephrostomy." WFUSM Division of Radiologic Sciences. May 8, 2003 [cited July 7, 2003]. <http://www.rad.bgsm.edu/patienteduc/percutaneous_nephrostomy.htm>.

Tish Davidson, AM
Monique Laberge, PhD

Neurosurgery

Definition

Neurosurgery is a specialized field of surgery for the treatment of diseases or conditions of the central nervous system (CNS) and spine.

Description

Neurosurgery is the specialized field of surgery that treats diseases that affect the CNS—the brain and the spine. A neurosurgeon is a medical doctor who has received extensive training in the surgical and medical management of neurological diseases. The field of neurosurgery is one of the most sophisticated surgical specialties and encompasses advanced surgical and imaging technology and new research in molecular neurosurgery and gene therapy. There are five general categories of neurosurgical diseases that are commonly managed by neurosurgeons: cerebrovascular (hemorrhage and aneurysms); traumatic head injury (THI)(traumatic injury caused by accident); degeneration diseases of the spine; tumors in the CNS; functional neurosurgery; surgery for congenital abnormalities; and neurosurgical management of the CNS.

Cerebrovascular diseases that usually require surgery include spontaneous intracranial hemorrhage, spontaneous subarachnoid hemorrhage, spontaneous intracerebral hemorrhage, cerebral aneurysms, hypertensive intracerebral hemorrhage, and angiomatous malformations.

Brain hemorrhage

Spontaneous intracranial hemorrhage (hemorrhage in the brain) is a condition characterized by hemorrhage in the brain (hemorrhagic stroke) that results in a sudden onset of neurologically worsening symptoms (that include focal neurologic deficits and loss of consciousness). **CT scans** are helpful in identifying the intracranial hemorrhage, of which there are two types—subarachnoid hemorrhage and intracerebral hematoma.

The subarachnoid space is an area that exists between two layers of coverings (membranes) that wrap around the brain. A spontaneous subarachnoid hemorrhage is defined as blood (not caused by trauma), in the subarachnoid space. The amount of blood in the subarachnoid space can be a focal (small area) amount or a larger, more diffuse hemorrhage, which can be further complicated by having an intraventricular hemorrhage or intracerebral hematoma at the same time. Subarachnoid hemorrhage can affect adults of all ages, but usually peaks in the fourth and fifth decades of life. Approximately 60% of patients are female.

The incidence of subarachnoid hemorrhage is 10 per 100,000 persons per year; approximately 30% of Americans will sustain a subarachnoid hemorrhage annually. The most frequent cause of spontaneous subarachnoid hemorrhage is rupture of an intracranial aneurysm. The symptoms of subarachnoid hemorrhage are characterized by a sudden onset of severe headache that worsens over time, and includes nausea, loss of consciousness (with or without seizure) and vomiting. Depending on the extent of the bleed, symptoms of subarachnoid hemorrhage can also include visual sensitivity to light (photophobia), a stiff neck, and minor (low grade) fever. Symptoms before rupture of the aneurysm occur in 40% of persons and are usually due to minor subarachnoid hemorrhage. These symptoms can also include headache or dizziness, and tend to go unnoticed.

Approximately 30% of subarachnoid hemorrhages occur during sleep. Smoking is a major factor in increasing the odds of sustaining a subarachnoid hemorrhage. After a subarachnoid hemorrhage, most patients are hypertensive and experience changes in cardiac rate and rhythm. CT scans are the best diagnostic tool for subarachnoid hemorrhage and are positive in the first 24 hours after the hemorrhage has been experienced in 90% of patients and in more than 50% in the first week. Spinal taps to sample the cerebrospinal fluid (CSF) may be required to evaluate some patients who have the potential to suffer a subarachnoid hemorrhage. This involves the insertion of a thin needle between the lumbar vertebral bodies (L–4 and L–5) to allow the removal of a small amount of fluid to look for either red or white blood cells (WBCs). Once the aneurysm has been identified, the patient is taken for surgery. A **craniotomy** is performed using microsurgical techniques. The operative microscope helps to identify the aneurysm, which is then clipped. Berry, or congenital aneurysm, is the reason for over half of all cases of spontaneous subarachnoid hemorrhage.

A spontaneous, intracerebral hemorrhage (SICH) is a blood clot in brain tissue that can arise abruptly and is strongly correlated with hypertension. There are approximately 40,000 new cases of SICH in the United States annually. Stroke is the third leading cause of death in the United States, and SICH accounts for 10% of all stroke cases. Advancing age is a major predisposing factor for SICH: The incidence of SICH is two per 1,000 persons per year by age 45, and a person aged 80 years or more has a 350 per 100,000 persons per year incidence. Hypertensive intracerebral hemorrhage can occur in different areas within the brain. Damage to some areas may be associated with a very high death rate. Treatment includes comprehensive ICU (**intensive care unit**) management of hypertension and maintenance of adequate cerebral perfusion (oxygenated blood going to the brain).

Accidents that result in head injury are a major public health problem. Trauma causes approximately 150,000 deaths annually in the United States; approximately half of these deaths were caused by fatal head trauma. Additionally, there are 10,000 new spinal cord injuries annually. The cost of disability (e.g., chronic long-term care, lost wages and work) is very high. Approximately 200,000 persons in the United States are living with disabilities associated with head and spinal cord trauma.

Severe head injury is defined as an injury that produces coma (patient will not open eyes even to painful stimulus; incapable of following simple commands; and inability to utter words). These clinical criteria are defined on the well-established Glasgow Coma Scale (GCS). A **physical examination** and neurologic assessment by a neurosurgeon and brain scan imaging (CT scan) is necessary for the initial evaluation. Additionally, a special catheter to monitor intracranial pressure

(due to brain swelling) is inserted. A large clot, larger than 25 to 30 cubic centimeters, is considered clinically large enough to cause progressive brain injury.

Tumors inside the brain (intracranial tumors) are typically of two types; primary and secondary intracranial tumors. Primary intracranial tumors (PICT) rarely metastasize and usually originate in the brain, coverings (membranes) of the brain, or the pituitary gland. The incidence of primary intracranial tumors is 11.5 per 100,000, or approximately 35,000 persons per year.

Secondary intracranial tumors arise from outside the brain coverings (meninges). Quite commonly, secondary intracranial tumors are blood-borne metastatic disease from primary malignant cancer outside the brain (i.e., cancer from some other location that has spread to the brain). Approximately 250,000 persons per year are affected by secondary intracranial tumors. A tumor in the brain can present clinically with symptoms of increased intracranial pressure, or with symptoms associated with compression of the brain (a tumor grows and compresses part of the brain against the skull). One common cause of increased intracranial pressure is growth of a tumor that obstructs the duct system of cerebrospinal fluid (CSF), which bathes and nourishes the brain and spinal cord. Common symptoms can include nausea, vomiting, headache that is worse in the morning, and a reduced level of consciousness that causes drowsiness. Tumors causing focal compression on or irritation of the brain usually result in loss of neurologic function. This progressive loss of neurologic function can manifest as tinnitus (ringing in the ears) or aphasia (language problems).

Technical improvements and advancement have made surgical removal of brain tumors more effective and safer. Surgical management of intracranial tumors focuses on diagnosis and reduction of tumor mass. Depending on tumor location and patient health status, the neurosurgeon may perform a needle biopsy (called image-directed stereotactic needle biopsy) or a craniotomy to extract a piece of tumor for pathologic analysis. Generally, if the tumor is located in an area where surgery can be performed, the neurosurgeon will remove the mass if the patient can tolerate general anesthesia. Exceptions to a surgical option may be exercised to treat malignant tumors that are very sensitive to chemotherapy or radiation therapy (i.e., to manage lymphoma or germinoma). One of the most common types of tumors is the glioma, which accounts for 50% of all primary brain tumors.

Degenerative disorders of the spine

Degenerative disorders of the spine are a common problem. Between 50% and 90% of the population will experience back pain at some point in their lifetime. However, most of these back pain symptoms subside on their own within a few weeks; the cost, however, results in decreased productivity and lost wages—a public health problem. Lower back pain (in the lumbar spine) is most common reason adults seek medical attention. In a normal person, the lumbar spine comprises five lumbar vertebra. The lumbar spine supports the weight of the entire column and, therefore, withstands a great load. Lower back disorders are among the most frequent reasons for referral to a neurosurgeon. Lumbar discs are very prone to herniation and desiccation (drying out) as a result of the heavy load they bear and the motion to which they are subject. Nerves that run from the vertebrae extend out to distant structures. Degeneration of the discs may change bony structures in such a manner that can cause nerve compression. Typically, persons with degenerative disorders of the spine may have pain, numbness, paresthesia (tingling), and restriction of neck movement (if the affected vertebrae is in the cervical spine, which is located in the back of the neck).

Surgery for congenital abnormalities

Congenital abnormalities occur during embryonic development. During development of the human embryo, important changes in growth and chemistry occur during the second week of gestation; these changes contribute to the development of the nervous system. Several different types of cells proliferate as they move together or separate into other structures according to an orchestrated, natural time clock. Defects can occur at different stages of development. The defects with which infants can be born include myelomeningoceles, encephaloceles, hydrocephalus, and craniosynostosis.

Central nervous system infections

Solitary or multiple brain abscesses can occur as a result of infection in the brain. Patients present with clinical symptoms such as focal (a specific area is affected) neurologic signs, seizures, altered mental status, and increased intracranial pressure. CT scans and **magnetic resonance imaging** (MRI) are helpful for identification of brain abscesses. Surgery is usually indicated if the abscess fails to resolve or worsens following antibiotic treatment, or if there are signs of mass effect and brain herniation. Although rare, a spinal epidural abscess can occur. Typically, bacteria can spread in patients who have acute bacterial meningitis (infection of the subarachnoid spaces and meninges). The specific type of bacteria varies according to the patient's age.

Functional neurosurgery

Functional neurosurgery is a special type of surgical procedure used to manage movement disorder, epilepsy, and pain. Stereotactic neurosurgery makes use of a coordinate system that provides accurate navigation to a specific point or region in the brain. This is usually done by placing and fixing into position a frame on the scalp (using four threaded pins that penetrate the outer skull to stabilize the frame in position) under local anesthesia. A special box and sterotactic arc are placed to precisely determine X, Y, and Z coordinates of any point within the frame.

Epilepsy surgery

Approximately 70 per 100,000 population in the United States take antiepileptic medications for seizure disorders. The risk of developing epilepsy over a lifetime is 3%, and there are 100,000 new cases per year. The majority of cases (approximately 60,000) are temporal lobe (the brain lobes located on the sides of the head) epilepsy. Approximately 25% of persons prescribed antiepileptic drugs for temporal lobe seizures are not controlled or the side effects of the drug are far too great and outweigh the therapeutic benefits. Approximately 5,000 new cases per year require epilepsy surgery (partial anterior temporal lobectomy). The patient and neurosurgeon should consider surgery if continual seizures cause injuries due to repeated falls; driving restrictions; limitation of social interactions; prob-

KEY TERMS

Angiomatous malformations—Tumors in blood vessels.

Cerebral aneurysms—A sac in a blood vessel in the brain that can rupture and cause bleeding in the brain.

Craniosynostosis—Premature closure of the skull, which results in skull deformities.

Craniotomy—Procedure to remove a lesion in the brain through an opening in the skull.

Desiccation—Tissue death.

Encephaloceles—Protrusion of the brain through a defect in the skull.

Germinoma—A tumor of germ cells (ovum and sperm cells that participate in production of the developing embryo).

Hydrocephalus—A defect characterized by an increase in cerebrospinal fluid (CSF), which bathes and nourishes the brain and spinal cord.

Intraventricular hemorrhage—Hemorrhage in the ventricles of the brain.

Lymphoma—A tumor of lymph glands or lymph tissues.

Meninges—Membranes that cover the brain.

Myelomeningoceles (MMC)—A protrusion in the vertebral column containing spinal cord and meninges.

Subarachnoid space—A space between membranes that covers and protects the brain.

---

into nerve cells and to redirect protein synthesis—to work toward reversing the disease process, in general.

Resources

BOOKS

Miller. E. *Anesthesia,* 5th Ed. Philadelphia, PA. Churchill Livingstone, Inc., 2000.

Townsend, C. Sabiston. *Textbook of Surgery,* 16th Ed. Philadelphia, PA. W. B. Saunders Company, 2001.

PERIODICALS

Freese, A., Simeone, F. "Ocular Surgery for the New Millennium." and "Treatment of Neurosurgical Disease in the New Millennium." *Ophthalmology Clinics of North America* 12, no.4 (December 1999).

ORGANIZATIONS

The American Board of Neurological Surgery. 6550 Fannin Street, Suite 2139 Houston, TX 77030. (713) 441-6015. <http://www.abns.org>.

Laith Farid Gulli, M.D.,M.S.
Miguel A. Melgar, M.D.,Ph.D.
Nicole Mallory, M.S.,PA-C

Nissen fundoplication *see*
Gastroesophageal reflux surgery

Nitrite test *see* **Urinalysis**

NMR *see* **Magnetic resonance imaging**

Nonmelanoma skin cancer surgery *see*
Curettage and electrosurgery

---

lems related to education and learning; and employment limitations.

The future of neurosurgery

Neurosurgery as a field is faced with many new opportunities and challenges, based on advanced technological approaches and molecular approaches to neurosurgical problems. Advances in technology have allowed the neurosurgeon to precisely locate abnormal tissue in the brain and spinal cord, thereby preserving normal tissues from surgical trauma. In addition to cardiovascular neurosurgery, functional neurosurgery, neuro-oncologic neurosurgery (surgical removal of brain tumors), and spinal surgery, the future holds many new research innovations. In the new millennium, the field of molecular neurosurgery can make it possible to introduce genetic material

---

Nonsteroidal anti-inflammatory drugs

Definition

Nonsteroidal anti-inflammatory drugs (NSAIDs) are medications other than **corticosteroids** that relieve pain, swelling, stiffness, and inflammation.

Purpose

Nonsteroidal anti-inflammatory drugs are prescribed for a variety of painful conditions, including arthritis, bursitis, tendinitis, gout, menstrual cramps, sprains, strains, and other injuries. They may be used for treatment of **post-surgical pain** that either is too mild to require narcotic **analgesics** or follows a period of use of stronger analgesics. Ketorolac (Toradol) may be used in place of narcotics for treatment of acute pain in patients who should not receive narcotics.

Description

The nonsteroidal anti-inflammatory drugs are a group of agents that inhibit prostaglandin synthetase, thereby reducing the process of inflammation. As a group, they are all effective analgesics. Some, including the salicylates, ibuprofen, and naproxene, are also useful antipyretics (fever-reducers).

Although NSAIDs fall into discrete chemical classes, they are usually divided into the nonselective NSAIDs and the COX-2 specific agents. Among the nonspecific NSAIDs are diclofenac (Voltaren), etodolac (Lodine), flurbiprofen (Ansaid), ibuprofen (Motrin, Advil, Rufen), ketorolac (Toradol), nabumetone (Relafen), naproxen (Naprosyn), naproxen sodium (Aleve, Anaprox, Naprelan), and oxaprozin (Daypro). The COX-2 specific drugs are celecoxib (Celebrex) and rofecoxib (Vioxx).

Nonselective NSAIDS inhibit both cyclooxygenase 1 and cyclooxygenase 2 (COX-2). Cyclooxygenase 1 is important for homeostatic maintenance such as platelet aggregation, the regulation of blood flow in the kidney and stomach, and the regulation of gastric acid secretion. The inhibition of cyclooxygenase 1 is considered the primary cause of NSAID toxicity, including gastric ulceration and bleeding disorders. COX-2 is the primary cause of pain and inflammation. Both celecoxib and rofecoxib are relatively selective, and may cause the same adverse effects as the nonselective drugs, although with somewhat reduced frequency.

The analgesic activity of NSAIDs has not been fully explained. Antipyretic activity may be caused by the inhibition of prostaglandin E2 (PGE2) synthesis.

Although not all NSAIDs have approved indications for all uses, as a class, they are used for:

- ankylosing spondylitis
- bursitis
- fever
- gout
- headache
- juvenile arthritis
- mild to moderate pain
- osteoarthritis
- PMS
- primary dysmennorhea
- rheumatoid arthritis
- tendinitis

Recommended dosage

Recommended doses vary, depending on the patient, the type of nonsteroidal anti-inflammatory drug prescribed, the condition for which the drug is prescribed, and the form in which it is used. The patient is advised to consult specific sources for detailed information or ask a physician.

Precautions

The most common hazard associated with NSAID use is gastrointestinal intolerance and ulceration. This may occur without warning and is a greater risk among patients over the age of 65. The risk appears to rise with increasing length of treatment and increasing dose. Patients should be aware of the warning signs of gastrointestinal (GI) bleeding.

Allergic reactions are rare, but may be severe. Patients who have allergic reactions to **aspirin** should not be treated with NSAIDs.

Because NSAID metabolites are eliminated by the kidney, renal toxicity should be considered. Clinicians should monitor kidney function before and during NSAID use.

Among the NSAIDs that are classed as pregnancy category B are ketoprofen, naproxen, naproxen sodium, flurbiprofen, and diclofenac. Etodolac, ketorolac, mefenamic acid, meloxicam, nabumetone, oxaprozin, tolmetin, piroxicam, rofecoxib, and celecoxib are category C. Breastfeeding is not advised while taking NSAIDs.

Many other rare but potentially serious adverse effects have been reported with NSAIDs. The consumer should consult specific references.

Interactions

Many drug interactions have been reported with NSAID therapy. The most serious are those that may affect the bleeding hazards associated with NSAIDs. Consumers are advised to consult specific references for further information. A partial list of interacting drugs follows:

- blood thinning drugs, such as warfarin (Coumadin)
- other nonsteroidal anti-inflammatory drugs
- heparin
- tetracyclines
- cyclosprorine
- digitalis drugs
- lithium
- phenytoin (Dilantin)
- zidovudine (AZT, Retrovir)

KEY TERMS

Bursitis—Inflammation of the tissue around a joint.

Homeostatic—The balance of all the different functions of the body to maintain itself.

Inflammation—Pain, redness, swelling, and heat that usually develop in response to injury or illness.

Metabolites—The chemicals produced in the body after nutrients, drugs, enzymes or other materials have been changed (metabolized).

Salicylates—A group of drugs that includes aspirin and related compounds; used to relieve pain, reduce inflammation, and lower fever.

Tendinitis—Inflammation of a tendon—a tough band of tissue that connects muscle to bone.

Resources

BOOKS

AHFS: Drug Information. Washington, DC: Amer Soc Health-systems Pharm, 2002.

Brody, T., J. Larner, K. P. Minneman, and H. C. Neu. *Human Pharmacology Molecular to Clinical.* 2nd edition. St Louis: Mosby Year-Book,1995.

Karch, A. M. *Lippincott's Nursing Drug Guide.* Springhouse, PA: Lippincott Williams & Wilkins, 2003.

Reynolds, J. E. F., ed. *Martindale, The Extra Pharmacopoeia.* 31st Edition. London: The Pharmaceutical Press, 1996.

Samuel D. Uretsky, PharmD

Norepinephrine *see* **Adrenergic drugs**

Nose job *see* **Rhinoplasty**

Nosocomial infections *see* **Hospital-acquired infections**

NSAIDs *see* **Nonsteroidal anti-inflammatory drugs**

Nuclear magnetic resonance *see* **Magnetic resonance imaging**

Nursing homes

Definition

A nursing home is a long-term care facility licensed by the state that offers 24-hour room and board and health care services, including basic and skilled nursing care, rehabilitation, and a full range of other therapies, treatments, and programs. People who live in nursing homes are referred to as residents.

Description

Slightly over 5% of people 65 years and older occupy nursing homes, congregate care, assisted living, and board-and-care homes. At any given time, approximately 4% of the population are in nursing homes with the rate of nursing home use increasing with age from 1.4% of the young-old to 24.5% of the oldest-old. Nearly 50% of those 95 years old and older live in nursing homes. Nursing homes must meet the physical, emotional, and social needs of its residents.

Required care plans

There are federal laws regarding the care given in a nursing home, and it is essential that staff members become aware of these regulations. It is required that staff conduct a thorough assessment of each new resident during the first two weeks following admission. The assessment includes the resident's ability to move, his or her rehabilitation needs, the status of the skin, any medical conditions that are present, nutritional state, and abilities regarding activities of daily living.

In some cases, the nursing home residents are unable to communicate their needs to the staff. Therefore, it is particularly important for nurses and other professionals to look for problems during their assessments. Signs of malnutrition and dehydration are especially important when assessing nursing home residents.

It is not normal for an elderly person to lose weight. However, some people lose their ability to taste and smell as they age and may lose interest in food. This can result in malnutrition, which can lead to confusion and impaired ability to fight off disease.

Older people are also more susceptible to dehydration. Their medications may lead to dehydration as a side effect, or they may limit fluids because they are too afraid of uncontrolled urination. It is very dangerous to be without adequate fluid, so the nurse and other staff must be able to recognize early signs of dehydration.

When the assessment is complete, a care plan is developed. This plan is subject to change as changes in the resident's condition occur.

Nursing homes are often the only alternative for patients who require nursing care over an extended period of time. They are too ill to remain at home, with families, or in less structured long-term facilities. These individuals are unable to live independently and need assistance with activities of daily living (ADL). Some nursing homes offer specialized care for certain medical conditions such as Alzheimer's disease.

Commonly, nursing home residents are no longer able to participate in the activities they once enjoyed. However, it is required by law that these facilities help residents achieve their highest possible quality of life. It is important for residents to have as much control as possible over their everyday lives. Laws and regulations exist to raise nursing home quality of life and care standards.

By law, nursing homes cannot use chemical or physical restraints unless they are essential for treating a medical problem. There are many dangers associated with the use of restraints, including the chance of a fall if a resident tries to walk while restrained. The devices may also lead to depression and decreased self-esteem. A doctor's order is necessary before restraints can be used in a nursing home.

Licensing

The Joint Commission on the Accreditation of Health Care Organizations (JCAHO) offers accreditation to nursing homes through the Long Term Care Accreditation Program established in 1966. This group helps nursing homes improve their quality of care. The JCAHO periodically surveys nursing homes to check on quality issues.

A nursing home may be certified by **Medicare** or **Medicaid** if it meets the criteria of these organizations. Families should be informed of the certifications a nursing home holds. Medicare and Medicaid are the main sources of financial income for nursing homes in the United States.

The state where a nursing home is located conducts inspections every nine to 15 months. Fines and other penalties may be enforced if the inspection reveals areas where the nursing home does not meet requirements set by that state and the federal government. Problem areas are noted in terms of scope and severity. The scope of a problem is how widespread it is, and the severity is the seriousness of its impact on the residents. When a nursing home receives an inspection report, it must post it in a place where it can be easily seen by residents and their guests.

Contract

When a resident checks into a nursing home, a contract is drawn up between the patient and the facility. This document includes information regarding the rights of the residents. It also provides details regarding services provided and discharge policies.

Resident decision-making

Decisions are made by each nursing home resident unless he or she has signed an advanced directive giving this authority to someone else. In order for health care decisions to be made by another person, the resident must have signed a document called a durable **power of attorney** for health care.

Costs

Nursing home care is costly. The rate normally includes room and board, housekeeping, bedding, nursing care, activities, and some personal items. Additional fees may be charged for haircuts, telephones, and other personal items.

Medicare covers the cost of some nursing home services, such as skilled nursing or rehabilitative care. This payment may be activated when the nursing home care is provided after a Medicare qualifying stay in the hospital for at least three days. It is common for nursing homes to have only a few beds available for Medicare or Medicaid residents. Residents relying solely on these types of coverage must wait for a Medicare or Medicaid bed to become available.

Medicare supplemental insurance, such as Medigap, assists with the payment of nursing home expenses that are not covered by Medicare.

Medicaid qualifications vary in each state. Families of potential residents should check with their state government to determine coverage options. According to a federal law, a nursing home that drops out of the Medicaid program cannot evict current residents whose care is supported by Medicaid.

Private insurance, such as long-term insurance, may cover costs associated with a nursing home. People may enroll in these plans through their employers or other group insurance policies.

In many cases, nursing homes are paid for by the residents' personal funds. When these funds are exhausted, the residents sometimes become eligible for Medicaid assistance.

Patients' rights

It is important for the professionals working in nursing homes to be aware of the residents' rights. Residents are informed of their rights when they are admitted. Residents have the right to:

• manage their finances

• privacy (for themselves and their belongings)

• make decisions (unless advanced directives or durable power of attorney exist)

- see visitors in private
- receive information regarding their medical care and treatments
- have social services
- leave the nursing home after giving the required amount of notice (A stay in a nursing home is normally considered voluntary; however, the facility will consider a variety of factors before discharging a resident. These factors include the resident's health, safety and potential danger to self or others, as well as the resident's payment for services. The contract will state how much notice is required before a resident may transfer to another facility, return home, or move in with a family member.)

Family involvement

In some cases, a nursing home is chosen after the family has only a short time to prepare for the change. For example, when a patient is unable to care for himself or herself due to a sudden illness or injury, the family must turn to nursing home care without having the luxury of researching this option over time. The nursing home's costs must be explained to the resident or family prior to admission. It is important for the nursing home staff to be willing to answer the family's questions and reassure them about the care their loved one will receive.

Nursing home professionals have an opportunity to continue to work closely with the resident's family and loved ones over the course of a resident's stay. In these facilities, concerned family members and friends of the resident are involved in his or her care, and may have guardianship or other decision-making responsibility. These individuals may voice their concerns through meetings between staff and family members. Those with legal guardianship are entitled to see a resident's medical records, care plans, and other related material.

Communication

As in other health care settings, communication among nursing home staff is very important. In nursing homes, the care is based on a team approach. Physicians, nurses, and allied health professionals work together to make sure the resident is able to experience the highest quality of life possible.

In many cases, physicians who have had a long-term relationship with a patient continue treatment after the patient has been admitted to a nursing home. It is important for the nursing home staff to leave blocks of time open in the schedule for physician visits. It is also the staff's duty to keep the personal physicians apprised of a resident's medical condition.

WHO PERFORMS THE PROCEDURE AND WHERE IS IT PERFORMED?

The nursing home staff may include an administrator, medical director, director of nursing, and directors for other allied health services. It is important for nursing home staff to understand the policies regarding care in these types of facilities.

The following professionals may provide care and treatments in nursing homes:

- physicians
- nurses
- nursing assistants
- dietitians
- physical, occupational, and speech therapists
- pharmacists
- social activities staff
- dentists
- social workers or psychological counselors
- other staff, such as custodians and office personnel

The resident, physician, and resident's legal guardian and family must be told immediately if any of the following situations arise: an accident involving the resident, the need for a major treatment change, and a decision regarding discharge or transfer. Unless an emergency arises, the nursing home must give 30 days written notice of discharge or transfer. The family may appeal the decision.

Results

The quality of care in nursing homes is an important issue. Quality issues include:

- Ratios of staff to patients. Advocacy groups are pushing for increased staff-to-patient ratios in nursing homes. The National Citizens' Coalition for Nursing Home Reform recommends one direct care staff (R.N., L.V.N., or C.N.A.) per five residents during the day shift, 10 residents during the evening shift, and 15 residents during the night shift.

- Elder abuse. It is important for nursing home personnel to look for signs of abuse or neglect when a resident checks in and during a resident's stay. Signs of abuse include bodily injuries that appear suspicious, visible harm to the wrist or ankles that may indicate the use of restraints, skin ulcers that seem neglected, poor hygiene, inadequate nutrition, unexplained dehydration, untreated medical problems, or personality disorders such as excessive nervousness or withdrawal. The nurse or allied health professional is to report any signs of abuse to the supervisor or physician.

• Reimbursement. Nursing home administrators report that reimbursements do not cover the expenses, while nursing home advocates would like a higher portion of revenues to be allocated for direct patient care.

Resources

BOOKS

Birkett, D. Peter, M.D., ed. *Psychiatry in the Nursing Home.* 2nd Edition. Binghamton, NY: Haworth Press Inc, 2001.

Hosley, Julie B. and Elizabeth A. Molle-Matthews (Editor). *Lippincott's Textbook of Clinical Medical Assisting* Philadelphia, PA: Lippincott, Williams & Wilkins, 1999.

Rhoades, Jeffrey A. *The Nursing Home Market: Supply and Demand for the Elderly (Garland Studies on the Elderly in America).* New York, NY: Garland Publishers, 1998.

ORGANIZATIONS

American Nurses Association. 600 Maryland Ave. SW, Ste. 100 West, Washington, DC 20024. (800) 274-4ANA. <http://www.nursingworld.org>.

Centers for Medicare & Medicaid Services. 7500 Security Boulevard, Baltimore, MD 21244-1850. (410) 786-3000. (877) 267-2323. <http://www.medicare.gov>.

e-Healthcare Solutions, Inc., 953 Route 202 North, Branchburg, N.J. 08876. (908) 203-1350. Fax: (908) 203-1307. info@e-healthcaresolutions.com. <http://www.digital healthcare.com/>.

Joint Commission on Accreditation of Health Care Organizations, One Renaissance Blvd., Oakbrook Terrace, IL 60181. (630) 792-5000. <http://www.jcaho.org>.

The U.S. Department of Health and Human Services, 200 Independence Avenue, SW, Washington, D.C. 20201. (202) 619-0257. (877)-696-6775. <http://www.hcfa.gov>.

OTHER

Coates, Karen J. *Senior Class.* May 2002 [cited March 1, 2003]. <http://www.nurseweek.com/news/features/02-05/senior.asp>.

Domrose, Cathryn. *Seasons of Change* May 2002 [cited March 1, 2003]. <http://www.nurseweek.com/news/features/02-05/longterm.asp>.

Rhonda Cloos, R.N.
Crystal H. Kaczkowski, M.Sc.

O

Obstetric and gynecologic surgery

Definition

Obstetric and gynecologic surgery refers to procedures that are performed to treat a variety of conditions affecting the female reproductive organs. The main structures of the reproductive system are the vagina, the uterus, the ovaries, and the fallopian tubes.

Description

Obstetrics is the branch of medicine that focuses on women during pregnancy, childbirth, and the postpartum period. Gynecology is a broader field, focusing on the general health care of women and treating conditions that affect the female reproductive organs. Medical doctors who choose to specialize in obstetrics and gynecology must undergo at least four years of post-medical school training (called a residency) in the areas of women's general health, pregnancy, labor and delivery, preconceptional and postpartum care, prenatal testing, and genetics. Obstetrician-gynecologists (also called OB-GYNs) may also subspecialize in the areas of gynecologic oncology (the treatment of cancers that affect the reproductive system), maternal-fetal medicine (the care of high-risk pregnancies), reproductive endocrinology and infertility (the study and treatment of the reproductive glands and hormones and the causes of infertility), and urogynecology (treatment of urinary tract and pelvic disorders).

Surgical procedures

There are a wide range of surgical procedures that have been developed to treat the various conditions that affect the female reproductive organs.

THE VAGINA. The vagina is the muscular canal that extends from the opening of the vulva (the external female genitals) to the cervix, the lower part of the uterus.

The vagina is the outlet for menstrual blood and is also where the penis is inserted during sexual intercourse.

Some common surgical procedures that are performed on the vagina include:

- Episiotomy. A surgical incision made in the perineum (the area between the vagina and anus) to expand the opening of the vagina to prevent tearing during delivery.

- Colporrhaphy. Surgical repair of the vagina may be necessary after childbirth, sexual assault, or other injuries.

- Colpotomy. This incision into the wall of the vagina may be used to excise ovarian cysts, perform **tubal ligation**, or remove uterine fibroids.

- Colposcopy. A colposcope is a specialized instrument used to visualize the vagina and cervix, to diagnose abnormalities, or to test for the presence of precancerous or cancerous cells.

THE UTERUS. The uterus is the hollow, muscular organ at the top of the vagina. The cervix is the neck-shaped opening at the lower part of the uterus, while the fundus is the rounded upper portion. The endometrium is the inner lining of the uterus; it is where a fertilized egg will implant during the early days of pregnancy. The endometrium normally sheds during each menstrual cycle if the egg released during ovulation has not been fertilized. The myometrium is the middle muscular layer of the uterus; it is the myometrium that rhythmically contracts during labor contractions.

Some common surgical procedures that are performed on the uterus include:

- Myomectomy. A procedure in which myomas (uterine fibroids) are surgically removed from the uterus.

- **Cesarean section**. A surgical procedure in which incisions are made through the woman's abdomen and uterus to deliver her baby.

- **Cervical cerclage**. The cervix is stitched closed to prevent a miscarriage or premature birth.

- Cervical cryosurgery. Cryosurgery freezes and destroys an area of the cervix in which precancerous cells have been found.

- Induced abortion. The intentional termination of a pregnancy before the fetus can live independently.

- Hysterectomy. The removal of part or all of the uterus may be done to treat uterine cancer, fibroid tumors, endometriosis, uterine prolapse, or other conditions of the uterus.

- Hysterotomy. This incision into the uterus is done during a cesarean section, open **fetal surgery**, and some second-trimester abortions.

- Dilatation and curettage. D&C is a gynecological procedure in which the cervix is dilated (expanded) and the lining of the uterus (endometrium) is scraped away.

THE OVARIES. The ovaries are egg-shaped structures located to each side of the uterus. It is within the ovaries that the female egg develops. A mature egg is released from one of the ovaries approximately every 28 days during a process called ovulation.

The surgical procedures that are performed on the ovaries include:

- Oophorectomy. One or both ovaries may be removed during this procedure to prevent or treat ovarian or other cancers, to remove large ovarian cysts, or to treat endometriosis.

- **Cystectomy**. An ovarian cystectomy may be used to remove part of an ovary to treat ovarian tumors or cysts.

THE FALLOPIAN TUBES. The fallopian tubes are the structures that carry a mature egg from the ovaries to the uterus. These tubes, which are about 4 in (10 cm) long and 0.2 in (0.5 cm) in diameter, are found on the upper outer sides of the uterus, and open into the uterus through small channels. It is within a fallopian tube that fertilization, the joining of the egg and the sperm, takes place.

Some common surgical procedures that are performed on the fallopian tubes include:

- Salpingostomy. An incision is made in the fallopian tube, often to excise an ectopic pregnancy.

- Salpingectomy. One or both fallopian tubes are removed in this procedure. It may be used to treat ruptured or bleeding fallopian tubes (as a result of ectopic pregnancy), infection, or cancer.

- Tubal ligation. A permanent form of birth control in which a woman's fallopian tubes are surgically cut or blocked off to prevent pregnancy.

THE VULVA. The external female genital organs (or vulva) include the labia majora, two lips or folds that enclose the labia minora. The labia minora, in turn, are two lips or folds that enclose the clitoris, a small sensitive organ with a high number of nerve endings.

Some examples of surgeries that affect the vulva are:

- Vulvectomy. The vulva may be partially or completely removed, as in the case of vulvar cancer.

- Laceration or hematoma repair. Vulvar hematoma (a localized collection of blood) or laceration may result from a "straddle" injury, sexual assault, or childbirth. Severe hematomas may need surgical drainage.

Obstetric and gynecologic anesthesia

There are a number of options available to women for pain relief during obstetric or gynecologic surgery. Pain medications given intravenously (into a vein) or intramuscularly (into a muscle) help to decrease the amount of pain during childbirth or certain procedures, although they will generally not completely eliminate pain.

Regional anesthesia, either a spinal or an epidural, is the preferred method of pain relief during childbirth and certain surgical procedures such as cesarean section, tubal ligation, cervical cerclage, and others that do not require the patient to be unconscious. The benefits of regional anesthesia include allowing the patient to be awake during the surgery, avoiding the risks of general anesthesia, and allowing early contact between mother and child in the case of a cesarean section. Spinal anesthesia involves inserting a needle into a region between the vertebrae of the lower back and injecting numbing medications. An epidural is similar to a spinal except that a catheter is inserted so that numbing medications may be administered as needed. Some women experience a drop in blood pressure when a regional anesthetic is administered; this can be countered with fluids and/or medications.

In some instances, use of general anesthesia may be indicated. General anesthesia can be more rapidly administered in the case of an emergency (e.g. severe fetal distress). If the mother has a coagulation disorder that would be complicated by a drop in blood pressure (a risk with regional anesthesia), general anesthesia is an alternative. General anesthesia is also used for some of the more complicated and prolonged obstetric and gynecologic surgeries.

Resources

BOOKS

Hammond, Charles B. "Gynecology: The Female Reproductive Organs." In *Sabiston Textbook of Surgery*. Philadelphia: W. B. Saunders Company, 2001.

KEY TERMS

Ectopic pregnancy—A pregnancy that occurs outside of the uterus, most often in the fallopian tubes.

Endometriosis—A condition in which the endometrium (lining of the uterus) grows outside of the uterus.

Ovarian cysts—Fluid-filled cavities on the surface of the ovary that may cause pain and bleeding if they become too large.

Uterine fibroids—Also called leiomyomas; benign growths in the smooth muscle of the uterus.

Uterine prolapse—A condition which the uterus descends into or beyond the vagina.

Hawkins, Joy L., David H. Chestnut, and Charles P. Gibbs. "Obstetric Anesthesia." In *Obstetrics: Normal & Problem Pregnancies.* Philadelphia: Churchill Livingstone, 2002.

ORGANIZATIONS

American Board of Obstetrics and Gynecology. 2915 Vine Street, Dallas, TX 75204. (214) 871-1619. <http://www.abog.org>.

American College of Obstetricians and Gynecologists. 409 12th St., SW, PO Box 96920, Washington, DC 20090-6920. <http://www.acog.org>.

Gynecologic Surgery Society. 2440 M Street, NW, Suite 801, Washington, DC 20037. (202) 293-2046. <http://www.gynecologicsurgerysociety.org>.

OTHER

"Atlas of the Body: Female Reproductive Organs." American Medical Association. January 28, 2002 [cited March 1, 2003]. <http://www.ama-assn.org/ama/pub/category/7163.html>.

Camaan, William, and Bhavani Shankar Kodali. "Pain Relief During Childbirth (Obstetrical Anesthesia)." Brigham & Women's Hospital Health and Information Services, November 22, 2002 [cited March 1, 2003]. <http://www.brighamandwomens.org/painfreebirthing>.

"Health Conditions and Medical Procedures." OBGYN.net [cited March 1, 2003]. <http://www.obgyn.net/women/conditions/conditions.asp>.

Magowan, Brian. "Diagnosis and Treatment, Obstetrics and Gynaecology." *Churchill's Pocketbook of Obstetrics and Gynaecology (2nd Edition),* 2000 [cited March 1, 2003]. <http://www.orgyn.com>.

Stephanie Dionne Sherk

Obstetric sonogram *see* **Pelvic ultrasound**

Omphalocele repair

Definition

An omphalocele is a congenital defect in which internal organs such as the liver, stomach, and intestines, are on the outside of the abdomen, at the umbilical cord, instead of being located inside the body. These abdominal cavity contents are enclosed in a thin, transparent, membranous sac that is actually formed inside the umbilical cord tissue. An omphalocele repair is a surgical procedure in which the organs are returned to the inside of the body, and the opening in the abdominal wall is closed. Whenever possible, a normal-looking belly button is created.

Purpose

The internal organs need to be enclosed inside the abdomen for protection against injury, and to ensure that the tissue remains properly hydrated. The omphalocele repair is necessary to return the tissue to the inside of the body.

Demographics

Omphaloceles usually occur in full-term infants, more frequently in boys than in girls. A recent study found that the ratio is two girls to three boys.

The presence of an omphalocele often occurs with other birth defects, including:

• heart defects, such as the tetralogy of Fallot

• imperforate anus, a malformation of the anorectal area of the gastrointestinal system

• urinary problems

• genetic disorders

• Beckwith-Wiedemann syndrome, with enlarged tongue, gigantism, and enlarged internal organs

• pentalogy of Cantrell, with malformations in the chest and abdominal area, including heart defects, and high mortality rate

To check for other congenital defects, x rays are usually taken of the heart, lungs, and diaphragm once the infant's condition has been stablized after birth.

Description

An omphalocele is a defect that can be viewed on sonogram during an ultrasound performed while the mother is pregnant. At about six to eight weeks of fetal development, the abdominal contents come out of the fetus's abdomen at the base of the umbilical cord. They return to the inside as development continues. If this process is interrupted in some way during the seventh to tenth week of fetal development, the contents remain on the outside, and an omphalocele develops. Because the abdominal contents are now on the outside of the body, the inside cavity may not develop properly. For this reason, a large omphalocele cannot simply be placed back inside because the cavity may be too small. The internal organs will need to be protected and kept hydrated while the inside is gradually stretched. Small amounts of the omphalocele are returned at any one time to allow the cavity to gradually stretch to accommodate them. If the sac surrounding the tissue has ruptured, or broken, there is a greater risk of infection, tissue damage, loss of body temperature, and dehydration.

The repair may be performed in stages. If the omphalocele is very small, it may be possible to return all of the contents to the inside, and surgically close the opening. If the omphalocele is too large to do this all at once, some contents will remain on the outside while a sterile pouch is created to protect the tissue that remains on the outside. To be sure that the tissue does not dry out, it will be covered with warm and moist sterile dressings. The infant can lose considerable body heat through the large amount of exposed surface area, so keeping him or her warm, and closely monitoring body temperature is a high priority. An antibacterial solution may be used to decrease the risk of infection. The infant will have a tube that goes in through the nose or mouth and down into the stomach, called a nasogastric tube. Suction is used to keep the stomach empty, avoiding the chance of vomiting, or of the fluid moving from the stomach up into the lungs. The contents of the sac will be carefully examined to make sure that none of the tissue is damaged or dead, and to check for signs of intestinal birth defects before being inserted into the body.

The omphalocele repair is a surgical procedure performed under general anesthesia. The infant will receive medication to relax his or her muscles, and to help the surgery move forward without causing any pain. A large omphalocele repair may be done in stages over several weeks. The contents of the sac are often swollen, which makes it impossible to return them into the small cavity all at once. The return of the sac contents into the abdominal cavity creates intra-abdominal pressure, which may cause the infant to have difficulty breathing. To help the infant breathe, a special breathing tube may be inserted. The tube is attached to a machine that regulates the length and frequency of the breaths. When the necessary surgeries have been completed, the suturing will be done in such a way as to leave, if possible, a somewhat normal-looking belly button. A large omphalocele repair can leave a large, unsightly scar. For cosmetic purposes, the scar may be operated on at a later date to make it less noticeable. Gastroesophageal reflux, which may require additional surgery, is common in patients with a repaired omphalocele.

Diagnosis/Preparation

The diagnosis of an omphalocele may take place during an ultrasound while the mother is still pregnant. A recent study found that 75% of omphaloceles were diagnosed by ultrasound, most commonly around week 18 of pregnancy. To avoid any injury to the omphalocele sac, a cesarean birth may be performed so that the infant does not travel through the birth canal. If the omphalocele has not been detected prior to birth, it is immediately noticeable upon birth.

Aftercare

The infant will need to spend some time after the surgery in the **intensive care unit**. Because infants are unable to properly regulate their temperature, they are placed in special beds that are kept warm. They will usually need oxygen and a breathing tube to help them breathe for a while. The breathing machine is referred to as **mechanical ventilation**, or a ventilator. This machine helps the baby breathe at the right depth and frequency for his or her age, allowing the infant to conserve energy for other functions. An infant that is struggling for air spends much energy on breathing, which slows the healing process.

Once the bowels are moving normally, feedings will be slowly started. Feedings are usually first done through a nasogastric tube so the infant does not need to use energy for sucking and swallowing. Sucking on a pacifier is avoided because this could cause the bowel to expand with air and slow down the healing process. Until the nasogastric tube is used, the infant will be fed intravenously. The intravenous line provides the infant with needed **antibiotics**, pain medication, and fluids.

Infants with an omphalocele may spend quite some time, perhaps several months, in the hospital before being discharged home. It may take them some time to learn to feed through normal infant sucking and swallowing. Their development may be delayed, and they may require help for months as they catch up to the physical and mental development that is normal for their age. If the parents do not live near the hospital, they should be encouraged to spend as much time with their infant as possible to ensure infant-parent bonding. When the repair is done in stages, it can be difficult for the parents to remain patient. The birth of a child with a birth defect can be quite emotionally difficult for the parents. Individuals trained to assist parents through this time should meet with them to provide information and support.

Risks

All surgery has risks, from the procedure itself as well as the anesthesia. Infection and bleeding are the two primary risks of surgery. Breathing problems and reactions to the anesthesics are the main risks from anesthesia. In addition to these standard surgical risks, an omphalocele repair has the associated risks of damage to the organs on the outside of the body, additional breathing problems from the added pressure inside the abdominal cavity when the contents are returned, infection of the abdominal cavity (peritonitis), and a slowing or paralysis of the bowels (paralytic ileus).

Normal results

The expected results depend on many factors, including:

- size of the omphalocele

- degree of development of the abdominal cavity

- presence and extent of other congenital defects

- damage to or loss of intestinal tissue

- whether the infant was full-term or premature at birth

Many omphaloceles can be completely corrected with excellent results.

Morbidity and mortality rates

An omphalocele occurs in about one in 5,000 live births. Other congenital defects are common. In one recent study, 50% of infants with omphalocele had other birth defects, primarily heart-related. On average, the infants spent three days on a ventilator, with about 45 total days spent in the hospital. The mortality rate was 8%, mostly due to heart problems.

Alternatives

There are no non-surgical alternatives to omphalocele repair. The abdominal contents need to be returned to the abdominal cavity, and the opening closed. While awaiting surgical repair, a sterile elastic bandage may be placed on the omphalocele to decrease edema (fluid accumulation).

Resources

BOOKS

Ashcraft, Keith W. *Pediatric surgery.* W. B. Saunders Company, 2000.

Pillitteri, Adele. *Maternal & Child Nursing: Care of the childbearing & childrearing family.* 3rd edition. Lippincott, 1999.

PERIODICALS

Barisic, I. et al. "Evaluation of Prenatal Ultrasound Diagnosis of Fetal Abdominal Wall Defects by 19 European Registries." *Ultrasound Obstet Gynecol* 18 (October 2001): 309–16.

Saxena, A. and G.H. Willital. "Omphalocele: Clinical Review and Surgical Experience Using Dura Patch Grafts." *Hernia* 6 (July 2002): 73–8

ORGANIZATIONS

National Library of Medicine: Medline Plus Health Information [cited July 7, 2003]. <http://www.nlm.nih.gov>

Esther Csapo Rastegari, R.N., B.S.N., Ed.M.

Onocology surgery *see* **Surgical oncology**

Oophorectomy

Definition

Unilateral oophorectomy (also called an ovariectomy) is the surgical removal of an ovary. If one ovary is removed, a woman may continue to menstruate and have children. If both ovaries are removed, a procedure called a bilateral oophorectomy, menstruation stops and a woman loses the ability to have children.

Purpose

Oophorectomy is performed to:

• remove cancerous ovaries

• remove the source of estrogen that stimulates some cancers

• remove a large ovarian cyst

• excise an abscess

• treat endometriosis

In an oophorectomy, one or a portion of one ovary may be removed or both ovaries may be removed. When an oophorectomy is done to treat ovarian cancer or other spreading cancers, both ovaries are removed (called a bilateral oophorectomy). Removal of the ovaries and fal-

---

lopian tubes is performed in about one-third of hysterectomies (surgical removal of the uterus), often to reduce the risk of ovarian cancer.

Oophorectomies are sometimes performed on premenopausal women who have estrogen-sensitive breast cancer in an effort to remove the main source of estrogen from their bodies. This procedure has become less common than it was in the 1990s. Today, chemotherapy drugs are available that alter the production of estrogen and tamoxifen blocks any of the effects any remaining estrogen may have on cancer cells.

Until the 1980s, women over age 40 having hysterectomies routinely had healthy ovaries and fallopian tubes removed at the same time. This operation is called a bilateral **salpingo-oophorectomy**. Many physicians reasoned that a woman over 40 was approaching menopause and soon her ovaries would stop secreting estrogen and releasing eggs. Removing the ovaries would eliminate the risk of ovarian cancer and only accelerate menopause by a few years.

In the 1990s, the thinking about routine oophorectomy began to change. The risk of ovarian cancer in women who have no family history of the disease is less than 1%. Meanwhile, removing the ovaries increases the risk of cardiovascular disease and accelerates osteoporosis unless a woman takes prescribed hormone replacements.

Under certain circumstances, oophorectomy may still be the treatment of choice to prevent breast and ovarian cancer in certain high-risk women. A study done at the University of Pennsylvania and released in 2000 showed that healthy women who carried the BRCA1 or BRCA2 genetic mutations that pre-disposed them to breast cancer had their risk of breast cancer drop from 80% to 19% when their ovaries were removed before age 40. Women between the ages of 40 and 50 showed less risk reduction, and there was no significant reduction of breast cancer risk in women over age 50. A 2002 study showed that five years after being identified as carrying

BRCA1 or BRCA2 genetic mutations, 94% of women who had received a bilateral salpingo-oophorectomy were cancer-free, compared to 79% of women who had not received surgery.

The value of ovary removal in preventing both breast and ovarian cancer has been documented. However, there are disagreements within the medical community about when and at what age this treatment should be offered. Preventative oophorectomy, also called prophylactic oophorectomy, is not always covered by insurance. One study conducted in 2000 at the University of California at San Francisco found that only 20% of insurers paid for preventive bilateral oophorectomy (PBO). Another 25% had a policy against paying for the operation, and the remaining 55% said that they would decide about payment on an individual basis.

Demographics

Overall, ovarian cancer accounts for only 4% of all cancers in women. But the lifetime risk for developing ovarian cancer in women who have mutations in BRCA1 is significantly increased over the general population and may cause an ovarian cancer risk of 30% by age 60. For women at increased risk, oophorectomy may be considered after the age of 35 if childbearing is complete.

Other factors that increase a woman's risk of developing ovarian cancer include age (most ovarian cancers occur after menopause), the number of menstrual periods a woman has had (affected by age of onset, pregnancy, breastfeeding, and oral contraceptive use), history of breast cancer, diet, and family history. The incidence of ovarian cancer is highest among Native American (17.5 cases per 100,000 population), white (15.8 per 100,000), Vietnamese (13.8 per 100,000), white Hispanic (12.1 per 100,000), and Hawaiian (11.8 per 100,000) women; it is lowest among Korean (7.0 per 100,000) and Chinese (9.3 per 100,000) women. African American women have an ovarian cancer incidence of 10.2 per 100,000 population.

Description

Oophorectomy is done under general or regional anesthesia. It is often performed through the same type of incision, either vertical or horizontal, as an abdominal **hysterectomy**. Horizontal incisions leave a less noticeable scar, but vertical incisions give the surgeon a better view of the abdominal cavity. After the incision is made, the abdominal muscles are stretched apart, not cut, so that the surgeon can see the ovaries. Then the ovaries, and often the fallopian tubes, are removed.

Oophorectomy can sometimes be done with a laparoscopic procedure. With this surgery, a tube containing a

QUESTIONS TO ASK THE DOCTOR

- Why is a oophorectomy being recommended?
- How will the procedure be performed?
- Will I have a remaining ovary (or portion of ovary)?
- What alternatives to oophorectomy are available to me?

tiny lens and light source is inserted through a small incision in the navel. A camera can be attached that allows the surgeon to see the abdominal cavity on a video monitor. When the ovaries are detached, they are removed though a small incision at the top of the vagina. The ovaries can also be cut into smaller sections and removed.

The advantages of abdominal incision are that the ovaries can be removed even if a woman has many adhesions from previous surgery. The surgeon gets a good view of the abdominal cavity and can check the surrounding tissue for disease. A vertical abdominal incision is mandatory if cancer is suspected. The disadvantages are that bleeding is more likely to be a complication of this type of operation. The operation is more painful than a laparoscopic operation and the recovery period is longer. A woman can expect to be in the hospital two to five days and will need three to six weeks to return to normal activities.

Diagnosis/Preparation

Before surgery, the doctor will order blood and urine tests, and any additional tests such as ultrasound or x rays to help the surgeon visualize the woman's condition. The woman may also meet with the anesthesiologist to evaluate any special conditions that might affect the administration of anesthesia. A colon preparation may be done, if extensive surgery is anticipated.

On the evening before the operation, the woman should eat a light dinner, then take nothing by mouth, including water or other liquids, after midnight.

Aftercare

After surgery a woman will feel discomfort. The degree of discomfort varies and is generally greatest with abdominal incisions, because the abdominal muscles must be stretched out of the way so that the surgeon can reach the ovaries. In order to minimize the risk of postoperative infection, **antibiotics** will be given.

When both ovaries are removed, women who do not have cancer are started on hormone replacement therapy to ease the symptoms of menopause that occur because estrogen produced by the ovaries is no longer present. If even part of one ovary remains, it will produce enough estrogen that a woman will continue to menstruate, unless her uterus was removed in a hysterectomy. To help offset the higher risks of heart and bone disease after loss of the ovaries, women should get plenty of **exercise**, maintain a low-fat diet, and ensure intake of calcium is adequate.

Return to normal activities takes anywhere from two to six weeks, depending on the type of surgery. When women have cancer, chemotherapy or radiation are often given in addition to surgery. Some women have emotional trauma following an oophorectomy, and can benefit from counseling and support groups.

Risks

Oophorectomy is a relatively safe operation, although, like all major surgery, it does carry some risks. These include unanticipated reaction to anesthesia, internal bleeding, blood clots, accidental damage to other organs, and post-surgery infection.

Complications after an oophorectomy include changes in sex drive, hot flashes, and other symptoms of menopause if both ovaries are removed. Women who have both ovaries removed and who do not take estrogen replacement therapy run an increased risk for cardiovascular disease and osteoporosis. Women with a history of psychological and emotional problems before an oophorectomy are more likely to experience psychological difficulties after the operation.

Complications may arise if the surgeon finds that cancer has spread to other places in the abdomen. If the cancer cannot be removed by surgery, it must be treated with chemotherapy and radiation.

Normal results

If the surgery is successful, the ovaries will be removed without complication, and the underlying problem resolved. In the case of cancer, all the cancer will be removed. A woman will become infertile following a bilateral oophorectomy.

Morbidity and mortality rates

Studies have shown that the complication rate following oophorectomy is essentially the same as that following hysterectomy. The rate of complications associated with hysterectomy differs by the procedure performed. Abdominal hysterectomy is associated with a

KEY TERMS

Cyst—An abnormal sac containing fluid or semi-solid material.

Endometriosis—A benign condition that occurs when cells from the lining of the uterus begin growing outside the uterus.

Fallopian tubes—Slender tubes that carry ova from the ovaries to the uterus.

Hysterectomy—Surgical removal of the uterus.

Osteoporosis—The excessive loss of calcium from the bones, causing the bones to become fragile and break easily.

higher rate of complications (9.3%), while the overall complication rate for vaginal hysterectomy is 5.3%, and 3.6% for laparoscopic vaginal hysterectomy. The risk of death is about one in every 1,000 women having a hysterectomy. The rates of some of the more commonly reported complications are:

- excessive bleeding (hemorrhaging): 1.8–3.4%
- fever or infection: 0.8–4.0%
- accidental injury to another organ or structure: 1.5–1.8%

Because of the cessation of hormone production that occurs with a bilateral oophorectomy, women who lose both ovaries also prematurely lose the protection these hormones provide against heart disease and osteoporosis. Women who have undergone bilateral oophorectomy are seven times more likely to develop coronary heart disease and much more likely to develop bone problems at an early age than are premenopausal women whose ovaries are intact.

Alternatives

Depending on the specific condition that warrants an oophorectomy, it may be possible to modify the surgery so at least a portion of one ovary remains, allowing the woman to avoid early menopause. In the case of prophylactic oophorectomy, drugs such as tamoxifen may be administered to block the effects that estrogen may have on cancer cells.

Resources

PERIODICALS

Kauff, N. D., J. M. Satagopan, M. E. Robson, et al. "Risk-Reducing Salpingo-oophorectomy in Women With a BRC1 or BRC2 Mutation." *New England Journal of Medicine* 346 (May 23, 2002): 1609–15.

ORGANIZATIONS

American Cancer Society. 1599 Clifton Road NE, Atlanta, GA 30329. (800) ACS-2345. <http://www.cancer.org>.

American College of Obstetricians and Gynecologists. 409 12th St., SW, PO Box 96920, Washington, DC 20090-6920. <http://www.acog.org>.

Cancer Information Service, National Cancer Institute. Building 31, Room 10A19, 9000 Rockville Pike, Bethesda, MD 20892. (800) 4-CANCER. <http://www.nci.nih.gov/cancerinfo/index.html>.

OTHER

"Ovarian Cancer: Detailed Guide." *American Cancer Society.* October 20, 2000 [cited March 14, 2003]. <http://www.cancer.org/downloads/CRI/CRC_-_OVARIAN_CANCER.pdf>.

"Prophylactic Oophorectomy." *American College of Obstetricians and Gynecologists.* September 7, 1999 [cited March 14, 2003]. <http://www.medem.com/MedLB/article_detaillb.cfm?article_ID=ZZZONIHKUJC&sub_cat=9>.

"Removing Ovaries Lowers Risk for Women at High Risk of Breast, Ovarian Cancer." *ACS News Today* November 8, 2000. [cited May 13, 2003]. <http://www.cancer.org>.

Surveillance, Epidemiology, and End Results. "Racial/Ethnic Patterns of Cancer in the United States: Ovary." *National Cancer Institute.* 1996 [cited March 14, 2003]. <http://seer.cancer.gov/publications/ethnicity/ovary.pdf>.

Tish Davidson, A.M.
Stephanie Dionne Sherk

Open decompression *see* **Laminectomy**

Open fracture reduction *see* **Fracture repair**

Open prostatectomy

Definition

Open prostatectomy is a procedure for removal of an enlarged prostate gland.

Purpose

The primary indication for open prostatectomy is benign prostatic hyperplasia (BPH), a condition whereby benign or noncancerous nodules grow in the prostate gland. The prostate gland is composed of smooth muscle cells, glandular cells, and cells that give the gland structure (stromal cells). A dense fibrous capsule surrounds the prostate gland. The glandular cells produce a milky fluid that mixes with seminal fluid and sperm to make semen. The prostate gland also produces a hormone (di-

hydrotestosterone) that has a major impact on the gland's development.

Description

The prostate gland undergoes several changes as a man ages. The pea size gland at birth grows only slightly during puberty, and reaches its normal adult shape and size (similar to a walnut) when a male is in his early twenties. The prostate gland remains stable until the mid-forties. At that time—in most men—the number of cells begins to multiply (cell multiplication), and the gland starts to enlarge. The enlargement—called hyperplasia—is due to an increase in the number of cells. Cell proliferation in the prostates of older men can cause symptoms (referred to as lower urinary tract symptoms, LUTS), which often include:

• straining when urinating

• hesitation before urine flow starts

• dribbling at the end of urination or leakage afterward

• weak or intermittent urinary strain

• painful urination

Other symptoms (called storage symptoms) sometime appear, and may include:

• urgent need to urinate

• bladder pain when urinating

• increased frequency of urination, especially at night

• bladder irritation during urination

The cause of BPH is not fully understood. Currently, it is thought to be caused by a hormone that the prostate gland synthesizes, called dihydrotestosterone (DHT). This hormone is synthesized from testosterone by a prostatic enzyme called 5-alpha reductase.

Surgery is generally indicated for persons with moderate to severe symptoms, particularly if urinary retention is intractable or if the enlarged prostate (BPH) is related to recurrent urinary tract infections, blood in the urine, bladder stones, or kidney problems.

Open prostatectomy is the treatment of choice for approximately 2–3% of BPH patients who have a very large prostate, a damaged bladder, or another serious related problem. Open prostatectomy is used when the prostate is so large (2.8–3.5 oz [80–100 g]) that **transurethral resection of the prostate** (TURP, a less strenuous surgical procedure to remove a smaller prostate) cannot be performed. Additionally, open prostatectomy is indicated for males with:

- recurrent or persistent urinary tract infections
- acute urinary distention
- bladder outlet obstructions
- recurrent gross hematuria (blood in urine) of prostate origin
- pathological changes in the bladder, ureters, or kidneys due to prostate obstruction

Contraindications to open prostatectomy include previous prostatectomy, prostate cancer, a small fibrous prostate gland, and previous pelvic surgery that may obstruct access to the prostate gland.

Demographics

The cause of BPH is not entirely known; however, the incidence increases with advancing age. Before 40 years of age, approximately 10% of males have BPH. A small amount of hyperplasia is present in 80% of males over 40 years old. Approximately 8–31% of males experience moderate to severe lower urinary tract symptoms (LUTS) in their fifties. By age 80, about 80% of men have LUTS. A risk factor is the presence of normally functioning testicles; research indicates that castration can minimize prostatic enlargement. It appears that the glandular tissues that multiply abnormally use male hormones produced in the testicles differently than the normal tissues do.

Approximately 5.5 million American males have BPH. It is more prevalent in the United States and Europe, and less common among Asians. BPH is more common in men who are married rather than single, and there is a strong genetic correlation. A man's chance for developing BPH is greater if three of more family members have the condition.

Description

Open prostatectomy can be performed by either the retropubic or suprapubic approach. The preferred anesthesia for open prostatectomy is a spinal or epidural nerve block. Regional anesthesia can help reduce blood loss during surgery, and lowers the risk of complications such as pulmonary embolus and postoperative deep vein thrombosis. General anesthesia may be used if the patient has an anatomic or medical contraindication for regional anesthesia.

Retropubic prostatectomy

The retropubic prostatectomy is accomplished through a direct incision of the anterior (front) prostatic capsule. The overgrowth of glandular cells (hyperplastic prostatic adenoma) is removed. These are the cells forming a mass in the prostate because of their abnormal multiplication.

A **cystoscopy** is performed prior to the open prostatectomy. The patient lies on his back on the operating table, and is prepared and draped for this procedure. Following the cystoscopy, the patient is changed to a Trendelenberg (feet higher than head) position. The surgical area is shaved, draped, and prepared. A catheter is placed in the urethra to drain urine. An incision is made from the umbilicus to the pubic area. The abdominal muscle (rectus abdominis) is separated, and a retractor is placed at the incision site to widen the surgical field. Further maneuvering is essential to clearly locate the veins (dorsal vein complex) and the bladder neck. Visualization of the bladder neck exposes the patient's main arterial blood supply to the prostate gland. Once the structures have been identified and the blood supply controlled, an incision is made deep into the level of the tumor. Scissors are used to dissect the prostatic tissue (prostatic capsule) from the underlying tissue of the prostatic tumor. The wound is closed after complete removal of the prostate tumor and hemostasis (stoppage of bleeding) occurs.

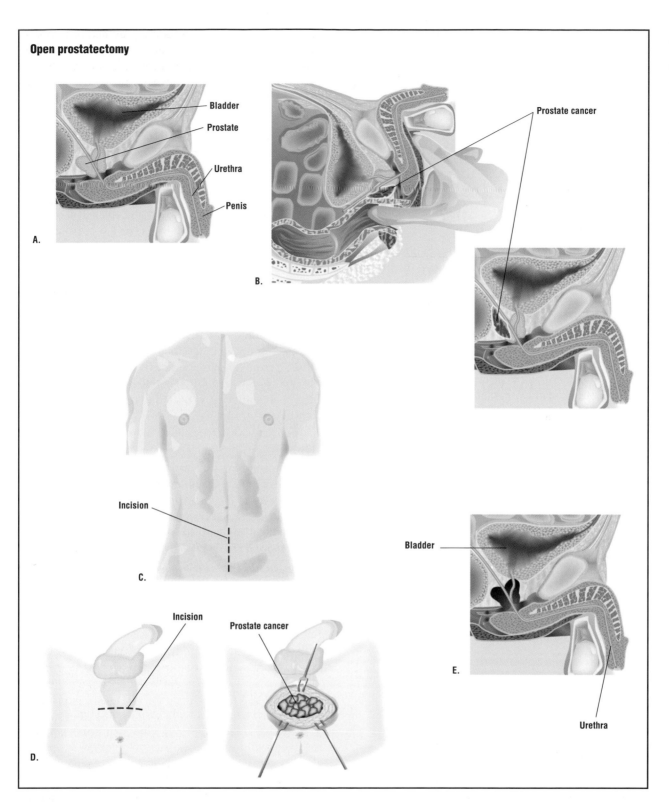

Open prostatectomy

During a digital rectal exam (B), the doctor may feel an enlargement of the prostate that can be benign or cancerous. If an open prostatectomy is needed, an incision may made the lower abdomen (C) or the perineal area (D). In either case, the prostate and any cancer is removed (E). *(Illustration by GGS Inc.)*

The advantages of the retropubic prostatectomy include:

• Direct visualization of the prostatic tumor.

• Accurate incisions in the urethra, which will minimize the complication of urinary continence.

• Excellent anatomic exposure and visualization of the prostate.

• Clear visualization to control bleeding after tumor removal.

• Little or no surgical trauma to the urinary bladder.

Suprapubic prostatectomy

Suprapubic prostatectomy (also called transvesical prostatectomy) is a procedure to remove the prostatic overgrowth via a different surgical route. The suprapubic approach utilizes an incision of the lower anterior (front) bladder wall. The primary advantage over the retropubic approach is that the suprapubic route allows for direct visualization of the bladder neck and bladder mucosa. Because of this, the procedure is ideally suited for persons who have bladder complications, as well as obese men. The major disadvantage is that visualization of the top part of the tumor is reduced. Additionally, with the suprapubic approach, hemostasis (stoppage of bleeding during surgery) may be more difficult due to poor visualization after removal of the tumor.

Using a scalpel, a lower midline incision is made from the umbilicus to the pubic area. A cystotomy (incision into the bladder) is made, and the bladder inspected. Using electrocautery (a special tool that produces heat at the tip, useful for hemostasis or tissue excision) and scissors, dissection proceeds until the prostatic tumor is identified and removed. After maintaining hemostasis and arterial blood supply to the prostate, the incisions to the bladder and abdominal wall are closed.

Diagnosis/Preparation

The presence of symptoms is indicative of the disease. Age also has an associated risk for an enlarged prostate, and can help establish diagnostic criteria.

Men must have a special blood test called the prostate specific antigen (PSA) and routine digital rectal examination (DRE) before surgery. If the PSA levels and DRE are suspiciously indicative of prostate cancer, a transrectal ultrasound guided needle biopsy of the prostate must be performed before open prostatectomy, to detect the presence of prostate cancer (carcinoma).

Additionally, preoperative patients should have lower urinary tract studies, including urinary flow rate and post void residual urine in the bladder. Because most patients are age 60 or older, preoperative evaluation should also include a detailed history and **physical examination**; standard blood tests; chest x ray; and electrocardiogram (EKG) to detect any possible preexisting conditions.

Aftercare

Open prostatectomy is a major surgical operation requiring an inpatient hospital stay of four to seven days. Blood transfusions are generally not required due to improvements in surgical technique. Immediately after the operation, the surgeon must closely monitor urinary output and fluid status. On the first day after surgery, most patients are given a clear liquid diet and asked to sit up four times. Morphine sulfate, given via a patient controlled analgesic pump (IV), is used to control pain.

On the second postoperative day, the urethral catheter is removed if the urine does not contain blood. Oral pain medications are begun if the patient can tolerate a regular diet.

On the third postoperative day, the pelvic drain is removed if drainage is less than 75ml/24 hr. The patient should gradually increase activity. Follow-up with the surgeon is necessary following **discharge from the hospital**. Full activity is expected to resume within four to six weeks after surgery.

Risks

Improvements in surgical technique have lowered blood loss to a minimal level. For several weeks after open prostatectomy, patients may have urgency and urge incontinence. The severity of bladder problems depends on the patient's preoperative bladder status. Erectile dysfunction occurs in 3–5% of patients undergoing this procedure. Retrograde (backward flow) ejaculation occurs in approximately 50–80% of patients after open prostatectomy. The most common non-urologic risks include pulmonary embolism, myocardial infarction (heart attack), deep vein thrombosis, and cerebrovascular accident (stroke). The incidence of any one of these potentially adverse effects is less than 1%.

Normal results

Normally, patients will not have the adverse effects of bleeding. Hematuria (blood in the urine) is typically resolved within two days after surgery. The patient should begin a regular diet and moderate increases in activity soon after surgery. His pre-surgical activity level should be restored within four to six weeks after surgery.

Morbidity and mortality rates

The overall rate of morbidity and mortality is extremely low. The overall mortality (death) rate for open prostatectomy is approximately zero.

KEY TERMS

Bladder mucosa—Mucous coat of the bladder.

Cerebrovascular accident—Brain hemorrhage, also known as a stroke.

Cystoscopy—Examination of the bladder using a special instrument to visualize the organ.

Cystotomy—An incision in the bladder.

Pulmonary embolus—A thrombi that typically detaches from a deep vein of a lower extremity.

Trendelenburg—Position in which the head is low and the body and legs are on an inclined plane.

Alternatives

For smaller prostates, treatment using medication may help to control abnormal prostatic growth. When the prostate gland is large (75 grams and bigger), surgery is indicated.

Resources

BOOKS

Walsh, P. *Campbell's Urology.* 8th Ed. St. Louis: Elsevier Science, 2002.

PERIODICALS

Dull, P., R. Reagan, R. Bahnson, "Practical Therapeutics: Managing Benign Prostatic Hyperplasia." *American Family Physician* 66 (July 1, 2002).

Miles, B., et al."Open Prostatectomy." eMedicine.com [cited July 7, 2003]. <http://www.emedicine.com/med/topic3041. htm>.

Laith Farid Gulli, M.D., M.S.
Alfredo Mori, M.B.B.S.
Abraham F. Ettaher, M.D.
Bilal Nasser, M.D.,M.S.

Operating room

Definition

An operating room (OR), also called surgery center, is the unit of a hospital where surgical procedures are performed.

Purpose

An operating room may be designed and equipped to provide care to patients with a range of conditions, or it may be designed and equipped to provide specialized care to patients with specific conditions.

Description

OR environment

Operating rooms are sterile environments; all personnel wear protective clothing called scrubs. They also wear shoe covers, masks, caps, eye shields, and other coverings to prevent the spread of germs. The operating room is brightly lit and the temperature is very cool; operating rooms are air-conditioned to help prevent infection.

The patient is brought to the operating room on a wheelchair or bed with wheels (called a gurney). The patient is transferred from the gurney to the operating table, which is narrow and has safety straps to keep him or her positioned correctly.

The monitoring equipment and anesthesia used during surgery are usually kept at the head of the bed. The anesthesiologist sits here to monitor the patient's condition during surgery.

Depending on the nature of the surgery, various forms of anesthesia or sedation are administered. The surgical site is cleansed and surrounded by a sterile drape.

The instruments used during a surgical procedure are different for external and internal treatment; the same tools are not used on the outside and inside of the body. Once internal surgery is started, the surgeon uses smaller, more delicate devices.

Operating room equipment

An operating room has special equipment such as respiratory and cardiac support, emergency resuscitative devices, patient monitors, and diagnostic tools.

Life support and emergency resuscitative equipment

Equipment for life support and emergency resuscitation includes the following:

- Heart-lung bypass machine, also called a cardiopulmonary bypass pump—takes over for the heart and lungs during some surgeries, especially heart or lung procedures. The heart-lung machine removes carbon dioxide from the blood and replaces it with oxygen. A tube is inserted into the aorta to carry the oxygenated blood from the bypass machine to the aorta for circulation to the body. The heart-lung machine allows the heart's beating to be stopped during surgery.

- Ventilator (also called a respirator)—assists with or controls pulmonary ventilation. Ventilators consist of a flexible breathing circuit, gas supply, heating/humidification mechanism, monitors, and alarms. They are microprocessor-controlled and programmable, and regulate the volume, pressure, and flow of respiration.

- Infusion pump—device that delivers fluids intravenously or epidurally through a catheter. Infusion pumps employ automatic, programmable pumping mechanisms to deliver continuous anesthesia, drugs, and blood infusions to the patient. The pump hangs from an intravenous pole that is located next to the patient's bed.

- Crash cart—also called resuscitation cart or code cart. A crash cart is a portable cart containing emergency resuscitation equipment for patients who are "coding" (i.e., **vital signs** are in a dangerous range). The emergency equipment includes a defibrillator, airway intubation devices, resuscitation bag/mask, and medication box. Crash carts are strategically located in the operating room for immediate accessibility if a patient experiences cardiorespiratory failure.

- Intra-aortic balloon pump—a device that helps reduce the heart's workload and helps blood flow to the coronary arteries for patients with unstable angina, myocardial infarction, or those awaiting organ transplants. Intra-aortic balloon pumps use a balloon placed in the patient's aorta. The balloon is on the end of a catheter that is connected to the pump's console, which displays heart rate, pressure, and electrocardiogram (ECG) readings. The patient's ECG is used to time the inflation and deflation of the balloon.

Patient monitoring equipment

Patient monitoring equipment includes the following:

- Acute care physiologic monitoring system—comprehensive patient monitoring systems that can be configured to continuously measure and display various parameters via electrodes and sensors connected to the patient. Parameters monitored may include the electrical activity of the heart via an ECG, respiratory (breathing) rate, blood pressure (noninvasive and invasive), body temperature, cardiac output, arterial hemoglobin oxygen saturation (blood oxygen level), mixed venous oxygenation, and end-tidal carbon dioxide.

- Pulse oximeter—monitors the arterial hemoglobin oxygen saturation (oxygen level) of the patient's blood with a sensor clipped over the finger or toe.

- Intracranial pressure monitor—measures the pressure of fluid in the brain in patients with head trauma or other conditions affecting the brain (such as tumors, edema, or hemorrhage). Intracranial pressure monitors are connected to sensors inserted into the brain through a cannula or bur hole. These devices signal elevated pressure and record or display pressure trends. Intracranial pressure monitoring may be a capability included in a physiologic monitor.

Diagnostic equipment

The use of diagnostic equipment may be required in the operating room. Mobile x ray units are used for bedside radiography, particularly of the chest. These portable units use a battery-operated generator that powers an x ray tube. Handheld portable clinical laboratory devices, called point-of-care analyzers, are used for blood analysis at the bedside. A small amount of whole blood is required, and blood chemistry parameters can be provided much faster than if samples were sent to the central laboratory.

Other operating room equipment

Disposable OR equipment includes urinary (Foley) catheters to drain urine during surgery, catheters used for arterial and central venous lines to monitor blood pressure during surgery or withdraw blood samples), Swan-Ganz catheters to measure the amount of fluid in the heart and to determine how well the heart is functioning, chest and endotracheal tubes, and monitoring electrodes.

New surgical techniques

Minimally invasive surgery, also called laparoscopic surgery, is an operative technique performed through a few small incisions, rather than one large incision. Through these small incisions, surgeons insert a laparoscope (viewing instrument that displays the surgery on a computer screen for easier viewing) and endoscopic instruments to perform the surgery.

Robot-assisted surgery allows surgeons to perform certain procedures through small incisions. In robotic surgery, a surgeon sits at a console several feet from the operating table and uses a joystick, similar to that used for video games, to guide the movement of robotic arms that hold endoscopic instruments and an endoscope (small camera). The robotic arms allow the surgeon to perform precise, fine hand movements, and provides access to parts of the body that are difficult to reach manually. In addition, robotic surgery provides a three-dimensional image, and the surgical field can be magnified to a greater extent than traditional or minimally invasive surgery. The goal of robotic surgery is to decrease incision size and length of hospital stay, while improving patient comfort and lessening recovery time.

Lasers are "scalpels of light" that may offer a new alternative for some surgical procedures. Lasers can be used to cut, burn, or destroy abnormal or diseased tissue; shrink or destroy lesions or tumors; sculpt tissue; and seal blood vessels. Lasers may help surgeons perform some procedures more effectively than other traditional methods. Because lasers cause minimal bleeding, the operative area may be more clearly viewed by

KEY TERMS

Advance directives—Legal documents that increase a patient's control over medical decisions. A patient may select medical treatment in advance, in the event that he or she becomes physically or mentally unable to communicate his or her wishes. Advance directives either state what kind of treatment the patient wants to receive (living will), or authorize another person to make medical decisions for the patient when he or she is unable to do so (durable power of attorney).

Anesthesiologist—A specially trained physician who administers anesthesia.

Arterial line—A catheter inserted into an artery and connected to a physiologic monitoring system to allow direct measurement of oxygen, carbon dioxide, and invasive blood pressure.

Catheter—A small, flexible tube used to deliver fluids or medications. A catheter may also be used to drain fluid or urine from the body.

Central venous line—A catheter inserted into a vein and connected to a physiologic monitoring system to directly measure venous blood pressure.

Chest tube—A tube inserted into the chest to drain fluid and air from around the lungs.

Critical care—The multidisciplinary healthcare specialty that provides care to patients with acute, life-threatening illness or injury.

Edema—An abnormal accumulation of fluids in intercellular spaces in the body; causes swelling.

Endotracheal tube—A tube inserted through the patient's nose or mouth that functions as an airway and is connected to a ventilator.

Foley catheter—A tube inserted into the bladder to drain urine into an external bag.

Gastrointestinal tube—A tube surgically inserted into the stomach for feeding a patient who is unable to eat by mouth.

Infectious disease team—A team of physicians and hospital staff who help control the hospital environment to protect patients against harmful sources of infection.

Inpatient surgery—Surgery that requires an overnight stay of one or more days in the hospital. The number of days spent in the hospital after surgery depends on the type of procedure performed.

Life support—Methods of replacing or supporting a failing bodily function, such as using mechanical ventilation to support breathing. In treatable or curable conditions, life support is used temporarily to aid healing until the body can resume normal functioning.

Nasogastric tube—A tube inserted through the nose and throat and into the stomach for directly feeding the patient.

NPO—Nothing by mouth. NPO refers to the time after which the patient is not allowed to eat or drink prior to a procedure or treatment.

Outpatient surgery—Also called same-day or ambulatory surgery. The patient arrives for surgery and returns home on the same day. Outpatient surgery can take place in a hospital, surgical center, or outpatient clinic.

Swan-Ganz catheter—Also called a pulmonary artery catheter. This is a type of tubing inserted into a large vessel in the neck or chest. It is used to measure the amount of fluid in the heart, and to determine how well the heart is functioning.

the surgeon. Lasers may also provide access to parts of the body that may not have been as easily reached manually.

Surgery centers

Freestanding surgery centers are available in many communities, primarily for the purpose of providing outpatient surgical procedures. The patient should make sure that the surgery center has been accredited by the Joint Commission on Accreditation of Healthcare Organizations (JCAHO), a professionally sponsored program that stimulates a high quality of patient care in health care facilities. There is also an accreditation option that is available for **ambulatory surgery centers**.

Choosing a surgery center with experienced staff is important. Here are some questions to consider when choosing a surgery center:

• How many surgeries are performed annually and what are the outcomes and survival rates for those procedures?

• How does the surgery center's outcomes compare with the national average?

- Does the surgery center offer procedures to treat a particular disease?

- Does the surgery center have experience treating patients in certain age groups?

- How much does surgery cost at this facility?

- Is financial assistance available?

- If the surgery center is far from the patient's home, will accommodations be provided for caregivers?

Resources

BOOKS

Deardoff, Ph.D., William and John Reeves, Ph.D. *Preparing for Surgery: A Mind-Body Approach to Enhance Healing and Recovery.* New Harbinger Publications, Oakland, CA: June 1997. (800) 748-6273. <http://www.newharbinger.com/>.

Furlong, Monica Winefryck. *Going Under: Preparing Yourself for Anesthesia: Your Guide to Pain Control and Healing Techniques Before, During and After Surgery.* Autonomy Publishing Company, November 1993.

Goldman, Maxine A. *Pocket Guide to the Operating Room* 2nd Edition. F.A. Davis Col, January 1996.

PERIODICALS

"Recommended practices for managing the patient receiving anesthesia." *AORN Journal* 75, no.4 (April 2002): 849.

ORGANIZATIONS

American Board of Surgery. 1617 John F. Kennedy Boulevard, Suite 860, Philadelphia, PA 19103. (215) 568-4000. <http://www.absurgery.org/>.

American College of Surgeons. 633 N. Saint Clair Street, Chicago, IL 60611-3211. (312) 202-5000. <http://www.facs.org/>.

American Society of Anesthesiologists. 520 N. Northwest Highway, Park Ridge, IL 60068-2573. (847) 825-5586. E-mail: mail@asahq.org. <http://www.asahq.org/>.

Association of Perioperative Registered Nurses (AORN, Inc.). 2170 South Parker Road. Suite 300, Denver, CO 80231. (800) 755-2676 or (303) 755-6304. <http://www.aorn.org/>.

National Heart, Lung and Blood Institute. Information Center. P.O. Box 30105, Bethesda, MD 20824-0105. (301) 251-2222. <http://www.nhlbi.nih.gov >.

National Institutes of Health. U.S. Department of Health and Human Services, 9000 Rockville Pike, Bethesda, MD 20892. (301) 496-4000. <http://www.nih.gov>.

OTHER

preSurgery.com. <http://www.presurgery.com>.

Reports of the Surgeon General. National Library of Medicine. <http://sgreports.nlm.nih.gov/NN/>.

SurgeryLinx. (surgery medical news and newsletters from top medical journals). MDLinx, Inc. 1025 Vermont Avenue, NW, Suite 810, Washington, DC 20005. (202) 543-6544. <http://sgreports.nlm.nih.gov/NN/>.

Surgical Procedures, Operative. (collection of links). <http://www.mic.ki.se/Diseases/e4.html>.

Angela M. Costello

Ophthalmologic surgery

Definition

Ophthalmologic surgery is a surgical procedure performed on the eye or any part of the eye.

Purpose

Surgery on the eye is routinely performed to repair retinal defects, remove cataracts or cancer, or to repair eye muscles. The most common purpose of ophthalmologic surgery is to restore or improve vision.

Demographics

Patients from the very young to very old have ocular conditions that warrant eye surgery. Two of the most common procedures are **phacoemulsification for cataracts** and elective refractive surgeries.

Cataract surgery is the most common ophthalmic procedure. More than 1.5 million cataract surgeries are performed in the United States each year. The National Eye Institute (NEI) recently reported that more than half of all United States residents age 65 and older have a cataract.

Elective refractive surgeries, especially **laser in-situ keratomileusis (LASIK)**, attract younger patients in their thirties and forties. Recently, the American Academy of Ophthalmology (AAO) estimated that 95% of the 1.8 million refractive surgery procedures performed in a year were LASIK.

Description

The surgeon, **operating room** nurses, and an anesthesiologist are present for ophthalmologic surgery. For many eye surgeries, only a local anesthetic is used, and the patient is awake but relaxed. The patient's eye area is scrubbed prior to surgery, and sterile drapes are placed over the shoulders and head. Heart rate and blood pressure are monitored throughout the procedure. The patient is required to lie still and for some surgery, especially refractive surgery, he or she is asked to focus on the light of the operating microscope. A speculum is placed in the eye to hold it open throughout surgery.

Common ophthalmologic surgery tools include scalpels, blades, forceps, speculums, and scissors. Many ophthalmologic surgeries now use lasers, which decrease the operating time as well as recovery time.

Surgeries requiring suturing can take as long as two to three hours. These intricate surgeries sometimes require the skill of a corneal or vitreo-retinal specialist, and require the patient to be put under general anesthesia.

Refractive surgeries

Refractive surgeries use an excimer laser to reshape the cornea. The surgeon creates a flap of tissue across the cornea with an instrument called a microkeratome, ablates the cornea for about 30 seconds, and then replaces the flap. The laser allows this surgery to take only minutes, without the use of stitches.

Trabeculectomy

Trabeculectomy surgery uses a laser to open the drainage canals or make an opening in the iris to increase outflow of aqueous humor. The purpose is to lower intraocular pressure in the treatment of glaucoma.

Laser photocoagulation

Laser photocoagulation is used to treat some forms of wet age-related macular degeneration. The procedure stops leakage of abnormal blood vessels by burning them to slow the progress of the disease.

Diagnosis/Preparation

Patients complaining of any ocular problem that requires surgery will receive a similar initial examination. A complete patient history is taken, including the chief complaint. The patient needs to disclose any allergies, medication usage, family eye and medical histories, and vocational and recreational vision requirements.

The diagnostic exam should include measurement of visual acuity under both low and high illumination, biomicroscopy with pupillary dilation, stereoscopic fundus examination with pupillary dilation, assessment of ocular motility and binocularity, visual fields, evaluation of pupillary responses to rule out afferent pupillary defects, refraction, and measurement of intraocular pressure (IOP).

Other examination procedures include corneal mapping, a keratometer reading to determine the curvature of the central part of the cornea, and a slit lamp exam to determine any damage to the cornea and evidence of glaucoma and cataracts. A fundus exam also will be performed to check for retinal holes, and macular degeneration and disease.

The patient's overall health must also be considered. Poor general health will affect the ophthalmologic surgery outcome. Surgeons may request a complete **physical examination**, in addition to the eye examination, prior to surgery.

Pre-surgery preparation

Patients having ophthalmologic surgery usually must stop taking **aspirin**, or aspirin-like products, 10 days before surgery unless directed otherwise by the surgeon. Patients taking blood thinners also must check with their physician to find out when they should stop taking the medication before surgery. A number of pain relievers may affect outcomes, making it important for patients to disclose all medication. The patient might have to ask about alternative medications if the surgeon requires that he or she stops taking the usual regime before the procedure. Some prescription medicines have been known to cause postsurgical scarring or flecks under the corneal flap after LASIK.

To reduce the chance of infection, the surgeon may request that the patient begin using antibiotic drops before surgery. Depending on the procedure, the patient may also be advised to discontinue contact lens wear and stop using creams, lotions, make-up, or perfume. Patients may also be asked to scrub their eyelashes for a period of time to remove any debris.

Patients are advised not to drink alcoholic beverages at least 24 hours before and after the ophthalmic procedure.

Patients must usually avoid eating or drinking anything after midnight on the day before the surgery; however, some patients may be allowed to have clear liquids in the morning. It is important for patients to ask their physician for a list of foods and medications permitted on the morning of surgery. Some patients may take morning medications (with physician approval) with the exclusion of **diuretics**, insulin, or diabetes pills. Patients are advised to dress comfortably for the surgery, and wear button-down shirts that will not have to pass over the head.

Presurgical tests sometimes are administered when the patient arrives for surgery. For refractive surgeries, this ensures the laser is set for the correct refractive error. Before cataract surgery, measurements help determine the refractive power of the intraocular lens (IOL). Other tests such as a chest x ray, blood work, or **urinalysis** may also be requested depending on the patient's overall health.

Most ophthalmic surgeries are done on an outpatient basis, and patients must arrange for someone to take them home after the procedure.

Before surgery, doctors will review the presurgical tests and instill any dilating eye drops, antibiotic drops, and a corticosteriod or nonsteroidal anti-inflammatory drops as needed. Anesthetic eye drops also will be administered. Many ophthalmologic surgeries are performed under a local anesthetic, and patients remain awake but in a relaxed state.

Aftercare

After surgery, the patient is monitored in a recovery area. For most outpatient procedures, the patient is advised to rest for at least 24 hours until he or she returns to the surgeon's office for follow-up care. Over-the-counter medications are usually advised for pain relief, but patients should check with their doctor to see what is recommended. Some pain relievers interfere with surgical outcomes. Patients may also use ice packs to help ease pain.

Some patients may experience slight drooping or bruising of the eye. This condition improves as the eye heals. Severe pain, nausea, or vomiting should be reported to the surgeon immediately.

After surgery, patients may be advised not to stoop, lift heavy objects, **exercise** vigorously, or swim. Patients may also be required to wear an eye shield while sleeping, and sunglasses or some type of protective lens during the day to avoid injury. Wearing make-up may be prohibited for weeks after surgery. The patient may be restricted from driving and air travel.

Patients usually have their first postoperative visit the day after the eye surgery. Subsequent exams are commonly scheduled at one, three, and six to eight weeks following surgery. This schedule depends on the patient's healing, and any complications he or she might experience.

Some patients will be required to instill eye drops for a number of weeks after surgery to prevent infection, pain, and to lessen inflammation. Eye drops also are used to lower intraocular pressure. In some cases, correct eye drop usage is critical to a successful surgery outcome.

Risks

Complications may occur during any surgery. Ophthalmologic surgery, however, is usually very safe.

Some risks include:

- Undercorrection or overcorrection in refractive surgery. Undercorrected refractive surgery patients usually can be treated with an enhancement, but overcorrected patients will need to use eyeglasses or contact lenses.

- Debilitating symptoms. These include glare, halos, double vision, and poor nighttime vision. Some patients may also lose contrast sensitivity. These symptoms may be temporary or permanent.

- Dry eye. Some patients are treated with artificial tears or punctal plugs.

- Retinal detachment. The retina can become detached by the surgery if this part of the eye has any weakness when the procedure is performed. This may not occur for weeks or months.

- Endophthalmitis. An infection in the eyeball is a complication that is less common today because of newer surgery techniques and **antibiotics**.

Other serious complications that may occur are blindness, glaucoma, or hemorrhage.

Normal results

Normal results include restored or improved vision, and a much improved quality of life. Specific improvements depend on the type of ophthalmologic surgery performed, and the type of ocular ailment being treated.

Morbidity and mortality rates

Death from ophthalmologic surgery is rare. However, complications can still arise from the use of general anesthesia. With most ophthalmic surgeries requiring only local anesthetic, that risk has been widely eliminated.

Blindness, which was sometimes caused by serious infection, has also been reduced because of more effective antibiotics.

Alternatives

Some medications can be used to treat certain ophthalmic conditions. For example, surgery for glaucoma is performed only in patients who do not respond to medication. Patients with myopia (nearsightedness), hyperopia (farsightedness), or presbyopia, can wear contact lenses or eyeglasses instead of having refractive surgery to improve their refractive errors.

Resources

BOOKS

Berkow, Robert, ed. *The Merck Manual of Medical Information.* Whitehorse Station, NJ: 1997.

Columbia University College of Physicians & Surgeons Complete Home Medical Guide 3rd Edition. New York, NY: Crown Publishers, 1995.

Daly, Stephen, ed. *Everything You Need to Know About Medical Treatments.* Springhouse, PA: Springhouse Corp., 1996.

ORGANIZATIONS

American Academy of Ophthalmology. PO Box 7424, San Francisco, CA 94120-7424. (415) 561-8500. <www.aao. org>.

American Optometric Association. 243 North Lindbergh Blvd., St. Louis, MO 63141. (314) 991-4100. <www.aoanet.org>.

American Society of Cataract and Refractive Surgery. 4000 Legato Road, Suite 850, Fairfax, VA 22033-4055. (703) 591-2220. E-mail: ascrs@ascrs.org; <www.ascrs.org>.

KEY TERMS

Ablation—During LASIK, the vaporization of eye tissue.

Cornea—The clear, curved tissue layer in front of the eye. It lies in front of the colored part of the eye (iris) and the black hole in the center of the iris (pupil).

Glaucoma—Disease of the eye characterized by increased pressure of the fluid inside the eye. Untreated, glaucoma can lead to blindness.

Macular degeneration—A condition usually associated with age in which the area of the retina called the macula is impaired due to hardening of the arteries (arteriosclerosis). This condition interferes with vision.

Retina—The inner, light-sensitive layer of the eye containing rods and cones; transforms the images it receives into electrical messages sent to the brain via the optic nerve.

National Eye Institute. 2020 Vision Place Bethesda, MD 20892-3655. (301) 496-5248. <www.nei.nih.gov>.

University of Michigan Kellogg Eye Center Department of Ophthalmology and Visual Sciences. 1000 Wall Street, Ann Arbor, MI 48105. (734) 763-1415. <www.kellogg. umich.edu>.

OTHER

"Conditions." *Vision Channel.* [cited April 12, 2003] <www.visionchannel.net>

"Surgical Procedures for Glaucoma." *Your Medical Source.* [cited April 12, 2003] <www.yourmedicalsource.com/library/glaucoma/GLC_surgery.html>

Mary Bekker

Opioid analgesics *see* **Analgesics, opioid**

Optional surgery *see* **Elective surgery**

Orchiectomy

Definition

Orchiectomy is the surgical removal of one or both testicles, or testes, in the human male. It is also called an orchidectomy, particularly in British publications. The

---

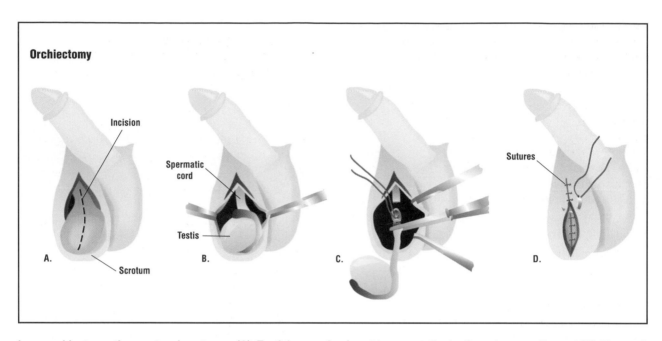

Orchiectomy

In an orchiectomy, the scrotum is cut open (A). Testicle covering is cut to expose the testis and spermatic cord (B). The cord is tied and cut, removing the testis (C), and the wound is repaired (D). *(Illustration by GGS Inc.)*

removal of both testicles is known as a bilateral orchiectomy, or castration, because the person is no longer able to reproduce. Emasculation is another word that is sometimes used for castration of a male. Castration in women is the surgical removal of both ovaries (bilateral **oophorectomy**).

Purpose

An orchiectomy is done to treat cancer or, for other reasons, to lower the level of testosterone, the primary male sex hormone, in the body. Surgical removal of a testicle is the usual treatment if a tumor is found within the gland itself, but an orchiectomy may also be performed to treat prostate cancer or cancer of the male breast, as testosterone causes these cancers to grow and metastasize (spread to other parts of the body). An orchiectomy is sometimes done to prevent cancer when an undescended testicle is found in a patient who is beyond the age of puberty.

A bilateral orchiectomy is commonly performed as one stage in male-to-female (MTF) gender reassignment surgery. It is done both to lower the levels of male hormones in the patient's body and to prepare the genital area for later operations to construct a vagina and external female genitalia.

Some European countries and four states in the United States (California, Florida, Montana, and Texas) allow convicted sex offenders to request surgical castration to help control their sexual urges. This option is considered controversial in some parts of the legal system. A small number of men with very strong sex drives request an orchiectomy for religious reasons; it should be noted, however, that official Roman Catholic teaching is opposed to the performance of castration for spiritual purity.

Demographics

Cancer

Cancers in men vary widely in terms of both the numbers of men affected and the age groups most likely to be involved. Prostate cancer is the single most common malignancy affecting American men over the age of 50; about 220,000 cases are reported each year. According to the Centers for Disease Control and Prevention (CDC), 31,000 men in the United States die every year from prostate cancer. African-American men are almost 70% more likely to develop prostate cancer than either Caucasian or Asian-American men; the reasons for this difference are not yet known. Other factors that increase a man's risk of developing prostate cancer include a diet high in red meat, fat, and dairy products, and a family history of the disease. Men whose father or brother(s) had prostate cancer are twice as likely as other men to develop the disease themselves. Today, however, there are still no genetic tests available for prostate cancer.

Testicular cancer, on the other hand, frequently occurs in younger men; in fact, it is the most common cancer diagnosed in males between the ages of 15 and

34. The rate of new cases in the United States each year is about 3.7 per 100,000 people. The incidence of testicular cancer has been rising in the developed countries at a rate of about 2% per year since 1970. It is not yet known whether this increase is a simple reflection of improved diagnostic techniques or whether there are other causes. There is some variation among racial and ethnic groups, with men of Scandinavian background having higher than average rates of testicular cancer, and African-American men having a lower than average incidence. Testicular cancer occurs most often in males in one of three age groups: boys 10 years old or younger; adult males between the ages of 20 and 40; and men over 60.

Other risk factors for testicular cancer include:

• Cryptorchidism, which is a condition in which a boy's testicles do not move down from the abdomen into the scrotum at the usual point in fetal development. It is also called undescended testicle(s). Ordinarily, the testicles descend before the baby is born; however, if the baby is born prematurely, the scrotal sac may be empty at the time of delivery. About 3–4% of full-term male infants are born with undescended testicles. Men with a history of childhood cryptorchidism are three to 14 times more likely to develop testicular cancer.

• Family history of testicular cancer.

• A mother who took diethylstilbestrol (DES) during pregnancy. DES is a synthetic hormone that was prescribed for many women between 1938 and 1971 to prevent miscarriage. It has since been found to increase the risk of certain types of cancer in the offspring of these women.

• Occupational and environmental factors. Separate groups of researchers in Germany and New Zealand reported in 2003 that firefighters have an elevated risk of testicular cancer compared to control subjects. The specific environmental trigger is not yet known.

Gender reassignment

Statistics for orchiectomies in connection with gender reassignment surgery are difficult to establish because most patients who have had this type of surgery prefer to keep it confidential. Persons undergoing the hormonal treatments and periods of real-life experience as members of the other sex that are required prior to genital surgery frequently report social rejection, job discrimination, and other negative consequences of their decision. Because of widespread social disapproval of surgical gender reassignment, researchers do not know the true prevalence of gender identity disorders in the general population. Early estimates were 1:37,000 males and 1:107,000 females. A recent study in the Netherlands,

however, maintains that a more accurate estimation is 1:11,900 males and 1:30,400 females. In any case, the number of surgical procedures is lower than the number of patients diagnosed with gender identity disorders.

Description

There are three basic types of orchiectomy: simple, subcapsular, and inguinal (or radical). The first two types are usually done under local or epidural anesthesia, and take about 30 minutes to perform. An inguinal orchiectomy is sometimes done under general anesthesia, and takes between 30 minutes and an hour to complete.

Simple orchiectomy

A simple orchiectomy is performed as part of gender reassignment surgery or as palliative treatment for advanced cancer of the prostate. The patient lies flat on an operating table with the penis taped against the abdomen. After the anesthetic has been given, the surgeon makes an incision in the midpoint of the scrotum and cuts through the underlying tissue. The surgeon removes the testicles and parts of the spermatic cord through the incision. The incision is closed with two layers of sutures and covered with a surgical dressing. If the patient desires, a prosthetic testicle can be inserted before the incision is closed to give the appearance of a normal scrotum from the outside.

Subcapsular orchiectomy

A subcapsular orchiectomy is also performed for treatment of prostate cancer. The operation is similar to a simple orchiectomy, with the exception that the glandular tissue is removed from the lining of each testicle rather than the entire gland being removed. This type of orchiectomy is done primarily to keep the appearance of a normal scrotum.

Inguinal orchiectomy

An inguinal orchiectomy, which is sometimes called a radical orchiectomy, is done when testicular cancer is suspected. It may be either unilateral, involving only one testicle, or bilateral. This procedure is called an inguinal orchiectomy because the surgeon makes the incision, which is about 3 in (7.6 cm) long, in the patient's groin area rather than directly into the scrotum. It is called a radical orchiectomy because the surgeon removes the entire spermatic cord as well as the testicle itself. The reason for this complete removal is that testicular cancers frequently spread from the spermatic cord into the lymph nodes near the kidneys. A long non-absorbable suture is left in the stump of the spermatic cord in case later surgery is necessary.

After the cord and testicle have been removed, the surgeon washes the area with saline solution and closes the various layers of tissues and skin with various types of sutures. The wound is then covered with sterile gauze and bandaged.

Diagnosis/Preparation

Diagnosis

CANCER. The doctor may suspect that a patient has prostate cancer from feeling a mass in the prostate in the course of a rectal examination, from the results of a transrectal ultrasound (TRUS), or from elevated levels of prostate-specific antigen (PSA) in the patient's blood. PSA is a tumor marker, or chemical, in the blood that can be used to detect cancer and monitor the results of therapy. A definite diagnosis of prostate cancer, however, requires a tissue biopsy. The tissue sample can usually be obtained with the needle technique. Testicular cancer is suspected when the doctor feels a mass in the patient's scrotum, which may or may not be painful. In order to perform a biopsy for definitive diagnosis, however, the doctor must remove the affected testicle by radical orchiectomy.

GENDER REASSIGNMENT. Patients requesting gender reassignment surgery must undergo a lengthy process of physical and psychological evaluation before receiving approval for surgery. The Harry Benjamin International Gender Dysphoria Association (HBIGDA), which is presently the largest worldwide professional association dealing with the treatment of gender identity disorders, has published standards of care that are followed by most surgeons who perform genital surgery for gender reassignment. HBIGDA stipulates that a patient must meet the diagnostic criteria for gender identity disorders as defined by either the *Diagnostic and Statistical Manual of Mental Disorders,* fourth edition *(DSM-IV)* or the *International Classification of Diseases–10 (ICD-10).*

Preparation

All patients preparing for an orchiectomy will have standard blood and urine tests before the procedure. They are asked to discontinue aspirin-based medications for a week before surgery and all non-steroidal anti-inflammatory drugs (NSAIDs) two days before the procedure. Patients should not eat or drink anything for the eight hours before the scheduled time of surgery.

Most surgeons ask patients to shower or bathe on the morning of surgery using a special antibacterial soap. They should take extra time to lather, scrub, and rinse their genitals and groin area.

Patients who are anxious or nervous before the procedure are usually given a sedative to help them relax.

CANCER. Patients who are having an orchiectomy as treatment for testicular cancer should consider banking sperm if they plan to have children following surgery. Although it is possible to father a child if only one testicle is removed, some surgeons recommend banking sperm as a precaution in case the other testicle should develop a tumor at a later date.

GENDER REASSIGNMENT. Most males who have requested an orchiectomy as part of male-to-female gender reassignment have been taking hormones for a period of several months to several years prior to surgery, and have had some real-life experience dressing and functioning as women. The surgery is not performed as an immediate response to the patient's request.

Because the standards of care for gender reassignment require a psychiatric diagnosis as well as a **physical examination**, the surgeon who is performing the orchiectomy should receive two letters of evaluation and recommendation by mental health professionals, preferably one from a psychiatrist and one from a clinical psychologist.

Aftercare

Patients who are having an orchiectomy in an ambulatory surgery center or other outpatient facility must have a friend or family member to drive them home after the procedure. Most patients can go to work the following day, although some may need an additional day of rest at home. Even though it is normal for patients to feel nauseated after the anesthetic wears off, they should start eating regularly when they get home. Some pain and swelling is also normal; the doctor will usually prescribe a pain-killing medication to be taken for a few days.

Other recommendations for aftercare include:

- Drinking extra fluids for the next several days, except for caffeinated and alcoholic beverages.

- Avoiding sexual activity, heavy lifting, and vigorous **exercise** until the follow-up appointment with the doctor.

- Taking a shower rather than a tub bath for a week following surgery to minimize the risk of absorbable stitches dissolving prematurely.

- Applying an ice pack to the groin area for the first 24–48 hours.

- Wearing a jock strap or snug briefs to support the scrotum for two weeks after surgery.

Some patients may require psychological counseling following an orchiectomy as part of their long-term aftercare. Many men have very strong feelings about any procedure involving their genitals, and may feel depressed or anxious about their bodies or their relationships after genital surgery. In addition to individual psychotherapy, support groups are often helpful. There are active networks of prostate cancer support groups in Canada and the United States as well as support groups for men's issues in general.

Long-term aftercare for patients with testicular cancer includes frequent checkups in addition to radiation treatment or chemotherapy. Patients with prostate cancer may be given various hormonal therapies or radiation treatment.

Risks

Some of the risks for an orchiectomy done under general anesthesia are the same as for other procedures. They include deep venous thrombosis, heart or breathing problems, bleeding, infection, or reaction to the anesthesia. If the patient is having epidural anesthesia, the risks include bleeding into the spinal canal, nerve damage, or a spinal headache.

Specific risks associated with an orchiectomy include:

- loss of sexual desire (This side effect can be treated with hormone injections or gel preparations.)

- impotence

- hot flashes similar to those in menopausal women, controllable by medication

- weight gain of 10–15 lb (4.5–6.8 kg)

- mood swings or depression

- enlargement and tenderness in the breasts

- fatigue

- loss of sensation in the groin or the genitals

- osteoporosis (Men who are taking hormone treatments for prostate cancer are at greater risk of osteoporosis.)

An additional risk specific to cancer patients is recurrence of the cancer.

Normal results

Cancer

Normal results depend on the location and stage of the patient's cancer at the time of surgery. Most prostate cancer patients, however, report rapid relief from cancer symptoms after an orchiectomy. Patients with testicular cancer have a 95% survival rate five years after surgery if the cancer had not spread beyond the testicle. Metastatic testicular cancer, however, has a poorer prognosis.

Gender reassignment

Normal results following orchiectomy as part of a sex change from male to female are a drop in testosterone levels with corresponding decrease in sex drive and gradual reduction of such masculine characteristics as beard growth. The patient may choose to have further operations at a later date.

Morbidity and mortality rates

Orchiectomy by itself has a very low rate of morbidity and mortality. Patients who are having an orchiecto-

KEY TERMS

Androgen—Any substance that promotes the development of masculine characteristics in a person. Testosterone is one type of androgen; others are produced in the adrenal glands located above the kidneys.

Bilateral—On both sides. A bilateral orchiectomy is the removal of both testicles.

Capsule—A general medical term for a structure that encloses another structure or body part. The capsule of the testicle is the membrane that surrounds the glandular tissue.

Castration—Removal or destruction by radiation of both testicles (in a male) or both ovaries (in a female), making the individual incapable of reproducing.

Cryptorchidism—A developmental disorder in which one or both testes fail to descend from the abdomen into the scrotum before birth.

Emasculation—Another term for castration of a male.

Epidural—A type of regional anesthetic delivered by injection into the area around the patient's lower spine. An epidural numbs the body below the waist but allows the patient to remain conscious throughout the procedure.

Gender identity disorder (GID)—A mental disorder in which a person strongly identifies with the other sex and feels uncomfortable with his or her biological sex. It occurs more often in males than in females.

Gender reassignment surgery—The surgical alteration and reconstruction of a person's sex organs to resemble those of the other sex as closely as possible; it is sometimes called sex reassignment surgery.

Inguinal—Referring to the groin area.

Metastasis—A process in which a malignant tumor transfers cells to a part of the body not directly connected to its primary site. A cancer that has spread from its original site to other parts of the body is said to be metastatic.

Oophorectomy—Removal of one or both ovaries in a woman.

Orchiectomy—Surgical removal of one or both testicles in a male. It is also called an orchidectomy.

Scrotum—The pouch of skin on the outside of the male body that holds the testes.

Spermatic cord—A tube-like structure that extends from the testicle to the groin area. It contains blood vessels, nerves, and a duct to carry spermatic fluid.

Subcapsular—Inside the outer tissue covering of the testicle. A subcapsular orchiectomy is a procedure in which the surgeon removes the inner glandular tissue of the testicle while leaving the outer capsule intact.

Testis (plural, testes)—The medical term for a testicle.

Testosterone—The major male sex hormone, produced in the testes.

Tumor marker—A circulating biochemical compound that indicates the presence of cancer. Tumor markers can be used in diagnosis and in monitoring the effectiveness of treatment.

Urology—The branch of medicine that deals with disorders of the urinary tract in both males and females, and with the genital organs in males.

my as part of cancer therapy have a higher risk of dying from the cancer than from testicular surgery.

The morbidity and mortality rates for persons having an orchiectomy as part of gender reassignment surgery are about the same as those for any procedure involving general or epidural anesthesia.

Alternatives

Cancer

There is no effective alternative to radical orchiectomy in the treatment of testicular cancer; radiation and chemotherapy are considered follow-up treatments rather than alternatives.

There are, however, several alternatives to orchiectomy in the treatment of prostate cancer:

• watchful waiting

• hormonal therapy (The drugs that are usually given for prostate cancer are either medications that oppose the action of male sex hormones [anti-androgens, usually flutamide or nilutamide] or medications that prevent the production of testosterone [goserelin or leuprolide acetate].)

- radiation treatment

- chemotherapy

Gender reassignment

The primary alternative to an orchiectomy for gender reassignment is hormonal therapy. Most patients seeking MTF gender reassignment begin taking female hormones (estrogens) for three to five months minimum before requesting genital surgery. Some persons postpone surgery for a longer period of time, often for financial reasons; others choose to continue on estrogen therapy indefinitely without surgery.

See also Orchiopexy.

Resources

BOOKS

"Breast Disorders: Breast Cancer in Men." Section 18, Chapter 242 in *The Merck Manual of Diagnosis and Therapy,* edited by Mark H. Beers and Robert Berkow. Whitehouse Station, NJ: Merck Research Laboratories, 1999.

"Congenital Anomalies: Renal and Genitourinary Defects." Section 19, Chapter 261 in *The Merck Manual of Diagnosis and Therapy,* edited by Mark H. Beers and Robert Berkow. Whitehouse Station, NJ: Merck Research Laboratories, 1999.

Morris, Jan. *Conundrum.* New York: Harcourt Brace Jovanovich, Inc., 1974.

"Principles of Cancer Therapy: Other Modalities." Section 11, Chapter 144 in *The Merck Manual of Diagnosis and Therapy,* edited by Mark H. Beers and Robert Berkow. Whitehouse Station, NJ: Merck Research Laboratories, 1999.

"Sexual and Gender Identity Disorders." In *Diagnostic and Statistical Manual of Mental Disorders,* 4th edition, text revision. Washington, DC: American Psychiatric Association, 2000.

PERIODICALS

Berruti, A., et al. "Background to and Management of Treatment-Related Bone Loss in Prostate Cancer." *Drugs and Aging,* 19 (2002): 899–910.

Dawson, C. "Testicular Cancer: Seek Advice Early." *Journal of Family Health Care,* 12 (2002): 3.

Elert, A., K. Jahn, A. Heidenreich, and R. Hofmann. "The Familial Undescended Testis." [in German] *Klinische Padiatrie,* 215 (January–February 2003): 40–45.

Geldart, T. R., P. D. Simmonds, and G. M. Mead. "Orchidectomy after Chemotherapy for Patients with Metastatic Testicular Germ Cell Cancer." *BJU International,* 90 (September 2002): 451–455.

Incrocci, L., W. C. Hop, A. Wijnmaalen, and A. K. Slob. "Treatment Outcome, Body Image, and Sexual Functioning After Orchiectomy and Radiotherapy for Stage I-II Testicular Seminoma." *International Journal of Radiation Oncology, Biology, Physics,* 53 (August 1, 2002): 1165–1173.

Landen, M., et al. "Donc Is Done—and Gone Is Gone. Sex Reassignment is Presently the Best Cure for Transsexuals." [in Swedish] *Lakartidningen,* 98 (July 25, 2001): 3322–3326.

Papanikolaou, Frank, and Laurence Klotz. "Orchiectomy, Radical." *eMedicine,,* October 3, 2001 [March 30, 2003]. <http://www.emedicine.com/med/topic3063.htm>.

Roberts, L. W., M. Hollifield, and T. McCarty. "Psychiatric Evaluation of a 'Monk' Requesting Castration: A Patient's Fable, with Morals." *American Journal of Psychiatry,* 155 (March 1998): 415–420.

Smith, M. R. "Osteoporosis and Other Adverse Body Composition Changes During Androgen Deprivation Therapy for Prostate Cancer." *Cancer and Metastasis Reviews,* 21 (2002): 159–166.

Stang, A., K. H. Jockel, C. Baumgardt-Elms, and W. Ahrens. "Firefighting and Risk of Testicular Cancer: Results from a German Population-Based Case-Control Study." *American Journal of Industrial Medicine,* 43 (March 2003): 291–294.

Stone, T. H., W. J. Winslade, and C. M. Klugman. "Sex Offenders, Sentencing Laws and Pharmaceutical Treatment: A Prescription for Failure." *Behavioral Sciences and the Law,* 18 (2000): 83–110.

Volm, M. D. "Male Breast Cancer." *Current Treatment Options in Oncology,* 4 (April 2003): 159–164.

ORGANIZATIONS

American Board of Urology (ABU). 2216 Ivy Road, Suite 210, Charlottesville, VA 22903. (434) 979-0059. <http://www.abu.org>.

American Cancer Society (ACS). (800) ACS-2345. <http://www.cancer.org>.

American Prostate Society. P. O. Box 870, Hanover, MD 21076. (800) 308-1106. <http://www.ameripros.org>.

Canadian Prostate Cancer Network. P. O. Box 1253, Lakefield, ON K0L 2H0 Canada. (705) 652-9200. <http://www.cpcn.org>.

Centers for Disease Control and Prevention (CDC) Cancer Prevention and Control Program. 4770 Buford Highway, NE, MS K64, Atlanta, GA 30341. (888) 842-6355. <http://www.cdc.gov/cancer/comments.htm>.

Harry Benjamin International Gender Dysphoria Association, Inc. (HBIGDA). 1300 South Second Street, Suite 180, Minneapolis, MN 55454. (612) 625-1500. <http://www.hbigda.org>.

National Cancer Institute (NCI). NCI Public Inquiries Office. Suite 3036A, 6116 Executive Boulevard, MSC8332, Bethesda, MD 20892-8322. (800) 4-CANCER or (800) 332-8615 (TTY). <http://www.nci.nih.gov>.

OTHER

Harry Benjamin International Gender Dysphoria Association (HBIGDA). *Standards of Care for Gender Identity Disorders,* 6th version, February, 2001 [April 1, 2003]. <http://www.hbigda.org/socv6.html>.

National Cancer Institute (NCI) Physician Data Query (PDQ). *Male Breast Cancer: Treatment,* December 9, 2002

[March 29, 2003]. <http://www.nci.nih.gov/cancerinfo/pdq/treatment/malebreast/healthprofessional>.

NCI PDQ. *Testicular Cancer: Treatment,* February 20, 2003 {March 29, 2003]. <http://www.nci.nih.gov/cancerinfo/pdq/treatment/testicular/healthprofessional>.

Rebecca Frey, PhD

Orchiopexy

Definition

Orchiopexy is a procedure in which a surgeon fastens an undescended testicle inside the scrotum, usually with absorbable sutures. It is done most often in male infants or very young children to correct cryptorchidism, which is the medical term for undescended testicles. Orchiopexy is also occasionally performed in adolescents or adults, and may involve one or both testicles. In adults, orchiopexy is most often done to treat testicular torsion, which is a urologic emergency resulting from the testicle's twisting around the spermatic cord and losing its blood supply.

Other names for orchiopexy include orchidopexy, inguinal orchiopexy, repair of undescended testicle, cryptorchidism repair, and testicular torsion repair.

Purpose

To understand the reasons for performing an orchiopexy in children, it is helpful to have an outline of the normal pattern of development of the testes in a male infant. The gubernaculum is an embryonic cord-like ligament that attaches the testes within the inguinal (groin) region of a male fetus up through the seventh month of pregnancy. Between the 28th and the 35th week of pregnancy, the gubernaculum migrates into the scrotum and creates space for the testes to descend. In normal development, the testes have followed the gubernaculum downward into the scrotum by the time the baby is born. The normal pattern may be interrupted by several possible factors, including inadequate androgen (male sex hormone) secretion, structural abnormalities in the boy's genitals, and defective nerves in the genital region.

Orchiopexy is performed in children for several reasons:

• To minimize the risk of infertility. Adult males with cryptorchidism typically have lower sperm counts and produce sperm of poorer quality than men with normal testicles. The risk of infertility rises with increasing age

at the time of orchiopexy and whether both testicles are affected. Men with one undescended testicle have a 40% chance of being infertile; this figure rises to 70% in men with bilateral cryptorchidism.

• To lower the risk of testicular cancer. The incidence of malignant tumors in undescended testes has been estimated to be 48 times the incidence in normal testes. Men with cryptorchidism have a 10% chance of eventually developing testicular cancer.

• To lower the risk of traumatic injury to the testicle. Undescended testicles that remain in the patient's groin area are vulnerable to sports injuries and pressure from car seat belts.

• To prevent the development of an inguinal hernia. An inguinal hernia is a disorder that occurs when a portion of the contents of the abdomen pushes through an abnormal opening in the abdominal wall. It is likely to occur in a male infant with cryptorchidism because a sac known as the processus vaginalis, which connects the scrotum and the abdominal cavity, remains open after birth. In normal development, the processus vaginalis closes shortly after the testes descend into the scrotum. If the sac remains open, a section of the child's intestine can extend into the sac. It may become trapped (incarcerated) in the sac, forming what is called a strangulated hernia. The portion of the intestine that is trapped in the sac may die, which is a medical emergency.

• To prevent testicular torsion in adolescence.

• To maintain the appearance of a normal scrotum. Orchiopexy is considered a necessary procedure for psychological reasons, as boys with only one visible testicle are frequently subjected to teasing and ridicule after they start school.

The primary reason for performing an orchiopexy in an adolescent or adult male is treatment of testicular torsion, rather than cryptorchidism. Testicles that have not descended by the time a boy reaches puberty are usually removed by a complete **orchiectomy**.

Demographics

Cryptorchidism

Cryptorchidism is the most common abnormality of the male genital tract, affecting 3–5% of full-term male infants and 30–32% of premature male infants. In most cases, the condition resolves during the first few months after delivery; only 0.8% of infants over three months of age still have undescended testicles. Because of the potentially serious consequences of cryptorchidism, however, doctors do not advise watchful waiting once the child is over six months old. Undescended testicles

Orchiopexy

An orchiopexy is used to repair an undescended testicle in childhood. An incision is made into the abdomen, the site of the undescended testicle, and another is made in the scrotum (A). The testis is detached from surrounding tissues (B) and pulled out of the abdominal incision attached to the spermatic cord (C). The testis is then pulled down into the scrotum (D) and stitched into place (E). *(Illustration by Argosy.)*

rarely come down into the scrotum of their own accord after that age.

Cryptorchidism is a frequent occurrence in prune belly syndrome (PBS) and a few other genetic disorders characterized by structural abnormalities of the genitourinary tract.

No variation in the incidence of cryptorchidism among different racial and ethnic groups has been reported.

Testicular torsion

Most American males suffering from testicular torsion are below age 30, with the majority between the

WHO PERFORMS THE PROCEDURE AND WHERE IS IT PERFORMED?

A pediatric surgeon or pediatric urologist is the specialist most likely to perform an orchiopexy in an infant or small child. In an adult patient, the procedure is usually performed by a urologist after referral from the patient's primary physician or the emergency care physician.

An orchiopexy can be performed in the surgical unit of a children's hospital or an ambulatory surgical center. Most orchiopexies in adults are performed as outpatient procedures.

ages of 12 and 18. The peak ages for an acute episode of testicular torsion are the first year of life and age 14. Testicular torsion occurs on the left side of the body slightly more often than on the right side, about 52% versus 48% of cases.

Description

Cryptorchidism

Some orchiopexies in children are relatively simple procedures; however, others are complicated by the location of the undescended testicle. In general, an orchiopexy for an undescended testicle that lies in front of the scrotum or just above it is a less complicated operation than one done to treat a non-palpable testicle. The procedure is usually done under general anesthesia.

If the undescended testis is in the groin area, the surgeon will make a small incision in the groin and a second small incision in the scrotum. The testis is moved downward from the groin without complete separation from the gubernaculum. It is then placed inside a small pouch created by the surgeon between the skin of the scrotum and a layer of muscle in the scrotum called the dartos muscle. The testicle is held in place with sutures that are eventually absorbed by the body.

The Fowler-Stephens technique is often used when the undescended testicle is located high above the scrotum or in the abdomen. It may be done in two stages scheduled several months apart. In the first stage, the surgeon moves the testicle downward and attaches it temporarily to the inside of the thigh. In the second stage, the testicle is transferred into the scrotum itself and sutured into place.

A third type of orchiopexy is called testicular auto-transplantation. The surgeon removes the undescended testicle completely from its present location and re-implants it in the scrotum by reattaching its surrounding tissues and blood vessels to nearby blood vessels. This technique minimizes the risk of an inadequate blood supply to the re-implanted testicle.

Testicular torsion

An orchiopexy done to treat testicular torsion is usually done under general or epidural anesthesia. The surgeon makes an incision in the patient's scrotum and untwists the spermatic cord. The affected testicle is inspected for signs of necrosis, or tissue death. If too much tissue has died due to loss of blood supply, the surgeon will remove the entire testicle. If the tissue appears to be healthy, the surgeon sutures the testicle to the wall of the scrotum and then closes the incision. In most cases, the surgeon will also attach the unaffected testicle to the scrotal wall as a preventive measure.

Diagnosis/Preparation

Cryptorchidism

The diagnosis of cryptorchidism is usually made when a pediatrician examines the newborn baby, although the condition can occur at any time before the boy reaches puberty. The first stage in diagnosis is an external **physical examination** of the child's genitals. If either testicle does not appear to be in the scrotum, the doctor will palpate, or touch, the groin area and abdomen to determine whether a testicle can be felt in any of those locations. If the testicle can be felt, the doctor will decide on the basis of its location whether it is an undescended testicle, a so-called ectopic testicle, or a retractile testicle. An ectopic testicle is one that has developed in a location outside the normal path of development in the inguinal canal. Ectopic testicles are most often discovered along the inner part of the thigh near the groin, at the base of the penis, or below the scrotum in the perineum (the area between the scrotum and the rectum). A retractile testicle is one that is readily pulled back out of the scrotum by an overly sensitive reflex called the cremasteric reflex; it is not a genuinely undescended testicle. It is important for the doctor to distinguish a retractile testicle from genuine cryptorchidism because retractile testicles do not need surgical treatment. At this point in the diagnostic workup, a general pediatrician will often consult a specialist in pediatric urology.

In about 20% of male infants with cryptorchidism, the missing testicle cannot be felt at all. It is known as a non-palpable testicle. The child may be given a hormone challenge test to help determine whether the testicle is located in the abdomen or whether it has failed to develop fully. If the testosterone level in the blood rises in response to the test, the doctor knows that there is a testis present somewhere in the child's body. In other cases, the testis has atrophied, or shriveled up due to an inadequate blood supply before birth. If neither testicle can be felt, the child should be examined further for evidence of inter-sexuality. The doctor may order an ultrasound to check for the presence of a uterus, particularly if the child's external genitals are ambiguous in appearance.

Surgery is the next step in searching for a non-palpable testicle. The surgeon may perform either an open inguinal procedure or a laparoscopic approach. In an open inguinal exploration, the surgeon makes an incision in the child's groin; if nothing is found, the incision may be extended into the lower abdomen. In a laparoscopic approach, the surgeon uses an instrument that looks like a small telescope with a light attached in order to see inside the groin or the abdominal cavity through a much smaller incision. If the surgeon is able to find the testicle, he or she may then proceed directly to perform an orchiopexy.

Testicular torsion

Testicular torsion is usually diagnosed in the emergency room. The doctor will usually suspect testicular torsion on the basis of sudden onset of severe pain on one side of the scrotum; it is unusual for pain to develop gradually in this disorder. The patient's history often indicates recent hard physical work, vigorous **exercise**, or trauma to the genital area; however, testicular torsion can also occur without any apparent reason. Other symptoms may include swelling of the scrotum, blood in the semen, nausea and vomiting, pain in the abdomen, and fever. A few patients feel the need to urinate frequently. When the doctor examines the patient's scrotum, the affected testicle is usually enlarged and is painful when the doctor touches it. It usually lies higher in the scrotum than the unaffected testicle and may be lying in a horizontal position.

Since testicular torsion is a medical emergency, most doctors will not risk permanent damage to the testicle by taking the time to perform imaging studies. If the diagnosis is unclear, however, the doctor may order a radionuclide scan or a color Doppler ultrasound to determine whether the blood flow to the testicle has been cut off. The patient will be given a mild pain medication and referred to a urologist for surgery as soon as possible.

Aftercare

Cryptorchidism

Aftercare in children depends partly on the complexity of the procedure. If the child has an uncomplicated orchiopexy, he can usually go home the same day. If the surgeon had to make an incision in the abdomen to

QUESTIONS TO ASK THE DOCTOR

- How often have you treated a child for cryptorchidism?
- What are the chances that the treatment will be successful?
- What should I tell my son about the operation?
- Are there likely to be any long-term aftereffects?

find a non-palpable testicle before performing the orchiopexy, the child may remain in the hospital for two or three days. The doctor will usually prescribe a pain medication for the first few days after the procedure.

After the child returns home, he should not bathe until the day after surgery. In addition, he should not ride a bicycle, climb trees, or do anything else that requires straddling for two or three weeks. An older boy should avoid sports or rough games that might result in injury to the genitals until he has a post-surgical checkup.

Most surgeons will schedule the child for a checkup one or two weeks after the orchiopexy, with a second checkup three months later.

Testicular torsion

Aftercare is similar to that for orchiopexy in a child. The area around the incision should be washed very gently the next day and a clean dressing applied. Medication will be prescribed for postoperative pain. The patient is advised to rest at home for several days after surgery, to remain in bed as much as possible, to drink extra fluids, and to elevate the scrotum on a small pillow to ease the discomfort. Vigorous physical and sexual activity should be avoided until the pain and swelling go away.

Risks

Cryptorchidism

The risks of orchiopexy in treating cryptorchidism include:

- infection of the incision
- bleeding
- damage to the blood vessels and other structures in the spermatic cord, leading to eventual loss of the testicle

KEY TERMS

Cremasteric reflex—A reflex in which the cremaster muscle, which covers the testes and the spermatic cord, pulls the testicles back into the scrotum. It is important for a doctor to distinguish between an undescended testicle and a hyperactive cremasteric reflex in small children.

Cryptorchidism—A developmental disorder in which one or both testes fail to descend from the abdomen into the scrotum before birth. It is the most common structural abnormality in the male genital tract.

Ectopic—Located in an abnormal site or tissue. An ectopic testicle is one that is located in an unusual position outside its normal line of descent into the scrotum.

Gonadotropins—Hormones that stimulate the activity of the ovaries in females and testes in males.

Hernia—The protrusion of a loop or piece of tissue through an incision or abnormal opening in other tissues.

Inguinal—Referring to the groin area.

Laparoscope—An instrument that allows a surgeon to look inside the abdominal cavity.

Non-palpable—Unable to be detected through the sense of touch. A non-palpable testicle is one that is located in the abdomen or other site where the doctor cannot feel it by pressing gently on the child's body.

Orchiectomy—Surgical removal of one or both testicles in a male; also called an orchidectomy.

Perineum—The area between the scrotum and the anus.

Peritoneum—The smooth, colorless membrane that lines the inner surface of the abdomen.

Prune belly syndrome (PBS)—A genetic disorder associated with abnormalities of human chromosomes 18 and 21. Male infants with PBS often have cryptorchidism along with other defects of the genitals and urinary tract. PBS is also known as triad syndrome and Eagle-Barrett syndrome.

Scrotum—The pouch of skin on the outside of the male body that holds the testes.

Spermatic cord—A tube-like structure that extends from the testicle to the groin area. It contains blood vessels, nerves, and a duct to carry spermatic fluid.

Testicular torsion—Twisting of the testicle around the spermatic cord, cutting off the blood supply to the testicle. It is considered a urologic emergency.

Testis (plural, testes)—The medical term for a testicle.

Urology—The branch of medicine that deals with disorders of the urinary tract in both males and females, and with the genital organs in males.

• failure of the testicle to remain in the scrotum (This problem can be repaired by a second operation.)

• difficulty urinating for a few days after surgery

Testicular torsion

The risks of orchiopexy as a treatment for testicular torsion include:

• infection of the incision

• bleeding

• loss of blood circulation in the testicle leading to loss of the testicle

• reaction to anesthesia

Normal results

In a normal orchiopexy, the testicle remains in the scrotum without re-ascending. If the procedure has been successful, there is no damage to the blood vessels supplying the testicle, no loss of fertility, and no recurrence of torsion.

Morbidity and mortality rates

Cryptorchidism

Orchiopexy is most likely to be successful in children when the undescended testicle is relatively close to the scrotum. The rate of failure for orchiopexy performed as a treatment for cryptorchidism is 8% if the testicle lies just above the scrotum; 10–20% if the testicle is located in the inguinal canal; and 25% if the testicle lies within the abdomen.

Testicular torsion

The mortality rate for orchiopexy in adults is very low because almost all patients are young males in good health. The procedure has a 99% rate of success in saving the testicle when the diagnosis is made promptly and treated within six hours. After 12 hours, however, the rate of success in saving the testicle drops to 2%. The average rate of testicular atrophy following orchiopexy for testicular torsion is about 27%.

Alternatives

Cryptorchidism

Hormonal therapy using gonadotropins to stimulate the production of more testosterone is effective in some children in causing the testes to descend into the scrotum without surgery. This approach, however, is usually successful only with undescended testes that are already close to the scrotum; its rate of success ranges from 10–50%. Undescended testes that are located higher almost never respond to hormonal therapy. In addition, treatment with hormones has several undesirable side effects, including aggressive behavior.

Some surgeons will, however, prescribe hormonal treatment before an orchiopexy in order to increase the size of the undescended testis and make it easier to identify during surgery.

Testicular torsion

Pain caused by testicular torsion can be relieved temporarily by manual detorsion. To perform this maneuver, the doctor stands at the patient's feet and gently rotates the affected testicle toward the outside of the patient's body in a sidewise direction. Manual detorsion is effective in relieving pain in 30–70% of patients; however, it is not considered an alternative to orchiopexy in preventing a recurrence of the torsion or loss of the testicle.

See also Orchiectomy; Urologic surgery.

Resources

BOOKS

"Congenital Anomalies: Renal and Genitourinary Defects." Section 19, Chapter 261 in *The Merck Manual of Diagnosis and Therapy,* edited by Mark H. Beers and Robert Berkow. Whitehouse Station, NJ: Merck Research Laboratories, 1999.

PERIODICALS

Baker, L. A., et al. "A Multi-Institutional Analysis of Laparoscopic Orchidopexy." *BJU International,* 87 (April 2001): 484–489.

Chang, B., L. S. Palmer, and I. Franco. "Laparoscopic Orchidopexy: A Review of a Large Clinical Series." *BJU International,* 87 (April 2001): 490–493.

Docimo, S. G., R. I. Silver, and W. Cromie. "The Undescended Testicle: Diagnosis and Management." *American Family Physician,* 62 (November 1, 2000): 2037–2044, 2047–2048.

Dogra, Vikram S., and Hamid Mojibian. "Cryptorchidism." *eMedicine,* June 21, 2002 [April 4, 2003]. <www.emedicine.com/radio/topic201.htm>.

Franco, Israel. "Prune Belly Syndrome." *eMedicine,* August 24, 2001 [April 4, 2003]. <www.emedicine.com/med/topic3055.htm>.

Jawdeh, Bassam Abu, and Samir Akel. "Cryptorchidism: An Update." *American University of Beirut Surgery,* (Summer 2002) [April 3, 2003]. <www.staff.aub.edu.lb/~websurgp/sc0a.html>.

Nair, S. G., and B. Rajan. "Seminoma Arising in Cryptorchid Testis 25 Years After Orchiopexy: Case Report." *American Journal of Clinical Oncology,* 25 (June 2002): 287–288.

Rupp, Timothy J., and Mark Zwanger. "Testicular Torsion." *eMedicine,* March 25, 2003 [April 4, 2003]. <www.emedicine.com/EMERG/topic573.htm>.

Sessions, A. E., et al. "Testicular Torsion: Direction, Degree, Duration, and Disinformation." *Journal of Urology,* 169 (February 2003): 663–665.

Shekarriz, B., and M. L. Stoller. "The Use of Fibrin Sealant in Urology." *Journal of Urology,* 167 (March 2002): 1218–1225.

Tsujihata, M., et al. "Laparoscopic Diagnosis and Treatment of Nonpalpable Testis." *International Journal of Urology,* 8 (December 2001): 692–696.

ORGANIZATIONS

American Academy of Pediatrics (AAP). 141 Northwest Point Boulevard, Elk Grove Village, IL 60007. (847) 434-4000. <http://www.aap.org>.

American Board of Urology (ABU). 2216 Ivy Road, Suite 210, Charlottesville, VA 22903. (434) 979-0059. <http://www.abu.org>.

National Organization for Rare Disorders (NORD). 55 Kenosia Avenue, P. O. Box 1968, Danbury, CT 06813-1968. (203) 744-0100. <http://www.rarediseases.org>.

Prune Belly Syndrome Network. P. O. Box 2125, Evansville, IN 47728-0125. <http://www.prunebelly.org>.

Rebecca Frey, PhD

Orthopedic surgery

Definition

Orthopedic (sometimes spelled orthopedic) surgery is an operation performed by a medical specialist such as an orthopedist or orthopedic surgeon, who is trained to assess and treat problems that develop in the bones, joints, and ligaments of the human body.

Purpose

Orthopedic surgery addresses and attempts to correct problems that arise in the skeleton and its attachments, the ligaments and tendons. It may also include some problems of the nervous system, such as those that arise from injury of the spine. These problems can occur at birth, through injury, or as the result of aging. They may be acute, as in an accident or injury, or chronic, as in many problems related to aging.

Orthopedics comes from two Greek words, *ortho*, meaning straight, and *pais*, meaning child. Originally, orthopedic surgeons treated skeletal deformities in children, using braces to straighten the child's bones. With the development of anesthesia and an understanding of the importance of **aseptic technique** in surgery, orthopedic surgeons extended their role to include surgery involving the bones and related nerves and connective tissue.

The terms orthopedic surgeon and orthopedist are used interchangeably today to indicate a medical doctor with special training and certification in orthopedics.

Many orthopedic surgeons maintain a general practice, while some specialize in one particular aspect of orthopedics such as **hand surgery**, joint replacements, or disorders of the spine. Orthopedists treat both acute and chronic disorders. Some orthopedic surgeons specialize in trauma medicine and can be found in emergency rooms and trauma centers, treating injuries. Others find their work overlapping with plastic surgeons, geriatric specialists, pediatricians, or podiatrists (foot care specialists). A rapidly growing area of orthopedics is sports medicine, and many sports medicine doctors are board certified in orthopedic surgery.

Demographics

The American Academy of Orthopedic Surgeons reports that in 2003, there are 15,853 active fellows, 1,829 resident members, and 2,240 candidate members, for a total of 19,922 orthopedic surgeons in the United States.

Description

The range of treatments provided by orthopedists is extensive. They include procedures such as **traction**,

amputation, hand reconstruction, **spinal fusion**, and joint replacements. They also treat strains and sprains, broken bones, and dislocations. Some specific procedures performed by orthopedic surgeons are listed as separate entries in this book, including **arthroplasty**, **arthroscopic surgery**, **bone grafting**, **fasciotomy**, **fracture repair**, **kneecap removal**, and traction.

In general, orthopedists are employed by hospitals, medical centers, trauma centers, or free-standing surgical centers where they work closely with a **surgical team**, including an anesthesiologist and surgical nurse. Orthopedic surgery can be performed under general, regional, or local anesthesia.

Much of the work of an orthopedic surgeon involves adding foreign material to the body in the form of screws, wires, pins, tongs, and prosthetics to hold damaged bones in their proper alignment or to replace damaged bone or connective tissue. Great improvements have been made in the development of artificial limbs and joints, and in the materials available to repair damage to bones and connective tissue. As developments occur in the fields of metallurgy and plastics, changes will take place in orthopedic surgery that will allow surgeons to more nearly duplicate the natural functions of bones, joints, and ligaments, and to more accurately restore damaged parts to their original ranges of motion.

Diagnosis/Preparation

Persons are usually referred to an orthopedic surgeon by a primary care physician, emergency room physician, or other doctor. Prior to any surgery, candidates undergo extensive testing to determine appropriate corrective procedures. Tests may include x rays, computed tomography (CT) scans, **magnetic resonance imaging** (MRI), myelograms, diagnostic arthroplasty, and blood tests. The orthopedist will determine the history of the disorder and any treatments that were previously tried. A period of rest to the injured part may be recommended before surgery is undertaken.

Surgical candidates undergo standard blood and urine tests before surgery and, for major procedures, may be given an electrocardiogram or other diagnostic tests prior to the operation. Individuals may choose to donate some of their own blood to be held in reserve for their use in major surgery such as **knee replacement**, during which heavy bleeding is common.

Aftercare

Rehabilitation from orthopedic injuries can require long periods of time. Rehabilitation is usually physically and mentally taxing. Orthopedic surgeons will work closely with physical therapists to ensure that patients receive treatment that will enhance the range of motion and return function to all affected body parts.

Risks

As with any surgery, there is always the risk of excessive bleeding, infection, and allergic reaction to anesthesia. Risks specifically associated with orthopedic surgery include inflammation at the site where foreign materials (pins, prostheses, or wires) are introduced into the body, infection as the result of surgery, and damage to nerves or to the spinal cord.

Normal results

Thousands of people have successful orthopedic surgery each year to recover from injuries or to restore lost function. The degree of success in individual recoveries depends on an individual's age and general health, the medical problem being treated, and a person's willingness to comply with rehabilitative therapy after the surgery.

Abnormal results from orthopedic surgery include persistent pain, swelling, redness, drainage or bleeding in the surgical area, surgical wound infection resulting in slow healing, and incomplete restoration of pre-surgical function.

Morbidity and mortality rates

Mortality from orthopedic surgical procedures is not common. The most common causes for mortality are adverse reactions to anesthetic agents or drugs used to control pain, post-surgical clot formation in the veins, and post-surgical heart attacks or strokes.

Alternatives

For the removal of diseased, non-functional, or non-vital tissue, there is no alternative to orthopedic surgery. Alternatives to orthopedic surgery depend on the condition being treated. Medications, acupuncture, or hypnosis are used to relieve pain. Radiation is an occasional alternative for shrinking growths. Chemotherapy may be used to treat bone cancer. Some foreign bodies may remain in the body without harm.

See also Elective surgery; Finding a surgeon.

Resources

BOOKS

Bland, K. I., W. G. Cioffi, and M. G. Sarr. *Practice of General Surgery.* Philadelphia: Saunders, 2001.

Canale, S. T. *Campbell's Operative Orthopedics.* St. Louis: Mosby, 2003.

Schwartz, S. I., J. E. Fischer, F. C. Spencer, G. T. Shires, and J. M. Daly. *Principles of Surgery, 7th Edition.* New York: McGraw Hill, 1998.

QUESTIONS TO ASK THE DOCTOR

- What tests will be performed prior to surgery?
- How will the procedure affect daily activities after recovery?
- Where will the surgery be performed?
- What form of anesthesia will be used?
- What will be the resulting appearance and level of function after surgery?
- Is the surgeon board certified by the American Academy of Orthopedic Surgeons?
- How many similar procedures has the surgeon performed?
- What is the surgeon's complication rate?

Townsend, C., K. L. Mattox, R. D. Beauchamp, B. M. Evers, and D. C. Sabiston. *Sabiston's Review of Surgery, 3rd Edition.* Philadelphia: Saunders, 2001.

PERIODICALS

Caprini, J. A., J. I. Arcelus, D. Maksimovic, C. J. Glase, J. G. Sarayba, and K. Hathaway. "Thrombosis Prophylaxis in Orthopedic Surgery: Current Clinical Considerations." *Journal of the Southern Orthopedic Association* 11, no.4 (2002): 190–196.

O'Brien, J. G. "Orthopedic Surgery: A New Frontier." *Mayo Clinic Proceedings* 78, no.3 (2003): 275–277.

Ribbans, W. J. "Orthopedic Care in Haemophilia." *Hospital Medicine* 64, no.2 (2003): 68–69.

Showstack, J. "Improving Quality of Care in Orthopedic Surgery." *Arthritis and Rheumatism* 48, no.2 (2003): 289–290.

ORGANIZATIONS

American Academy of Orthopedic Surgeons. 6300 North River Road Rosemont, IL 60018-4262. (847) 823-7186 or (800) 346-2267. <http://www.aaos.org/wordhtml/home2.htm>.

American College of Sports Medicine. 401 West Michigan Street, Indianapolis, IN 46202-3233 (Mailing Address: P.O. Box 1440, Indianapolis, IN 46206-1440). (317) 637-9200, Fax: (317) 634-7817. <http://www.acsm.org>.

American College of Surgeons. 633 North Saint Claire Street, Chicago, IL 60611. (312) 202-5000. <http://www.facs.org/>.

American Society for Bone and Mineral Research 2025 M Street, NW, Suite 800, Washington, DC 20036-3309. (202) 367-1161. <http://www.asbmr.org/>.

Orthopedic Trauma Association. 6300 N. River Road, Suite 727, Rosemont, IL 60018-4226. (847) 698-1631. <http://www.ota.org/links.htm>.

OTHER

American Osteopathic Association. [cited April 7, 2003] <http://www.aoa-net.org/Certification/orthopedsurg.htm>.

Brigham and Woman's Hospital (Harvard University School of Medicine). [cited April 7, 2003] <http://splweb.bwh.harvard.edu:8000/pages/projects/ortho/ortho.html>.

Martindale's Health Science Guide, 2003. [cited April 7, 2003] <http://www-sci.lib.uci.edu/HSG/MedicalSurgery.html>.

Thomas Jefferson University Hospital. [cited April 7, 2003] <http://www.jeffersonhospital.org/e3front.dll?durki=4529>.

University of Maryland College of Medicine. [cited April 7, 2003] <http://www.umm.edu/surg-ortho/>.

L. Fleming Fallon, Jr, MD, DrPH

Orthopedic x rays *see* **Bone x rays**

Orthotopic transplantation *see* **Liver transplantation**

Osteotomy, hip *see* **Hip osteotomy**

Osteotomy, knee *see* **Knee osteotomy**

Otolaryngologic surgery *see* **Ear, nose, and throat surgery**

Otoplasty

Definition

Otoplasty refers to a group of plastic surgery procedures done to correct deformities of or disfiguring injuries to the external ear. It is the only type of plastic surgery that is performed more often in children than adults.

Purpose

Otoplastic surgery may done for the following reasons:

- To reconstruct an external ear in children who are born with a partially or completely missing auricle (the visible part of the external ear). This type of birth defect is called microtia; it occurs in such disorders as hemifacial microsomia and Treacher Collins syndrome. Most cases of microtia, however, involve only one ear.

- To correct the appearance of protruding or prominent ears. This procedure is also known as setback otoplasty or pinback otoplasty.

- To correct major disparities in the size or shape of a patient's ears.

- To reshape deformed ears. One congenital type of deformity is known as Stahl's ear, which is characterized by a pointed upper edge produced by the flattening of the ear rim and folding of the cartilage. Stahl's deformity is also known as Vulcan ear or Spock ear because it resembles the ears of the well-known *Star Trek* character.

- To repair or reconstruct the auricle after traumatic injuries or cancer surgery.

Otoplasty is considered reconstructive rather than cosmetic surgery. Consequently, it is often covered by health insurance. People who are considering otoplasty for themselves or their children should check with their insurance carrier about coverage. The average surgeon's fee for an otoplasty in the United States in 2001 was $2,168.

Otoplasty is not done to correct hearing difficulties related to the structures of the middle and inner ear. Hearing problems are treated surgically by otolaryngologists (physicians who specialize in ear, nose, and throat procedures).

Demographics

Statistics for congenital deformities of the external ear are difficult to obtain because the causes are so diverse. Such genetic disorders as Treacher Collins syndrome and hemifacial microsomia affect between one in 3,500 and one in 10,000 children. In addition, microtia has been associated with certain medications taken during pregnancy—particularly anticonvulsants, which are drugs given to treat epilepsy, and isotretinoin, a drug prescribed for severe acne.

Stahl's deformity is found more often among Asian Americans than among Caucasian or African Americans. As of 2003, it is thought to be a hereditary disorder.

Setback or pinback otoplasty is the most frequently performed procedure for reconstruction of prominent or protruding ears. According to the American Society of Plastic Surgeons, 33,107 setback otoplasties were performed in the United States in 2001. This figure represents about 2% of all plastic surgical procedures. There

Otoplasty

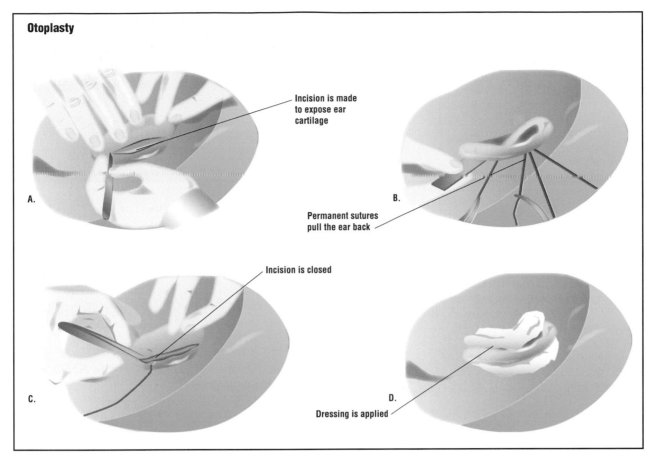

A. Incision is made to expose ear cartilage

B. Permanent sutures pull the ear back

C. Incision is closed

D. Dressing is applied

During a setback otoplasty, an incision is made in the back of the ear, exposing cartilage (A). Permanent sutures in the cartilage pull the ear back closer to the skull (B). The incision is closed (C), and dressings are applied (D). *(Illustration by GGS Inc.)*

are no exact statistics on the incidence of protruding ears in the general population, although about 8% of patients treated for this deformity have a family history of it. Large or protruding ears appear to be equally common in males and females; however, it is easier for girls and women to avoid social discomfort by styling their hair to cover their ears. This factor may explain why a slight majority (53%) of setback otoplasties is done on boys. Although most setback otoplasties are performed in children between the ages of four and 14, the second largest group of patients in this category is women in their 20s and 30s.

The most common cause of trauma requiring otoplasty is human and animal bites. Although exact figures are not known because many bite cases are not reported, a large percentage of dog and human bites cause wounds on the head and neck. With regard to human bites, the single most common injury requiring medical treatment is auricular avulsion, or tearing of the external ear. In the United States, 93% of patients treated for ear injuries caused by human bites are males between the ages of 15 and 25. Most cases of auricular avulsion in children, however, are caused by dog bites, which are likely to cause crushing as well as tearing of the tissues. Although statistics cover bites on all parts of the body, it is still noteworthy that plastic surgeons in the United States performed 43,687 operations to repair injuries caused by animal bites in 2001.

Description

Otoplasty in children is performed under general anesthesia; in adults, it may be done under either general anesthesia or local anesthesia with sedation. Most otoplasties take about two or three hours to complete. Many plastic surgeons prefer to use absorbable sutures when performing an otoplasty in order to minimize the risk of disturbing the shape of the ear by removing stitches later.

Otoplasty for microtia

Otoplasty for microtia requires a series of three or four separate operations. In the first operation, a piece of cartilage is removed from the child's rib cage on the side opposite the affected ear, so that the surgeon can use the natural curve of the cartilage in fashioning the new ear. The surgeon works from a template derived from photographs and computer models when he or she carves the cartilage into the desired shape. The cartilage is then carefully positioned under the skin on the side of the face. The skin will shape itself to fit the cartilage framework of the new ear. The second and third operations are done to shape the ear lobe and to raise the new ear into its final position.

Otoplasty for protruding ears

There is no universally accepted single technique for performing a setback otoplasty. Variations in the procedure are due partly to the different causes of ear protrusion. The patient's ear may have a large concha (the shell-like hollow of the external ear); the angle of the fold in the ear cartilage may cause the ear to protrude; or the ear lobe may be unusually large.

After the patient has been anesthetized, the surgeon makes an incision behind the ear in the fold of skin where the ear meets the head. In one technique, the surgeon exposes the ear cartilage beneath the skin and reshapes it or removes a small piece. The cartilage is bent back toward the head and secured in place with non-re-

movable sutures. Removal of cartilage is sometimes referred to as a conchal resection.

Another procedure for protruding ears involves the removal of skin and suturing the cartilage back on itself. This technique reshapes the ear without the need to remove cartilage; it is sometimes called a cartilage-sparing otoplasty.

After the surgeon has finished reshaping the ear and carefully drying the area, the incision is closed. The surgeon covers the ear with a cotton dressing moistened with mineral oil or other soft dressing.

Diagnosis/Preparation

Congenital abnormalities of the ear

Diagnosis of microtia is made by the obstetrician or pediatrician at the time of the child's birth. The diagnosis of prominent or protruding ears, however, is somewhat more complex because the deformity is a matter of shape and proportion rather than the absence or major malformation of a body part. The head of a newborn infant is larger in proportion to its body than is the case in adults, and as a result, the shape of the ears may not concern the parents until the child is two or three years old.

Otoplasty to correct microtia is usually started when the child is at least five years old. The surgeon must remove a portion of rib cartilage in order to construct a framework for the missing ear, and children younger than five may not have enough cartilage. In addition, it is easier for the surgeon to use the child's normal ear as a model for the size and shape of the reconstructed ear when the child is five or seven years old. Otoplasty for microtia is preceded by consultations between the surgeon and the child's parents. Following the diagnosis, a comprehensive treatment plan is made that includes long-term psychosocial as well as surgical follow-up. The reconstruction of a missing ear must be done in several stages because the surgeon must allow for changes in the proportions of the child's face and skull as he or she matures as well as attempt to make the new ear look as normal as possible.

As of 2003, there is some debate among plastic surgeons concerning the best age for performing a setback otoplasty. Many recommend the operation when the child is between five and seven years old. One reason is that the human ear has attained 85–90% of its adult size by this age, and therefore the surgeon can estimate the final size and shape of the ear with considerable accuracy. In addition, the cartilage in the ear is still relatively soft and easier for the surgeon to reshape. Another reason for performing an otoplasty in children in the early elementary school years is psychological; name-calling and teasing by peers can be emotionally destructive for children in this age bracket. On the other hand, some surgeons have reported performing setback otoplasties on children as young as nine months with no disturbances in the growth of the ear or recurrence of the problem.

Preparation for otoplasty in children should include an assessment of the child's feelings about the procedure. Some surgeons consider opposition on the child's part to be a contraindication for surgery, as well as unrealistic expectations on the part of the parents. In general, a positive attitude is associated with faster recovery and better overall results.

Preparation for otoplasty in adults includes a **physical examination** and standard blood tests. Patients are usually advised to discontinue taking **aspirin** and any other medications that thin the blood for two weeks prior to surgery. Plastic surgeons strongly urge adult patients to quit smoking before the surgery, because smoking delays and complicates the healing process. Adult patients are also asked to shower and shampoo their hair thoroughly on the morning of the procedure. Men should have a haircut or trim a day or two before surgery; women should braid or pin their hair close to the head.

Trauma

Avulsion injuries caused by bites, thermal or chemical burns resulting from industrial accidents, and other traumatic injuries of the auricle are diagnosed by emergency physicians.

Plastic surgery for traumatic injuries of the auricle is preceded by thorough cleansing of the wound and **debridement** of damaged tissue. It is important to treat ear injuries promptly because the ears are not well supplied with blood vessels. This characteristic makes it easier for infection to develop in parts of the auricle where the skin has been torn open or crushed. In some cases, plastic surgery is postponed for a few days and the patient is given oral penicillin to prevent infection.

Aftercare

After an otoplasty, the patient's head is wrapped with a turban-type bandage that is worn for four or five days following surgery. The patient is instructed to wear a ski-type headband over the ears continuously for about a month after the turban is removed, and then at night for an additional two months. Warm compresses should be applied to the ears two or three times a day for two weeks after the turban is removed.

Patients should follow the surgeon's instructions about washing their hair, and avoid holding hot-air blow dryers too close to the ear.

QUESTIONS TO ASK THE DOCTOR

• How long will it take for the ear to assume its final shape?
• How much change in the shape of the ear can be reasonably expected?
• Would my child benefit from ear molding rather than surgery?
• How many otoplasties have you performed?

Patients should also avoid contact sports for at least three months after otoplasty. An anti-inflammatory medication (Kenalog) can be applied to the ear in the event of abnormal scar formation.

Risks

Some risks associated with otoplasties are common to all operations performed under general anesthesia. They include bleeding or infection of the incision; numbness or loss of feeling in the area around the incision; and a reaction to the anesthesia.

Specific risks associated with otoplasties include the following:

• Formation of abnormal scar tissue. This complication can usually be corrected later; plastic surgeons advise waiting at least six months for revision surgery.
• Hematoma, which is a collection of blood within a body organ or tissue caused by leakage from broken blood vessels. In the case of the ear, a hematoma can damage the results of plastic surgery because it creates tension and pressure that distort the final shape of the ear. Careful drying of the ear at the end of the procedure and application of a pressure bandage can reduce the risk of a hematoma. In the event that one develops, it is treated by reopening the incision and draining the collected blood.
• Distortion of the shape of the ear caused by overcorrection of deformed features.
• Reappearance of ear protrusion (in setback otoplasty). This complication is most likely to occur in the first six months after surgery.

Normal results

The normal result of an otoplasty is a reconstructed or reshaped ear that resembles a normal ear (or the patient's other ear) more closely. In a setback otoplasty, the normal result is an ear that lies closer to the patient's head without an overcorrected, "pinned-back" look.

KEY TERMS

Auricle—The portion of the external ear that is not contained inside the head. It is also called the pinna.

Avulsion—A type of injury caused by ripping or tearing. Most ear injuries requiring otoplasty are avulsion injuries.

Concha—The hollow shell-shaped portion of the external ear.

Congenital—Present at the time of birth.

Ear molding—A non-surgical method for treating ear deformities shortly after birth with the application of a mold held in place by tape and surgical glue.

Hematoma—A localized collection of blood in an organ or tissue due to broken blood vessels.

Hemifacial microsomia (HFM)—A term used to describe a group of complex birth defects characterized by underdevelopment of one side of the face.

Microtia—The partial or complete absence of the auricle of the ear.

Pinna—Another name for the auricle; the visible portion of the external ear.

Setback otoplasty—A surgical procedure done to reduce the size or improve the appearance of large or protruding ears; it is also known as pinback otoplasty.

Stahl's deformity—A congenital deformity of the ear characterized by a flattened rim and pointed upper edge caused by a fold in the cartilage; it is also known as Vulcan ear or Spock ear.

Treacher Collins syndrome—A disorder that affects facial development and hearing, thought to be caused by a gene mutation on human chromosome 5. Treacher Collins syndrome is sometimes called mandibulofacial dysostosis.

Morbidity and mortality rates

The mortality rate in otoplasty is extremely low and is almost always associated with anesthesia reactions. The most common complication reported is asymmetrical ears (18.4%), followed by skin irritation (9.8%); increased sensitivity to cold (7.5%); soreness when the ear is touched (5.7%); abnormal shape to the ear (4.4%); loss of feeling in the ear (3.9%); bleeding (2.6%); and hematoma (0.4%).

Alternatives

Some ear deformities in children, including protruding ears and Stahl's deformity, can be treated with ear molding in the early weeks of life, when the cartilage in the ear can be reshaped by the application of splints and Steri-Strips. One technique involves making a mold in the shape desired for the child's ear from dental compound and attaching it to the ear with methylmethacrylate glue. The ear and the mold are held in place with surgical tape and covered with a tubular bandage or ear wrap for reinforcement. The mold and tape must be worn constantly for six weeks, with a change of dressing every two weeks. Ear molding is reported to be about 85% effective when it is started within six weeks after the baby's birth. It costs less than surgery—about $600—and is considerably less painful. The chief disadvantage of ear molding is its ineffectiveness in treating ear deformities characterized by the absence of skin and cartilage rather than distorted shape.

There are no effective alternatives to otoplasty in treating ear deformities or injuries in adults; however, some plastic surgeons use custom-made silicone molds to help maintain the position of the ears in adult patients for several weeks after surgery.

See also Craniofacial reconstruction; Pediatric surgery.

Resources

BOOKS

"Chromosomal Abnormalities." Section 19, Chapter 261 in *The Merck Manual of Diagnosis and Therapy,* edited by Mark H. Beers and Robert Berkow. Whitehouse Station, NJ: Merck Research Laboratories, 1999.

"Drugs in Pregnancy." Section 18, Chapter 249 in *The Merck Manual of Diagnosis and Therapy,* edited by Mark H. Beers and Robert Berkow. Whitehouse Station, NJ: Merck Research Laboratories, 1999.

"External Ear: Trauma." Section 7, Chapter 83 in *The Merck Manual of Diagnosis and Therapy,* edited by Mark H. Beers and Robert Berkow. Whitehouse Station, NJ: Merck Research Laboratories, 1999.

Sargent, Larry. *The Craniofacial Surgery Book.* Chattanooga, TN: Erlanger Health System, 2000.

PERIODICALS

Aygit, A. C. "Molding the Ears After Anterior Scoring and Concha Repositioning: A Combined Approach for Protruding Ear Correction." *Aesthetic Plastic Surgery,* 27 (March 14, 2003) [e-publication ahead of print].

Bauer, B. S., D. H. Song, and M. E. Aitken. "Combined Otoplasty Technique: Chondrocutaneous Conchal Resection as the Cornerstone to Correction of the Prominent Ear." *Plastic and Reconstructive Surgery,* 110 (September 15, 2002): 1033–1040.

Caouette-Laberge, L., N. Guay, P. Bortoluzzi, and C. Belleville. "Otoplasty: Anterior Scoring Technique and Results in 500 Cases." *Plastic and Reconstructive Surgery,* 105 (February 2000): 504–515.

Furnas, D. W. "Otoplasty for Prominent Ears." *Clinics in Plastic Surgery,* 29 (April 2002): 273–288.

Gosain, A. K., and R. F. Recinos. "Otoplasty in Children Less than Four Years of Age: Surgical Technique." *Journal of Craniofacial Surgery,* 13 (July 2002): 505–509.

McNamara, Robert M. "Bites, Human." *eMedicine,* April 25, 2001 [April 7, 2003]. <www.emedicine.com/emerg/topic 61.htm>.

Manstein, Carl H. "Ear, Congenital Deformities." *eMedicine,* June 20, 2002 [April 6, 2003]. "www.emedicine.com/plastic/topic207.htm>.

Peker, F., and B. Celikoz. "Otoplasty: Anterior Scoring and Posterior Rolling Technique in Adults." *Aesthetic Plastic Surgery,* 26 (July–August 2002): 267–273.

Vital, V., and A. Printza. "Cartilage-Sparing Otoplasty: Our Experience." *Journal of Laryngology and Otology,* 116 (September 2002): 682–685.

Yugueros, P., and J. A. Friedland. "Otoplasty: The Experience of 100 Consecutive Patients." *Plastic and Reconstructive Surgery,* 108 (September 15, 2001): 1045–1051.

ORGANIZATIONS

American Academy of Facial Plastic and Reconstructive Surgery (AAFPRS). 310 South Henry Street, Alexandria, VA 22314. (703) 299-9291. <www.facemd.org>.

American Society of Plastic Surgeons (ASPS). 444 East Algonquin Road, Arlington Heights, IL 60005. (847) 228-9900. <www.plasticsurgery.org>.

FACES: The National Craniofacial Association. P. O. Box 11082, Chattanooga, TN 37401. (800) 332-2373. <www.faces-cranio.org>.

National Organization for Rare Disorders (NORD). 55 Kenosia Avenue, P. O. Box 1968, Danbury, CT 06813-1968. (203) 744-0100.

OTHER

American Academy of Facial Plastic and Reconstructive Surgery. *2001 Membership Survey: Trends in Facial Plastic Surgery.* Alexandria, VA: AAFPRS, 2002.

American Academy of Facial Plastic and Reconstructive Surgery. *Procedures: Understanding Otoplasty Surgery,* [April 6, 2003]. <www.facial-plastic-surgery.org/patient/procedures/otoplasty.html>.

American Society of Plastic Surgeons. *Procedures: Otoplasty,* [April 5, 2003]. <www.plasticsurgery.org/public_education/procedures/Otoplasty.cfm>.

Rebecca Frey, PhD

Otosclerosis surgery *see* **Stapedectomy**

Outpatient surgery

Definition

Outpatient surgery, also referred to as ambulatory surgery, is surgery that does not require an overnight hospital stay. Patients may go home after being released following surgery and time spent in the **recovery room**.

Purpose

Mounting pressure to keep hospitalization costs down and improved technology have increased the frequency of outpatient surgery, with shorter medical procedure duration, fewer complications, and less cost.

Description

Due to improved pain control, advanced medical techniques—including those that reduce recovery time—and cost-cutting considerations, more and more surgeries are being performed on an outpatient basis. Surgeries suited to a non-hospital setting generally are those with a low percentage of postoperative complications, which would require serious attention by a physician or nurse. Outpatient surgery continues to mushroom: in 1984, roughly 400,000 outpatient surgeries were performed. By 2000, the number had risen to 8.3 million. A 2002 study reports that 65% of all surgical procedures did not involve a hospital stay. This statistic also reflects the fact that many patients (especially children) prefer to recover at home or in a familiar setting.

With increased technological advances in instruments such as the arthroscope and laparoscope, more physicians are performing surgery in their offices or in other outpatient settings, primarily ambulatory clinics and surgical centers, or surgicenters. Among the most frequently performed outpatient surgeries are tonsillectomies, arthroscopy, cosmetic surgery, removal of cataracts, gynecological, urological and orthopedic procedures, wound and hernia repairs, and gallbladder removals. Even such procedures as microscopically controlled surgery under local anesthesia (Mohs) for skin cancer have been recommended on an outpatient basis.

Preparation

While many outpatient surgeries are covered by insurance plans, many are not. Candidates for such surgeries should check in advance with their insurance carrier concerning whether their procedures are covered on an outpatient basis.

Preparing for outpatient surgery varies, of course, with the surgical procedure to be performed. There are, however, guidelines common to most outpatient surgeries. Patients should be in good health before undergoing ambulatory surgery. Colds, fever, chills, or flu symptoms are all reasons to postpone a procedure, and surgical candidates should notify their primary health care physicians if such conditions exist.

Patients should check with their physician for all information covering preparation for outpatient procedures. A near-universal requirement is to have a family member or friend take charge of delivering the outpatient to surgery, either to wait there or to arrive in time to pick up the patient on release from recovery. The evening before, a light meal is recommended to preoperative patients, with no alcohol taken for a full day before surgery. Nothing is to be taken by mouth after midnight of the day preceding surgery. Smokers should stop or cut back on smoking prior to surgery. Loose-fitting clothing is recommended, and it is advised to bring enough money along to cover postoperative prescription drugs.

This same information applies if the outpatient is a child. If children are permitted clear liquids on the day of outpatient surgery, parents will be told when the child must stop taking them. Surgery will be cancelled or delayed if these requirements are not met.

Results

The benefits of outpatient surgery include lower medical costs (one study sets them at 60–75% lower than comparable hospital procedures), tighter scheduling—because patients are not subject to the potential delays encountered in hospital operating rooms—and what many patients would consider a less stressful environment than a hospital setting. Recovery time spent in one's own home, either with familiar caregivers or home nurses, is a choice many postoperative patients prefer.

Complications related to surgery occur less than 1% of the time in outpatient settings. However, in terms of patient safety, non-hospital settings are not as regulated as are hospitals, so patients should inquire about potential risks concerning outpatient surgery that arise in ambulatory clinics, surgical centers, and physicians' offices. There are guidelines for surgery in outpatient settings, but oversight and enforcement may vary. In 2002, though 20 states required ambulatory surgical facilities to be accredited by one of three existing accreditation organizations, only half of these 20 states issued regulations on office-based procedures, and fewer still have established a system for reporting events in outpatient settings. Patients may wish to find out whether their outpatient center is licensed or certified as a medical facility, or is accredited, in the states that require this. The latter may be accomplished by contacting the

---

KEY TERMS

Ambulatory surgery—Surgery done on an outpatient basis; the patient goes home the same day.

Ambulatory surgery center—An outpatient facility with at least two operating rooms, either connected or not connected to a hospital.

Outpatient procedures—Surgery that is performed on an outpatient basis, involving less recovery time and fewer expected complications.

Joint Commission on Accreditation of Healthcare Organizations.

Among problems encountered during outpatient surgery are those concerning anesthesia administration, infection, bleeding that calls for a **transfusion**, and respiratory and resuscitation events.

Resources

PERIODICALS

Lewis, C. "Sizing up Surgery." *FDA Consumer Magazine* (November–December, 1998). <http://www.fda.gov/fdac/features/1998/698_surg.html>.

ORGANIZATIONS

Joint Commission on Accreditation of Healthcare Organizations. (630) 792-5000. <http://www.jcaho.org/>.
Questions To Ask Your Doctor Before You Have Surgery. Agency for Health Care Research and Quality. <http://www.ahcpr.gov/consumer/surgery.htm#head2/>.

OTHER

Wax, C. M. *Preparation for Surgery.* <http://www.HealthIsNumberOne.com>.

Nancy McKenzie, PhD

Ovary and fallopian tube removal *see* **Salpingo-oophorectomy**

Ovary removal *see* **Oophorectomy**

Oxygen therapy

Definition

Oxygen may be classified as an element, a gas, and a drug. Oxygen therapy is the administration of oxygen

---

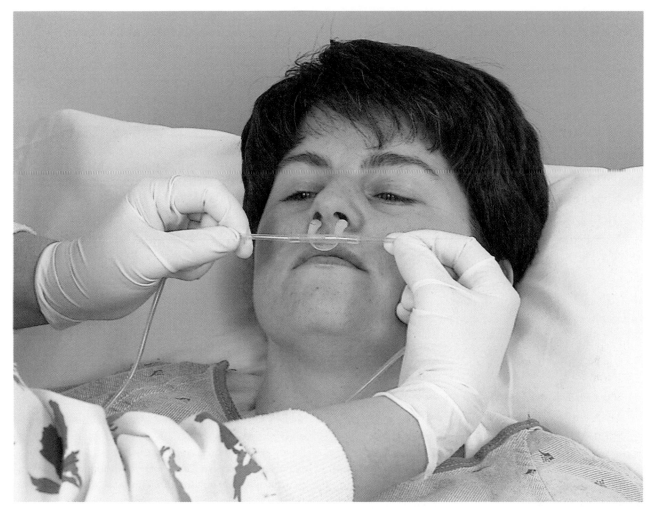

Insertion of nasal cannula. The cannula delivers oxygen directly into the patient's nose. *(From Fundamentals of Nursing, Standards & Practice, 1st edition by DELAUNE. (c) 1998. Reprinted with permission of Delmar Learning, a division of Thomson Learning: www.thomsonrights.com. Fax: 800-730-2215.)*

at concentrations greater than that in room air to treat or prevent hypoxemia (not enough oxygen in the blood). Oxygen delivery systems are classified as stationary, portable, or ambulatory. Oxygen can be administered by nasal cannula, mask, and tent. Hyperbaric oxygen therapy involves placing the patient in an airtight chamber with oxygen under pressure.

Purpose

The body is constantly taking in oxygen and releasing carbon dioxide. If this process is inadequate, oxygen levels in the blood decrease, and the patient may need supplemental oxygen. Oxygen therapy is a key treatment in respiratory care. The purpose is to increase oxygen saturation in tissues where the saturation levels are too low due to illness or injury. Breathing prescribed oxygen increases the amount of oxygen in the blood, reduces the

extra work of the heart, and decreases shortness of breath. Oxygen therapy is frequently ordered in the **home care** setting, as well as in acute (urgent) care facilities.

Some of the conditions oxygen therapy is used to treat include:

- documented hypoxemia
- severe respiratory distress (e.g., acute asthma or pneumonia)
- severe trauma
- chronic obstructive pulmonary disease (COPD, including chronic bronchitis, emphysema, and chronic asthma)
- pulmonary hypertension
- cor pulmonale
- acute myocardial infarction (heart attack)
- short-term therapy, such as post-anesthesia recovery

Oxygen may also be used to treat chronic lung disease patients during **exercise**.

Hyperbaric oxygen therapy is used to treat the following conditions:

- gas gangrene
- decompression sickness
- air embolism
- smoke inhalation
- carbon monoxide poisoning
- cerebral hypoxic event

Helium-oxygen therapy is a treatment that may be used for patients with severe airway obstruction. The combination of helium and oxygen, known as heliox, reduces the density of the delivered gas, and has been shown to reduce the effort of breathing and improve ventilation when an airway obstruction is present. This type of treatment may be used in an emergency room for patients with acute, severe asthma.

Description

Oxygen delivery (other than mechanical ventilators and hyperbaric chambers)

In the hospital, oxygen is supplied to each patient room via an outlet in the wall. Oxygen is delivered from a central source through a pipeline in the facility. A flow meter attached to the wall outlet accesses the oxygen. A valve regulates the oxygen flow, and attachments may be connected to provide moisture. In the home, the oxygen source is usually a canister or air compressor. Whether in home or hospital, plastic tubing connects the oxygen source to the patient.

Oxygen is most commonly delivered to the patient via a nasal cannula or mask attached to the tubing. The nasal cannula is usually the delivery device of choice since it is well tolerated and doesn't interfere with the patient's ability to communicate, eat, or drink. The concentration of oxygen inhaled depends upon the prescribed flow rate and the ventilatory minute volume (MV).

Another delivery option is transtracheal oxygen therapy, which involves a small flexible catheter inserted in the trachea or windpipe through a tracheostomy tube. In this method, the oxygen bypasses the mouth, nose, and throat, and a humidifier is required at flow rates of 1 liter (2.1 pt) per minute and above. Other oxygen delivery methods include tents and specialized infant oxygen delivery systems.

TYPES OF OXYGEN DELIVERY SYSTEMS. The types of oxygen delivery systems include:

- Compressed oxygen—oxygen that is stored as a gas in a tank. A flow meter and regulator are attached to the oxygen tank to adjust oxygen flow. Tanks vary in size from very large to smaller, portable tanks. This system is generally prescribed when oxygen is not needed constantly (e.g., when it is only needed when performing physical activity).

- Liquid oxygen—oxygen that is stored in a large stationary tank that stays in the home. A portable tank is available that can be filled from the stationary tank for trips outside the home. Oxygen is liquid at very cold temperatures. When warmed, liquid oxygen changes to a gas for delivery to the patient.

- Oxygen concentrator—electric oxygen delivery system approximately the size of a large suitcase. The concentrator extracts some of the air from the room, separates the oxygen, and delivers it to the patient via a nasal cannula. A cylinder of oxygen is provided as a backup in the event of a power failure, and a portable tank is available for trips outside the home. This system is generally prescribed for patients who require constant supplemental oxygen or who must use it when sleeping.

- Oxygen conserving device, such as a demand inspiratory flow system or pulsed-dose oxygen delivery system—uses a sensor to detect when inspiration (inhalation) begins. Oxygen is delivered only upon inspiration, thereby conserving oxygen during exhalation. These systems can be used with either compressed or liquid oxygen systems, but are not appropriate for all patients.

Preparation

A physician's order is required for oxygen therapy, except in emergency use. The need for supplemental oxygen is determined by inadequate oxygen saturation, indicated in blood gas measurements, pulse oximetry, or clinical observations. The physician will prescribe the specific amount of oxygen needed by the patient. Some patients require supplemental oxygen 24 hours a day, while others may only need treatments during exercise or sleep. No special patient preparation is required to administer oxygen therapy.

Patient education

SELECTING AN OXYGEN SYSTEM. A health care provider will meet with the patient to discuss the oxygen systems available. A system recommendation will be made, based on the patient's overall condition and personal needs, as well as the system's ease of use, reliability, cost, range of oxygen delivery, and features. The health care provider can give the patient a list of medical supply companies that stock home oxygen equipment and supplies. The patient can meet with home care representatives from these companies to evaluate the product lines that best fit his or her needs. Patients in the home setting are directed to notify the vendors when replacement oxygen supplies are needed.

OXYGEN SAFETY. Patients will receive instructions about the safe use of oxygen in the home. Patients must be advised not to change the flow rate of oxygen unless directed to do so by the physician.

Oxygen supports combustion, therefore no open flame or combustible products should be permitted when oxygen is in use. These include petroleum jelly, oils, and aerosol sprays. A spark from a cigarette, electric razor, or other electrical device could easily ignite oxygen-saturated hair or bedclothes around the patient. Explosion-proof plugs should be used for vaporizers and humidifier attachments. The patient should be sure to have a functioning smoke detector and fire extinguisher in the home at all times.

Care must be taken with oxygen equipment used in the home or hospital. The oxygen system should be kept clean and dust-free. Cylinders should be kept in carts, or have collars for safe storage. If not stored in a cart, smaller canisters may be lain on the floor. Knocking cylinders together can cause sparks, so bumping them should be avoided. In the home, the oxygen source must be placed at least 6 ft (1.8 m) away from flames or other sources of ignition, such as a lit cigarette. Oxygen tanks should be kept in a well–ventilated area. Oxygen tanks should not be kept in the trunk of a car. "No Smoking—Oxygen in Use" signs should be used to warn visitors not to smoke near the patient.

Special care must be given when administering oxygen to premature infants because of the danger of high oxygen levels causing retinopathy of prematurity, or contributing to the construction of ductus arteriosis. PaO_2 (partial pressure of oxygen) levels greater than 80 mm Hg should be avoided.

Patients who are undergoing a laser **bronchoscopy** should receive concurrent administration of supplemental oxygen to avoid burns to the trachea.

Insurance clearance

The patient should check with his or her insurance provider to determine if the treatment is covered and what out-of-pocket expenses may be incurred. Oxygen therapy is usually fully or partially covered by most insurance plans, including **Medicare**, when prescribed according to specific guidelines. Usually test results indicating the medical necessity of the supplemental oxygen are needed before insurance clearance is granted.

Travel guidelines

Traveling with oxygen requires advanced planning. The patient needs to obtain a letter from his or her health care provider that verifies all medications, including oxygen. In addition, a copy of the patient's oxygen prescription must be shown to travel personnel. Home health care companies can help the patient make travel plans, and can arrange for oxygen when the patient arrives at his or her destination. Patients cannot bring or use their own oxygen tanks on an airplane; therefore the patient must leave his or her portable oxygen tank at the airport before boarding. Oxygen suppliers can pick up the oxygen unit from the airport if necessary, or a family member can take it home.

Aftercare

Once oxygen therapy is initiated, periodic assessment and documentation of oxygen saturation levels is required. Follow-up monitoring includes blood gas measurements and pulse oximetry tests. If the patient is using a mask or a cannula, gauze can be tucked under the tubing to prevent irritation of the cheeks or the skin behind the ears. Water-based lubricants can be used to relieve dryness of the lips and nostrils.

Risks

Oxygen is not addictive and causes no side effects when used as prescribed. Complications from oxygen therapy used in appropriate situations are infrequent. Respiratory depression, oxygen toxicity, and absorption atelectasis are the most serious complications of oxygen overuse.

A physician should be notified and emergency services may be required if the following symptoms develop:

• frequent headaches
• anxiety
• cyanotic (blue) lips or fingernails
• drowsiness
• confusion
• restlessness
• slow, shallow, difficult, or irregular breathing

Oxygen delivery equipment may present other problems. Perforation of the nasal septum as a result of using a nasal cannula and non–humidified oxygen has been reported. In addition, bacterial contamination of nebulizer and humidification systems can occur, possibly leading to the spread of pneumonia. High-flow systems that employ heated humidifiers and aerosol generators, especially when used by patients with artificial airways, also pose a risk of infection.

KEY TERMS

Arterial blood gas test—A blood test that measures oxygen and carbon dioxide in the blood.

Atelectasis—Partial or complete collapse of the lung, usually due to a blockage of the air passages with fluid, mucus or infection.

Breathing rate—The number of breaths per minute.

Cannula—Also called nasal cannula. A small, light-weight plastic tube with two hollow prongs that fit just inside the nose. Nasal cannulas are used to supply supplemental oxygen through the nose.

Cyanosis—Blue, gray, or dark purple discoloration of the skin caused by a deficiency of oxygen.

Ductus arteriosis—A fetal blood vessel that connects the pulmonary artery to the aorta; normally closes at birth.

Flow meter—Device for measuring the rate of a gas (especially oxygen) or liquid.

Hypoxemia—Oxygen deficiency, defined as an oxygen level less than 60 mm Hg or arterial oxygen saturation of less than 90%. Different values are used for infants and patients with certain lung diseases.

Oxygenation—Saturation with oxygen.

Peak expiratory flow rate—A test used to measure how fast air can be exhaled from the lungs.

Pulmonary function tests—A series of tests that measure how well air is moving in and out of the lungs and carrying oxygen to the bloodstream.

Pulmonary rehabilitation—A program that helps patients learn how to breathe easier and improve their quality of life. Pulmonary rehabilitation includes treatment, exercise training, education, and counseling.

Pulmonologist—A physician who specializes in caring for people with lung diseases and breathing problems.

Pulse oximetry—A non-invasive test in which a device that clips onto the finger measures the oxygen level in the blood.

Residual volume—The volume of air remaining in the lungs, measured after a maximum expiration.

Respiratory failure—The sudden inability of the lungs to provide normal oxygen delivery or normal carbon dioxide removal.

Respiratory therapist—A health care professional who specializes in assessing, treating, and educating people with lung diseases.

Total lung capacity test—A test that measures the amount of air in the lungs after a person has breathed in as much as possible.

Vital capacity—Maximal breathing capacity; the amount of air that can be expired after a maximum inspiration.

Normal results

A normal result is a patient that demonstrates adequate oxygenation through pulse oximetry, blood gas tests, and clinical observation. Signs and symptoms of inadequate oxygenation include cyanosis, drowsiness, confusion, restlessness, anxiety, or slow, shallow, difficult, or irregular breathing. Patients with obstructive airway disease may exhibit "aerophagia" (air hunger) as they work to pull air into the lungs. In cases of carbon monoxide inhalation, the oxygen saturation can be falsely elevated.

Resources

BOOKS

Branson, Richard, et al. *Respiratory Care Equipment* 2nd. ed. Philadelphia: Lippincott Williams and Wilkins Publishers, 1999.

Hyatt, Robert E., Paul D. Scanlon, Masao Nakamura,. *Interpretation of Pulmonary Function Tests: A Practical Guide,* 2nd ed. Philadelphia: Lippincott Williams and Wilkins Publishers, 2003.

Wilkins, Robert, et al. *Clinical Assessment in Respiratory Care,* 2nd ed. St. Louis: Mosby, 2000.

Wilkins, Robert, et al. *Egan's Fundamentals of Respiratory Care,* 8th ed. St. Louis: Mosby, 2003.

Yutsis, Pavel I. *Oxygen to the Rescue: Oxygen Therapies and How They Help Overcome Disease, Promote Repair, and Improve Overall Function.* Basic Health Publications, Inc., 2003.

PERIODICALS

Crockett, A. J., J.M. Cranston, et al. "A Review of Long-term Oxygen Therapy for Chronic Obstructive Pulmonary Disease." *Respiratory Medicine* 95 (June 2001): 437-43.

Eaton, T.E., et al. "An Evaluation of Short-term Oxygen Therapy: The Prescription of Oxygen to Patients with Chronic Lung Disease Hypoxic at Discharge." *Respiratory Medicine* 95 (July 2001): 582-7.

Kelly, Martin G., et al. "Nasal Septal Perforation and Oxygen Cannulae." *Hospital Medicine* 62, no.4 (April 2001): 248.

Ruiz-Bailen M, M.C. Serrano-Corcoles, J.A. Ramos-Cuadra "Tracheal Injury Caused by Ingested Paraquat." *Chest* 119, no.6 (June 2001): 1956-7.

ORGANIZATIONS

American Association for Cardiovascular and Pulmonary Rehabilitation (AACVPR). 7600 Terrace Avenue, Suite 203, Middleton, Wisconsin 53562. (608) 831-6989. E-mail: aacvpr@tmahq.com. <http://www.aacvpr.org>.

American Association for Respiratory Care, 11030 Ables Lane, Dallas, Texas 75229. (972) 243-2272. E-mail: info@aarc.org. <http://www.aarc.org>.

American College of Chest Physicians. 3300 Dundee Road, Northbrook, Illinois 60062-2348. (847) 498-1400. <http://www.chcstnct.org>.

American Lung Association and American Thoracic Society. 1740 Broadway, New York, NY 10019-4374. (800) LUNG-USA or (800) 586-4872. <http://www.lungusa.org>.

National Heart, Lung and Blood Institute. Information Center. P.O. Box 30105, Bethesda, Maryland 20824. (301) 251-2222. <http://www.nhlbi.nih.gov/nhlbi/>.

National Jewish Medical and Research Center. Lung-Line. 14090 Jackson Street, Denver, Colorado 80206. <http://www.nationaljewish.org>.

OTHER

Daily Lung. <http://www.dailylung.com>. A full-feature magazine covering lung disease and related health topics.

National Lung Health Education Program. <http://www.nlhep.org>.

The Pulmonary Paper. P.O. Box 877, Ormond Beach, Florida 32175. (800) 950-3698. <http://www.pulmonarypaper.org>. Not-for-profit newsletter supporting people with chronic lung problems.

Maggie Boleyn, R.N., B.S.N.
Angela M. Costello

Oxytocin *see* **Uterine stimulants**